ESSENTIALS OF
Nursing Research

APPRAISING EVIDENCE FOR NURSING PRACTICE

Tenth Edition

T0175318

ESSENTIALS OF
Nursing Research

APPRAISING EVIDENCE FOR NURSING PRACTICE

Tenth Edition

Denise F. Polit, PhD, FAAN

President, Humanalysis, Inc.
Saratoga Springs, New York
Adjunct Professor, Griffith University School of Nursing
Brisbane, Australia
www.denisepolit.com

Cheryl Tatano Beck, DNSc, CNM, FAAN

Distinguished Professor, School of Nursing
University of Connecticut
Storrs, Connecticut

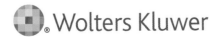

. Wolters Kluwer

Philadelphia • Baltimore • New York • London
Buenos Aires • Hong Kong • Sydney • Tokyo

Not authorised for sale in United States, Canada, Australia, New Zealand, Puerto Rico, or U.S. Virgin Islands.

Vice President, Nursing Segment: Julie K. Stegman
Manager, Nursing Education and Practice Content: Jamie Blum
Acquisitions Editor: Michael Kerns
Senior Development Editor: Meredith L. Brittain
Editorial Coordinator: Julie Kostelnik
Marketing Manager: Brittany Clements
Editorial Assistant: Molly Kennedy
Production Project Manager: Barton Dudlick
Design Coordinator: Steve Druding
Art Director: Jennifer Clements
Manufacturing Coordinator: Karin Duffield
Prepress Vendor: Absolute Service, Inc.

Tenth edition

Copyright © 2022 Wolters Kluwer.

Copyright © 2018 Wolters Kluwer. Copyright © 2014, 2010 by Wolters Kluwer Health | Lippincott Williams & Wilkins. Copyright © 2006, 2001 by Lippincott Williams & Wilkins. Copyright © 1997 Lippincott-Raven Publishers. Copyright © 1993, 1989, 1985 J. B. Lippincott Company. All rights reserved. This book is protected by copyright. No part of this book may be reproduced or transmitted in any form or by any means, including as photocopies or scanned-in or other electronic copies, or utilized by any information storage and retrieval system without written permission from the copyright owner, except for brief quotations embodied in critical articles and reviews. Materials appearing in this book prepared by individuals as part of their official duties as U.S. government employees are not covered by the above-mentioned copyright. To request permission, please contact Wolters Kluwer at Two Commerce Square, 2001 Market Street, Philadelphia, PA 19103, via email at permissions@lww.com, or via our website at shop.lww.com (products and services).

9 8 7 6 5 4 3 2 1

Printed in China

Library of Congress Cataloging-in-Publication Data

Library of Congress Control Number: 2020945965

This work is provided "as is," and the publisher disclaims any and all warranties, express or implied, including any warranties as to accuracy, comprehensiveness, or currency of the content of this work.

This work is no substitute for individual patient assessment based on health care professionals' examination of each patient and consideration of, among other things, age, weight, gender, current or prior medical conditions, medication history, laboratory data, and other factors unique to the patient. The publisher does not provide medical advice or guidance, and this work is merely a reference tool. Health care professionals, and not the publisher, are solely responsible for the use of this work including all medical judgments and for any resulting diagnosis and treatments.

Given continuous, rapid advances in medical science and health information, independent professional verification of medical diagnoses, indications, appropriate pharmaceutical selections and dosages, and treatment options should be made and health care professionals should consult a variety of sources. When prescribing medication, health care professionals are advised to consult the product information sheet (the manufacturer's package insert) accompanying each drug to verify, among other things, conditions of use, warnings, and side effects and identify any changes in dosage schedule or contraindications, particularly if the medication to be administered is new, infrequently used, or has a narrow therapeutic range. To the maximum extent permitted under applicable law, no responsibility is assumed by the publisher for any injury and/or damage to persons or property, as a matter of products liability, negligence law or otherwise, or from any reference to or use by any person of this work.

CCS1220

TO

Our families and friends

The heroes on the front lines of health care

Those who are working to address social and health inequities

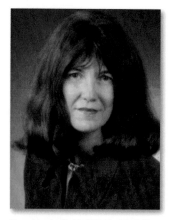

Denise F. Polit, PhD, FAAN

Denise F. Polit, PhD, FAAN, is an American health care researcher who is recognized internationally as an authority on research methods, statistics, and measurement. She received her Bachelor's degree from Wellesley College and her PhD from Boston College. She is the president of a research consulting company, Humanalysis, Inc., in Saratoga Springs, New York, and an adjunct professor at Griffith University, Brisbane, Australia. She has published in numerous journals and has written several award-winning textbooks, including a groundbreaking book on measurement in health, *Measurement and the Measurement of Change: A Primer for the Health Professions*, and a book on statistical analysis, *Statistics and Data Analysis for Nursing Research*. Her research methods books with Dr. Cheryl Tatano Beck have been translated into French, Spanish, Portuguese, German, Chinese, and Japanese. She has been invited to give lectures and presentations in many countries, including Australia, India, Ireland, Denmark, Norway, South Africa, Turkey, Sweden, and the Philippines.

Denise has lived in Saratoga Springs for 33 years and is active in the community. She has assisted numerous nonprofit organizations in designing surveys and analyzing survey data. Currently, she serves on the board of directors of the Saratoga Foundation and the New Leaf Coalition, an organization dedicated to addressing the complex needs of formerly incarcerated people in New York City.

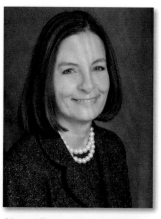

Cheryl Tatano Beck, DNSc, CNM, FAAN

Cheryl Tatano Beck, DNSc, CNM, FAAN, is a distinguished professor at the University of Connecticut, School of Nursing, with a joint appointment in the Department of Obstetrics and Gynecology at the School of Medicine. She received her master's degree in maternal–newborn nursing from Yale University and her doctor of nursing science degree from Boston University. She has received numerous awards such as the Association of Women's Health, Obstetric and Neonatal Nursing's Distinguished Professional Service Award; Eastern Nursing Research Society's Distinguished Researcher Award; the Distinguished Alumna Award from Yale University School of Nursing; and the Marcé Medal from the International Marcé Society for Perinatal Mental Health in recognition of her program of research. She was recently inducted into the Sigma Theta Tau International Nurse Researcher Hall of Fame.

Over the past 35 years, Cheryl has focused her research efforts on developing a research program on postpartum mood and anxiety disorders. Based on the findings from her series of qualitative studies, Cheryl developed the Postpartum Depression Screening Scale (PDSS), which is published by Western Psychological Services. She is a prolific writer who has published over 150 journal articles. In addition to coauthoring award-winning research methods books with Denise Polit, Cheryl coauthored with Dr. Jeanne Driscoll *Postpartum Mood and Anxiety Disorders: A Clinician's Guide*, which received the 2006 *American Journal of Nursing* Book of the Year Award. In addition, Cheryl has published five other books: *Traumatic Childbirth*, *Routledge International Handbook of Qualitative Nursing Research*, *Developing a Program of Research in Nursing*, *Secondary Qualitative Analysis in the Health and Social Sciences*, and *Introduction to Phenomenology: Focus on Methodology*.

Essentials of Nursing Research, 10th edition, helps students learn how to read and critically appraise research reports and to develop an appreciation of research as a path to enhancing nursing practice.

We continue to enjoy updating this book with important innovations in research methods and with examples of nurse researchers' use of emerging research strategies. Feedback from our loyal adopters has inspired several important changes to the content and organization of this book. We are convinced that these revisions introduce important improvements—while at the same time retaining many features that have made this book a classic best-selling textbook throughout the world. The 10th edition of this book, its study guide, and its online resources will make it easier and more satisfying for nurses to pursue a professional pathway that incorporates thoughtful appraisals of evidence.

LEGACY OF *ESSENTIALS OF NURSING RESEARCH*

This edition, like its predecessors, is focused on the art—and science—of critically appraising studies conducted by nurses and other health care professionals. The textbook offers guidance to students who are learning to assess research reports and to use research findings in practice.

Among the basic principles that helped to shape this and earlier editions of this book are the following:

1. Confidence in the idea that competence in doing and appraising research is critical to the nursing profession
2. A conviction that research inquiry is intellectually and professionally rewarding to nurses
3. An unswerving belief that learning about research methods need be neither intimidating nor dull

Consistent with these principles, we have tried to present research fundamentals in a way that both facilitates understanding and arouses curiosity and interest. We hope that, for some, it will arouse passion for the pursuit of research-based knowledge to guide practice.

NEW TO THIS EDITION

New Organization

A lot has happened in the world of research since the ninth edition. A particularly salient issue is patient (and other stakeholder) involvement in identifying important questions and translating research evidence into local settings. Relatedly, standard methods of appraising evidence for the **rigor** of study methods (which has been a focus of evidence-based practice, or EBP, initiatives) are being supplemented by a new emphasis on the **relevance** and **applicability** of research evidence for individual patients or small groups of patients (as espoused by the movement for **practice-based evidence** and **patient-centered research**). This new perspective led us to reorganize the content on EBP. In this edition, basic EBP concepts are woven into Chapter 1 (rather than Chapter 2). Evidence-based practice and practice-based evidence are given broader attention in the final chapter of the book, Chapter 18. We believe that this new organization will better facilitate the use of research evidence in nursing practice.

Manageable Text for One-Semester Course

We have streamlined the text even further in this edition to make it more manageable for use in a one-semester course. We reduced the length by organizing content differently and by keeping essential information in the text while moving background/advanced content to online supplements.

Enhanced Accessibility

To make this edition even more user-friendly than in the past, we have made a concerted effort to simplify the presentation of complex topics. For example, we reduced and simplified the coverage of statistical information. In addition, throughout the book we have used more straightforward, concise language.

New Content

New ideas and concepts have been threaded throughout this 10th edition. In addition to updating the book with new information on conventional research methods and recent examples of nursing studies, we have added content on the following topics:

- **Quality improvement (QI)** projects play an increasingly important role in the practice of most health care professionals. In this edition, we describe how QI projects are distinct from research studies and how they can be undertaken with rigor. The expanded content on quality improvement is found in Chapter 12.
- **Clinical significance** is a seldom mentioned but important topic that has gained prominence among researchers in other health care fields that has only recently gained traction among nurse researchers. Expanded coverage on this topic is found in Chapter 14.
- **Comparative effectiveness research (CER)**, which emphasizes patient centeredness, is an important manifestation of emerging directions in health care research. CER is discussed in Chapters 12 and 18.
- **Systematic reviews** serve as critical sources of state-of-the-art evidence for health care practitioners. We have expanded the coverage of this topic (Chapter 17) and have introduced the **GRADE system** for evaluating reviewers' confidence in the review's conclusions.

THE TEXT

The content of this edition is as follows:

- **Part 1, Overview of Nursing Research and Its Role in Evidence-Based Practice**, introduces fundamental concepts in nursing research. Chapter 1 summarizes the background of nursing research, discusses the philosophical underpinnings of qualitative research versus quantitative research, describes major purposes of nursing research, and introduces key concepts relating to evidence-based practice. Chapter 2 introduces readers to key research terms and presents an overview of steps in the research process for both quantitative and qualitative studies. Chapter 3 focuses on research journal articles, explaining what they are and how to read them. Chapter 4 discusses ethics in nursing studies.
- **Part 2, Preliminary Steps in Quantitative and Qualitative Research**, further sets the stage for learning about the research process by considering aspects of a study's conceptualization.

Chapter 5 focuses on the development of research questions and the formulation of research hypotheses. Chapter 6 discusses how to retrieve research evidence (especially in electronic bibliographic databases) and the role of research literature reviews. Chapter 7 presents information about theoretical and conceptual frameworks for nursing studies.

- **Part 3, Designs and Methods for Quantitative and Qualitative Nursing Research,** presents material on the design and conduct of all types of nursing studies. Chapter 8 describes fundamental design principles and discusses many specific aspects of quantitative research design, including efforts to enhance rigor. Chapter 9 introduces the topics of sampling and data collection in quantitative studies. Concepts relating to quality in measurements—reliability and validity—are introduced in this chapter. Chapter 10 describes the various qualitative research traditions that have contributed to the growth of constructivist inquiry and presents the basics of qualitative design. Chapter 11 covers sampling and data collection methods used in qualitative research, describing how these differ from approaches used in quantitative studies. Chapter 12 provides an overview of several distinctive types of research, with a special emphasis on mixed methods research. This chapter also discusses other special types of research such as surveys, comparative effectiveness studies, evaluation research, and outcomes research. Methods of undertaking quality improvement projects are also described.

- **Part 4, Analysis, Interpretation, and Application of Nursing Research,** presents tools for making sense of—and using—research data. Chapter 13 reviews methods of statistical analysis. The chapter assumes no prior instruction in statistics and focuses primarily on helping readers to understand why statistics are useful, what test might be appropriate in a given situation, and what statistical information in a research article means. Chapter 14 discusses approaches to interpreting statistical results, including interpretations linked to assessments of clinical significance. Chapter 15 discusses qualitative analysis, with an emphasis on ethnographic, phenomenologic, and grounded theory studies. In this edition, we offer an expanded discussion of the coding of qualitative data. Chapter 16 elaborates on criteria for appraising trustworthiness and integrity in qualitative studies. Chapter 17 describes systematic reviews, including how to understand and appraise meta-analyses and metasyntheses—and how the GRADE system works in the context of systematic reviews. Finally, Chapter 18 describes key steps in evidence-based practice and also explains emerging ideas about how to improve EBP by striving for evidence that is more practice-based and patient-centered—that is, how to enhance the applicability of evidence to individual patients or well-defined subgroups of patients.

- At the end of the book, we offer students additional support for critical appraisal. **In the appendices, we offer full-length research articles**—two quantitative, one qualitative, and one mixed methods—that students can read, analyze, and appraise. Some of the Critical Thinking Exercises in each chapter focus on these four studies. We also have included our critical appraisal of one of these studies (the one in Appendix D), which can be used as a model. A **glossary** at the end of the book provides additional support for those needing to look up the meaning of a methodologic term.

FEATURES OF THE TEXT

We have retained many of the classic features that were successfully used in previous editions to assist those learning to read and apply evidence from nursing research:

- **Clear, User-Friendly Style.** Our writing style is easily digestible and nonintimidating—and we have worked even harder in this edition to write clearly and simply. Concepts are introduced carefully, difficult ideas are presented thoughtfully, and readers are assumed to have no prior knowledge of technical terms.

- **Critical Appraisal Guidelines.** Each chapter includes guidelines for conducting a critical appraisal of various aspects of a research report. The guidelines sections provide a list of questions that walk students through a study, drawing attention to aspects of the study that are amenable to evaluation by research consumers.
- **Research Examples and Critical Thinking Exercises.** Each chapter concludes with summaries of one or two research examples designed to highlight important points made in the chapter and to sharpen the reader's critical thinking skills. In addition, many research examples are used to illustrate key points in the text and to stimulate students' thinking about areas of research inquiry. We have chosen many international examples to communicate to students that nursing research is growing in importance worldwide. Some of the Critical Thinking Exercises focus on the full-length articles in the four appendices.
- **Tips for Students.** The textbook is filled with practical guidance and tips on how to translate the abstract notions of research methods into more concrete applications. In these tips, we have paid special attention to helping students *read* research reports, which are often daunting to those without specialized research training.
- **Graphics.** Colorful graphics—in the form of supportive tables, figures, and examples—reinforce the text and offer visual stimulation.
- **Chapter Objectives.** Learning objectives are identified in the chapter opener to focus students' attention on critical content.
- **Key Terms.** Each chapter opener includes a list of new research terms. In the text, new terms are defined in context (and bolded) when used for the first time; terms of lesser importance are italicized. Key terms are also defined in our glossary.
- **Bulleted Summary Points.** A succinct list of summary points that focus on salient chapter content is provided at the end of each chapter.

A COMPREHENSIVE PACKAGE FOR TEACHING AND LEARNING

To further facilitate teaching and learning, a carefully designed ancillary package has been developed to assist faculty and students.

Resources for Instructors

Tools to assist with teaching this text are available upon its adoption on thePoint° at http://thePoint.lww.com/PolitEssentials10e.

- NEW! **Test Generator Questions** are completely new and written by the book's authors for the 10th edition. Hundreds of multiple-choice questions aid instructors in assessing their students' understanding of the chapter content.
- **An Instructor's Manual** offers guidance to improve the teaching experience. We have recognized the need for strong support for instructors in teaching a course that can be quite challenging. Part of the difficulty stems from students' anxiety about the course content and their concern that research methods might not be relevant to their nursing practice. We offer numerous suggestions on how to make learning about—and teaching—research methods more rewarding. The contents of the Instructor's Manual include the following for each chapter:
  - ○ **Statement of Intent.** Discover the authors' goals for each chapter.
  - ○ **Special Class Projects.** Find numerous ideas for interesting and meaningful class projects. Check out the icebreakers and activities relating to the Great Cookie Experiment and "How Do You Feel" icebreakers.

○ **Test Questions and Answers.** True/false questions, plus important application questions, test students' comprehension and their ability to put their new appraisal skills to use. The application questions focus on a brief summary of a study and include several short-answer questions (with our answers), plus essay questions. These application questions are intended to assess students' knowledge about methodologic concepts and their critical appraisal skills.

○ **Answers to Critical Thinking Exercises.** These are provided for selected questions related to the studies in the appendices of the textbook.

● **Two sets of PowerPoint Slides:**

○ **"Test Yourself!" PowerPoint Slides.** For each chapter, a slide set of five multiple-choice "Test Yourself!" questions relating to key concepts in the chapter are followed by answers to the questions. (A few chapters have two sets of "Test Yourself!" slides.) The aim of these slides is not to evaluate student performance. We recommend these slides be given to students for self-testing, or they can be used in the classroom with iClicker to assess students' grasp of important concepts. To enhance the likelihood that students will see the relevance of the concepts to clinical practice, all the questions are application-type questions. We hope instructors will use the slides to clarify any misunderstandings and, just as importantly, to reward students with immediate positive feedback about newly acquired skills.

○ **PowerPoint Presentations** offer traditional summaries of key points in each chapter for use in class presentations. These slides are available in a format that permits easy adaptation and also include audience response questions that can be used on their own or are compatible with iClicker and other audience response programs and devices.

● **An Image Bank** includes figures from the text.

● **A Sample Syllabus** is provided for a 14-week course.

● **A QSEN Map** shows how the book content integrates QSEN competencies.

● **A BSN Essentials Competencies Map** shows how the book content integrates American Association of Colleges of Nursing (AACN) Essentials of Baccalaureate Education for Professional Nursing Practice competencies.

● **Learning Management System Course Cartridges.**

● **Access to all student resources previously discussed.**

Resources for Students

An exciting set of resources is available to help students review material and become even more familiar with vital concepts. Students can access all these resources on thePoint at http://thePoint.lww.com/PolitEssentials10e, using the codes printed on the inside front cover of their textbooks.

● **Supplements for Each Chapter** further students' exploration of specific topics. A full list of the supplements appears on page xx. These supplements can be assigned to provide additional background or to offer advanced material to meet students' specific needs.

● **Hundreds of Student Review Questions** help students to identify areas of strength and areas needing further study.

● **Answers to Critical Thinking Exercises** are provided for selected questions related to the studies in the appendices of the textbook.

● **Journal Articles**—18 full articles from Wolters Kluwer journals (one corresponding to each chapter)—are provided for additional critical appraisal opportunities. Some of these are the full journal articles for studies used as the end-of-chapter Research Examples. All journal articles that appear on thePoint are identified in the text with ☀ and are called out in the References lists for appropriate chapters with a double asterisk (**).

● **Internet Resources with relevant and useful websites** related to chapter content can be clicked on directly without having to retype the URL and risk a typographical error.

This edition also includes **links to all open-access articles cited in the textbook;** these articles are called out in the References lists for appropriate chapters with a single asterisk (*).

● **Critical Appraisal Guidelines** and **Learning Objectives** from the textbook are available in Microsoft Word for students' convenience.

STUDY GUIDE

The accompanying *Study Guide for Essentials of Nursing Research*, 10th edition, is available for separate purchase and augments the text, providing students with opportunities to apply their learning.

● **Critical appraisal opportunities** abound in the *Study Guide*, **which includes eight research articles in their entirety.** The studies represent a range of nursing topics and research approaches, including a randomized controlled trial, a correlational/mixed methods study, an EBP project, two qualitative studies (ethnographic and grounded theory studies), a quality improvement project, a meta-analysis, and a metasynthesis. The **Application Exercises** in each chapter guide students in reading, understanding, and appraising these eight studies.

● Answers to the "Questions of Fact" section in the Application Exercises in each chapter are presented in Appendix I of the *Study Guide* so that students can get immediate feedback about their responses.

● Although critical appraisal skills are emphasized in the *Study Guide*, other included activities support students' learning of fundamental research terms and principles, such as fill-in-the-blank exercises, matching exercises, and focused study questions. Answers to those questions that have an objective answer are provided in Appendix I.

A COMPREHENSIVE, DIGITAL, INTEGRATED COURSE SOLUTION: LIPPINCOTT® COURSEPOINT

The same trusted solution, innovation, and unmatched support that you have come to expect from *Lippincott CoursePoint* is now enhanced with more engaging learning tools and deeper analytics to help prepare students for practice. This powerfully integrated, digital learning solution combines learning tools, case studies, real-time data, and the most trusted nursing education content on the market to make curriculum-wide learning more efficient and to meet students where they're at in their learning. The solution connects learning to real-life application by integrating content from *Essentials of Nursing Research* with video cases, interactive modules, and research journal articles. Ideal for active, case-based learning, this powerful solution helps students develop higher level cognitive skills and asks them to make decisions related to simple-to-complex scenarios. And now, it's easier than ever for instructors and students to use, giving them everything they need for course and curriculum success! To learn more about this solution, contact your local Wolters Kluwer representative.

Lippincott CoursePoint for Polit & Beck: Essentials of Nursing Research, 10th edition includes the following:

● **Leading Content in Context**, with digital content from *Essentials of Nursing Research*, 10th edition, is embedded in our powerful tools, engaging students and encouraging interaction and learning on a deeper level.

○ The complete interactive e-book provides students with anytime, anywhere access on multiple devices.

○ Full online access to *Stedman's Medical Dictionary for the Health Professions and Nursing* ensures students work with the best medical dictionary available.

- Engaging course content provides a variety of learning tools to engage students of all learning styles.
- A more **personalized learning approach** gives students the content and tools they need at the moment they need it, giving them data for more focused remediation and helping to boost their confidence and competence.
- **Powerful tools** help students learn the critical thinking and clinical judgment skills to help them become practice-ready nurses, including the following:
  - **Video Cases** show how nursing research and evidence-based practice relate to real-life nursing practice. By watching the videos and completing related activities, students will flex their nursing research skills and build a spirit of inquiry.

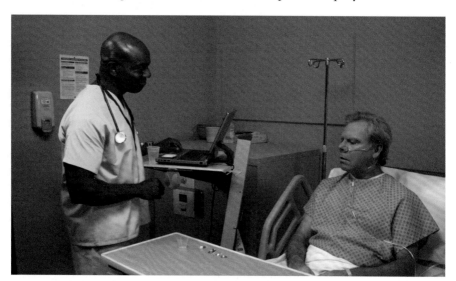

  - **Interactive Modules** help students quickly identify what they do and do not understand, so they can study smartly. With exceptional instructional design that prompts students to discover, reflect, synthesize, and apply, students actively learn. Remediation links to the digital textbook are integrated throughout.
- Unparalleled reporting provides in-depth dashboards with several data points to track student progress and help identify strengths and weaknesses.
- Unmatched support includes training coaches, product trainers, and nursing education consultants to help educators and students implement CoursePoint with ease.

CLOSING NOTE

It is our hope and expectation that the content, style, and organization of this 10th edition of *Essentials of Nursing Research* will be helpful to those students who want to become skillful, thoughtful readers of nursing studies and to those wishing to enhance their clinical performance based on research findings. We also hope that this textbook will help to develop an enthusiasm for the kinds of discoveries and knowledge that research can produce.

Denise F. Polit, PhD, FAAN
Cheryl Tatano Beck, DNSc, CNM, FAAN

Learning Objectives focus students' attention on critical content →

Learning Objectives

On completing this chapter, you will be able to:

- Describe the logic of sampling for qualitative studies
- Identify and describe several types of sampling approaches in qualitative studies
- Evaluate the appropriateness of the sampling method and sample size used in a qualitative study
- Identify and describe methods of collecting unstructured self-report data
- Identify and describe methods of collecting and recording unstructured observational data
- Critically appraise a qualitative researcher's decisions regarding the data collection plan
- Define new terms in the chapter

Key Terms alert students to important terminology →

Key Terms

- Data saturation
- Diary
- Field notes
- Focus group interview
- Key informant
- Log
- Maximum variation sampling
- Participant observation
- Photo elicitation
- Photovoice
- Purposive (purposeful) sampling
- Semi-structured interview
- Snowball sampling
- Theoretical sampling
- Topic guide
- Unstructured interview

Examples help students apply content to real-life research →

Example of a convergent design •••••••••••••••••••••••••••••••••
Kalanlar and Kuru Alici (2020) used a convergent design to study the effect of care burden on formal caregivers' quality of work life. Structured questionnaires were used to obtain quantitative data about the key constructs. In-depth interviews were also undertaken with some caregivers, who were asked such questions as, "What are the most challenging situations while giving care?" and "How does your care burden affect your home life?"

Tip boxes describe what is found in actual research articles →

TIP When a quantitative study is based on a theory or model, the research article typically states this fact early—often in the abstract or the title. Some reports also have a subsection of the introduction called "Theoretical Framework." The report usually includes a brief overview of the theory so that all readers can understand, in a broad way, the conceptual context of the study.

How-to-Tell Tip boxes explain confusing issues in actual research articles →

HOW-TO-TELL TIP How can you tell if a study is experimental? Researchers usually indicate in the method section of their reports that they used an experimental or randomized design (RCT). If such terms are missing, you can conclude that a study is experimental if the article says that the study purpose was to *test the effects of* an intervention AND if participants were put into groups at random.

Critical Appraisal Guidelines boxes lead students through key issues in a research article

Box 9.1 Guidelines for Critically Appraising Quantitative Sampling Plans

1. Was the population identified? Were eligibility criteria specified?
2. What type of sampling design was used? Was the sampling plan one that could be expected to yield a representative sample?
3. How many participants were in the sample? Was the sample size affected by high rates of refusals or attrition? Was the sample size large enough to support statistical conclusion validity? Was the sample size justified on the basis of a power analysis or other rationale?
4. Were key characteristics of the sample described (e.g., mean age, percentage of female)?
5. To whom can the study results reasonably be generalized?

Research Examples highlight critical points made in the chapter and sharpen critical thinking skills

RESEARCH EXAMPLES WITH CRITICAL THINKING EXERCISES

This section presents an example of a study that described its theoretical links. Read the summary and then answer the critical thinking questions, referring to the full research report if necessary. Answers to the questions for Exercise 1 are available to instructors on thePoint. The critical thinking questions for Exercises 2 and 3 are based on the studies that appear in their entirety in Appendices A and B of this book. Our comments for these exercises are in the Student Resources section on thePoint.

EXAMPLE 1: SOCIAL COGNITIVE THEORY IN A QUANTITATIVE STUDY

Study: Predicting engagement with online walking promotion among metropolitan and rural cancer survivors (Frensham et al., 2020)

Statement of Purpose: The purpose of the study was to evaluate the effectiveness of a 12-week online intervention (Steps Toward Improving Diet and Exercise or STRIDE) that was designed to promote walking and other health-promoting behaviors among cancer survivors living in rural and urban areas of Australia.

Critical Thinking Exercises provide opportunities to practice critically appraising research articles

Critical Thinking Exercises

1. Answer the relevant questions from Box 7.1 regarding this study.
2. Also consider the following targeted question: Is there another model or theory that was described in this chapter that could have been used to study the effect of this intervention?
3. If the results of this study are valid and generalizable, what might be some of the uses to which the findings could be put in clinical practice?

Summary Points review chapter content to ensure success

Summary Points

- A **research problem** is a perplexing or troubling situation that a researcher wants to address through disciplined inquiry.
- Researchers usually identify a broad *topic*, narrow the scope of the problem, and then identify research questions consistent with a paradigm of choice.
- Researchers communicate their aims in research articles as problem statements, statements of purpose, research questions, or hypotheses.
- A **problem statement** articulates the problem and an *argument* that explains the need for a study. Problem statements typically include several components: problem identification; background, scope, and consequences of the problem; knowledge gaps; and possible solutions to the problem.
- A **statement of purpose**, which summarizes the overall study goal, identifies the key concepts (variables) and the study group or population. Purpose statements often communicate, through the choice of verbs and other key terms, aspects of the study design, or the research tradition.

Special icons alert students to important content found on thePoint and in the accompanying Study Guide

- **Research questions** are the specific queries researchers want to answer in addressing the research problem.
- A **hypothesis** states predicted relationships between two or more variables—that is, the anticipated association between independent and dependent variables.
- **Directional hypotheses** predict the direction of a relationship; **nondirectional hypotheses** predict the existence of relationships, not their direction.
- **Research hypotheses** predict the existence of relationships; **null hypotheses**, which express the absence of relationships, are the hypotheses subjected to statistical testing.
- Hypotheses are never proved or disproved—they are accepted or rejected, supported or not supported by the data.

Vera C. Brancato, EdD, MSN, BSN, RN, CNE
Professor of Nursing
Alvernia University
Reading, Pennsylvania

Angeline Bushy, PhD, RN, FAAN
Professor, Bert Fish Chair
University of Central Florida
College of Nursing
Daytona Beach, Florida

E.B. Dowdell, PhD, RN, FAAN
Professor
Villanova University College of Nursing
Villanova, Pennsylvania

Amanda J. Flagg, PhD, RN, EdM/MSN, ACNS, CNE
Associate Professor
Middle Tennessee State University School of Nursing
Murfreesboro, Tennessee

Mary Gergis, PhD, MSN, BSN, RN
Assistant Professor
Towson University
Towson, Maryland

Natalie Heywood, MSN-Ed, BSN, RN
Nursing Faculty
Arizona State University
Phoenix, Arizona

Donald Johnston, PhD, RN-MHS, RRT
Assistant Professor of Nursing
Northwestern State University
Natchitoches, Louisiana

Sherri Marlow, DNP, RN, CNE
Associate Professor
Cabarrus College of Health Sciences
Concord, North Carolina

Karen May, PhD, RN, CNE
Assistant Professor
Widener University
Chester, Pennsylvania

Wendy J. Waldspurger Robb, PhD, RN, CNE
Dean and Professor
Cedar Crest College School of Nursing
Allentown, Pennsylvania

Dulce Anne Santacroce, DNP, RN, CCM
Assistant Professor
Touro University Nevada
Henderson, Nevada

Peggy Z. Shipley, PhD, RN
Assistant Professor
Bloomsburg University
Bloomsburg, Pennsylvania

Megan Smith, MSN
Assistant Professor
Viterbo University
La Crosse, Wisconsin

Brent W. Thompson, PhD, RN
Associate Professor
West Chester University of Pennsylvania
Exton, Pennsylvania

Laura Pruitt Walker, DHEd, MSN, RN, CNE, COI, CCTP
Associate Professor
Jacksonville State University
Jacksonville, Alabama

Robin Wilson, EdD, MSN, RNC
Assistant Professor of Nursing
Lincoln Memorial University
Harrogate, Tennessee

Theresa R. Wyatt, PhD, RN, CCM, CFN, CCRE, FACFEI
Assistant Professor
University of Detroit Mercy
Detroit, Michigan

ACKNOWLEDGMENTS

This 10th edition, like the previous nine editions, depended on the contribution of many generous people. To all of the many faculty and students who used the text and have made invaluable suggestions for its improvement, we are very grateful. Suggestions were made to us both directly in personal interactions (mostly at the University of Connecticut and Griffith University in Australia) and via e-mail correspondence. We would like in particular to thank Valori Banfi, nursing librarian at the University of Connecticut, and Carrie Morgan Eaton, a faculty member at the University of Connecticut.

Other individuals made specific contributions. Although it would be impossible to mention all, we note with thanks the nurse researchers who shared their work with us as we developed examples, including work that in some cases was not yet published. We also extend our warm thanks to those who helped to turn the manuscript into a finished product. The staff at Wolters Kluwer has been of tremendous assistance in the support they have given us over the years. We are indebted to Michael Kerns, Meredith L. Brittain, Barton Dudlick, and all the others behind the scenes for their fine contributions.

Finally, we thank our families, our loved ones, and our friends, who provided ongoing support and encouragement throughout this endeavor and who were tolerant when we worked long into the night, over weekends, and during holidays to get this 10th edition finished.

CONTENTS

Chapter Supplements Available on thePoint°

1 Introducing Nursing Research for Evidence-Based Practice

Learning Objectives

On completing this chapter, you will be able to:

- Describe why research is important in nursing and discuss the importance of evidence-based practice
- Describe broad historical trends and future directions in nursing research
- Describe alternative sources of evidence for nursing practice
- Describe major characteristics of the positivist and constructivist paradigm and discuss similarities and differences between the traditional scientific method (quantitative research) and constructivist methods (qualitative research)
- Identify several purposes of qualitative and quantitative nursing research
- Understand sources of information for evidence-based practice
- Describe evidence hierarchies and level of evidence scales
- Identify a well-worded clinical question for evidence-based practice
- Define new terms in the chapter

Key Terms

- Applicability
- Assumption
- Cause-probing research
- Clinical nursing research
- Clinical significance
- Constructivist paradigm
- Empirical evidence
- Evidence-based practice
- Evidence hierarchy
- Generalizability
- Journal club
- Level of evidence scale
- Meta-aggregation
- Meta-analysis
- Metasynthesis
- Mixed methods research
- Mixed studies review
- Nursing research
- Paradigm
- Patient centeredness
- PICO format
- Positivist paradigm
- Primary study
- Qualitative research
- Quantitative research
- Research
- Research methods
- Scientific method
- Systematic review

NURSING RESEARCH IN PERSPECTIVE

We know that most readers are not reading this book because they plan to become nurse researchers. Yet, we are confident that many of you *will* participate in research-related activities during your careers, and virtually all of you will be expected to be research-savvy at a basic level. We hope that you will come to see the value of nursing research and will be inspired by the efforts of the thousands of nurse researchers now working worldwide to improve patient care. You are embarking on a lifelong voyage in which research will play a role. We hope to help you enjoy the journey.

What Is Nursing Research?

Research is systematic inquiry that relies on disciplined methods to answer questions and solve problems. The ultimate goal of research is to gain knowledge that can benefit many people. **Nursing research** is systematic inquiry designed to develop evidence about issues of importance to nurses and their clients. Nurses undertake research to address problems relating to nursing education and nursing administration, but in this book, we emphasize **clinical nursing research**—that is, research designed to guide nursing practice and to improve the health and quality of life of nurses' clients. Clinical nursing research typically begins with questions stemming from practice problems—problems you may have already encountered.

Examples of nursing research questions •
- Does a massage intervention reduce post-operative pain in infants with complex congenital heart disease? (Harrison et al., 2020)
- What is it like to cope with the fear of cancer recurrence among ovarian cancer survivors? (Galica et al., 2020)

 TIP You may think that research is too abstract to have a bearing on patient care. But nursing research focuses on *real* people with *real* problems, and studying those problems offers opportunities to address them through improvements to nursing care.

The Importance of Research to Evidence-Based Nursing

Nursing has experienced profound changes in the past few decades. Nurses are increasingly expected to understand research and to base their practice on evidence from research—that is, to adopt an **evidence-based practice (EBP)**. EBP involves using the best evidence in making patient care decisions, and such evidence typically comes from research conducted by nurses and other health care professionals. Nurse leaders recognize the need to base specific nursing decisions on evidence indicating that the decisions are clinically appropriate, resulting in positive client outcomes, as well as cost-effective. We discuss EBP in greater detail later in this chapter.

In some countries, research plays a role in nursing credentialing and status. For example, the American Nurses Credentialing Center—an arm of the American Nurses Association—has developed a Magnet Recognition Program to recognize health care organizations that provide high-quality nursing care. To achieve Magnet status, practice environments must demonstrate a sustained commitment to EBP; the 2019 Magnet application manual incorporated revisions that strengthen evidence-based requirements. Changes to nursing practice are happening every day because of EBP efforts.

Example of evidence-based practice •
Many clinical practice changes reflect the impact of research. For example, "kangaroo care," the holding of diaper-clad preterm infants skin to skin, chest to chest by parents, is now widely practiced in neonatal intensive care units (NICUs), but before 2000, only a minority of NICUs offered kangaroo care options. Expanded adoption of this practice resulted from mounting evidence that early skin-to-skin contact has clinical benefits without negative side effects. Some of that evidence came from rigorous studies conducted by nurse researchers (e.g., Bastani et al., 2017; Billner-Garcia et al., 2018; Cho et al., 2016; Lowson et al., 2015; Xie et al., 2020).

Roles of Nurses in Research

Most nurses are likely to engage in one or more activity along a continuum of research participation. At one end of the continuum are *consumers of nursing research*—nurses who read research reports to keep up-to-date on findings that may affect their practice. EBP depends on well-informed nursing research consumers.

At the other end of the continuum are the *producers of nursing research*—nurses who actively undertake studies. Research is increasingly being conducted by practicing nurses who want to find what works best for their clients.

Between these two end points on the continuum lie a variety of research activities in which nurses engage. Even if you never carry out a study, you may do one of the following:

1. Contribute an idea for a study.
2. Gather information from those taking part in a study.
3. Advise clients about participating in a study.
4. Search for research evidence to address a practice problem.
5. Discuss the implications of a study in a **journal club** in your practice setting, which involves meetings (in groups or online) to discuss research articles.

In all these possible research-related activities, nurses who have some research skills are better able than those without them to make a contribution to nursing and to EBP.

Nursing Research: Past and Present

Most people agree that research in nursing began with Florence Nightingale in the 1850s. Based on her skillful analysis of factors affecting soldier mortality and morbidity during the Crimean War, she was successful in bringing about changes in nursing care and in public health. After Nightingale's work, however, research disappeared from the nursing literature until the early 1900s, but most studies at that time concerned nurses' education.

In the 1950s, research by nurses began to accelerate. Increased numbers of nurses with advanced degrees, the growth in research funding, and the establishment of the journal *Nursing Research* helped to propel nursing research at mid-20th century. During the 1960s, practice-oriented research began to emerge, and research-oriented journals started publication in several countries. During the 1970s, there was a change in research emphasis from areas such as teaching and nurses' characteristics to improvements in client care. Nurses also began to pay attention to the utilization of research findings in nursing practice.

In 1986, the National Center for Nursing Research (NCNR) was established at the National Institutes of Health (NIH) in the United States. A key purpose of NCNR was to promote and financially support research relating to patient care. In 1993, nursing research was strengthened when NCNR was promoted to full institute status within the

NIH: The *National Institute of Nursing Research* (NINR) was created. NINR helped put nursing research into the mainstream of activities enjoyed by other health disciplines. Funding opportunities for nursing research also expanded in other countries. The 1990s witnessed the birth of several more journals for nurse researchers.

 TIP   For those interested in learning more about the history of nursing research, we offer an expanded summary in the supplement to this chapter on thePoint® website.

Current and Future Directions for Nursing Research

Nursing research continues to develop at a rapid pace and will undoubtedly flourish throughout the 21st century as research findings grow. In 1986, NCNR had a budget of $16 million, whereas NINR funding in fiscal year 2020 was approximately $170 million. Among the trends we foresee for the near future are the following:

- *Continued focus on EBP.* Nurses' use of research findings in their practice will continue to be encouraged. This means that improvements will be needed in nurses' skills in locating, understanding, critically appraising, and using relevant study results.
- *Ongoing growth of research syntheses.* Systematic reviews, which are a cornerstone of EBP, rigorously integrate research information on a topic so that conclusions about the state of evidence can be reached.
- *Increased emphasis on patient centeredness.* **Patient centeredness** has become a central concern in health care and in research. Efforts are increasing to ensure that research is relevant to patients and that patients play a role in setting research priorities.
- *Relatedly, greater interest in the* **applicability** *of research.* More attention is being paid to figuring out how study results can be applied to individual patients or subgroups of patients. A limitation of the current EBP model is that evidence typically is based on the *average effects* of health care interventions implemented under ideal circumstances.
- *Expanded local research and quality improvement efforts in health care settings.* Small studies designed to solve local problems are increasing. This trend will be reinforced as more hospitals apply for (and are recertified for) Magnet status in the United States and other countries. Mechanisms are being developed to ensure that evidence from local projects becomes available to others facing similar problems.
- *Increased focus on health disparities.* Health disparities continue to be a crucially important concern, and this in turn has raised consciousness about the cultural sensitivity of health interventions. Research (and health care more generally) must be sensitive to the beliefs, life experiences, barriers, and values of racially, culturally, and linguistically diverse populations.
- *Growing interest in defining and ascertaining* **clinical significance**. Research findings increasingly must meet the test of being clinically significant, and patients have taken center stage in efforts to define clinical significance.

What are nurse researchers likely to be studying in the future? Although there is tremendous diversity in research interests, research priorities have been articulated by NINR, Sigma Theta Tau International, and other nursing organizations. For example, the primary areas of interest articulated in the 2016 NINR strategic plan were the following:

- Symptom science: promoting personalized health strategies
- Wellness: promoting health and preventing disease
- Self-management: improving quality of life for individuals with chronic illness
- End-of-life and palliative care: the science of compassion

TIP All websites cited in this chapter, plus additional websites with useful content relating to the foundations of nursing research, are in the Internet Resources on thePoint® website. This will allow you to simply use the "Control/Click" feature to go directly to the website, without having to type in the URL and risk a typographical error. Websites corresponding to the content of all chapters of the book are on thePoint®.

KNOWLEDGE SOURCES FOR NURSING PRACTICE

Nurses make clinical decisions based on a large repertoire of knowledge. As a nursing student, you are gaining skills in nursing practice from your instructors, textbooks, and clinical placements. When you become a registered nurse (RN), you will continue to learn from other nurses and health care professionals. Because evidence is constantly evolving, learning about best-practice nursing will be an ongoing quest throughout your career.

Some of what you have learned thus far is based on systematic research, but much of it is not. Where does knowledge for nursing practice come from? Until fairly recently, knowledge was based primarily on clinical experience, trial and error, tradition, and expert opinion. These alternative sources of knowledge are different from research-based information.

Tradition and "Experts"

Some nursing decisions are based on untested traditions and "unit culture" rather than on sound evidence. One analysis suggested that some "sacred cows" (ineffective customs) persist even in a health care center recognized as a leader in EBP (Hanrahan et al., 2015). Another common source of knowledge is an authority, a person with specialized expertise. Reliance on experts (such as nursing faculty, mentors, or textbook authors) is unavoidable. Experts, however, are not infallible—particularly if their expertise is based primarily on personal experience or outdated information; yet, their knowledge is often unchallenged.

 TIP The consequences of *not* using research-based evidence can be devastating. For example, from 1956 through the 1980s, Dr. Benjamin Spock published several editions of *Baby and Child Care*, a parental guide that sold over 19 million copies worldwide. Dr. Spock wrote the following advice: "I think it is preferable to accustom a baby to sleeping on his stomach from the beginning if he is willing" (Spock, 1979, p. 164). Research has demonstrated that this sleeping position is associated with heightened risk of sudden infant death syndrome (SIDS). In their systematic review of evidence, Gilbert and colleagues (2005) wrote, "Advice to put infants to sleep on the front for nearly half a century was contrary to evidence from 1970 that this was likely to be harmful" (p. 874). They estimated that if medical advice had been guided by research evidence, over 60,000 infant deaths might have been prevented.

Clinical Experience and Trial and Error

Clinical experience is a functional source of knowledge—indeed, it is a component of the EBP model. Yet, personal experience has limitations as a source of evidence for practice because each nurse's experience is too narrow to be generally useful, and personal experiences are often colored by biases. Trial and error—alternatives tried successively until a solution to a problem is found—can be practical but the method tends to be haphazard and solutions may be idiosyncratic.

Disciplined Research

Disciplined research is considered the best method of acquiring reliable knowledge. Evidence-based health care compels nurses to base their clinical practice to the extent possible on rigorous research-based findings rather than on tradition, authority, or personal experience—although nursing will always remain a rich blend of art and science.

PARADIGMS AND METHODS FOR NURSING RESEARCH

The questions that nurse researchers ask, and the strategies they use to answer their questions, spring from a researcher's view of how the world "works." In research parlance, a **paradigm** is a worldview, a general perspective on the world's complexities.

Disciplined inquiry in nursing has been conducted mainly within two paradigms. The paradigm that dominated nursing research for decades is called the **positivist paradigm**. Positivism, rooted in 19th century thought, is a reflection of a broad cultural movement that emphasizes the rational and scientific. The **constructivist paradigm** (sometimes called the *naturalistic paradigm*) began as a countermovement to positivism and is a major alternative system for conducting research in nursing.

This section describes the two paradigms and outlines the research methods associated with them. **Research methods** are the techniques researchers use to structure a study and to gather and analyze relevant information. The two paradigms are associated with different methods of developing evidence.

The Positivist Paradigm

An **assumption** is a principle that is believed to be true without verification. Paradigms are associated with a set of assumptions that have implications for the kinds of research questions that researchers ask and the methods they use to answer them.

Worldview of the Positivist Paradigm

A fundamental assumption of positivists is that there is a reality *out there* that can be studied and known. Positivists assume that nature is ordered and regular, and that a reality exists independent of human observation. The assumption of *determinism* refers to the positivists' belief that phenomena are not haphazard but rather have antecedent causes. Within the positivist paradigm, research activity is often aimed at understanding the underlying causes of natural phenomena. Because of their belief in a factual reality, positivists prize objectivity. Their approach involves the use of orderly, disciplined procedures with tight controls over the research situation to test hunches about the nature of phenomena being studied and relationships among them.

 TIP   What do we mean by *phenomena*? In a research context, *phenomena* are those things in which researchers are interested—such as a health event (e.g., a patient fall), a health outcome (e.g., pain), or a health experience (e.g., living with chronic pain).

Strict positivist thinking has been challenged. *Postpositivists* recognize the impossibility of total objectivity, but they view objectivity as a goal and strive to be as unbiased as possible. Postpositivists also appreciate the barriers to knowing reality with certainty and therefore seek *probabilistic* evidence—i.e., learning what the true state of a phenomenon *probably* is. This modified positivist position remains a dominant force in nursing research. For the sake of simplicity, we refer to it as positivism.

The Scientific Method and Quantitative Research

The traditional, positivist **scientific method** involves using orderly procedures to gather primarily quantitative information. Quantitative researchers typically move in a systematic fashion from the definition of a problem to a solution. By *systematic*, we mean that investigators progress through a series of steps, according to a prespecified plan. Quantitative researchers use methods designed to control the research situation with the goal of minimizing *bias* and maximizing validity.

Quantitative researchers gather **empirical evidence**—evidence that is rooted in objective reality and gathered through the senses rather than through personal beliefs. Evidence for a study using the traditional scientific method is gathered systematically, using instruments to collect needed information. Usually, the information is *quantitative*—numeric information that results from some type of formal measurement and that is analyzed statistically. Quantitative researchers strive to go beyond the specifics of a situation; the ability to generalize research findings to individuals who did not take part in the study (referred to as **generalizability**) is an important goal.

The traditional scientific method has been used productively by nurse researchers studying a wide range of questions. Yet, there are important limitations. For example, quantitative researchers must deal with problems of *measurement*. To study a phenomenon, scientists must measure it, that is, attach numeric values that express quantity. For example, if the phenomenon of interest were patient stress, researchers would want to assess if stress was high or low, or higher under certain conditions. Physiologic phenomena like blood pressure and temperature can be measured with accuracy and precision, but the same cannot be said of psychological phenomena, such as stress, resilience, or pain.

Nursing research focuses on human beings, who are inherently complicated and diverse. Quantitative studies typically focus on only a few concepts (e.g., weight gain, depression). Complexities tend to be controlled and, if possible, eliminated rather than studied directly, and this narrowness of focus can sometimes obscure insights. Quantitative research within the positivist paradigm has been criticized for failing to capture the full breadth of human experience.

Example of a quantitative study •
Tung and colleagues (2020) examined the effect of meridian cuffing exercises on functional fitness and cardiopulmonary functioning in community-dwelling older adults. The researchers measured such outcomes as upper body flexibility, handgrip strength, lung capacity, and aerobic endurance among people who either did or did not receive the exercise intervention.

 TIP Students often find quantitative studies more intimidating than qualitative ones. Try not to worry too much about the jargon at first—remember that each study has a *story* to tell, and grasping the main point of the story is what is initially important.

The Constructivist Paradigm

This section describes the assumptions and research methods associated with the constructivist paradigm.

Worldview of the Constructivist Paradigm

For the naturalistic inquirer, reality is not a fixed entity but rather a construction of the people participating in the research; reality exists within a context, and many constructions are possible. Constructivists take the position of relativism: If there are multiple interpretations of reality that exist in people's minds, then there is no process by which the ultimate truth or falsity of the constructions can be determined.

The constructivist paradigm assumes that knowledge is maximized when the distance between the inquirer and participants in the study is minimized. The voices and interpretations of those under study are crucial to understanding the phenomenon of interest, and subjective interactions are the best way to access them. Findings from a constructivist inquiry are the product of the interaction between the inquirer and the participants.

Constructivist Methods and Qualitative Research

Researchers in the constructivist versus the positivist paradigm rely on different research methods (Table 1.1). Researchers in constructivist traditions emphasize the inherent complexity of humans, their ability to shape their own experiences, and the idea that truth is a composite of realities. Consequently, constructivist studies are focused on understanding the human experience as it is lived, through the careful collection and analysis of *qualitative* materials that are narrative and subjective.

Qualitative researchers believe that a major limitation of the traditional scientific method is that it is *reductionist*—that is, it reduces human experience to the few concepts under investigation, and those concepts are defined in advance rather than emerging from the experiences of those under study. Constructivist researchers tend to emphasize the dynamic, holistic, and individual aspects of human life and try to capture those aspects in their entirety, within the context of those who are experiencing them.

Flexible, evolving procedures are used to capitalize on findings that emerge during the study, which typically is undertaken in naturalistic settings. The collection and analysis of information usually progress concurrently. As researchers sift through information, insights are gained, new questions emerge, and further evidence is sought to confirm the insights. Through an inductive process (going from specifics to the general), researchers integrate information to develop a theory or description that illuminates the phenomena under observation.

Constructivist studies yield rich, in-depth information that can potentially clarify the dimensions of a complicated phenomenon. The findings are grounded in the real-life experiences of people with firsthand knowledge of a phenomenon. Nevertheless, the approach has several limitations. Human beings are used directly as the instrument through which information is gathered, and humans are highly intelligent—but fallible—tools.

TABLE 1.1 **Key Methodologic Differences in the Positivist and Constructivist Paradigms**

Positivist Paradigm (Quantitative Research)	Constructivist Paradigm (Qualitative Research)
Deductive processes → hypothesis testing	Inductive processes → hypothesis generation
Emphasis on discrete, specific concepts	Emphasis on the entirety of a phenomenon; holistic
Focus on the objective and quantifiable	Focus on the subjective and nonquantifiable
Outsider knowledge—researcher is external, separate	Insider knowledge—researcher is part of the process
Fixed, prespecified research design	Flexible, emergent research design
Controls over context	Context-bound
Large, representative samples	Small, information-rich samples
Measured (quantitative) information	Narrative (unstructured) information
Statistical analysis	Qualitative analysis
Seeks generalizations	Seeks in-depth understanding

Another issue involves the subjectivity of constructivist inquiry, which can raise concerns about the idiosyncratic nature of the judgments. Would two constructivist researchers studying the same phenomenon in similar settings arrive at comparable conclusions? The problem is exacerbated by the fact that most constructivist studies involve a small number of participants. Thus, the generalizability of findings from constructivist inquiries is a potential concern.

Example of a qualitative study •
Drageset and colleagues (2020) conducted an in-depth study to explore breast cancer survivors' coping experiences 9 years after they had primary breast cancer surgery.

 TIP Researchers seldom discuss or even mention the underlying paradigm of their studies in their reports. The paradigm shapes the inquiry without being explicitly referenced.

Multiple Paradigms and Nursing Research

Paradigms are lenses that help to sharpen researchers' focus on phenomena of interest. The availability of alternative paradigms for studying nursing problems can maximize the breadth of new evidence for practice. Nursing is enriched by the use of diverse methods—methods that are often complementary in their strengths and limitations.

We have emphasized differences between the two paradigms and associated methods so that distinctions would be easy to understand. It is equally important, however, to note that the two paradigms have many features in common, some of which are mentioned here:

- *Ultimate goals.* The ultimate aim of disciplined research, regardless of paradigm, is to answer questions and solve problems. All researchers seek to capture the truth with regard to the phenomena in which they are interested.
- *External evidence.* The word *empiricism* is often associated with the scientific method, but qualitative researchers also gather and analyze evidence gathered empirically, that is, through their senses.
- *Reliance on human cooperation.* Human cooperation is essential in both qualitative and quantitative research. To understand people's characteristics and experiences, researchers must persuade them to participate in the study and to speak candidly.
- *Ethical constraints.* Regardless of paradigms or methods, research with human beings is guided by ethical principles that sometimes conflict with research goals.
- *Fallibility.* Virtually, all studies have limitations. The fallibility of any single study makes it important to understand and critically appraise researchers' methods when evaluating evidence quality.

Thus, despite philosophic and methodologic differences, researchers using the traditional scientific or constructivist methods face many similar challenges. The selection of an appropriate method depends not only on researchers' worldview but also on the research question. If a researcher asks, "What are the effects of cryotherapy on oral mucositis in patients undergoing chemotherapy?" the researcher needs to examine effects through a careful quantitative assessment of patient outcomes. On the other hand, if a researcher asks, "What is the process by which parents learn to cope with the death of a child?" the researcher would be hard pressed to quantify the process. Personal worldviews of researchers help to shape the questions they ask.

In reading about the alternative paradigms, you likely were more attracted to one of the two paradigms—the one that corresponds to your view of the world. It is important, however, to learn about and value both approaches to disciplined inquiry and to recognize their respective strengths and limitations. This book will hopefully help you to become *methodologically bilingual*—a skill that is increasingly important because many nurse researchers are now undertaking **mixed methods research** that involves the collection and analysis of both qualitative and quantitative data in a single study, as we discuss in Chapter 12.

 HOW-TO-TELL TIP How can you quickly tell if a study is qualitative or quantitative? As you progress through this book, you should be able to identify most studies as qualitative versus quantitative based on terms in the introductory summary or on the report title. At this point, though, it may be easiest to distinguish the two types of studies based on how many *numbers* appear in the article, especially in tables. Qualitative studies may have no tables with quantitative information, or only one numeric table describing participants' characteristics (e.g., the percentage who were male or female). Quantitative studies typically have several tables with numbers and statistical information. Qualitative studies often have "word tables" or diagrams and figures illustrating processes inferred from the narrative information gathered.

THE PURPOSES OF NURSING RESEARCH

Why do nurses do research? Several systems have been devised to classify research goals.

Research for Varying Levels of Explanation

One classification system concerns the extent to which studies provide explanatory information. The descriptive/explanatory continuum includes studies whose purposes are identification, description, exploration, prediction/control, and explanation of health-related phenomena. For each purpose, various types of question are addressed—some more amenable to qualitative than to quantitative inquiry, and vice versa. Here are some examples of questions researchers ask related to these purposes, with a designation of whether the inquiry would most likely be quantitative (Quan) or qualitative (Qual):

- *Identification*: What is this phenomenon? What is its name? (Qual)
- *Description*: How prevalent is the phenomenon? (Quan) What are the dimensions or characteristics of the phenomenon? (Qual)
- *Exploration*: What factors are related to the phenomenon? (Quan) What is the full nature of the phenomenon? (Qual)
- *Prediction/control*: If phenomenon X occurs, will phenomenon Y follow? Can the phenomenon be prevented? (Quan)
- *Explanation*: What is the underlying cause of the phenomenon? (Quan) What does the phenomenon mean? (Qual)

 TIP Specific study goals can range along a descriptive/explanatory continuum, but a fundamental distinction is between studies whose primary intent is to *describe* phenomena and those that are **cause-probing**—i.e., designed to illuminate the underlying causes of phenomena. Questions in the prediction/control and explanation categories are cause-probing.

Research Purposes Linked to Evidence-Based Practice

Another system for classifying studies has emerged in efforts to communicate EBP-related purposes (e.g., Guyatt et al., 2015; Melnyk & Fineout-Overholt, 2019). In this classification scheme, most purposes can best be addressed with quantitative research.

Therapy/Intervention

Therapy/intervention questions are addressed by health care researchers who want to learn the benefits of specific actions, treatments, products, or processes. Studies with a therapy purpose seek to identify effective treatments for ameliorating or preventing health problems. Such studies range from evaluations of highly specific treatments (e.g., comparing two types of cooling blankets for febrile patients) to complex multicomponent interventions designed to result in behavioral changes (e.g., testing a nurse-led smoking cessation intervention). Therapy questions are foundational for evidence-based decision making; evidence for changes to nursing practice comes from studies that have tested the effects of intervening in a particular way.

Example of a study aimed at Therapy •
Is an Avatar application effective in teaching heart attack recognition and response in patients with acute coronary syndrome (Tongpeth et al., 2020)?

Diagnosis and Assessment

Many nursing studies concern the rigorous development and testing of formal instruments to screen, diagnose, and assess patients and to measure clinical outcomes—that is, they address **Diagnosis/assessment questions**. High-quality instruments with documented accuracy are essential for clinical practice and for research.

Example of a study aimed at Diagnosis/assessment •
Resnick and colleagues (2020) developed and rigorously evaluated the Checklist for Function-Focused Care in Service Plans, using data from 242 people living in assisted living facilities. The checklist was designed to assess whether service plans were helping to optimize physical activity and function.

Prognosis

Researchers who ask **Prognosis questions** strive to understand the outcomes associated with a disease or a health problem (i.e., its consequences), to estimate the probability they will occur, and to predict the types of people for whom the outcomes are most likely. Such studies facilitate the development of long-term care plans for patients. They also provide valuable information for guiding patients to make beneficial lifestyle choices or to be vigilant for key symptoms.

Example of a study aimed at Prognosis •
Yoo and colleagues (2020) studied the effect of physical function limitations in patients with end-stage renal disease on 1-year kidney transplant outcomes (graft success and patient survival).

Etiology (Causation)/Prevention of Harm

It is difficult to prevent harm or treat health problems if we do not know what causes them—and this is the focus of **Etiology questions**. For example, there would be no smoking cessation programs if research had not provided firm evidence that smoking cigarettes causes or contributes to many health problems. Thus, determining the factors and exposures that affect or cause illness, mortality, or morbidity is an important purpose of many studies.

Example of a study aimed at Etiology/prevention of harm ••••••••••••••
Tang and coresearchers (2020) did a study to identify factors associated with reductions in functional status among older intensive care unit (ICU) survivors who were discharged 6 months earlier. The risk factors included delirium, impaired mobility while in the ICU, and use of mechanical ventilation during the ICU stay.

Description

Description questions are not in a category typically identified in EBP-related classification schemes, but so many nursing studies have a descriptive purpose that we include it here. Examples of phenomena that nurse researchers have described include patients' pain, physical function, confusion, and levels of depression. Quantitative description focuses on the prevalence, size, intensity, and measurable attributes of phenomena. Qualitative researchers, by contrast, describe the dimensions or the evolution of phenomena.

Example of a quantitative study aimed at Description ••••••••••••••••••
Porter and coresearchers (2020) did a study to describe Code Blue activations in a regional Australian health care service. They found, for example, that activation was highest on Tuesdays (19%) and that the emergency department was the most common clinical setting for a Code Blue event (28%). About half the patients (49%) survived the activations.

Example of a qualitative study aimed at Description ••••••••••••••••••
Niela-Vilen and colleagues (2020) undertook a study to describe the perspectives of both health care professionals and pregnant women with high-risk pregnancies regarding remote monitoring in maternity care versus being a "Google mom."

Meaning and Processes

Many health care activities (e.g., motivating people to comply with treatments, designing appealing interventions) can benefit from gaining insight into the clients' perspectives, using qualitative research methods that address **Meaning/process questions**. Research that offers evidence about what health and illness mean to clients, what barriers they face to positive health practices, and what processes they experience in a transition through a health care crisis are important to evidence-based nursing practice.

Example of a study aimed at Meaning/process ••••••••••••••••••••••••
Neris and colleagues (2020) studied the experiences and journey of self-discovery throughout the urologic cancer survival trajectory of men in Brazil.

 TIP   Several EBP-related purposes involve *cause-probing* research. Therapy/intervention research focuses on whether an intervention *causes* improvements in key outcomes. Prognosis research examines whether a disease or health condition *causes* subsequent adverse consequences. Etiology research seeks explanations about the underlying *causes* of health problems.

TABLE 1.2 Different Categories of Question Relating to Cigarette Smoking

Type of Question	Example of a Research Question on Cigarette Smoking
Therapy/intervention	Does a nurse-led smoking cessation program for young adults reduce smoking?
Diagnosis/assessment	Is our Smoking Susceptibility Index a valid and reliable measure of teenagers' propensity to initiate smoking?
Prognosis	Is a diagnosis of smoking-related lung cancer associated with increased risk of suicidal ideation?
Etiology (causation)/prevention of harm	Does being a smoker increase the risk of a fatality among people infected with the novel coronavirus?
Description	What percentage of high school students smoke ≥1 pack of cigarettes per week?
Meaning/process	What is it like for long-term smokers to attempt and fail at quitting?

Links Between Study Purposes and Evidence-Based Practice

Studies that address Therapy/intervention questions provide the most direct evidence for EBP. If we want to know, for example, whether wedge-shaped foam cushions are more effective in preventing heel pressure ulcers than standard foam pillows, we would need to look for rigorous studies that have addressed this Therapy question.

Other questions also play a role in improving the quality of nursing care, albeit in different ways. Table 1.2 presents examples of different questions relating to cigarette smoking, using the EBP-related purpose categories. The findings from studies relating to only one of these questions is directly *actionable*—the Therapy question. If there is good evidence that nurse-led smoking cessation programs are effective in reducing smoking among young adults, we might consider initiating such a program in our own community.

Strong evidence from studies addressing the other questions in Table 1.2 could also guide efforts to improve nursing practice—but not as directly. For example, evidence about suicide ideation from the Prognosis question might prompt us to develop a program of emotional support for patients with lung cancer. Results from the Etiology study might lead us to launch a smoking-cessation initiative in communities hit hard by coronavirus infections. The stories from long-term smokers who failed to quit despite efforts to do so (the Meaning question) could lead us to involve them in the design of an intervention for persistent smokers.

Nurse researchers are making strides in addressing all types of questions about important health problems—but evidence regarding what "works" to improve nursing practice comes from studies addressing Therapy questions. Evidence about the scope of a problem, factors affecting the problem, the consequences of the problem, and the meaning of the problem can, however, play a crucial role in efforts to design better interventions, to aim resources at those in greatest need, and to provide appropriate guidance to clients in everyday practice.

BASICS OF EVIDENCE-BASED NURSING PRACTICE

In this section, we describe some basic principles of EBP. We elaborate on EBP issues in Chapter 18.

Definition of Evidence-Based Practice

Dozens of definitions of EBP have been proposed. Most definitions describe EBP as a *decision-making* (or *problem-solving*) *process*. Most definitions also include the idea that EBP

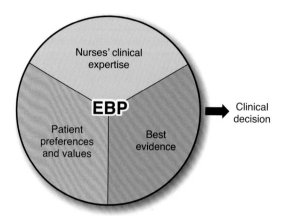

Figure 1.1 Model of evidence-based nursing practice.

is built on a "three-legged stool," each "leg" of which is essential to the process: *best evidence*, *patient preferences and values*, and *clinical expertise*. Figure 1.1 depicts these concepts.

Best Evidence

A basic feature of EBP as a clinical problem-solving strategy is that it de-emphasizes decisions based on tradition or expert opinion. The emphasis is on identifying and evaluating the best available research evidence as a tool for solving problems. There continues to be debate about what qualifies as "best" evidence. As we discuss in the next section, evidence is often evaluated in relation to *evidence hierarchies* that rank evidence sources according to the degree to which the evidence is unbiased. Evidence, however, whether "best" or not, is never by itself a sufficient basis for clinical decision making.

Patient Preferences and Values

Patient input encompasses several concepts, including patient preferences for type of treatment, preferences for being involved in decision making, social or cultural values, preferences about involving family members in health care decisions, priorities regarding quality of life issues, and spiritual or religious values. EBP decisions also require understanding patients' circumstances, such as the resources at their disposal. Nurses thus need the skills to elicit and understand patient preferences and their situations.

Nurses' Clinical Expertise

Decision making in clinical practice also relies on clinicians' expertise, which is an amalgam of academic knowledge gained during training and continuing education, experiences with patient care, and interdisciplinary sharing of new knowledge. David Sackett, the pioneer of evidence-based medicine, strongly advocated for the importance of clinical expertise in making decisions because even very strong research evidence is seldom appropriate for all patients.

Sources of "Best" Research Evidence

Thousands of studies of relevance to nurses are published every month in professional journals. **Primary studies** must be critically appraised to determine if the evidence is sufficiently rigorous to warrant consideration in nursing practice. Finding evidence useful for practice is often facilitated by the availability of evidence that is preprocessed (synthesized) and sometimes pre-appraised. For example, several evidence-based journals publish synopses of original research (e.g., *Evidence-Based Nursing*, *The Online Journal of Knowledge Synthesis for Nursing*), and the synopses are occasionally accompanied by commentary about the clinical utility of the evidence.

Syntheses that integrate evidence from multiple studies on a given topic are an especially important resource for EBP. The most widely respected type of synthesis is the systematic review. A **systematic review** is not just a literature review—it is a methodical, scholarly inquiry that summarizes and evaluates current evidence on a research question. Systematic reviews are the basis for most clinical practice guidelines.

Systematic reviewers sometimes integrate findings from quantitative studies using statistical methods, in what is called a **meta-analysis**. Meta-analysts treat the findings from a study as one piece of information. The findings from multiple studies on the same topic are combined and analyzed statistically. Meta-analysis is an objective method of integrating a body of findings and of observing patterns that might otherwise have gone undetected (see Chapter 17).

Systematic reviews of qualitative studies often take the form of metasyntheses. A **metasynthesis** is less about combining information and more about amplifying and interpreting it. For certain qualitative questions, an aggregative (rather than interpretive) approach to systematic synthesis called **meta-aggregation** may be appropriate. Strategies have also been developed for systematic **mixed studies review**, which are efforts to integrate and synthesize both quantitative and qualitative evidence on a topic.

Evidence Hierarchies and Level of Evidence Scales

Judgments about what evidence is "best" are often guided by evidence hierarchies. **Evidence hierarchies** rank evidence sources in terms of their risk of bias, focusing mainly on risk of bias in studies addressing Therapy questions. Most evidence hierarchies are represented as pyramids, with the highest ranking sources—those presumed to have the least bias for making inferences about the effects of an intervention—at the top. The hierarchies form **level of evidence (LOE) scales** that rank order types of evidence. Level I evidence usually is considered the best (least biased) type of evidence.

Figure 1.2 shows our eight-level evidence hierarchy for Therapy/intervention questions. In our scheme, the Level I evidence source is a systematic review of studies called *randomized controlled trials* (RCTs), which are the "gold standard" type of study for Therapy questions. An individual RCT is a Level II evidence source. Going down the "rungs" of the evidence hierarchy for Therapy questions results in evidence with a higher risk of bias in answering questions about "what works." (Technical terms in Figure 1.2, such as "quasi-experiment," are explained later in the book.)

 TIP Sometimes, evidence hierarchies are used to "level" or grade evidence sources, with the implication that higher levels provide better quality evidence. As pointed out by Levin (2014), however, an evidence hierarchy "is not meant to provide a quality rating for evidence retrieved in the search for an answer" (p. 6). She noted that "leveling" a study is not a substitute for a critical appraisal of the evidence.

Asking Well-Worded Clinical Questions for Evidence-Based Practice

In Chapter 18, we describe a five-step process for putting research to use in clinical settings—the "5A" process: Ask, Acquire, Appraise, Apply, and Assess. Here, we focus on the first step.

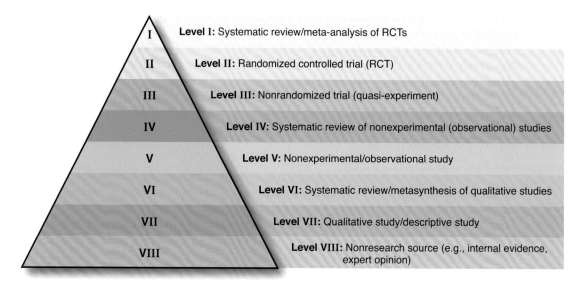

I	**Level I:** Systematic review/meta-analysis of RCTs
II	**Level II:** Randomized controlled trial (RCT)
III	**Level III:** Nonrandomized trial (quasi-experiment)
IV	**Level IV:** Systematic review of nonexperimental (observational) studies
V	**Level V:** Nonexperimental/observational study
VI	**Level VI:** Systematic review/metasynthesis of qualitative studies
VII	**Level VII:** Qualitative study/descriptive study
VIII	**Level VIII:** Nonresearch source (e.g., internal evidence, expert opinion)

Figure 1.2 Polit–Beck Evidence Hierarchy/Level of Evidence Scale for Therapy questions.

The first activity in EBP involves asking well-worded clinical questions that can be answered with research evidence. For example, we may wonder, "Is a fish oil–enhanced nutritional supplement effective in stabilizing weight in cancer patients with cachexia?" The answer to such a Therapy question may provide "best evidence" on how to address the needs of patients with cachexia.

Most guidance for EBP uses the acronyms PIO and **PICO** to help practitioners develop well-worded questions. In the PICO form, the clinical question is worded to identify four components:

P: the *Population* or *patients* (What are key characteristics of the patients or people?)
I: the *Intervention, influence,* or *exposure* (What is the intervention or therapy of interest? or, What is a potentially beneficial—or harmful—influence?)
C: an explicit *Comparison* to the "I" component (With what is the intervention or influence being compared?)
O: the *Outcome* (What is the outcome in which we are interested?)

Applying this scheme to our question about cachexia, our *population* (P) is cancer patients with cachexia; the *intervention* (I) is fish oil–enhanced nutritional supplements; and the *outcome* (O) is weight stabilization. In this question, the *comparison* is not formally stated, but the implied "C" is the *absence* of fish oil–enhanced supplements—the question is in a PIO format. However, when there is an explicit comparison of interest, the full PICO format is used. For example, we might be interested in learning whether fish oil–enhanced supplements (I) are better than melatonin (C) in stabilizing weight (O) in patients with cachexia (P).

For questions that can best be answered with qualitative information (e.g., about the meaning of an experience or health problem), two components are most relevant:

The *population* (What are the characteristics of the patients or clients?)
The *situation* (What conditions, experiences, or circumstances are we interested in understanding?)

For example, suppose our question was, "What is it like to suffer from cachexia?" In this case, the question calls for rich qualitative information; the *population* is patients with advanced cancer, and the *situation* is the experience of cachexia.

TABLE 1.3 **Question Templates for Clinical Questions: PIO and PICO**

Type of Question	PIO Question Template (Questions Without an Explicit Comparison)	PICO Question Template (Questions With an Explicit Comparison)
Therapy/treatment/intervention	In _____ (Population), what is the effect of _____ (Intervention) on _____ (Outcome)?	In _____ (Population), what is the effect of _____ (Intervention), in comparison to _____ (Comparative/alternative intervention), on _____ (Outcome)?
Diagnosis/assessment	For _____ (Population), does _____ (Identifying tool/procedure) yield accurate and appropriate diagnostic/assessment information about _____ (Outcome)?	For _____ (Population), does _____ (Identifying tool/procedure) yield more accurate or more appropriate diagnostic/assessment information than _____ (Comparative tool/procedure) about _____ (Outcome)?
Prognosis	In _____ (Population), does _____ (Influence/exposure to disease or condition) increase the risk of _____ (Outcome)?	In _____ (Population), does _____ (Influence/exposure to disease or condition), relative to _____ (Comparative disease/condition OR absence of the disease/condition) increase the risk of _____ (Outcome)?
Etiology/harm	In _____ (Population), does _____ (Influence/exposure/characteristic) increase the risk of _____ (Outcome)?	In _____ (Population), does _____ (Influence/exposure/characteristic) compared to _____ (Comparative influence/exposure OR lack of influence or exposure) increase the risk of _____ (Outcome)?
Description (prevalence/incidence)	In _____ (Population), how prevalent is _____ (Outcome)?	*Explicit comparisons are not typical, except to compare different populations.*
Meaning or process	What is it like for _____ (Population) to experience (condition, illness, circumstance)? OR What is the process by which _____ (Population) cope with, adapt to, or live with _____ (condition, illness, circumstance)?	*Explicit comparisons are not typical in these types of questions.*

Table 1.3 offers question templates for asking well-framed clinical questions for specific types of questions. The right-hand column includes questions with an explicit comparison (PICO questions), whereas the middle column does not (PIO). The questions are categorized according to the EBP purposes described earlier.

 TIP Although EBP has had a powerful and beneficial impact on health care practices, recent concerns have emerged regarding the applicability of evidence from systematic reviews for individual patients. In Chapter 18, we elaborate on new ideas for creating *practice-based evidence* that enhances *applicability* to individuals, small groups of people, and local contexts.

Box 1.1 Questions for a Preliminary Overview of a Research Report

1. How relevant is the research problem to the practice of nursing?
2. Was the study quantitative or qualitative?
3. What was the underlying purpose (or purposes) of the study—Therapy/intervention, Diagnosis/Assessment, Prognosis, Etiology/harm, Description, or Meaning?
4. What might be some clinical implications of this research? To what type of people and settings is the research most relevant? If the findings were accurate, how might *I* use the results of this study?

ASSISTANCE FOR CONSUMERS OF NURSING RESEARCH

We hope that this book will help you develop skills that will allow you to read, appraise, use, and appreciate nursing studies. In each chapter, we present information about methods that nurse researchers use to conduct their studies and provide guidance in several ways. First, we offer tips that often explain what you can expect to find in actual research articles, identified by the icon ☞ . There are also special "how-to-tell" tips (identified with the icon ☞) that help with some potentially confusing issues in research articles.

Second, we include guidelines for critically appraising various aspects of a study in every chapter. The guiding questions in Box 1.1 are designed to assist you in using the information in this chapter in a preliminary assessment of a research article.

And third, we offer opportunities to apply your new skills. The critical thinking exercises at the end of each chapter guide you through appraisals of real examples of qualitative and quantitative studies. These activities also challenge you to think about how the findings from these studies could be used in nursing practice. Answers to some of these questions are in the Student Resources on thePoint° website, and the answers to others are in the Instructor Resources on thePoint° website. Four journal articles for the critical thinking exercises are found in the appendices to this book. The full journal article for studies identified with ** in the references of each chapter are also available on thePoint° website. ☀

RESEARCH EXAMPLES WITH CRITICAL THINKING EXERCISES

This section presents examples of studies with different purposes. Read the research summaries for Examples 1 and 2 and then answer the critical thinking questions that follow, referring to the full research reports if necessary. Answers to these questions are available to instructors on thePoint°. The critical thinking questions for Exercises 3 and 4 are based on the studies that appear in their entirety in Appendices A and B of this book. Our comments for these questions are in the Student Resources section on thePoint°. ☀

EXAMPLE 1: QUANTITATIVE RESEARCH

Study: Effect of inhalation aromatherapy on pain, anxiety, comfort, and cortisol levels during trigger point injection (Kasar et al., 2020)

Study Purpose: The purpose of the study was to test whether lavender oil inhalation had a positive effect on the pain, comfort, anxiety, and cortisol levels of people with myofascial pain syndrome (MPS) during trigger point injection.

Study Methods: A total of 66 patients who were admitted to a hospital clinic in Turkey for trigger point injections were included in the study. The patients were assigned to one of three groups, with 22 patients per group: (1) those receiving lavender oil inhalation during the injections, (2) those receiving inhalation of an odorless organic baby oil, and (3) those not receiving any inhalation application. All study participants were assessed for pain, comfort, and anxiety before and after the injections, and saliva samples were collected for cortisol level measurements.

Key Findings: The researchers found that patients who received the lavender oil inhalation had lower pain and anxiety and higher levels of comfort than patients who did not receive the aromatherapy. The intervention had no effect on saliva cortisol levels.

Conclusions: The researchers "recommended that aromatherapy, which is low cost, noninvasive, and easily applicable, be applied to individuals with MPS during trigger point injection because of its anxiety and stress-reducing effects" (p. 62).

Critical Thinking Exercises

1. Answer questions 1 to 3 in Box 1.1 regarding this study.
2. Also consider the following targeted questions which may assist you in assessing aspects of the study's merit:
   a. Why do you think the researchers used three groups rather than just two to assess the effects of the aromatherapy intervention?
   b. Could this study have been undertaken as a qualitative study? Why or why not?

EXAMPLE 2: QUALITATIVE RESEARCH

Study: Health and disability among young black men (Ricks et al., 2020)

Study Purpose: The purpose of this study was to explore how young Black men in the United Stated experienced the onset of chronic disabling conditions while at the same time negotiating health-promoting activities. The central questions were, What is the essence of losing abilities among young black men in Western societies? and What is the context of learning health promotion among Black men living with disabilities?

Study Methods: Eleven self-identified Black men were screened for functional limitations and were subsequently interviewed twice. The goal of the interviews, which were audiorecorded and later transcribed, was to "gain descriptions of how the men remembered times of socially channeled incapacity" (p. 14). Interviews, which were scheduled 2 to 4 weeks apart, lasted between 30 and 120 minutes. The interviewer maintained detailed field notes about the participants' attire, body language, facial expressions, and demeanor.

Key Findings: Four recurring themes described how masculinity couples with the male body to drive health promotion and health-related decisions: (1) maintaining manhood, (2) economic constraints, (3) the "risk" of health care, and (4) health promotion. Here is an excerpt from an interview that illustrates the third theme on perceived risks: "Most of us don't wanna go to the doctor, man. We're afraid of what they're going to tell us. It's almost like, man, . . . we know . . . we're going to get diagnosed with something. So, oh well, I might as well just live my life and just die not knowing there's something" (p. 19).

Conclusions: The researchers concluded that knowledge of the men's experiences and perspectives contributes to the understanding of their personal challenges and health needs.

Critical Thinking Exercises

1. Answer questions 1 to 3 in Box 1.1 regarding this study.
2. Also consider the following targeted questions, which may assist you in assessing aspects of the study's merit:
   a. Why do you think that the researchers audiorecorded and transcribed their in-depth interviews with study participants?
   b. Do you think it would have been appropriate for the researchers to conduct this study using quantitative research methods? Why or why not?

EXAMPLE 3: QUANTITATIVE RESEARCH IN APPENDIX A

1. Read the abstract and the introduction from Swenson and colleagues' study ("Parents' use of praise and criticism in a sample of young children seeking mental health services") in Appendix A of this book and then answer questions 1 to 3 in Box 1.1.
2. Also consider the following targeted questions:
   a. Could this study have been undertaken as a qualitative study? Why or why not?
   b. Who helped to pay for this research? (This information appears on the first page of the report.)
   c. What might a Prognosis question for this study be?

EXAMPLE 4: QUALITATIVE RESEARCH IN APPENDIX B

1. Read the abstract and the introduction from Beck and Watson's study ("Posttraumatic growth after birth trauma") in Appendix B of this book and then answer questions 1 to 3 in Box 1.1.
2. Also consider the following targeted questions:
   a. Was Beck and Watson's study conducted within the positivist paradigm or the constructivist paradigm? Provide a rationale for your choice.
   b. What was the phenomenon that Beck and Watson were studying? How was it defined?

WANT TO KNOW MORE?

A wide variety of resources to enhance your learning and understanding of this chapter is available on thePoint.

- Chapter Supplement on The History of Nursing Research
- Answers to the Critical Thinking Exercises for Examples 3 and 4
- Internet Resources with useful websites for Chapter 1
- A Wolters Kluwer journal article on a topic related to this chapter

Additional study aids, including eight journal articles and related questions, are also available in *Study Guide for Essentials of Nursing Research, 10e.*

Summary Points

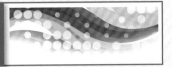

- **Nursing research** is systematic inquiry undertaken to develop evidence on problems of importance to nurses.

- Nurses in various settings are adopting an **evidence-based practice (EBP)** that incorporates research findings into their decisions and interactions with clients.

- Knowledge of nursing research enhances the professional practice of all nurses—including both *consumers of research* (who read and evaluate studies) and *producers of research* (who design and undertake studies).

- Nursing research began with Florence Nightingale but developed slowly until its rapid acceleration in the 1950s. Since the 1980s, a major focus has been on **clinical nursing research**—that is, on problems relating to clinical practice.

- The National Institute of Nursing Research (NINR), established at the U.S. National Institutes of Health in 1993, affirms the stature of nursing research in the United States.

- Contemporary issues in nursing research include the growth of EBP, expansion of local research and quality improvement efforts, research synthesis through systematic reviews, **patient centeredness**, interest in the **applicability** of research to individual patients or groups, and efforts to measure the **clinical significance** of research results.

- Disciplined research stands in contrast to other knowledge sources for nursing practice, such as tradition, authority, personal experience, and trial and error.

- Disciplined inquiry in nursing is conducted mainly within two **paradigms**—worldviews with underlying **assumptions** about reality: the positivist paradigm and the constructivist paradigm.

- In the **positivist paradigm**, it is assumed that there is an objective reality and that natural phenomena are regular and orderly. The assumption of *determinism* refers to the belief

that phenomena result from prior causes and are not haphazard.

- **Quantitative research** (associated with positivism) involves the collection and analysis of numeric information. Quantitative research is typically conducted within the traditional **scientific method**, which is systematic and controlled. Quantitative researchers base their findings on **empirical evidence** (evidence collected by way of the human senses) and strive for **generalizability** beyond a single setting or situation.

- In the **constructivist paradigm**, it is assumed that reality is not a fixed entity but is rather a construction of human minds—and thus "truth" is a composite of multiple constructions of reality.

- Constructivist researchers emphasize understanding human experience as it is lived through the collection and analysis of subjective, narrative materials using flexible procedures; this paradigm is associated with **qualitative research**.

- A fundamental distinction that is especially relevant in quantitative research is between studies whose primary intent is to *describe* phenomena and those that are **cause-probing**—i.e., designed to illuminate underlying causes of phenomena. Specific purposes on a description/explanation continuum include identification, description, exploration, prediction/control, and explanation.

- Nursing studies can also be classified in terms of EBP-related aims: Therapy/intervention, Diagnosis/assessment, Prognosis, Etiology (causation)/prevention of harm, Description, and Meaning/processes. Therapy questions are foundational for evidence-based decision making.

- EBP is the conscientious integration of current best evidence and other factors in making clinical decisions. The three "legs" of EBP are (1) best research evidence, (2) patient preferences and values, and (3) nurses' own clinical experience and knowledge.

- **Primary studies** of original research published in professional journals are one source of evidence for EBP, but preprocessed (synthesized) evidence is especially useful in addressing clinical queries. Systematic reviews, considered the cornerstone of EBP, are important sources of evidence.

- **Systematic reviews** are rigorous integrations of research evidence from multiple studies on a topic. Systematic reviews can involve either narrative approaches to integration (including **metasynthesis** and **meta-aggregation** of qualitative studies) or quantitative approaches (**meta-analysis**) that integrate findings statistically by using individual studies as the unit of analysis.

- There has been a proliferation of **evidence hierarchies** that provide a preliminary guide for finding "best" evidence—evidence with the lowest risk of bias. Evidence hierarchies reflect **level of evidence (LOE) scales** that rank order types of evidence source—primarily for Therapy/intervention questions. In LOEs for Therapy questions, systematic reviews of *randomized controlled trials* (RCTs) are considered Level I sources.

- EBP efforts typically start by asking a well-worded clinical question for which evidence is then sought. A widely used scheme for asking well-worded clinical questions involves four primary components, an acronym for which is **PICO**: Population or patients (P), Intervention or influence (I), Comparison (C), and Outcome (O).

REFERENCES FOR CHAPTER 1

Bastani, F., Rajai, N., Farsi, Z., & Als, H. (2017). The effects of kangaroo care on the sleep-wake states of preterm infants. *Journal of Nursing Research, 25*, 231–239.

Billner-Garcia, R., Spilker A., & Goyal, D. (2018). Skin to skin contact: Newborn temperature stability in the operating room. *MCN: American Journal of Maternal/Child Nursing, 43*, 158–163.

Cho, E., Kim, S., Kwon, M., Cho, H., Kim, E., Jun, E., & Lee, S. (2016). The effects of kangaroo care in the neonatal intensive care unit on the physiological functions of preterm infants, maternal-infant attachment, and maternal stress. *Journal of Pediatric Nursing, 31*, 430–438.

Drageset, S., Lindstrøm, T., & Ellingsen, S. (2020). "I have both lost and gained." Norwegian survivors' experiences of coping 9 years after primary breast cancer surgery. *Cancer Nursing, 43*, E30–E37.

Galica, J., Giroux, J., Francis, J., & Maheu, C. (2020). Coping with fear of cancer recurrence among ovarian cancer survivors living in small urban and rural settings: A qualitative descriptive study. *European Journal of Oncology Nursing, 44*, 101705.

*Gilbert, R., Salanti, G., Harden, M., & See, S. (2005). Infant sleeping position and the sudden infant death syndrome: Systematic review of observational studies and historical review of recommendations from 1940 to 2002. *International Journal of Epidemiology, 34*, 874–887.

Guyatt, G., Rennie, D., Meade, M., & Cook, D. (2015). *Users' guide to the medical literature: Essentials of evidence-based clinical practice* (3rd ed.). New York, NY: McGraw Hill.

Hanrahan, K., Wagner, M., Matthews, G., Stewart, S., Dawson, C., Greiner, J., . . . Williamson, A. (2015). Sacred cow gone to pasture: A systematic evaluation and integration of evidence-based practice. *Worldviews on Evidence-Based Nursing, 12*, 3–11.

Harrison, T., Brown, R., Duffey, T., Frey, C., Bailey, J., Nist, M., . . . Fitch, J. (2020). Effects of massage on post-operative pain in infants with complex congenital heart disease. *Nursing Research.* Advance online publication. doi: 10.1097/NNR.0000000000000459.

Kasar, K., Yildirim, Y., Aykar, F., Uyar, M., Sagin, F., & Atay, S. (2020). Effect of inhalation aromatherapy on pain, anxiety, comfort, and cortisol levels during trigger point injection. *Holistic Nursing Practice, 34*, 57–64.

Levin, R. F. (2014). Levels, grades, and strength of evidence: "What's it all about, Alfie?" *Research and Theory for Nursing Practice, 28*, 5–8.

*Lowson, K., Offer, C., Watson, J., McGuire, B., & Renfrew, M. (2015). The economic benefits of increasing kangaroo skin-to-skin care and breastfeeding in neonatal units: Analysis of a pragmatic intervention in clinical practice. *International Breastfeeding Journal, 10*, 11.

Melnyk, B. M., & Fineout-Overholt, E. (2019). *Evidence-based practice in nursing and healthcare: A guide to best practice* (4th ed.). Philadelphia, PA: Lippincott Williams & Wilkins.

*National Institute of Nursing Research. (2016). *The NINR strategic plan: Advancing science, improving lives.* Bethesda, MD: Author.

Neris, R., Leite, A., Nascimento, L., García-Vivar, C., & Zago, M. (2020). "What I was and what I am": A qualitative study of survivors' experience of urological cancer. *European Journal of Oncology Nursing, 44*, 101692.

Niela-Vilen, H., Rahmani, A., Liljeberg, P., & Axelin, A. (2020). Being 'A Google Mom' or securely monitored at home: Perceptions of remote monitoring in maternity care. *Journal of Advanced Nursing, 76*, 243–252.

Porter, J., Peck, B., McNabb, T., & Missen, K. (2020). A review of Code Blue activations in a single regional Australian healthcare service. *Journal of Clinical Nursing, 29*, 221–227.

Resnick, B., Galik, E., Boltz, M., Holmes, S., Fix, S., Lewis, R., & Vigne, E. (2020). Reliability and validity of the Checklist for Function-Focused Care in Service Plans. *Clinical Nursing Research, 29*, 21–30.

**Ricks, T., Frederick, A., & Harrison, T. (2020). Health and disability among young black men. *Nursing Research, 69*, 13–21.

Spock, B. (1979). *Baby and child care.* New York, NY: Dutton.

Tang, H., Tang, H., Chang, C., Su, P., & Chen, C. (2020). Functional status in older intensive care unit survivors. *Clinical Nursing Research, 29*, 5–12.

Tongpeth, J., Du, H., Barry, T., & Clark, R. (2020). Effectiveness of an Avatar application for teaching heart attack recognition and response: A pragmatic randomized control trial. *Journal of Advanced Nursing, 76,* 297–311.

Tung, H., Lai, C., Chen, K., & Tsai, H. (2020). Meridian cuffing exercises improved functional fitness and cardiopulmonary functioning of community older adults. *Clinical Nursing Research, 29,* 37–47.

Xie, X., Chen, X., Sun, P., Cao, A., Zhuang, Y., Xiong, X., & Yang, C. (2020). Kangaroo mother care reduces non-invasive ventilation and total oxygen support duration in extremely low birth weight infants. *American Journal of Perinatology,* Advance online publication. doi:10.1055/s-0039-3402717.

Yoo, J., Park, C., & Ryan, C. (2020). Impact of physical function on 1-year kidney transplant outcomes. *Western Journal of Nursing Research, 42,* 50–56.

*A link to this open-access article is provided in the Internet Resources section on thePoint° website.

**This journal article is available on thePoint° for this chapter.

2 Understanding Key Concepts and Steps in Quantitative and Qualitative Research

Learning Objectives

On completing this chapter, you will be able to:

- Define new terms presented in the chapter and distinguish terms associated with quantitative and qualitative research
- Distinguish experimental and nonexperimental research
- Identify three main disciplinary traditions for qualitative nursing research
- Describe the flow and sequence of activities in quantitative and qualitative research and discuss how and why they differ

Key Terms

- Associative relationship
- Cause-and-effect (causal) relationship
- Clinical trial
- Concept
- Conceptual definition
- Construct
- Data
- Dependent variable
- Emergent design
- Ethnography
- Experimental research
- Gaining entrée
- Grounded theory
- Hypothesis
- Independent variable
- Informant
- Intervention protocol
- Literature review
- Nonexperimental research
- Observational study
- Operational definition
- Outcome variable
- Phenomenology
- Population
- Qualitative data
- Qualitative descriptive research
- Quantitative data
- Relationship
- Research design
- Sample
- Saturation
- Statistical analysis
- Study participant
- Subject
- Theme
- Theory
- Variable

THE BUILDING BLOCKS OF RESEARCH

Research, like any discipline, has its own language—its own *jargon* that can sometimes be intimidating. We readily admit that the jargon is plentiful and can be confusing. Some research jargon used in nursing research has its roots in the social sciences, but sometimes, different terms are used in medical research. Also, some terms are used by both qualitative and quantitative researchers, but others are used mainly by one or the other group. Please bear with us as we cover key terms that you will likely encounter in the research literature.

TABLE 2.1 Key Terms in Quantitative and Qualitative Research

Concept	Quantitative Term	Qualitative Term
Person contributing information	Subject Study participant —	— Study participant Informant, key informant
Person undertaking the study	Researcher Investigator	Researcher Investigator
That which is being investigated	— Concepts Constructs Variables	Phenomena Concepts — —
Information gathered	Data (numerical values)	Data (narrative descriptions)
Connections between concepts	Relationships (cause-and-effect, associative)	Patterns of association
Logical reasoning processes	Deductive reasoning	Inductive reasoning

The Faces and Places of Research

When researchers address a research question, they are doing a *study* (or an *investigation*). Studies with humans involve two sets of people: those who do the research and those who provide the information. In a quantitative study, the people being studied are called **subjects** or **study participants**, as shown in Table 2.1. In a qualitative study, the people cooperating in the study are called study participants or **informants**. The person who conducts the research is the *researcher* or *investigator*. Studies are often undertaken by a research team rather than by a single researcher.

 HOW-TO-TELL TIP How can you tell if an article appearing in a nursing journal is a *study*? In journals that specialize in research (e.g., the journal *Nursing Research*), most articles are original research reports, but in specialty journals, there is usually a mix of research and nonresearch articles. Sometimes you can tell by the title, but sometimes you cannot. You can tell, however, by looking at the major headings of an article. If there is no heading called "Method" or "Research Design" (the section that describes what a researcher *did*) and no heading called "Findings" or "Results" (the section that describes what a researcher *learned*), then it is probably not a study.

Research can be undertaken in a variety of *settings* (the types of place where information is gathered), such as clinics, homes, or other community settings. A *site* is the broad location for the research—it could be an entire community (e.g., a Haitian neighborhood in Miami) or an institution (e.g., a nursing home in Seattle). Researchers sometimes do *multisite studies* because the use of multiple sites yields a larger and often more diverse group of participants.

Concepts, Constructs, and Theories

Research addresses real-world problems, but studies are conceptualized in abstract terms. For example, *pain*, *fatigue*, and *obesity* are abstractions of human attributes. These abstractions are called *phenomena* (especially in qualitative studies) or **concepts**.

Researchers sometimes use the term **construct**, which also refers to an abstraction, but often one that is deliberately invented (or constructed). For example, *self-care* in Orem's model of health maintenance is a construct. The terms *construct* and *concept* are sometimes used interchangeably, but a construct often refers to a more complex abstraction than a concept.

A **theory** is an explanation of some aspect of reality. In a theory, concepts are knitted together into a coherent system to describe or explain some aspect of the world. Theories play a role in both qualitative and quantitative research. In a quantitative study, researchers sometimes start with a theory and, using deductive reasoning, make predictions about how phenomena would behave in the real world *if the theory were valid*. The specific predictions are then tested. In qualitative studies, theory often is the *product* of the research: The investigators use information from study participants inductively to develop a theory rooted in the participants' experiences.

 TIP The reasoning process of *deduction* is associated with quantitative research, and *induction* is associated with qualitative research. The supplement for Chapter 2 on thePoint® website explains and illustrates the distinction.

Variables

In quantitative studies, concepts are called **variables**. A variable, as the name implies, is something that varies. Weight, anxiety, and nausea are all variables—they vary from one person to another. Most human characteristics are variables. If everyone weighed 150 pounds, weight would not be a variable, it would be a *constant*. But it is precisely because people and conditions *do* vary that most research is conducted. Quantitative researchers seek to understand how or why things vary and to learn how differences in one variable relate to differences in another. For example, in lung cancer research, lung cancer is a variable because not everybody has this disease. Researchers have studied factors that might be linked to lung cancer, such as cigarette smoking. Smoking is also a variable because not everyone smokes. A variable, then, is any quality of a person, group, or situation that varies or takes on different values. Variables are the central building blocks of quantitative studies.

 TIP Every study focuses on one or more phenomena, concepts, or variables, but these terms per se are not necessarily used in research reports. For example, a report might say, "The purpose of this study is to examine the effect of nurses' workload on hand hygiene compliance." Although the researcher did not explicitly label anything a variable, the variables under study are *workload* and *hand hygiene compliance*. Key concepts or variables are often indicated in the study title.

Characteristics of Variables

Variables are often inherent human traits, such as age or weight, but sometimes researchers *create* a variable. For example, if a researcher tests the effectiveness of patient-controlled analgesia compared to intramuscular analgesia in relieving pain after surgery, some patients would be given one type of analgesia and some would receive the other. In the context of this study, method of pain management is a variable because different patients are given different methods.

Some variables take on a wide range of values than can be represented on a continuum (e.g., a person's age or weight). Other variables take on only a few values; sometimes such variables convey quantitative information (e.g., number of children), but others simply involve placing people into categories (e.g., blood type A, B, AB, or O).

Dependent and Independent Variables

As noted in Chapter 1, many studies seek to understand causes of phenomena. Does a nursing intervention *cause* improvements in patient outcomes? Does smoking *cause* lung cancer? The presumed cause is the **independent variable**, and the presumed effect is the

dependent or **outcome variable**. The dependent variable is the outcome that researchers want to understand, explain, or predict. In terms of the PICO scheme discussed in Chapter 1, the dependent variable corresponds to the "O" (outcome). The independent variable corresponds to the "I" (the intervention, influence, or exposure), plus the "C" (the comparison).

 TIP In *searching* for evidence, a nurse might want to learn about the effects of an intervention or influence (I), compared to *any* alternative, on an outcome (O) of interest. In a cause-probing study, however, researchers must always specify the comparator (the "C").

The terms *independent variable* and *dependent variable* also can be used to indicate *direction of influence* rather than cause and effect. For example, suppose we compared levels of depression among men and women diagnosed with pancreatic cancer and found men to be more depressed. We could not conclude that depression was *caused* by gender. Yet the direction of influence clearly runs from gender to depression: It makes no sense to suggest that patient's depression influenced their gender. In this situation, it is appropriate to consider depression as the dependent variable and gender as the independent variable.

 TIP Few research reports explicitly label variables as dependent and independent. Moreover, variables (especially independent variables) are sometimes not fully spelled out. Take the following research question: What is the effect of exercise on heart rate? In this example, heart rate is the dependent variable. Exercise, however, is not in itself a variable. Rather, exercise versus something else (e.g., no exercise) is a variable; "something else" is implied rather than stated in the research question.

Most outcomes have multiple causes or influences. If we were studying factors that influence people's body mass index, the independent variables might be height, physical activity, and diet. And, two or more outcome variables often are of interest. For example, a researcher may compare the effects of alternative dietary interventions on participants' weight, lipid profile, and self-esteem. It is common to design studies with multiple independent and dependent variables.

Variables are not *inherently* dependent or independent. A dependent variable in one study could be an independent variable in another. For example, a study might examine the effect of an exercise intervention (the independent variable) on osteoporosis (the dependent variable) to answer a Therapy question. Another study might investigate the effect of osteoporosis (the independent variable) on bone fracture incidence (the dependent variable) to address a Prognosis question. In short, whether a variable is independent or dependent is a function of the role that it plays in a particular study.

Example of independent and dependent variables •
Research question (Etiology/Harm question): Is vitamin D deficiency associated with poor sleep quality in African American and Hispanic pregnant women? (Woo et al., 2020)
Independent variable: Vitamin D deficiency (versus no Vitamin D deficiency)
Dependent variable: Sleep quality

Conceptual and Operational Definitions

The concepts of interest to researchers are abstractions, and researchers' worldview shapes how those concepts are defined. A **conceptual definition** is the theoretical meaning of a concept. Researchers need to conceptually define even seemingly straightforward terms. A classic example is the concept of *caring*. Morse and colleagues (1990) examined how researchers and theorists defined *caring* and identified five categories of conceptual definitions: a human trait, a moral imperative, an affect, an interpersonal relationship, and a therapeutic intervention. More recently, Andersson and colleagues (2015) found that nurses offered multiple interpretations of caring. Researchers undertaking studies of caring need to clarify how they conceptualized it.

In qualitative studies, conceptual definitions of key phenomena may be a major end product, reflecting an intent to have concepts explained by those being studied. In quantitative studies, however, researchers must define concepts at the outset because they must decide how the variables will be measured. An **operational definition** specifies what the researchers must do to measure the concept and collect needed information.

Readers of research articles may not agree with how researchers conceptualized and operationalized variables. However, definitional precision is important in communicating what concepts mean within the context of the study.

Example of conceptual and operational definitions •••••••••••••••••••••••••

Webel and colleagues (2020) studied the relationships among social capital, HIV self-management, and substance use in women. *Social capital* was conceptually defined as "the aggregation of potential resources, linked to a durable network of relationships of mutual acquaintance or recognition . . . components of social capital include reciprocity, trust, safety, social agency, social networks, value of life, and employment connections" (p. 5). The construct of social capital was operationalized using a measure with 36 questions, called the Social Capital Scale.

Data

Research **data** (singular, datum) are the pieces of information gathered in a study. In quantitative studies, researchers identify and define their variables and then collect relevant data from participants. The actual *values* of the study variables constitute the data. Quantitative researchers collect primarily **quantitative data**—information in numeric form. For example, if we conducted a quantitative study in which a key variable was *depression*, we would need to measure how depressed participants were. We might ask, "Thinking about the past week, how depressed would you say you have been on a scale from 0 to 10, where 0 means 'not at all' and 10 means 'the most possible'?" Box 2.1 presents quantitative data for three fictitious people. Subjects provided a number on the 0 to 10 continuum corresponding to their degree of depression—9 for subject 1 (a high level of depression), 0 for subject 2 (no depression), and 4 for subject 3 (mild depression).

In qualitative studies, researchers collect primarily **qualitative data**, that is, narrative descriptions. Narrative data can be obtained by conversing with participants, by making notes about their behavior in naturalistic settings, or by obtaining narrative records, such

Box 2.1 Example of Quantitative Data

Question:	Thinking about the past week, how depressed would you say you have been on a scale from 0 to 10, where 0 means "not at all" and 10 means "the most possible"?
Data:	9 (Subject 1)
	0 (Subject 2)
	4 (Subject 3)

Box 2.2 Example of Qualitative Data

Question: Tell me about how you've been feeling lately—have you felt sad or depressed at all, or have you generally been in good spirits?

Data: "Well, actually, I've been pretty depressed lately, to tell you the truth. I wake up each morning and I can't seem to think of anything to look forward to. I mope around the house all day, kind of in despair. I just can't seem to shake the blues and I've begun to think I need to go see a shrink." (Participant 1)

"I can't remember ever feeling better in my life. I just got promoted to a new job that makes me feel like I can really get ahead in my company. And I've just gotten engaged to a really great guy who is very special." (Participant 2)

"I've had a few ups and downs the past week but basically things are on a pretty even keel. I don't have too many complaints." (Participant 3)

as diaries. Suppose we were studying depression qualitatively. Box 2.2 presents qualitative data for three participants responding conversationally to the question, "Tell me about how you've been feeling lately—have you felt sad or depressed at all, or have you generally been in good spirits?" Here, the data consist of rich narrative descriptions of participants' emotional state. In reports on qualitative studies, researchers include excerpts from their narrative data to support their interpretations.

Relationships

Researchers usually study phenomena in relation to other phenomena—they examine relationships. A **relationship** is a connection between phenomena; for example, researchers repeatedly have found that there is a *relationship* between frequency of turning bedridden patients and the incidence of pressure ulcers. Qualitative and quantitative researchers examine relationships in different ways.

In quantitative studies, relationships are often explicitly expressed in quantitative terms, such as *more than* or *less than*. For example, consider a person's weight as our outcome variable. What variables are related to (associated with) a person's weight? Some possibilities include height, caloric intake, and exercise. For each independent variable, we can make a prediction about its relationship to the outcome:

Height: Tall people will weigh more than short people.
Caloric intake: People with high caloric intake will be heavier than those with low caloric intake.
Exercise: The lower the amount of exercise, the greater will be the person's weight.

Each statement expresses a predicted relationship between weight (the outcome) and a measurable independent variable. Most quantitative research is conducted to assess whether relationships exist among variables and to measure how strong the relationship is.

 TIP Relationships are expressed in two basic forms. First, relationships can be expressed as "if more of Variable X, then more of (or less of) Variable Y." For example, there is a relationship between height and weight: With greater height, there tends to be greater weight, i.e., tall people tend to weigh more than short people. The second form involves relationships expressed as group differences. For example, there is a relationship between gender and height: Men tend to be taller than women.

Variables can be related to one another in different ways, including **cause-and-effect** (or **causal**) **relationships**. Within the positivist paradigm, natural phenomena are assumed to have antecedent causes that are discoverable. For example, we might speculate that there is a causal relationship between caloric intake and weight: All else being equal, eating more calories causes greater weight. As noted in Chapter 1, many quantitative studies are *cause-probing*—they seek to illuminate the causes of phenomena.

Example of a study of causal relationships •
Chen and colleagues (2020) studied whether the use of virtual reality for children during intravenous injections would *cause* improvements in the children's pain and fear and shorten time for intravenous insertions.

Not all relationships can be interpreted as causal. There is a relationship, for example, between a person's pulmonary artery and tympanic temperatures: People with high readings on one tend to have high readings on the other. We cannot say, however, that pulmonary artery temperature *caused* tympanic temperature, or vice versa. This type of relationship is sometimes referred to as an **associative** (or *functional*) **relationship** rather than a causal one.

Example of a study of associative relationships •
Kwon and colleagues (2020) studied factors associated with adolescents' Internet use and suicide ideation. In their sample of over 60,000 adolescents, they found that a higher percentage of suicide ideation was reported by girls than by boys. Gender was also associated with a different amount of Internet use by those with suicide ideation.

Qualitative researchers are not concerned with quantifying relationships nor in testing and confirming causal relationships. However, qualitative researchers may seek patterns of association as a way of illuminating the underlying meaning and dimensionality of phenomena of interest. Patterns of interconnected concepts are identified as a means of understanding the whole.

Example of a qualitative study of patterns •
Epstein and colleagues (2020) explored newly graduated nurses' strategies for, and experiences of, sleep problems when starting shiftwork. They reported that for these new nurses, sleep problems were common, especially during "quick returns"—an evening shift followed by a morning shift—and that high workload on the evening shift worsened the problem.

MAJOR CLASSES OF QUANTITATIVE AND QUALITATIVE RESEARCH

Researchers usually work within a paradigm that is consistent with their worldview and that gives rise to the types of question that excite their curiosity. In this section, we briefly describe broad categories of quantitative and qualitative research.

Quantitative Research: Experimental and Nonexperimental Studies

A basic distinction in quantitative studies is between experimental and nonexperimental research. In **experimental research**, researchers actively introduce an intervention or treatment—usually to address Therapy questions. In **nonexperimental research**, on the other hand, researchers are bystanders—they collect data without introducing treatments (most often, to address Etiology, Prognosis, Diagnosis, or Description questions). For example, if a researcher gave bran flakes to one group of subjects and prune juice to another to evaluate which method facilitated elimination more effectively, the study would be experimental because the researcher intervened. If, on the other hand, a researcher compared elimination patterns of two groups whose regular eating patterns differed, the study would be nonexperimental because there is no intervention. In medical and epidemiological research, experimental studies usually are called **clinical trials**, and nonexperimental inquiries are called **observational studies**.

Experimental studies are explicitly designed to test causal relationships—to test whether an intervention *causes* changes in the outcome. Sometimes, nonexperimental studies also explore causal relationships, but causal inferences in nonexperimental research are tricky and less conclusive, for reasons we explain in a later chapter.

Example of experimental research •
Kim and coresearchers (2020) tested whether the time of postoperative feeding after total hip arthroplasty affected such gastrointestinal outcomes as nausea, vomiting, abdominal pain, and time to defecation. Some participants had early postoperative feeding (4 hours postoperatively) or late postoperative feeding (8+ hours postoperatively).

In this example, the researchers intervened by designating that some patients would be fed their first postoperative meal at 4 hours after the procedure and others would be fed 8 hours or more after the procedure. In other words, the researcher *controlled* the independent variable, which in this case was the timing of the postoperative meal to see if timing affected important outcomes.

Example of nonexperimental research •
Matsunaga-Myoji and colleagues (2020) did a 3-year follow-up study of patients who had undergone total hip arthroplasty. They examined changes over time in the patients' physical activity, physical function, and quality of life. They also examined factors associated with improved outcomes (e.g., the patients' age).

In this nonexperimental study to address a Prognosis question, the researchers did not intervene in any way. They were interested in a similar population as in the previous example (people who had a hip arthroplasty), but their intent was to study patterns of improvement or decline after the arthroplasty and associated factors.

Qualitative Research: Disciplinary Traditions

The majority of qualitative nursing studies can best be described as **qualitative descriptive research**. Many qualitative studies, however, are rooted in research traditions that originated in anthropology, sociology, and psychology. Three such traditions are briefly described here. Chapter 10 provides a fuller discussion of these and other traditions and the methods associated with them.

Grounded theory research seeks to describe and understand key social psychological processes. Grounded theory was developed in the 1960s by two sociologists, Glaser and Strauss (1967). The focus of most grounded theory studies is on a developing social experience—the social and psychological processes that characterize an event or situation. A major component of grounded theory is the discovery of a *core variable* that is central in explaining what is going on in that social scene. Grounded theory researchers strive to generate explanations of phenomena that are grounded in reality.

Example of a grounded theory study •••••••••••••••••••••••••••••••••••••

Bloxsome and colleagues (2020) used grounded theory methods to understand why midwives in Western Australia choose to remain in their profession. The researchers' analysis of their in-depth data revealed that the core variable was *I love being a midwife; it's who I am.*

Phenomenology is concerned with the lived experiences of humans. Phenomenology is an approach to thinking about what people's life experiences are like and what they mean. Phenomenological researchers ask the questions: What is the *essence* of this phenomenon as experienced by these people? or, What is the meaning of the phenomenon to those who experience it?

Example of a phenomenological study •••••••••••••••••••••••••••••••••

Celia and colleagues (2020) conducted in-depth interviews to explore the lived experiences of parents caring for their autistic children and their experiences with safety for these children.

Ethnography, the primary research tradition in anthropology, provides a framework for studying the patterns and lifeways of a defined cultural group in a holistic fashion. Ethnographers typically engage in extensive *fieldwork*, often participating to the extent possible in the life of the culture under study. Ethnographers strive to learn from members of a cultural group, to understand their worldview, and to describe their customs and norms.

Example of an ethnographic study •••••••••••••••••••••••••••••••••••••

Chaaban and colleagues (2020) conducted an ethnographic study of the culture of French nursing homes to understand nurses' influence on prescribing antibiotics for the treatment of suspected infections.

MAJOR STEPS IN A QUANTITATIVE STUDY

In quantitative studies, researchers move from the beginning point of a study (posing a question) to the end point (obtaining an answer) in a reasonably linear sequence of steps that is broadly similar across studies (Fig. 2.1). This section describes that flow, and the next section describes how qualitative studies differ.

Phase 1: The Conceptual Phase

The early steps in a quantitative study typically involve activities with a strong conceptual element. During this phase, researchers rely on creativity, deductive reasoning, and a grounding in research evidence on the focal topic.

Step 1: Formulating and Delimiting the Problem

Quantitative researchers begin by identifying an interesting research problem and formulating *research questions*. The research questions identify what the study variables are. In developing questions, nurse researchers must attend to substantive issues (Is this problem important?), theoretical issues (Is there a conceptual framework for this problem?), clinical issues (Will findings be useful in clinical practice?), methodologic issues (How can this

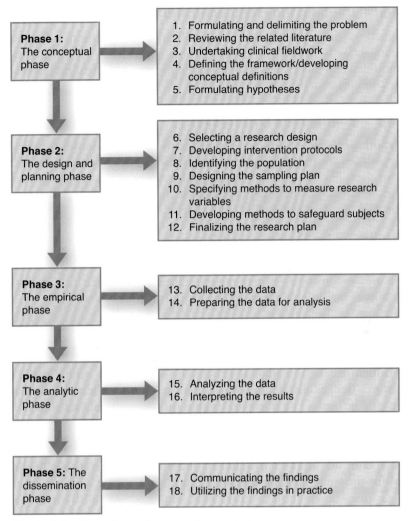

Figure 2.1 Flow of steps in a quantitative study.

question be answered to yield high-quality evidence?), and ethical issues (Can this question be addressed in an ethical manner?).

Step 2: Reviewing the Related Literature

Quantitative research is conducted within the context of previous knowledge. Quantitative researchers typically strive to understand what is already known about a topic by undertaking a thorough **literature review** before any data are collected.

Step 3: Undertaking Clinical Fieldwork

Researchers embarking on a clinical study often benefit from spending time in relevant clinical settings (in the *field*), discussing the topic with clinicians and observing current practices. Such clinical fieldwork can provide perspectives on clinicians' and clients' viewpoints.

Step 4: Defining the Framework and Developing Conceptual Definitions

When quantitative research is performed within the context of a theoretical framework, the findings may have broader significance and utility. Even when the research question is not embedded in a theory, researchers should have a conceptual rationale and a clear vision of the concepts under study.

Step 5: Formulating Hypotheses

Hypotheses state researchers' expectations about relationships between study variables. Hypotheses are predictions of the relationships that researchers expect to observe in the study data. The research question identifies the concepts of interest and asks how the concepts might be related; a hypothesis is the predicted answer. Most quantitative studies are designed to test hypotheses through statistical analysis.

Phase 2: The Design and Planning Phase

In the second major phase of a quantitative study, researchers decide on the methods they will use to address the research question. Researchers make many methodological decisions that have crucial implications for the quality of study evidence.

Step 6: Selecting a Research Design

The **research design** is the overall plan for obtaining answers to the research questions. Quantitative designs tend to be structured and controlled, with the goal of minimizing bias. Research designs also indicate how often data will be collected and what types of comparisons will be made. The research design is the architectural backbone of the study.

Step 7: Developing Protocols for the Intervention

In experimental research, researchers introduce an intervention. An **intervention protocol** for the study must be developed, specifying exactly what the intervention will entail (e.g., who will administer it, over how long a period will the treatment last, and so on) *and* what the comparative condition will be. In nonexperimental research, this step is not necessary.

Step 8: Identifying the Population

Quantitative researchers need to specify what characteristics study participants should possess—that is, they must identify the population to be studied. A **population** is *all* the individuals or objects with common, defining characteristics (the "P" component in PICO questions).

Step 9: Designing the Sampling Plan

Researchers collect data from a **sample**, which is a subset of the population. The researcher's *sampling plan* specifies how the sample will be selected and how many participants there will be. The goal is to have a sample that adequately reflects the population's traits.

Step 10: Specifying Methods to Measure Research Variables

Quantitative researchers must find methods to measure their research variables accurately. A variety of quantitative data collection approaches exist; the primary methods are *self-reports* (e.g., interviews and questionnaires), *observations* (e.g., watching and recording people's be-havior), and *biophysiological measures (biomarkers)*. The task of measuring research variables and developing a *data collection plan* is complex and challenging.

Step 11: Developing Methods to Safeguard Human/Animal Rights

Most nursing research involves humans, although some involve animals. In either case, procedures need to be developed to ensure that the study adheres to ethical principles.

Step 12: Reviewing and Finalizing the Research Plan

Before collecting data, researchers often undertake assessments to ensure that procedures will work smoothly. For example, they may evaluate the *readability* of written materials to see if participants with low reading skills can comprehend them. Researchers usually have their research plan critiqued by reviewers to obtain clinical or methodological feedback. Researchers seeking financial support submit a *proposal* to a funding source.

Phase 3: The Empirical Phase

The third phase of quantitative research involves collecting the data. This phase is often the most time-consuming part of the study. Data collection often requires months or years of work.

Step 13: Collecting the Data

The actual collection of data in a quantitative study often proceeds according to a prees-tablished plan. The plan typically spells out procedures for training data collection staff, for implementing the sampling plan and collecting data (e.g., where and when the data will be gathered), and for recording information.

Step 14: Preparing the Data for Analysis

Data collected in a quantitative study must be prepared for analysis. For example, one pre-liminary step is *coding*, which involves translating verbal data into numeric form (e.g., coding gender information as "1" for females, "2" for males, and "3" for other).

Phase 4: The Analytic Phase

Quantitative data must be subjected to analysis and interpretation, which occur in the fourth major phase of a project.

Step 15: Analyzing the Data

To answer research questions and test hypotheses, researchers analyze their data in a systematic fashion. Quantitative data are analyzed through **statistical analyses**, which include some simple procedures (e.g., computing an average) as well as more complex methods.

Step 16: Interpreting the Results

Interpretation involves making sense of study results and examining their implications. Re-searchers attempt to explain the findings in light of prior evidence, theory, and clinical ex-perience—and in light of the adequacy of the methods they used in the study. Interpretation also involves coming to conclusions about the *clinical significance* of the new evidence.

Phase 5: The Dissemination Phase

In the analytic phase, researchers come full circle: The questions posed at the outset are answered. The researchers' job is incomplete, however, until study results are disseminated.

Step 17: Communicating the Findings

A study cannot contribute evidence to nursing practice if the results are not communicated. Another—and often final—task of a research project is the preparation of a *research report* that can be shared with others. We discuss research reports in the next chapter.

Step 18: Putting the Evidence Into Practice

Ideally, the concluding step of a high-quality study is to plan for its use in practice settings. Although nurse researchers may not implement a plan for using research findings, they can contribute to the process by developing recommendations on how the evidence could be used in practice, by ensuring that adequate information has been provided for a meta-analysis, and by pursuing opportunities to disseminate the findings to practicing nurses.

ACTIVITIES IN A QUALITATIVE STUDY

Quantitative research involves a fairly linear progression of tasks—researchers plan what steps to take and then follow those steps. In qualitative studies, by contrast, the progression is closer to a circle than to a straight line. Qualitative researchers continually examine and interpret data and make decisions about how to proceed based on what has been discovered (Fig. 2.2).

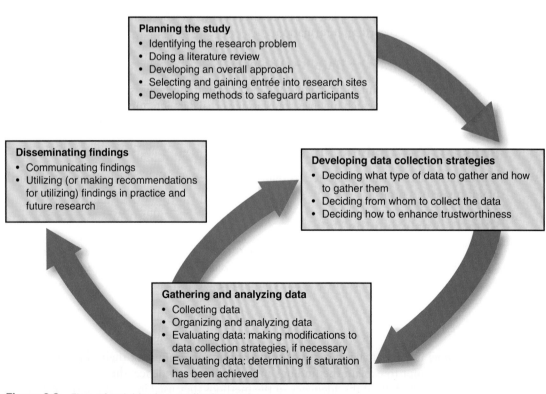

Figure 2.2 Flow of activities in a qualitative study.

Because qualitative researchers have a flexible approach, we cannot show the flow of activities precisely—the flow varies from one study to another, and researchers themselves may not know in advance how the study will unfold. We provide a general sense of qualitative studies by describing major activities and indicating when they might be performed.

Conceptualizing and Planning a Qualitative Study

Identifying the Research Problem

Qualitative researchers usually begin with a general topic, often focusing on an aspect about which little is known. Qualitative researchers often proceed with a fairly broad initial question that allows the focus to be sharpened and delineated more clearly once the study is underway.

Doing a Literature Review

Some qualitative researchers avoid consulting the literature before collecting data. They worry that prior studies might influence the conceptualization of the phenomenon under study, which they believe should be based on participants' viewpoints rather than on prior findings. Others believe that researchers should conduct at least a brief literature review at the outset. In any case, qualitative researchers typically find a relatively small body of relevant previous work because of the type of questions they ask.

Selecting and Gaining Entrée Into Research Sites

Before going into the field, qualitative researchers must identify an appropriate site. For example, if the topic is the health beliefs of the urban poor, an inner-city neighborhood with a concentration of low-income residents must be identified. In some cases, researchers may have access to the selected site, but in others they need to gain entrée into it. **Gaining entrée** typically involves negotiations with *gatekeepers* who have the authority to permit entry into their world.

 TIP The process of gaining entrée is usually associated with doing fieldwork in qualitative studies, but quantitative researchers often need to gain entrée into sites for collecting data as well.

Developing an Overall Approach

Quantitative researchers do not collect data before finalizing their research design. Qualitative researchers, by contrast, use an **emergent design** that materializes during data collection. Certain design features are guided by the study's qualitative tradition, but qualitative studies rarely have rigid designs that prohibit changes while in the field.

Addressing Ethical Issues

Qualitative researchers must also develop plans for addressing ethical issues—and, indeed, there are special concerns in qualitative studies because of the more intimate nature of the relationship that typically develops between researchers and participants.

Conducting a Qualitative Study

In qualitative studies, the tasks of sampling, data collection, data analysis, and interpretation typically take place iteratively. Qualitative researchers often begin by talking with people who have firsthand experience with the phenomenon of interest. The discussions are loosely structured, allowing participants to express a full range of beliefs, feelings, and behaviors. Analysis and interpretation are ongoing activities that guide choices about "next steps."

The process of data analysis involves clustering related narrative information into a coherent scheme. Through inductive reasoning, researchers identify **themes** and categories, which are used to build a rich description or theory of the phenomenon. Data gathering becomes increasingly purposeful: As conceptualizations develop, researchers seek participants who can confirm and enrich theoretical understandings, as well as participants who can potentially challenge them.

Quantitative researchers decide in advance how many people to include in the study, but qualitative researchers' sampling decisions are guided by the data. Many qualitative researchers use the principle of **saturation**, which occurs when participants' accounts of their experiences become redundant, such that no new thematic development can occur from further data collection.

Quantitative researchers seek to collect high-quality data by measuring their variables with instruments that have been demonstrated to be accurate and valid. Qualitative researchers, by contrast, *are* the main data collection instrument and must take steps to demonstrate the *trustworthiness* of the data. The central feature of these efforts is to confirm that the findings accurately reflect the viewpoints of participants, rather than researchers' perceptions. One confirmatory activity, for example, involves going back to participants, sharing preliminary interpretations with them, and asking them to evaluate whether the researcher's thematic analysis is consistent with their experiences.

Qualitative nursing researchers also strive to share their findings at conferences and in journal articles. Qualitative studies help to shape nurses' perceptions of a problem, their conceptualizations of potential solutions, and their understanding of patients' concerns and experiences.

GENERAL QUESTIONS IN REVIEWING A STUDY

Box 2.3 presents some further suggestions for performing a preliminary overview of a research report, drawing on concepts explained in this chapter. These guidelines supplement those presented in Box 1.1, Chapter 1.

Box 2.3 Additional Questions for a Preliminary Review of a Study

1. What was the study all about? What were the main phenomena, concepts, or constructs under investigation?
2. If the study was quantitative, what were the independent and dependent variables?
3. Did the researcher examine relationships or patterns of association among variables or concepts? Did the report imply the possibility of a causal relationship?
4. Were key concepts defined, both conceptually and operationally?
5. What type of study does it appear to be, in terms of types described in this chapter—experimental or nonexperimental/observational? Grounded theory, phenomenological, or ethnographic?
6. Did the report provide information to suggest how long the study took to complete?

RESEARCH EXAMPLES WITH CRITICAL THINKING EXERCISES

In this section, we illustrate the progression of activities and discuss the time schedule of a study conducted by the second author of this book. Read the summary and then answer the critical thinking questions that follow, referring to the full research report as necessary. Answers to Example 1 are available to instructors on thePoint® website. The critical thinking questions for Exercises 2 and 3 are based on the studies that appear in their entirety in Appendices A and B of this book. Our comments for these exercises are in the Student Resources section on thePoint®.

EXAMPLE 1: PROJECT SCHEDULE FOR A QUALITATIVE STUDY

Study: Mothers' experiences interacting with their infants after traumatic childbirth (Beck & Watson, 2019)

Study Purpose: The purpose of this study was to describe the meaning of mothers' experiences interacting with their infants after a traumatic childbirth.

Study Methods: This study required 3 years and 5 months to complete. Key activities and methodologic decisions included the following:

Phase 1. Conceptual Phase: 3 Months. Beck and Watson had conducted several qualitative studies on traumatic childbirth and the negative consequences for mothers (e.g., the impact of the traumatic birth on breastfeeding experiences). In the earlier studies, mothers had hinted at difficulty bonding with their infants. Beck and Watson were familiar with published research in this area so they did not need much time to review the literature.

Phase 2. Design and Planning Phase: 3 Months. Beck and Watson chose a descriptive phenomenological design for this study. They had conducted several phenomenological studies using the methods of Colaizzi for data analysis. This time they chose a different descriptive phenomenological method, and so they needed time to learn more about this method before their proposal was submitted to the university's ethics committee for approval.

Phase 3. Empirical/Analytic Phrases: 23 Months. A recruitment notice was placed on the website of Trauma and Birth Stress, a charitable trust in New Zealand. A link was provided for mothers to learn more about the study and to participate in the electronic survey. Eighteen mothers sent narratives about their experiences interacting with their infants after their traumatic births. It took 20 months to recruit the sample and collect the data. Analysis of the mothers' stories took an additional 3 months. The data analysis revealed four main themes (components): (1) feelings of numbness and detachment, (2) crying and anger, (3) distressing cognitive changes, and (4) limited outside interactions.

Phase 4. Dissemination Phase: 12 Months. It took approximately 3 months to prepare the manuscript reporting this study. It was submitted to the *MCN: The American Journal of Maternal/Child Nursing* on March 7, 2019. This journal had an unusually rapid response and a little more than 1 month later, on April 12, 2019, Beck and Watson received a "revise-and-resubmit" decision from the journal. Only minor revisions were needed, and so on April 24, 2019, the authors submitted their revised manuscript. Only 1 day later, on April 25, 2019, Beck and Watson received notification that their manuscript had been accepted for publication. The article was published in the December 2019 issue of *MCN*.

Critical Thinking Exercises

1. Answer the relevant questions from Box 2.3 regarding this study.
2. Also consider the following targeted questions:
   a. Do you think an appropriate amount of time was allocated to the various phases and steps in this study?
   b. Would it have been appropriate for the researchers to address the research question using quantitative research methods? Why or why not?
3. If the results of this study are valid, what might be some of the uses to which the findings could be put in clinical practice?

EXAMPLE 2: QUANTITATIVE RESEARCH IN APPENDIX A

1. Read the abstract and the introduction of Swenson and colleagues' study ("Parents' use of praise and criticism in a sample of young children seeking mental health services") in Appendix A of this book and then answer the relevant questions in Box 2.3.
2. Also consider the following targeted questions:
   a. Comment on the composition of the research team for this study.
   b. Did this report present any actual *data* from the study participants?
   c. Would it have been possible for the researchers to use an experimental design for this study?

EXAMPLE 3: QUALITATIVE RESEARCH IN APPENDIX B

1. Read the abstract and the introduction from Beck and Watson's study ("Posttraumatic growth after birth trauma") in Appendix B of this book and then answer the relevant questions in Box 2.3.
2. Also consider the following targeted questions:
   a. Did this report present any actual *data* from the study participants? What is an example?
   b. What information is provided in the article about the schedule for this project?

WANT TO KNOW MORE?

A wide variety of resources to enhance your learning and understanding of this chapter is available on thePoint°. ⚡

- Chapter Supplement on Deductive and Inductive Reasoning
- Answers to the Critical Thinking Exercises for Examples 2 and 3
- Internet Resources with useful websites for Chapter 2
- A Wolters Kluwer journal article on a topic related to this chapter

Additional study aids, including eight journal articles and related questions, are also available in *Study Guide for Essentials of Nursing Research, 10e.*

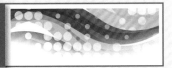

Summary Points

- The people who provide information to the researchers in a **study** are called **subjects** or **study participants** in quantitative research, and study participants or **informants** in qualitative research; collectively, they comprise the study **sample**.

- The *site* is the location for the research; researchers sometimes engage in *multisite studies*.

- Researchers investigate **concepts** and *phenomena* (or **constructs**), which are abstractions inferred from people's behavior or attributes.

- Concepts are the building blocks of **theories**, which are systematic explanations of some aspect of the real world.

- In quantitative studies, concepts are called variables. A **variable** is a characteristic or quality that takes on different values (i.e., varies from one person or object to another).

- The **dependent** (or **outcome**) **variable** is the behavior, characteristic, or outcome the researcher is interested in explaining, predicting, or affecting (the "O" in the PICO format). The **independent variable** is the presumed cause of or influence on the dependent variable. The independent variable corresponds to the "I" and the "C" components in the PICO scheme.

- A **conceptual definition** describes the abstract meaning of a concept being studied. An **operational definition** specifies how a variable will be measured.

- **Data**—the information collected during the course of a study—may take the form of narrative information (**qualitative data**) or numeric values (**quantitative data**).

- A **relationship** is a connection or pattern of association between variables. Quantitative researchers study the relationship between independent variables and outcome variables.

- When the independent variable is a cause of the dependent variable, the relationship is a **cause-and-effect** (or **causal**) **relationship**. In an **associative** (*functional*) **relationship**, variables are related in a noncausal manner.

- A key distinction in quantitative studies is between **experimental research**, in which researchers actively intervene to test an intervention or therapy, and **nonexperimental** (or **observational**) **research**, in which researchers collect data about phenomena without intervening.

- Qualitative research sometimes is rooted in research traditions that originate in other disciplines. Three such traditions are grounded theory, phenomenology, and ethnography.

- **Grounded theory** seeks to describe and understand key social psychological processes that occur in a social setting.

- **Phenomenology** focuses on the lived experiences of humans and is an approach to gaining insight into what the life experiences of people are like and what they mean.

- **Ethnography** provides a framework for studying the meanings, patterns, and lifeways of a culture in a holistic fashion.

- In a quantitative study, researchers usually progress in a series of linear steps, from asking research questions to answering them. The main phases in a quantitative study are the conceptual, planning, empirical, analytic, and dissemination phases.

- The *conceptual phase* involves (1) defining the problem to be studied, (2) doing a **literature review**, (3) engaging in *clinical fieldwork* for clinical studies, (4) developing a framework and conceptual definitions, and (5) formulating **hypotheses** to be tested.

- The *planning phase* entails (6) selecting a **research design**, (7) developing **intervention protocols** if the study is experimental, (8) specifying the **population** (the "P" in the PICO format), (9) developing a *sampling plan*, (10) specifying a *data collection plan* and methods to measure variables, (11) developing strategies to safeguard participants' rights, and (12) finalizing the research plan.

- The *empirical phase* involves (13) collecting data and (14) preparing data for analysis (e.g., *coding* data).

- The *analytic phase* involves (15) performing **statistical analyses** and (16) interpreting the results.

- The *dissemination phase* entails (17) communicating the findings and (18) promoting the use of the study evidence in nursing practice.

- The flow of activities in a qualitative study is flexible and less linear than in a quantitative study. Qualitative studies typically involve an **emergent design** that evolves during data collection.

- Qualitative researchers begin with a broad question regarding a phenomenon of interest, often focusing on a little-studied aspect. In the early phase of a qualitative study, researchers select a site and seek to **gain entrée** into it, which typically involves enlisting the cooperation of *gatekeepers* within the site.

- Once in the field, qualitative researchers select informants, collect data, and then analyze and interpret them in an iterative fashion; experiences during data collection help in an ongoing fashion to shape the design of the study.

- Early analysis in qualitative research leads to refinements in sampling and data collection, until **saturation** (redundancy of information) is achieved. Analysis typically involves a search for critical **themes** or categories in the data.

- Both qualitative and quantitative researchers disseminate their findings, most often by publishing their research reports in professional journals.

REFERENCES FOR CHAPTER 2

*Andersson, E., Willman, A., Sjöström-Strand, A., & Borglin, G. (2015). Registered nurses' descriptions of caring: A phenomenographic interview study. *BMC Nursing, 14*, 16.

**Beck, C., & Watson, S. (2019). Mothers' experiences interacting with infants after traumatic childbirth. *MCN: The American Journal of Maternal Child Nursing, 44*, 338–344.

Bloxsome, D., Bayes, S., & Ireson, D. (2020). "I love being a midwife; it's who I am": A Glaserian grounded theory study of why midwives stay in midwifery. *Journal of Clinical Nursing, 29*, 208–220.

Celia, T., Freysteinson, W., Fredland, N., & Bowyer, P. (2020). Battle weary/battle ready: A phenomenological study of parents' lived experiences caring for children with autism and their safety concerns. *Journal of Advanced Nursing, 76*, 221–233.

*Chaaban, T., Ahouah, M., Lombrail, P., Le Febvre, H., Mourad, A., Morvillers, J., & Rothan-Tondeur, M. (2020). Decisional issues in antibiotic prescribing in French nursing homes: An ethnographic study. *Journal of Public Health Research, 8*, 1533.

Chen, Y., Cheng, S., Lee, P., Lai, C., Hou, I., & Chen, C. (2020). Distraction using virtual reality for children during intravenous injections in an emergency department: A randomised trial. *Journal of Clinical Nursing, 29*, 503–510.

Epstein, M., Söderström, M., Jirwe, M., Tucker, P., & Dahlgren, A. (2020). Sleep and fatigue in newly graduated nurses—Experiences and strategies for handling shiftwork. *Journal of Clinical Nursing, 29*, 184–194.

Glaser, B. G., & Strauss, A. L. (1967). *The discovery of grounded theory: Strategies for qualitative research*. Chicago, IL: Aldine.

Kim, J., Park, Y., Kim, J., Jang, E., & Ha, Y. (2020). The optimal time of postoperative feeding after total hip arthroplasty: A prospective, randomized, controlled trial. *Clinical Nursing Research, 29*, 31–36.

*Kwon, M., Kim, S., & So, W. (2020). Factors associated with adolescents' Internet use duration by suicidal ideation. *International Journal of Environmental Research and Public Health, 17*, 433.

Matsunaga-Myoji, Y., Fujita, K., Makimoto, K., Tabuchi, Y., & Matawari, M. (2020). Three-year follow-up study of physical activity, physical function, and health-related quality of life after total hip arthroplasty. *The Journal of Arthroplasty, 35*, 198–203.

Morse, J. M., Solberg, S. M., Neander, W. L., Bottorff, J. L., & Johnson, J. L. (1990). Concepts of caring and caring as a concept. *ANS. Advances in Nursing Science, 13*, 1–14.

Webel, A., Smith, C., Perazzo, J., Phillips, J., Al Battashi, H., & Dawson-Rose, C. (2020). The relationships among social capital, HIV self-management, and substance use in women. *Western Journal of Nursing Research, 42*, 4–13.

Woo, J., Penckofer, S., Giurgescu, C., & Yeatts, P. (2020). Vitamin D deficiency and sleep quality in minority pregnant women. *MCN: The American Journal of Maternal Child Nursing, 45*, 155–160.

*A link to this open-access article is provided in the Internet Resources section on the Point® website.

**This journal article is available on the Point® for this chapter.

3 Reading and Critically Appraising Research Articles

Learning Objectives

On completing this chapter, you will be able to:

- Identify and describe the major sections of a research journal article
- Characterize the style used in quantitative and qualitative research reports
- Read a research article and broadly grasp its "story"
- Describe aspects of a critical appraisal of a study
- Understand the many challenges researchers face and identify some tools they use to address methodological challenges
- Define new terms in the chapter

Key Terms

- Abstract
- Bias
- Blinding
- Confounding variable
- Credibility
- Critical appraisal
- Findings
- IMRAD format

- Inference
- Journal article
- Level of significance
- *p*
- Placebo
- Randomness
- Reflexivity
- Reliability

- Research control
- Scientific merit
- Statistical significance
- Statistical test
- Transferability
- Triangulation
- Trustworthiness
- Validity

Evidence from nursing studies is communicated through research reports that describe what was studied, how it was studied, and what was found. Research reports are often daunting to readers without research training. This chapter aims to make research reports more accessible and provides some guidance regarding critical appraisals of research reports.

TYPES OF RESEARCH REPORTS

Nurses are most likely to find research evidence in journals or at nursing conferences. Research **journal articles** are descriptions of studies published in professional journals. Competition for journal space is keen, so research articles are brief—generally only 10 to 20 double-spaced pages. This means that researchers must condense a lot of information about the study into a short report.

Usually, manuscripts are reviewed by two or more *peer reviewers* (other researchers) who make recommendations to the journal editor about accepting or requesting revisions to the manuscript. Reviews are usually *blind*—reviewers are not told researchers' names, and authors are not told reviewers' names. Consumers thus have some assurance that journals articles have been vetted by impartial nurse researchers. Nevertheless, publication does not mean that the findings can be uncritically accepted. Research methods courses help nurses to evaluate the quality of evidence reported in journal articles.

At conferences, research findings are presented as oral presentations or poster sessions. In an *oral presentation*, researchers are typically allotted 10 to 20 minutes to describe key features of their study to an audience. In *poster sessions*, many researchers simultaneously present visual displays summarizing their studies, and conference attendees walk around the room looking at the displays. Conferences offer an opportunity for dialogue: Attendees can ask questions to help them better understand what the findings mean; moreover, they can offer and receive suggestions relating to clinical implications of the study. Thus, professional conferences are a valuable forum for clinical audiences.

THE CONTENT OF RESEARCH JOURNAL ARTICLES

Many research articles are structured using the **IMRAD format**. This format organizes content into four main sections—**I**ntroduction, **M**ethod, **R**esults, **and D**iscussion. The paper starts with a title and an abstract and concludes with references.

The Title and Abstract

Research reports have titles that succinctly convey key information. In qualitative studies, the title normally includes the central phenomenon and group under investigation. In quantitative studies, the title communicates key variables and the population (in other words, PICO components).

The **abstract** is a brief description of the study placed at the beginning of the article. The abstract answers questions like the following: What were the research questions? What methods were used to address those questions? What were the findings? and What are the implications for nursing practice? Readers can review an abstract to judge whether to read the full report.

The Introduction

The introduction to a research article acquaints readers with the research problem and its context. This section usually describes the following:

- The central phenomena, concepts, or variables under study
- The study purpose and research questions or hypotheses
- A brief review of related literature
- The theoretical or conceptual framework
- The significance of and need for the study

Thus, the introduction lets readers understand the problem the researcher sought to address.

> **Example of introductory material** •
> Older adults with chronic obstructive pulmonary disease (COPD) are at increased risk for deconditioning during hospitalization and diminished functional status at discharge. COPD pathology produces impaired gas exchange and air trapping, causing baseline shortness of breath that worsens with physical activity. Physical activity may become more challenging in the presence of acute illness and hospitalization, leading to decreased mobility and deconditioning . . . The purpose of this study was to examine correlations between in-hospital mobility activities and indicators of functional status in hospitalized older adults with COPD (Shay et al., 2020, p. 13; references removed).

In this paragraph, the researchers described the population of interest (older adults with COPD), the central concepts of the study (mobility activities and functional status among older COPD patients who were hospitalized), and the study purpose.

> **TIP** The introduction section of most reports is not specifically labeled "Introduction." The introduction immediately follows the abstract.

The Method Section

The method section describes the methods used to answer the research questions. In a quantitative study, the method section usually describes the following, which may be presented in labeled subsections:

- The research design
- The sampling plan
- Methods of measuring variables and collecting study data
- Study procedures, including procedures to protect human rights
- Data analysis methods

Qualitative researchers discuss many of the same issues, but with different emphases. For example, a qualitative study often provides more information about the research setting and the study context. Reports of qualitative studies also describe the researchers' efforts to enhance the integrity of the study.

The Results Section

The results section presents the **findings** that were obtained by analyzing the study data. The text presents a narrative summary of key findings, often accompanied by more detailed tables. Virtually all results sections contain descriptive information, including a description of the participants (e.g., average age, percent married or unmarried).

In quantitative studies, the results section usually reports the following information relating to statistical tests performed:

- *The names of statistical tests used.* Researchers test their hypotheses and assess the probability that the results are reliable using **statistical tests**. For example, if the researcher finds that the average birth weight of drug-exposed infants in the sample is lower than the birth weight of infants not exposed to drugs, how probable is it that the same would be true for the population of infants? A statistical test helps answer the question, Is the relationship between prenatal drug exposure and infant birth weight *real*, and would it likely be observed with a new sample from the same population? Statistical tests are based on common principles; you do not have to know the names of all statistical tests to comprehend the findings.
- *The value of the calculated statistic.* Computers are used to calculate a numeric value for the particular statistical test used. The value allows researchers to reach conclusions about their hypotheses. The *actual* value of the statistic, however, is not inherently meaningful and need not concern you.
- *Statistical significance.* A critical piece of information is whether the statistical tests were significant (not to be confused with clinically important). If a researcher reports that the results are **statistically significant**, it means the findings are probably true and replicable. Research reports also indicate the **level of significance**, which is an index of how *probable* it is that the findings are reliable. For example, if a report indicates that a finding was significant at the .05 probability level (symbolized as p), this means that only 5 times out of 100 (5 ÷ 100 = .05) would the obtained result be spurious. In other words, 95 times

out of 100, similar results would be obtained with a new sample. Readers can thus have a high degree of confidence—but not total assurance—that the results are accurate.

> **Example from the results section of a quantitative study** •••••••••••••••••
> Chang, Tsai, and colleagues (2020) tested the effects of a nurse-led exercise program on exercise capacity and quality of life among cancer survivors after esophagectomy. The findings indicated that, compared to patients who did not received the intervention, those receiving the special program had fewer symptoms of fatigue ($t = 4.37$, $p < .001$), appetite loss ($t = 4.56$, $p < .001$), and pain ($t = 2.82$, $p < .01$).

In this example, the researchers stated that fatigue, appetite loss, and pain were significantly better among those who received the intervention. The differences between the groups were not likely to have been haphazard and probably would be replicated with a new sample. These findings are very reliable. For example, with regard to fatigue, it was found that a group difference of the magnitude obtained would occur just as a "fluke" less than 1 time in 1,000 ($p < .001$). Note that to comprehend this finding, you do not need to understand what a t statistic is, nor do you need to concern yourself with the actual value of the t statistic, 4.37.

 TIP Results are *more* reliable if the p value is *smaller*. For example, there is a higher probability that the results are accurate when $p = .01$ (1 in 100 chance of a spurious result) than when $p = .05$ (5 in 100 chances of a spurious result). Researchers sometimes report an exact probability (e.g., $p = .03$) or a probability below conventional thresholds (e.g., $p < .05$—less than 5 in 100).

In qualitative reports, researchers often organize findings according to the major themes, processes, or categories that were identified in the data. The results section of qualitative reports sometimes has several subsections, the headings of which correspond to the researcher's labels for the themes. Excerpts from the *raw data* (the actual words of participants) are presented to support and provide a rich description of the thematic analysis. The results section of qualitative studies may also present the researcher's emerging theory about the phenomenon under study.

> **Example from the results section of a qualitative study** ••••••••••••••••••••
> Clutter (2020) explored the experiences and viewpoints of birth fathers regarding open adoption. The analysis of the in-depth interviews with 10 birth fathers revealed six themes, one of which was positive views about open adoption: "Birth fathers were unanimously positive about openness in their adoptions . . . Openness began because birth parents thought it was the best for their birth child. One explained that '*if they are not in the spot where they can have a child, keep him or her safe, and provide, open adoption is the way to go because you get to pick the family. It has changed my life and I'm walking proof of it*'" (p. 29).

The Discussion Section

In the discussion, the researcher presents conclusions about the meaning and implications of the findings, i.e., what the results mean, why things turned out the way they did, how the findings fit with other evidence, and how the results can be used in practice. The discussion in both qualitative and quantitative reports may include the following elements:

- An interpretation of the results
- Clinical and research implications
- Study limitations and ramifications for the believability of the results

Researchers are in the best position to point out deficiencies in their studies. A discussion section that presents the researcher's grasp of study limitations demonstrates to readers that the authors were aware of the limitations and likely took them into account in interpreting the findings.

References

Research articles conclude with a list of the articles and books that were referenced. If you are interested in learning more about a topic, the reference list of a recent study is a good place to begin.

THE STYLE OF RESEARCH JOURNAL ARTICLES

Research reports tell a story. However, the style in which many research journal articles are written—especially for quantitative studies—makes it difficult for some readers to understand or become interested in the story.

Why Are Research Articles so Hard to Read?

To unaccustomed audiences, research reports may seem bewildering. Four factors contribute to this impression:

1. *Compactness.* Journal space is limited, so authors compress a lot of information into a small space. Interesting, personalized aspects of the investigation cannot be reported, and, in qualitative studies, only a handful of supporting quotes can be included.
2. *Jargon.* The authors of research articles use research terms that may seem esoteric.
3. *Objectivity.* Quantitative researchers tend to avoid any impression of subjectivity, and so they tell their research stories in a way that makes them sound impersonal. Most quantitative research articles are written in the passive voice, which tends to make the articles less inviting and lively. Qualitative reports are often written in a more conversational style.
4. *Statistical information.* In quantitative reports, numbers and statistical symbols may intimidate readers who do not have statistical training.

A goal of this textbook is to assist you in understanding the content of research reports and in overcoming anxieties about jargon and statistical information.

 HOW-TO-TELL TIP   How can you tell if the voice is active or passive? In the active voice, the article would say what the researchers *did* (e.g., "We used a mercury sphygmomanometer to measure blood pressure"). In the passive voice, the article indicates what *was done*, without indicating who did it, although it is implied that the researchers were the agents (e.g., "A mercury sphygmomanometer *was used* to measure blood pressure").

Tips on Reading Research Articles

As you progress through this book, you will acquire skills for evaluating research articles, but the skills involved in critical appraisal take time to develop. The first step is to comprehend research articles. Here are some hints on digesting research reports.

- Grow accustomed to the style of research articles by reading them frequently, even though you may not yet understand the technical points.
- Read journal articles slowly. It may be useful to skim the article first to get the major points and then read the article more carefully a second time.

- On the second reading, train yourself to become an *active* reader. Reading actively means constantly monitoring yourself to verify that you understand what you are reading. If you have difficulty, you can ask someone for help. In most cases, that "someone" will be your instructor, but also consider contacting the researchers themselves.
- Keep this textbook with you as a reference when you read articles so that you can look up unfamiliar terms in the glossary or index.
- Try not to get bogged down in (or scared away by) statistical information. Try to grasp the gist of the story without letting symbols and numbers frustrate you.

CRITICALLY APPRAISING RESEARCH REPORTS

A critical reading of a research article involves a careful appraisal of the researcher's major conceptual and methodologic decisions. It would be difficult to assess these decisions at this point, but your skills will improve as you progress through this book.

Research Critiques and Critical Appraisals

A distinction is sometimes made between a research *critique* and a **critical appraisal**. The latter term is favored by those focusing on the evaluation of evidence for nursing practice. The term *critique* is more often used when individual studies are being evaluated for their scientific merit—for example, when a manuscript is reviewed by *peer reviewers* who make recommendations about publishing the paper in a journal. In both cases, the goal is to apply knowledge about research methods, theory, and substantive issues to draw conclusions about the validity and relevance of the findings.

Both critiques and critical appraisals involve objective assessments of a study's strengths and limitations, but they vary in scope and aims. Peer reviewers who are asked to prepare a written critique for a manuscript submitted to a journal may evaluate the strengths and weaknesses in terms of substantive issues (Was the research problem significant to nursing?), theoretical issues (Were the conceptual underpinnings sound?), methodological decisions (Were the methods rigorous, yielding believable evidence?), interpretive (Did the researcher reach defensible conclusions?), ethics (Were participants' rights protected?), and style (Is the report clear, grammatical, and well organized?). In short, peer reviewers do a comprehensive review to provide feedback to the researchers and to journal editors about the merit of both the study and the report and typically offer suggestions for revisions.

Critical appraisals designed to inform evidence-based nursing practice are seldom comprehensive. For example, it is of little consequence to evidence-based practice (EBP) that an article is ungrammatical. An appraisal of the clinical utility of a study focuses on whether the evidence is accurate, sound, and clinically relevant—the focus is on appraising the research methods and the findings themselves.

Students taking a research methods course also may be asked to appraise a study. Such appraisals are often intended to cultivate critical thinking and to induce students to apply newly acquired skills in research methods.

Critical Appraisal Support in This Textbook

We provide several types of support for the critical appraisal of individual studies. First, suggestions for appraising relevant aspects of a study are included at the end of each chapter. Second, it is always illuminating to have a good model, so we prepared an appraisal of a quantitative study. Both the report and the appraisal are in Appendix D.

Third, we offer key appraisal guidelines for quantitative and qualitative reports in this chapter, in Tables 3.1 and 3.2, respectively. The questions in the guidelines concern the rigor

TABLE 3.1 Guide to a Focused Critical Appraisal of Evidence Quality in a Quantitative Research Report

Aspect of the Report	Critical Appraisal Questions	Detailed Appraisal Guidelines
Method Research design	• What was the level of evidence for the study, and was the level the highest possible for the study purpose? • Were appropriate comparisons made to enhance interpretability of the findings? • Was the number of data collection points appropriate? Was the period of follow-up (if any) adequate? • Did the design minimize biases and threats to the validity of the study (e.g., was blinding used, was attrition low)?	Box 8.1, page 135
Population and sample	• Was the population of interest clearly identified? Was the sample adequately described? • Was the best possible sampling design used to enhance the sample's representativeness? Were sampling biases minimized? • Was the sample size adequate? Was a power analysis used to estimate sample size needs?	Box 9.1, page 146
Data collection and measurement	• Were key variables operationalized using the best possible method (e.g., interviews, observations, biomarkers)? • Were clinically important and patient-centered outcomes measured? Were the specific instruments adequately described? • Did the report provide evidence that the data collection methods yielded data that were reliable and valid?	Box 9.2, page 156
Procedures	• If there was an intervention, was it adequately described, and was it properly implemented? Did most participants allocated to the intervention group actually receive it? • Were data collected in a manner that minimized bias?	Box 8.1, page 135; Box 9.2, page 156
Results Data analysis	• Were appropriate statistical methods used? • Was the most powerful analytic method used (e.g., did the analysis control for confounding variables)? • Were Type I and Type II errors avoided or minimized?	Box 13.1, page 233
Findings and interpretation	• Was information about statistical significance presented? • Was information about effect size and precision of estimates (confidence intervals) presented? • Was the clinical significance of the findings discussed? • Did the design and analysis enhance the applicability of the study results?	Box 14.1, page 252
Summary assessment	• Despite any limitations, do the study findings appear to be valid—do you have confidence in the *truth* value of the results? • Does the study contribute any meaningful evidence that can be used in nursing practice or that is useful to the nursing discipline?	

TABLE 3.2 Guide to a Focused Critical Appraisal of Evidence Quality in a Qualitative Research Report

Aspect of the Report	Critical Appraisal Questions	Detailed Appraisal Guidelines
Method Research design and research tradition	• Is the identified research tradition (if any) congruent with the methods used to collect and analyze data? • Was an adequate amount of time spent in the field or with study participants? • Was there evidence of reflexivity in the design?	Box 10.1, page 171
Sample and setting	• Was the group or population of interest adequately described? • Were the setting and sample described in sufficient detail? • Was the best possible method of sampling used to enhance information richness? • Was the sample size adequate? Was saturation achieved?	Box 11.1, page 180
Data collection	• Were appropriate methods used to gather data? Were data gathered through two or more methods to achieve triangulation? • Were the data of sufficient depth and richness?	Box 11.2, page 185
Procedures	• Do data collection and recording procedures appear appropriate? • Were data collected in a manner that minimized bias?	Box 11.2, page 185
Enhancement of trustworthiness	• Did the researchers use effective strategies to enhance the trustworthiness/integrity of the study? • Was there "thick description" of the context, participants, and findings? • Do the researchers' clinical and methodologic experience enhance confidence in the findings and their interpretation?	Box 16.1, page 286
Results Data analysis	• Was the data analysis strategy compatible with the research tradition and with the nature and type of data gathered? • Did the analysis yield an appropriate "product" (e.g., a theory, taxonomy, thematic pattern?	Box 15.1, page 269
Findings	• Were the findings effectively summarized, with good use of excerpts from the data and strong supporting arguments? • Did the analysis yield an insightful, provocative, authentic, and meaningful picture of the phenomenon under investigation? • Were the findings interpreted within an appropriate social or cultural context?	Box 15.1, page 269
Summary assessment	• Do the study findings appear to be trustworthy—do you have confidence in the *truth* value of the results? • Does the study contribute any meaningful evidence that can be used in nursing practice or that is useful to the nursing discipline?	

with which the researchers dealt with critical research challenges, some of which we describe in the next section.

> **TIP** For those undertaking a comprehensive appraisal, we offer broader guidelines in the supplement to this chapter on thePoint° website.

The second columns of Tables 3.1 and 3.2 lists some important appraisal questions, and the third column cross-references the more detailed guidelines in the various chapters of the book. We know that most of the questions are too difficult for you to answer at this point, but your methodological and appraisal skills will develop as you progress through this book.

The question wording in these guidelines calls for a yes or no answer (although it may well be that the answer sometimes will be "Yes, *but...*"). In all cases, the desirable answer is *yes*; a *no* suggests a possible limitation, and a *yes* suggests a strength. Therefore, the more *yeses* a study gets, the stronger it is likely to be. Cumulatively, then, these guidelines can suggest a global assessment: A study with 10 *yeses* is likely to be superior to one with only 2. However, these guidelines are not intended to yield a formal quality "score."

We acknowledge that our guidelines have shortcomings. In particular, they are generic even though appraisals cannot use a one-size-fits-all list of questions. Important questions that are relevant to certain studies (e.g., those that have a Therapy purpose) do not fit into a set of general questions for all quantitative studies. Thus, you need to use some judgment about whether the guidelines are sufficiently comprehensive for the type of study you are appraising. We also note that there are questions in these guidelines for which there are no totally objective answers. Even experts sometimes disagree about methodological strategies.

> **TIP** Just as a careful clinician seeks research evidence that certain practices are or are not effective, you as a reader should demand evidence that the researchers' methodological decisions were sound.

Critical Appraisal With Key Research Challenges in Mind

In appraising a study, it is useful to be aware of the challenges that confront researchers. For example, they face ethical challenges (e.g., Can the study achieve its goals without infringing on human rights?), practical challenges (Will I be able to recruit enough participants?), and methodological challenges (Will the methods I use yield results that can be trusted?). Most of this book provides guidance relating to the last question, and this section highlights key methodological challenges. This section offers us an opportunity to introduce important terms and concepts that are relevant in a critical appraisal. The worth of a study's evidence for nursing practice often relies on how well researchers deal with these challenges.

Inference

Inference is an integral part of doing and appraising research. An **inference** is a conclusion drawn from the study evidence using logical reasoning and taking into account the methods used to generate that evidence.

Inference is necessary because researchers use proxies that "stand in" for things that are fundamentally of interest. A sample of participants is a proxy for an entire population. A control group that does not receive an intervention is a proxy for what would happen to the people who received the intervention if they had *not* received it.

Researchers face the challenge of using methods that yield good and persuasive evidence in support of inferences that they wish to make. Readers must draw their own inferences based on an appraisal of methodological decisions.

Reliability, Validity, and Trustworthiness

Researchers want their inferences to correspond to the *truth*. Research cannot contribute evidence to guide clinical practice if the findings are inaccurate, biased, or fail to represent the experiences of the target group.

Quantitative researchers use several criteria to assess the quality of a study, sometimes referred to as its **scientific merit**. Two especially important criteria are reliability and validity. **Reliability** refers to the accuracy and consistency of information obtained in a study. The term is most often associated with the methods used to measure variables. For example, if a thermometer measures Alan's temperature as 98.1°F one minute and as 102.5°F the next minute, the thermometer is not reliable.

Validity is a more complex concept that broadly concerns the *soundness* of the study's evidence. Like reliability, validity is an important criterion for evaluating methods to measure variables. In this context, the validity question is whether the methods are really measuring the concepts that they purport to measure. Is a paper-and-pencil measure of depression *really* measuring depression? Or is it measuring something else, such as loneliness or stress? Researchers strive for solid conceptual definitions of research variables and valid methods to operationalize them.

Another aspect of validity concerns the quality of evidence about the relationship between the independent variable and the dependent variable. Did a nursing intervention *really* bring about improvements in patients' outcomes—or were other factors responsible for patients' progress? Researchers make numerous methodological decisions that can influence this type of study validity.

Qualitative researchers use different criteria and terminology in evaluating a study's integrity. In general, qualitative researchers pursue methods of enhancing the **trustworthiness** of the study's data and findings (Lincoln & Guba, 1985). Trustworthiness encompasses several different dimensions—credibility, transferability, confirmability, dependability, and authenticity—which are described in Chapter 16.

Credibility is an especially important aspect of trustworthiness. Credibility is achieved to the extent that the research methods inspire confidence that the results are truthful and accurate. Credibility in a qualitative study can be enhanced in several ways, but one strategy merits early discussion because it has implications for the design of all studies, including quantitative ones. **Triangulation** is the use of multiple sources or referents to draw conclusions about what constitutes the truth. In a quantitative study, this might mean having two ways to measure an outcome, to assess whether results are consistent. In a qualitative study, triangulation might involve efforts to understand the complexity of a phenomenon by using multiple data collection methods to converge on the truth (e.g., having in-depth discussions with participants as well as watching their behavior in natural settings). Nurse researchers are also beginning to triangulate across paradigms—that is, to integrate both qualitative and quantitative data in a single study to enhance the validity of the conclusions in *mixed methods research* (see Chapter 12).

Example of triangulation •
Tanaka (2020) studied the depression-linked beliefs among older Japanese adults diagnosed with depression and being treated in a psychiatric ward. Data were gathered from 19 patients, using multiple in-depth interviews and observations of the patients on multiple occasions during their hospital stay.

Nurse researchers need to design their studies to minimize threats to the reliability, validity, and trustworthiness of their studies, and users of research must evaluate the extent to which they were successful.

 TIP In reading and appraising research articles, it is appropriate to have a "show me" attitude—that is, to expect researchers to build and present a solid case for the merit of their inferences. They do this by providing evidence that the findings are reliable and valid or trustworthy.

Bias

Bias can threaten a study's validity and trustworthiness. A **bias** is a distortion or influence that results in an error in inference. Bias can be caused by various factors, including researchers' preconceptions, faulty methods of collecting data, or participants' lack of candor.

Some bias is haphazard and affects only small segments of the data. As an example, a few study participants might provide inaccurate information because they were tired at the time of data collection. *Systematic bias* results when the bias is consistent or uniform. For example, if a scale consistently measured people's weight as being 2 pounds heavier than their true weight, there would be systematic bias in the data on weight.

Rigorous research methods aim to eliminate or minimize bias, using a variety of strategies. Triangulation is one such approach, the idea being that multiple sources of information or points of view offer avenues to identify biases. In quantitative research, methods to combat bias often entail research control.

Research Control

In most quantitative studies, researchers strive to control aspects of the research. **Research control** usually involves holding constant influences on the outcome so that the relationship between the independent and dependent variables can be understood. In other words, research control attempts to eliminate contaminating factors that might cloud the relationship between the variables that are of central interest.

Contaminating factors, often called **confounding** (or *extraneous*) **variables**, can best be illustrated with an example. Suppose we were studying whether urinary incontinence (UI) leads to depression. Prior evidence suggests that this might be the case, but previous studies have not clarified the nature of the relationship. The question is whether UI itself (the independent variable) contributes to higher levels of depression, or whether there are other factors that can account for the relationship between UI and depression. We need to design a study that controls other determinants of the outcome—determinants that are also related to the independent variable, UI.

One confounding variable here is age. Levels of depression tend to be higher in older people, and people with UI tend to be older than those without this problem. In other words, perhaps age is the *real* cause of higher depression in people with UI. If age is not controlled, then any observed relationship between UI and depression could be caused by UI, or by age.

Three possible explanations might be portrayed schematically as follows:

1. UI→depression
2. Age→UI→depression
3.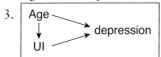

The arrows symbolize a causal mechanism or influence. In model 1, UI directly affects depression, independently of other factors. In model 2, UI is a *mediating variable*—the effect of age on depression is *mediated* by UI. According to this representation, age affects depression *through* the effect that age has on UI. In model 3, both age and UI have separate effects on depression, and age also increases the risk of UI. Some research is specifically designed to test paths of mediation and multiple causation, but in the present example, age is extraneous to the research question. We want to design a study that tests the first explanation. Age must be controlled if our goal is to explore the validity of model 1, which posits that, no matter what a person's age, having UI makes a person more vulnerable to depression.

How can we impose such control? There are a number of ways, as we discuss in Chapter 8, but the general principle underlying each alternative is that the confounding variable must be *held constant*. The confounding variable must somehow be handled so that, in the context of the study, it is not related to the independent variable or the outcome. As an example, let us say we wanted to compare the average scores on a depression scale for those with and without UI. We would want to design a study in such a way that the ages of those in the UI and non-UI groups are comparable, even though, in general, the groups are not comparable in terms of age.

By exercising control over age, we would be taking a step toward understanding the relationship between UI and depression. The world is complex, and many variables are interrelated in complicated ways. The evidence in quantitative studies is often affected by how well researchers controlled confounding influences.

Research rooted in the constructivist paradigm does not impose controls. With their emphasis on holism and individual human experience, qualitative researchers typically believe that imposing controls removes some of the meaning of reality.

Bias Reduction: Randomness and Blinding

For quantitative researchers, a powerful tool for eliminating bias involves **randomness**—having certain features of the study established by chance rather than by researcher preference. When people are selected *at random* to participate in a study, for example, each person in the initial pool has an equal chance of being selected. This in turn means that there are no systematic biases in the make-up of the sample. Men and women have an equal chance of being selected, for example. Similarly, if participants are allocated *at random* to groups that will be compared (e.g., special intervention and "usual care" groups), then there are no biases in the groups' composition. Randomness is a compelling method of controlling confounding variables and reducing bias.

Another bias-reducing strategy is called **blinding** (or *masking*), which is used in some quantitative studies to prevent biases stemming from people's awareness. Blinding involves concealing information from participants, data collectors, or care providers to enhance objectivity. For example, if study participants are aware of whether they are getting an experimental drug or a sham drug (a **placebo**), then their outcomes could be influenced by their expectations of the new drug's efficacy. Blinding involves withholding information about participants' status in the study (e.g., whether they are in a certain group) or about study hypotheses.

Example of randomness and blinding •
Chang, Lee, and colleagues (2020) tested the effect of heart rate variability biofeedback on autonomic dysfunction, cognitive impairment, and psychological distress in patients with acute ischemic stroke (AIS). Patients with AIS were randomly assigned to receive either the biofeedback intervention or usual care. An investigator who was blinded to the group assignments collected follow-up measurements at 1 and 3 months after the intervention.

Qualitative researchers do not consider randomness or blinding desirable tools for understanding phenomena. A researcher's judgment is viewed as an indispensable vehicle for uncovering the complexities of the phenomena of interest.

Reflexivity

Qualitative researchers are also interested in discovering the truth about human experience. Qualitative researchers often rely on reflexivity to guard against personal bias and preconceptions. **Reflexivity** is the process of reflecting critically on the self and of analyzing and noting personal values and beliefs that could affect data collection and interpretation. Qualitative researchers are trained to explore these issues, to be reflective about decisions made during the inquiry, and to record their thoughts in personal diaries and memos.

Example of reflexivity •
Bellens and colleagues (2020) explored how nurses in Belgian hospitals and in home care experience their involvement with patients requesting euthanasia. They described their approach to reflexivity and minimizing the impact of their own views about euthanasia on the analysis of their data. "Before the start of the interviews, we individually noted our personal thoughts about the subject. Regular critical self-reflection and discussion in team about our feelings and attitudes helped us to foster an open attitude to listen to and interpret the experiences of the respondents" (p. 495).

 TIP Reflexivity can be a useful tool in quantitative as well as qualitative research—self-awareness and introspection can enhance the quality of any study.

Generalizability and Transferability

Nurses increasingly rely on research evidence to guide their clinical practice. EBP is based on the assumption that study findings are not unique to the people, places, or circumstances of the original research.

As noted in Chapter 1, *generalizability* in quantitative studies refers to the extent to which the findings can be applied to other groups and settings. How do researchers enhance the generalizability of a study? First and foremost, they must design studies strong in reliability and validity. There is little point in wondering whether results are generalizable if they are not accurate or valid. In selecting participants, researchers must also give thought to the types of people to whom results might be generalized—and then select participants accordingly. If a study is intended to have implications for adult male and female patients, then men and women should be included in the sample.

Qualitative researchers do not specifically aim for generalizability, but they do want to generate knowledge that might be useful in other situations. Lincoln and Guba (1985), in their influential book on naturalistic inquiry, discuss the concept of **transferability**, the extent to which qualitative findings can be transferred to other settings, as another aspect of trustworthiness. An important mechanism for promoting transferability is the amount of rich descriptive information qualitative researchers provide about study contexts.

RESEARCH EXAMPLES WITH CRITICAL THINKING EXERCISES

Abstracts for a quantitative and a qualitative nursing study are presented in the following sections. Read the abstracts for Examples 1 and 2 and then answer the critical thinking questions that follow. Answers to these questions are available to instructors on thePoint*. The critical thinking questions for Exercises 3 and 4 are based on the studies that appear in their entirety in Appendices A and B of this book. Our comments for these exercises are in the Student Resources section on thePoint*.

EXAMPLE 1: QUANTITATIVE RESEARCH

Study: Two HEmostasis Methods After Transradlal Catheterization: THEMATIC randomized clinical trial (Dos Santos et al., 2020)

Objective: The aim of this study was to compare the effect of two hemostasis devices on the incidence of radial artery occlusion (RAO) after transradial cardiac catheterization.

Background: Radial artery occlusion is the most prevalent ischemic complication after radial artery catheterization. There is still no predictive pattern of vessel patency assessment, and the comparative effectiveness of different hemostasis techniques has yet to be established.

Methods: This study used a randomized clinical trial of adult patients undergoing transradial cardiac catheterization. Participants were randomized into an intervention group (hemostasis with the TR Band device) and a control group (hemostasis with a conventional pressure dressing). The primary end point was the incidence of RAO (at discharge and at 30 days postcatheterization).

Results: Among the 600 patients included (301 in the intervention group and 299 controls), immediate RAO occurred in 24 (8%) in the TR Band group and 19 (6%) in the pressure-dressing group; at 30 days, RAO was present in 5 patients (5%) in the TR Band group and 7 (6%) in the pressure-dressing group. In multivariate analysis, peripheral vascular disease was the only independent predictor of RAO at discharge and at 30 days.

Conclusions: The incidence of RAO was similar in patients who received hemostasis with a TR Band versus a pressure dressing after transradial cardiac catheterization.

Critical Thinking Exercises

1. Consider the following targeted questions:
   a. What were the independent and dependent variables in this study? What are the PICO components?
   b. Is this study experimental or nonexperimental?
   c. How, if at all, was *randomness* used in this study?
   d. How, if at all, was *blinding* used in this study?
   e. Did the researchers use any statistical tests? If yes, were any of the results statistically significant?
2. If the results of this study are valid and generalizable, what might be some of the uses to which the findings could be put in clinical practice?

EXAMPLE 2: QUALITATIVE RESEARCH

Study: Adolescents and young adult cancer survivors' perspectives of disconnectedness from healthcare providers during cancer treatment (Phillips & Haase, 2020)

Background: Adolescent/young adult (AYA) cancer survivors experience greater psychosocial distress than younger or older adults. To address their psychosocial distress, it is important that health care providers (HCPs) foster connectedness with AYAs; however, some HCPs' words and behaviors may actually create a sense of disconnectedness with AYAs.

Objective: The aim of this study was to describe AYA cancer survivors' experiences of disconnectedness from HCPs during cancer treatment.

Methods: This empirical phenomenological study sample included nine AYA cancer survivors (aged 20 to 23 years) diagnosed during adolescence. In-person interviews were conducted using a broad data-generating question and analyzed using an adapted Colaizzi's method.

Results: Health care providers' behaviors that create disconnectedness include (1) exhibiting a lack of appreciation for AYAs' personhood, (2) inflicting unnecessary harm or discomfort, (3) being apathetic of needs and preferences, (4) treating AYAs like they have minimal rights, (5) speaking in a patronizing manner, (6) ignoring their requests, and (7) failing to be vigilant for basic needs. When AYAs experience disconnectedness, they feel dehumanized, powerless, and a lack of self-determination.

Conclusion: Findings highlight disturbing HCP behaviors that create AYA disconnectedness. Despite generally feeling connected to HCPs, AYA cancer survivors" experiences of disconnectedness leave lingering feelings of anger and resentment, even after treatment ends. Preventing disconnectedness behaviors must be a priority.

Implications for Practice: AYA cancer survivors' can benefit from having the opportunity to share their experiences of disconnectedness and having the chance to be autonomous in their care. Bringing awareness to HCPs about what behaviors cause disconnectedness is essential in preventing the behaviors.

Critical Thinking Exercises

1. Consider the following targeted questions:
   a. On which qualitative research tradition, if any, was this study based?
   b. Is this study experimental or nonexperimental?
   c. How, if at all, was *randomness* to used in this study?
   d. Is there any indication in the abstract that *triangulation* was used? *Reflexivity*?
2. If the results of this study are trustworthy and transferable, what might be some of the uses to which the findings could be put in clinical practice?

EXAMPLE 3: QUANTITATIVE RESEARCH IN APPENDIX A

1. Read the abstract and the introduction of Swenson and colleagues' study ("Parents' use of praise and criticism in a sample of young children seeking mental health services") in Appendix A of this book. Then, answer the following targeted questions:
   a. Did this article follow a traditional IMRAD format? Where does the introduction to this article begin and end?
   b. How, if at all, was *randomness* used in this study?
   c. How, if at all, was *blinding* used?
   d. Comment on the possible generalizability of the study findings.

EXAMPLE 4: QUALITATIVE RESEARCH IN APPENDIX B

1. Read the abstract and the introduction of Beck and Watson's study ("Posttraumatic growth after birth trauma") in Appendix B of this book. Then, answer the following targeted questions:
   a. Where does the introduction to this article begin and end?
   b. How, if at all, was *randomness* used in this study?
   c. Is there any indication in the abstract that *triangulation* was used? *Reflexivity*?
   d. Comment on the possible transferability of the study findings.

WANT TO KNOW MORE?

A wide variety of resources to enhance your learning and understanding of this chapter is available on the Point.

- Chapter Supplement on Guide to an Overall Critical Appraisal of a Quantitative Research Report and Guide to an Overall Critical Appraisal of a Qualitative Research Report
- Answers to the Critical Thinking Exercises for Examples 3 and 4
- Internet Resources with useful websites for Chapter 3
- A Wolters Kluwer journal article on a topic related to this chapter

Additional study aids, including eight journal articles and related questions, are also available in *Study Guide for Essentials of Nursing Research, 10e.*

Summary Points

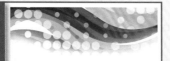

- Both qualitative and quantitative researchers disseminate their findings, most often by publishing reports of their research as **journal articles**, which concisely describe what researcher did and what they found.

- Journal articles often consist of an **abstract** (a synopsis of the study) and four major sections that often follow the **IMRAD format**: an **I**ntroduction (the research problem and its context), **M**ethods (the strategies used to answer research questions), **R**esults (study findings), **a**nd **D**iscussion (interpretation and implications of the findings).

- Research reports are often difficult to read because they are dense, concise, and contain jargon. Quantitative research reports may be intimidating at first because, compared to qualitative reports, they are more impersonal and report on statistical tests.

- **Statistical tests** are used to test hypotheses and to evaluate the reliability of the findings. Findings that are **statistically significant** have a high probability of being "real."

- A goal of this book is to help students to prepare **critical appraisals** of the strengths and limitations of a study, to assess the worth of the evidence for nursing practice.

- Researchers face numerous challenges, the solutions to which must be appraised because they affect the inferences that can be made.

- An **inference** is a conclusion drawn from the study evidence, taking into account the methods used to generate that evidence. Researchers strive to have their inferences correspond to the *truth*.

- **Reliability** (a key challenge in quantitative research) refers to the accuracy of information obtained in a study. **Validity** broadly concerns the *soundness* and rigor of the study's methods—that is, whether the evidence is convincing and well grounded.

- **Trustworthiness** in qualitative research encompasses several different dimensions, including credibility, dependability, confirmability, transferability, and authenticity.

- **Credibility** is achieved to the extent that the methods engender confidence in the truth of the data and in the researchers' interpretations. **Triangulation**, the use of multiple sources to draw conclusions about the truth, is one approach to enhancing credibility.

- A **bias** is an influence that produces a distortion in the study results. In quantitative studies, research control is an approach to addressing bias. **Research control** is used to *hold constant* outside influences on the dependent variable so that the relationship between the independent and dependent variables can be better understood.

- Researchers seek to control **confounding** (or *extraneous*) **variables**—variables that are extraneous to the purpose of a specific study.

- For quantitative researchers, **randomness**—having certain features of the study established by chance—is a powerful tool to eliminate bias.

- **Blinding** (or *masking*) is sometimes used to avoid biases stemming from participants' or research agents' awareness of study hypotheses or research status.

- **Reflexivity**, the process of reflecting critically on the self and of scrutinizing personal values that could affect data collection and interpretation, is an important tool in qualitative research.

- Generalizability in a quantitative study concerns the extent to which the findings can be applied to members of a population who were not included in the study sample.

- A similar concept in qualitative studies is **transferability**, the extent to which qualitative findings can be transferred to other settings. One mechanism for promoting transferability is a rich and thorough description of the research context so that others can make inferences about contextual similarities.

REFERENCES FOR CHAPTER 3

Bellens, M., Debien, E., Claessens, F., Gastmans, C., & de Casterlé, B. (2020). "It is still intense and not unambiguous." Nurses' experiences in the euthanasia care process 15 years after legalisation. *Journal of Clinical Nursing, 29*, 492–502.

Chang, W., Lee, J., Li, C., Davis, A., Yang, C., & Chen, U. (2020). Effects of heart rate variability biofeedback in patients with acute ischemic stroke: A randomized controlled trials. *Biological Research for Nursing, 22*, 33–44.

Chang, Y., Tsai, Y., Hsu, C., Chao, Y., Hsu, C., & Lin, K. (2020). The effectiveness of a nurse-led exercise and health education informatics program on exercise capacity and quality of life among cancer survivors after esophagectomy: A randomized controlled trial. *International Journal of Nursing Studies, 101*, 103418.

**Clutter, L. (2020). Perceptions of birth fathers about their open adoptions. *MCN: The American Journal of Maternal Child Nursing, 45*, 26–32.

Dos Santos, S., Wainstein, R., Valle, F., Corrêa, C., Aliti, G., Ruschel, K., . . . Rabelo-Silca, E. (2020). Two HEmostasis Methods After TransradIal Catheterization: THEMATIC randomized clinical trial. *The Journal of Cardiovascular Nursing, 35*, 217–222.

Lincoln, Y. S., & Guba, E. G. (1985). *Naturalistic inquiry.* Newbury Park, CA: Sage.

Phillips, C., & Haase, J. (2020). Like prisoners in a war camp: Adolescents and young adult cancer survivors' perspectives of disconnectedness from healthcare providers during cancer treatment. *Cancer Nursing, 43*, 69–77.

Shay, A., Fulton, J., & O'Malley, P. (2020). Mobility and functional status among hospitalized COPD patients. *Clinical Nursing Research, 29*, 13–20.

Tanaka, K. (2020). Depression-linked beliefs in older adults with depression. *Journal of Clinical Nursing, 29*, 228–229.

**This journal article is available on thePoint° for this chapter.

4 Attending to Ethics in Research

Learning Objectives

On completing this chapter, you will be able to:

- Discuss the historical background that led to the creation of various codes of ethics
- Understand the potential for ethical dilemmas stemming from conflicts between ethical requirements and research goals
- Identify the three primary ethical principles articulated in the *Belmont Report* and the dimensions encompassed by each
- Identify procedures for adhering to ethical principles and protecting study participants
- Identify vulnerable groups who may require extra protections in participating in research
- Given sufficient information, evaluate the ethical dimensions of a research report
- Define new terms in the chapter

Key Terms

- Anonymity
- Assent
- *Belmont Report*
- Beneficence
- Certificate of Confidentiality
- Code of ethics
- Confidentiality
- Consent form
- Debriefing
- Ethical dilemma
- Full disclosure
- Informed consent
- Institutional Review Board (IRB)
- Minimal risk
- Risk/benefit assessment
- Stipend
- Vulnerable group

ETHICS AND RESEARCH

In research with humans or animals, researchers must take ethical issues into consideration. Ethical concerns are prominent in nursing research because the line between what constitutes the expected practice of nursing and the collection of research data sometimes gets blurred. This chapter discusses ethical principles that should be kept in mind when reading about a study.

Historical Background

We might like to think that violations of moral principles among researchers occurred centuries ago rather than recently, but this is not the case. The Nazi medical experiments of the 1930s and 1940s are the most famous example of recent disregard for ethical conduct.

The Nazi program of research involved using prisoners of war and "racial enemies" in medical experiments. The studies were unethical not only because they exposed people to harm but also because subjects could not refuse participation.

There are more recent examples. For instance, between 1932 and 1972, the Tuskegee Syphilis Study, sponsored by the U.S. Public Health Service, investigated the effects of syphilis among 400 poor African American men. Medical treatment was deliberately withheld to study the course of the untreated disease. It was revealed in 1993 that U.S. federal agencies had sponsored radiation experiments since the 1940s on hundreds of people, many of them prisoners or elderly hospital patients. And, in 2010, it was revealed that a U.S. doctor who worked on the Tuskegee study inoculated prisoners in Guatemala with syphilis in the 1940s. Other examples of studies with ethical transgressions have emerged to give ethical concerns the high visibility they have today.

Codes of Ethics

In response to human rights violations, various **codes of ethics** have been developed. The ethical standards known as the Nuremberg Code were developed in 1949 in response to the Nazi atrocities. Several other international standards have been developed, including the Declaration of Helsinki, which was adopted in 1964 by the World Medical Association and was most recently revised in 2013.

Most disciplines, such as medicine and nursing, have established their own code of ethics. In the United States, the American Nurses Association (ANA) issued *Ethical Guidelines in the Conduct, Dissemination, and Implementation of Nursing Research* in 1995 (Silva, 1995). The ANA, which declared 2015 the Year of Ethics, published a revised *Code of Ethics for Nurses with Interpretive Statements*, a document that not only covers ethical issues for practicing nurses primarily but also includes principles that apply to nurse researchers. In Canada, the Canadian Nurses Association published a revised version of *Code of Ethics for Registered Nurses* in 2017. And, the International Council of Nurses (ICN) developed the *ICN Code of Ethics for Nurses*, updated in 2012 but it is currently being revised (Stievano & Tschudin, 2019).

 TIP Many useful websites are devoted to ethics and research, links to some of which are listed in the Internet Resources for this chapter on thePoint website. ☀—

Government Regulations for Protecting Study Participants

Governments throughout the world fund research and establish rules for adhering to ethical principles. In the United States, an important code of ethics was adopted by the National Commission for the Protection of Human Subjects of Biomedical and Behavioral Research. The commission issued a report in 1978, known as the *Belmont Report*, which provided a model for many guidelines adopted by disciplinary organizations in the United States. The *Belmont Report* also served as the basis for regulations affecting research sponsored by the U.S. government, including studies supported by National Institute of Nursing Research (NINR). The U.S. ethical regulations that have been codified at Title 45 Part 46 of the Code of Federal Regulations and were revised most recently in 2018.

Ethical Dilemmas in Conducting Research

Research that violates ethical principles typically occurs because a researcher believes that knowledge is potentially beneficial in the long run. For some research problems, participants' rights and study quality are put in direct conflict, posing **ethical dilemmas** for researchers.

Here are examples of research problems in which the desire for rigor conflicts with ethical considerations:

1. *Research question:* Does a new medication prolong life in patients with AIDS?
   Ethical dilemma: The best way to test the effectiveness of an intervention is to administer the intervention to some participants but withhold it from others to see if the groups have different outcomes. However, if the intervention is untested (e.g., a new drug), the group receiving the intervention may be exposed to potentially hazardous side effects. On the other hand, the group *not* receiving the drug may be denied a beneficial treatment.

2. *Research question:* Are nurses equally empathic in their care of male and female patients in the intensive care unit (ICU)?
   Ethical dilemma: Ethics require that participants be aware of their role in a study. Yet, if the researcher informs nurse participants that their empathy in caring for male and female ICU patients will be scrutinized, will their behavior be "normal?" If the nurses' usual behavior is altered because of the known presence of research observers, then the findings will be inaccurate.

3. *Research question:* How do parents cope when their children have a terminal illness?
   Ethical dilemma: To answer this question, the researcher may need to probe into parents' psychological state at a vulnerable time; yet, knowledge of the parents' coping mechanisms might help to design effective ways of addressing parents' grief and stress.

4. *Research question:* What is the process by which adult children adapt to the day-to-day burden of caring for a parent with Alzheimer's disease?
   Ethical dilemma: Sometimes, especially in qualitative studies, a researcher may get so close to participants that they become willing to share "secrets" and privileged information. Interviews can become confessions—sometimes of unseemly or illegal behavior. In this example, suppose a woman admitted to physically abusing her mother—how does the researcher respond to that information without undermining a pledge of confidentiality? And, if the researcher divulges the information to authorities, how can a pledge of confidentiality be given in good faith to other participants?

As these examples suggest, researchers are sometimes in a bind. Their goal is to develop high-quality evidence for practice, but they must also protect human rights. Another dilemma may arise if nurse researchers face conflict-of-interest situations, in which their expected behavior as nurses conflicts with standard research behavior (e.g., deviating from a research protocol to assist a patient). It is precisely because of such dilemmas that codes of ethics are needed to guide researchers' efforts.

ETHICAL PRINCIPLES FOR PROTECTING STUDY PARTICIPANTS

The **Belmont Report** articulated three primary ethical principles on which standards of ethical research conduct are based: beneficence, respect for human dignity, and justice. We briefly discuss these principles and then describe methods researchers use to comply with them.

Beneficence

Beneficence imposes a duty on researchers to minimize harm and maximize benefits. Human research should be intended to produce benefits for participants, or—more typically—for others. This principle covers multiple aspects.

The Right to Freedom From Harm and Discomfort

Researchers have an obligation to prevent or minimize harm in studies with humans. Participants must not be subjected to unnecessary risks of harm or discomfort, and their participation in research must be necessary for achieving societally important aims. In research with humans, *harm* and *discomfort* can be physical (e.g., injury), emotional (e.g., stress), social (e.g., loss of social support), or financial (e.g., expenses incurred). Ethical researchers must use strategies to minimize all types of harms and discomforts, even temporary ones.

Protecting human beings from physical harm is often straightforward, but psychological consequences are often hard to discern. For example, participants may be asked questions about their personal lives that lead them to reveal deeply personal information. The need for sensitivity may be especially great in qualitative studies, which often involve in-depth exploration of highly personal experiences.

The Right to Protection From Exploitation

Involvement in a study should not place participants at a disadvantage. Participants need to be assured that their participation, or information they provide, will not be used against them. For example, people reporting illegal drug use should not fear being reported for a crime.

Study participants enter into a special relationship with researchers, and this relationship should not be exploited. Nurse researchers may have a nurse–patient (in addition to a researcher–participant) relationship, and so special care may be needed to avoid exploiting that bond. Patients' consent to participate in a study may result from their understanding of the researcher's role as *nurse*, not as *researcher*.

In qualitative research, psychological distance between researchers and participants often declines as the study progresses. The emergence of a pseudotherapeutic relationship is not uncommon, which could create additional risks that exploitation could inadvertently occur. On the other hand, qualitative researchers often are in a better position than quantitative researchers to *do good*, rather than just to avoid doing harm, because of the close relationships they develop with participants.

> **Example of therapeutic research experiences** •
> Cheryl Beck has conducted many qualitative studies in which study participants commented that telling their experiences was therapeutic for them. For example, one of the participants in Beck and Casavant's (2020) study on vicarious posttraumatic growth in NICU nurses wrote the researchers the following: "Thank you for heading up this study and know that just acknowledging us and allowing this research to take place is healing and will help many nurses for futures to come."

Respect for Human Dignity

Respect for human dignity is the second ethical principle in the *Belmont Report*. This principle includes the right to self-determination and the right to full disclosure.

The Right to Self-Determination

The principle of *self-determination* means that prospective participants have the right to decide voluntarily whether to participate in a study, without risk of prejudicial treatment. It also means that people have the right to ask questions, refuse answering questions, and drop out of the study.

A person's right to self-determination includes freedom from coercion. *Coercion* involves explicit or implicit threats of penalty from failing to participate in a study or excessive rewards from agreeing to participate. The issue of coercion requires careful thought when researchers are in a position of authority or influence over potential participants, as might be the case in a nurse–patient relationship. Coercion can be subtle. For example, a generous monetary incentive (or **stipend**) to encourage the participation of a low-income group (e.g., the homeless) might be considered mildly coercive because such an incentive might pressure prospective participants to cooperate.

The Right to Full Disclosure

Respect for human dignity encompasses people's right to make informed decisions about study participation, which requires full disclosure. **Full disclosure** means that the researcher has fully described the study, the person's right to refuse participation, and potential risks and benefits. The right to self-determination and the right to full disclosure are the two elements on which informed consent—discussed later in this chapter—is based.

Full disclosure is not always straightforward because it can result in biases and sample recruitment problems. Suppose we were testing the hypothesis that high school students with a high absentee rate are more likely to be substance abusers than students with good attendance. If we approached potential participants and fully explained the study's purpose, some students might refuse to participate, and nonparticipation would be selective; students who are substance abusers—the group of primary interest—might be least likely to participate. Moreover, by knowing the study purpose, those who participate might not give candid responses. In such a situation, full disclosure could undermine the study.

In such situations, researchers sometimes use *covert data collection* (*concealment*), which is collecting data without participants' knowledge and thus without their consent. This might happen if a researcher wanted to observe people's behavior and was worried that doing so openly would change the behavior of interest. Researchers might choose to obtain needed information through concealed methods, such as observing while pretending to be engaged in other activities.

A more controversial technique is the use of *deception*, which can involve deliberately withholding information about the study, or providing participants with false information. For example, in studying high school students' use of drugs, we might describe the research as a study of students' health practices, which is a mild form of misinformation.

Deception and concealment are problematic ethically because they interfere with people's right to make truly informed decisions about personal costs and benefits of participation. Some people think that deception is never justified, but others believe that if the study involves minimal risk yet offers benefits to society, then slight deceptiveness may be acceptable.

Full disclosure has emerged as a concern in connection with data collected from the Internet (e.g., analyzing the content of messages posted to blogs or social media sites). The issue is whether such messages can be used as data without the authors' consent. Some researchers believe that anything posted electronically is in the public domain, but others feel that the same ethical standards must apply in cyberspace research and that researchers must carefully protect the rights of individuals who are participants in "virtual" communities.

Justice

The third principle articulated in the *Belmont Report* concerns justice, which includes participants' right to fair treatment and their right to privacy.

The Right to Fair Treatment

One aspect of justice concerns the equitable distribution of benefits and burdens of research. The selection of participants should be based on research requirements and not on people's vulnerabilities. For example, groups with lower social standing (e.g., prisoners) have sometimes been selected as study participants, raising ethical concerns.

Potential discrimination is another aspect of distributive justice. During the 1990s, it was found that women and minorities were being *ex*cluded from many clinical studies. In the United States, this led to regulations requiring that researchers who seek funding from the National Institutes of Health (including NINR) include women and minorities as study participants.

The right to fair treatment encompasses other obligations. For example, researchers must treat people who decline to participate in a study in a nonprejudicial manner, honor all agreements made with participants, show respect for the beliefs of people from different backgrounds, and treat participants courteously and tactfully at all times.

The Right to Privacy

Research with humans involves intrusions into people's lives. Researchers should ensure that their research is not more intrusive than it needs to be and that privacy is maintained. Participants have the right to expect that any data they provide will be kept in strict confidence.

Privacy issues have become even more salient in the U.S. health care community since the passage of the Health Insurance Portability and Accountability Act of 1996 (HIPAA), which articulates federal standards to protect patients' medical records and health information. For health care providers who transmit health information electronically, compliance with HIPAA regulations (the Privacy Rule) has been required since 2003.

PROCEDURES FOR PROTECTING STUDY PARTICIPANTS

Now that you are familiar with ethical principles for conducting research, you need to understand the procedures researchers use to adhere to them. It is compliance with these procedures that should be evaluated in critically appraising the ethical aspects of a study.

 TIP Information about ethical considerations is usually presented in the method section of a research report, often in a subsection labeled *procedures.*

Risk/Benefit Assessments

One strategy that researchers use to protect participants is to conduct a **risk/benefit assessment**. Such an assessment is designed to evaluate whether the benefits of participating in a study are in line with the costs—i.e., whether the *risk/benefit ratio* is acceptable. Box 4.1 summarizes major costs and benefits of research participation to study participants. Benefits to society and to nursing should also be taken into account. The selection of a significant topic that has the potential to improve patient care is the first step in ensuring that research is ethical.

 TIP In evaluating the risk/benefit ratio of a study, you might want to consider how comfortable *you* would have felt about being a study participant.

Sometimes risks are negligible. **Minimal risk** is a risk expected to be no greater than those ordinarily encountered in daily life or during routine procedures. When the risks are not minimal, researchers must proceed with caution, taking every step possible to reduce risks and maximize benefits.

Box 4.1 Potential Benefits and Risks of Research to Participants

Major Potential Benefits to Participants
- Access to a potentially beneficial intervention that might otherwise be unavailable
- Relief in being able to discuss their situation or problem with a friendly, objective person
- Increased knowledge about themselves or their conditions
- Escape from normal routine
- Satisfaction that information they provide may help others with similar problems
- Direct gains through stipends or other incentives

Major Potential Risks to Participants
- Physical harm, including unanticipated side effects
- Physical discomfort, fatigue, or boredom
- Emotional distress from self-disclosure, discomfort with strangers, embarrassment relating to questions being asked
- Social risks, such as the risk of stigma, negative effects on personal relationships
- Loss of privacy
- Loss of time
- Monetary costs (e.g., for transportation, childcare, time lost from work)

Informed Consent

An important procedure for safeguarding participants involves obtaining their informed consent. **Informed consent** means that participants have adequate information about the study, comprehend the information, and can consent to or decline participation voluntarily.

Researchers usually document informed consent by having participants sign a **consent form**. This form includes information about the study purpose, specific expectations regarding participation (e.g., how much time will be required), the voluntary nature of participation, and potential costs and benefits.

 TIP The chapter supplement on thePoint® website provides additional information about the content of informed consent forms, as well as an actual example from a study by one of the book's authors (Beck).

Example of informed consent
Alvariza and coresearchers (2020) explored palliative care nurses' work experiences caring for patients at the end of life in private homes. Participant-generated photographs were used in follow-up interviews with 10 palliative home care nurses. The nurses signed informed consent forms. Additionally, because photographs of their work environments included images of patients and others, the nurses obtained informed consent from the people who were photographed to use the photos of them and their homes in the research.

Researchers may not obtain written informed consent when data collection is through self-administered questionnaires. Researchers often assume *implied consent* (i.e., returning a completed questionnaire implies the person's consent to participate).

In qualitative studies that involve repeated data collection, it may be difficult to obtain meaningful consent at the outset. Because the design emerges during the study, researchers may not know what the risks and benefits will be. In such situations, consent may be an ongoing process, called *process consent*, in which consent is continuously renegotiated.

Confidentiality Procedures

Study participants have the right to expect that the data they provide will be kept in strict confidence. Participants' right to privacy is protected through confidentiality procedures.

Anonymity

Anonymity, the most secure means of protecting confidentiality, occurs when the researcher cannot link participants to their data. For example, if questionnaires were distributed to nursing home residents and were returned without identifying information, responses would be anonymous.

> **Example of anonymity** •
> Schnall and colleagues (2020) conducted a study of the symptoms experienced by persons living with HIV in the Deep South of the United States. People receiving services at a community outreach program for people with HIV were asked to complete a questionnaire on an iPad. No identification information was collected.

Confidentiality in the Absence of Anonymity

When anonymity is not possible, other confidentiality procedures need to be implemented. A promise of **confidentiality** is a pledge that any information participants provide will not be publicly reported in a manner that identifies them and will not be made accessible to others.

Researchers can take a number of steps to ensure that a *breach of confidentiality* does not occur. These include maintaining identifying information in locked files, substituting *identification (ID) numbers* for participants' names on records, and reporting only aggregate data for groups of participants.

Confidentiality is especially salient in qualitative studies because of their in-depth nature: Anonymity is rarely possible. Qualitative researchers also face the challenge of adequately disguising participants in their reports. Because the number of respondents is small and because rich descriptive information is presented, qualitative researchers must be especially vigilant in safeguarding participants' identity.

 TIP As a means of enhancing individual and institutional privacy, researchers frequently avoid giving information about the study locale. For example, a report might say that data were collected in a 200-bed, private nursing home, without mentioning its name or location.

Confidentiality sometimes creates tension between researchers and legal authorities, especially if participants engage in criminal activity such as substance abuse. To avoid the forced disclosure of information (e.g., through a court order), researchers in the United States can apply for a **Certificate of Confidentiality** from the National Institutes of Health. The certificate allows researchers to refuse to disclose information on study participants in any legal proceeding.

> **Example of confidentiality procedures** •
> Strandås and colleagues (2019) conducted a focused ethnography to gain a deeper understanding of nurse–patient relationships in Norwegian public home care. Participants (who were observed interacting with nurses and interviewed) received information about the researchers and the study, including rights to withdraw. Oral informed consent was obtained from patients who were included in observations. Data were anonymized by removing names and locations and by changing some details. Interview transcripts and audiotapes were kept in locked files.

Debriefings and Referrals

Researchers should show respect for participants during the interactions they have with them—they should be polite and make evident their tolerance of cultural, linguistic, and lifestyle diversity. Formal strategies for communicating respect are also available. For example, it is sometimes advisable to offer **debriefing** sessions following data collection so that participants can ask questions or express concerns. Researchers can also demonstrate their interest in participants by offering to share study findings with them after the data have been analyzed. Researchers also may need to assist participants by making referrals to appropriate health, social, or psychological services.

Example of referrals •
Jones and colleagues (2020) studied first responders' perceptions of mental health problems and of barriers and facilitators to seeking mental health care. To address the potential risk of mental or emotional distress during interviews, the researchers obtained permission from various mental health providers to designate them as available resources.

Treatment of Vulnerable Groups

Adherence to ethical standards is often straightforward, but special **vulnerable groups** may need extra protections. Vulnerable populations may be incapable of giving fully informed consent, (e.g., cognitively impaired people) or may be at high risk of unintended side effects (e.g., pregnant women). You should pay particular attention to ethical aspects of a study when people who are vulnerable are involved. Among the groups that should be considered vulnerable are the following:

- *Children.* Legally and ethically, children do not have the competence to give informed consent, and so the consent of children's parents or guardians should be obtained. However, it is appropriate—especially if the child is at least 7 years of age—to obtain the child's assent as well. **Assent** refers to the child's affirmative agreement to participate.
- *Mentally or emotionally disabled people.* Individuals whose disability makes it impossible for them to make informed decisions (e.g., people in a coma) also cannot legally provide informed consent. In such cases, researchers should obtain the consent of a legal guardian.
- *Severely ill or physically disabled people.* For patients who are very ill or undergoing certain treatments (e.g., mechanical ventilation), it might be necessary to assess their ability to make reasoned decisions about study participation.
- *The terminally ill.* Terminally ill people seldom benefit personally from research, and thus, the risk/benefit ratio needs to be carefully assessed.
- *Institutionalized people.* Nurses often conduct studies with hospitalized or institutionalized people (e.g., prisoners) who might feel that their care would be jeopardized by failure to cooperate. Researchers studying institutionalized groups need to emphasize the voluntary nature of participation.
- *Pregnant women.* The U.S. government has issued additional requirements governing research with pregnant women and fetuses. These requirements reflect a desire to safeguard both the pregnant woman, who may be at heightened physical or psychological risk, and the fetus, who cannot give informed consent.

Example of research with a vulnerable group •
Pu et al. (2020) conducted an in-depth study of people with dementia who had participated in a test of an intervention involving interactions with a therapeutic robot (PARO). Informed written consent was obtained from the study participants, where possible, or from their family carer. Assent from the people with dementia was obtained at every intervention session.

External Reviews and the Protection of Human Rights

Researchers may not be objective in developing procedures to protect participants' rights. Biases may arise from their commitment to an area of knowledge and their desire to conduct a rigorous study. Because a biased self-evaluation is possible, the ethical dimensions of a study are usually subjected to external review.

Most hospitals, universities, and other institutions where research is conducted have established formal committees for reviewing research plans. These committees are sometimes called *human subjects committees* or (in Canada) *Research Ethics Boards*. In the United States, the committee is often called an **Institutional Review Board (IRB)**. Before undertaking a study, researchers must submit research plans to the IRB and must also undergo formal IRB training. An IRB can approve the proposed plans, require modifications, or disapprove them.

Example of IRB approval •
Suchting and colleagues (2020) studied the effect of transcranial direct current stimulation on inflammation in older adults with knee osteoarthritis. The procedures and protocols for the study were approved by the Institutional Review Board of the University of Florida.

Ethical Issues in Using Animals in Research

Some nurse researchers who focus on biophysiologic phenomena use animals as their subjects. Ethical considerations are clearly different for animals; for example, *informed consent* is not relevant. In the United States, the Public Health Service has issued a policy statement on the humane care and use of animals. The guidelines articulate principles for the proper care and treatment of animals used in research, covering such issues as the transport of research animals, pain and distress in animal subjects, the use of appropriate anesthesia, and euthanizing animals under certain conditions during or after the study.

Example of research with animals •
Kupferschmid and colleagues (2020) studied sickness responses and spatial learning in aging Brown Norway rats following recurrent administration of lipopolysaccharide to model infection. The University of Michigan's Institutional Animal Care and Use Committee approved all procedures.

CRITICALLY APPRAISING THE ETHICAL ASPECTS OF A STUDY

Guidelines for appraising the ethical aspects of a study are presented in Box 4.2. Members of an IRB or human subjects committee are provided with sufficient information to answer all these questions, but research articles do not always include detailed information about ethics because of space constraints in journals. Thus, it may be difficult to evaluate researchers' adherence to ethical guidelines. Nevertheless, we offer a few suggestions for considering ethical issues.

Many research reports do acknowledge that the study procedures were reviewed by an IRB or human subjects committee. When a report mentions a formal review, it is usually safe to assume that a panel of concerned people thoroughly reviewed ethical issues in a proposed study.

You can also come to some conclusions based on a description of the study methods. There may be sufficient information to judge, for example, whether study participants were

Box 4.2 Guidelines for Critically Appraising the Ethical Aspects of a Study

1. Was the study approved and monitored by an Institutional Review Board, Research Ethics Board, or other similar ethics review committee?
2. Were study participants subjected to any physical harm, discomfort, or psychological distress? Did the researchers take appropriate steps to remove or prevent harm?
3. Did the benefits to participants outweigh any potential risks or actual discomfort they experienced? Did the benefits to society outweigh the costs to participants?
4. Was any type of coercion or undue influence used to recruit participants? Did they have the right to refuse to participate or to withdraw without penalty?
5. Were participants deceived in any way? Were they fully aware of participating in a study, and did they understand the purpose and nature of the research?
6. Were appropriate informed consent procedures used with participants? If not, was there a justifiable rationale?
7. Were adequate steps taken to safeguard participants' privacy? How was confidentiality maintained? Was a Certificate of Confidentiality obtained—and, if not, should one have been obtained?
8. Were vulnerable groups involved in the research? If yes, were special precautions instituted because of their vulnerable status?
9. Were groups omitted from the inquiry without a justifiable rationale, such as women (or men), or minorities?

subjected to harm or discomfort. Reports do not always state whether informed consent was secured, but you should be alert to situations in which the data could not have been gathered as described if participation were purely voluntary (e.g., if data were gathered unobtrusively).

In thinking about the ethical aspects of a study, you should also consider who the study participants were. For example, if the study involves vulnerable groups, there should be more information about protective procedures. You might also need to attend to who the study participants were *not*. For example, there has been considerable concern about the omission of certain groups (e.g., minorities) from clinical research.

RESEARCH EXAMPLES WITH CRITICAL THINKING EXERCISES

A brief summary focusing on the ethical aspects of a qualitative nursing study is presented in the following sections. Read the summary and then answer the critical thinking questions that follow, referring to the full research report if necessary. Answers to Example 1 are available to instructors on thePoint® website. The critical thinking questions for Exercises 2 and 3 are based on the studies that appear in their entirety in Appendices A and B of this book. Our comments for these exercises are in the Student Resources section on thePoint®.

EXAMPLE 1: ETHICAL ASPECTS OF A QUALITATIVE STUDY

Study: Health-related street outreach: Exploring the perceptions of homeless people with experience of sleeping rough (Ungpakorn & Rae, 2020)

Study Purpose: The purpose of the study was to understand how health-related street outreach by health professionals is perceived by homeless people with experience of sleeping rough—defined as living on the street, in doorways, parks, tents, stairways, or other places not designed for habitation.

Study Methods: The researchers used a qualitative description design. They recruited a sample of 10 homeless people with experience of sleeping rough. Each participant was interviewed face-to-face, and the interviews were audiorecorded. The interviews began with broad questions about perceptions of health-related street outreach and ended with more specific questions about the provision of items on the street.

Ethics-Related Procedures: The researchers recruited participants in three drop-in centers in London. Potential participants were approached, given information about the study, asked questions to determine if they were eligible for the study, and then interviewed the same day if they gave consent. Because of the potential for low levels of literacy, the participant information form was read aloud. It stated that access to services would not be compromised by refusal to participate. In the event of any participant distress, the nurse on duty at the drop-in center would have been asked to provide needed support. Based on the advice of a local peer advocate, a cash stipend of £10 was given to every participant at the end of the interview, which was conducted in a private room at the drop-in center. In the report, the researchers used pseudonyms to protect the identity of participants. A university ethics committee approved the protocol for this study.

Key Findings: The findings suggested that homeless people with experience of sleeping rough saw health-related street outreach as being able to offer a human connection to reduce their sense of isolation and exclusion.

Critical Thinking Exercises

1. Answer the relevant questions from Box 4.2 regarding this study.
2. Also consider the following targeted questions:
   a. The researchers offered a stipend—comment on whether you think this was ethically appropriate. Was it sufficiently large?
   b. Comment on the appropriateness of the location of the interview.
3. If the results of this study are trustworthy and transferable, what might be some of the uses to which the findings could be put in clinical practice?

EXAMPLE 2: QUANTITATIVE STUDY IN APPENDIX A

1. Read the method section of Swenson and colleagues' study ("Parents' use of praise and criticism in a sample of young children seeking mental health services") in Appendix A of this book and then answer relevant questions in Box 4.2.
2. Also consider the following targeted questions:
   a. Where was information about ethical issues located in this report?
   b. What additional information regarding the ethical aspects of their study could the researchers have included in this article?

EXAMPLE 3: QUALITATIVE STUDY IN APPENDIX B

1. Read the method section from Beck and Watson's study ("Posttraumatic growth after birth trauma") in Appendix B of this book and then answer relevant questions in Box 4.2.
2. Also consider the following targeted questions:
   a. Where was information about the ethical aspects of this study located in the report?
   b. What additional information regarding the ethical aspects of Beck and Watson's study could the researchers have included in this article?

WANT TO KNOW MORE?

A wide variety of resources to enhance your learning and understanding of this chapter is available on the Point®.

- Chapter Supplement on Informed Consent
- Answers to the Critical Thinking Exercises for Examples 2 and 3
- Internet Resources with useful websites for Chapter 4
- A Wolters Kluwer journal article on a topic related to this chapter

Additional study aids, including eight journal articles and related questions, are also available in *Study Guide for Essentials of Nursing Research, 10e.*

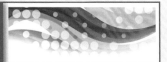

Summary Points

- Because research has not always been conducted ethically and because of genuine **ethical dilemmas** that researchers face in designing studies that are both ethical and rigorous, **codes of ethics** have been developed to guide researchers.

- Three major ethical principles from the *Belmont Report* are incorporated into many ethical guidelines: beneficence, respect for human dignity, and justice.

- **Beneficence** involves the performance of some good and the protection of participants from physical and psychological harm and exploitation.

- Respect for human dignity involves the participants' right to self-determination, which includes participants' right to participate in a study voluntarily.

- **Full disclosure** means that researchers have fully described to prospective participants their rights and the study's costs and benefits. When full disclosure poses the risk of biased results, researchers sometimes use *concealment* (the collection of information without participants' knowledge) or *deception* (withholding information or providing false information).

- *Justice* includes the right to fair treatment and the right to privacy. In the United States, privacy has become a major issue because of the Privacy Rule regulations that resulted from the Health Insurance Portability and Accountability Act (HIPAA).

- Procedures have been developed to safeguard study participants' rights, including the performance of a risk/benefit assessment, the implementation of informed consent procedures, and methods to safeguard participants' confidentiality.

- In a **risk/benefit assessment**, the potential benefits of the study to individual participants and to society are weighed against the costs to individuals.

- **Informed consent** procedures, which provide prospective participants with information needed to make a reasoned decision about participation, normally involve signing a **consent form** to document voluntary and informed participation.

- Privacy can be maintained through **anonymity** (wherein not even researchers know participants' identities) or through formal **confidentiality** procedures that safeguard the participants' data.

- Some U.S. researchers obtain a **Certificate of Confidentiality** that protects them against the forced disclosure of confidential information through a court order.

- Researchers sometimes offer **debriefing** sessions after data collection to provide participants with more information or an opportunity to air complaints.

- **Vulnerable groups** require additional protection. These people may be vulnerable because they are not able to make an informed decision about study participation (e.g., children), because of diminished autonomy (e.g.,

prisoners), or because their circumstances heighten the risk of harm (e.g., pregnant women, the terminally ill).

- External review of the ethical aspects of a study by a human subjects committee or **Institutional Review Board (IRB)** is highly desirable and is often required by universities and organizations from which participants are recruited.

REFERENCES FOR CHAPTER 4

Alvariza, A., Mjörnberg, M., & Goliath, I. (2020). Palliative care nurses' strategies when working in private homes—a photo-elicitation study. *Journal of Clinical Nursing, 29*, 139–151.

American Nurses Association. (2015). *Code of ethics for nurses with interpretive statements* (2nd ed.). Silver Spring, MD: Author.

Beck, C. T., & Casavant, S. (2020). Vicarious posttraumatic growth in NICU nurses. *Advances in Neonatal Care, 20*, 324–332.

*Canadian Nurses Association. (2017). *Code of ethics for registered nurses*. Ottawa, Canada: Author.

Jones, S., Agud, K., & McSweeney, J. (2020). Barriers and facilitators to seeking mental health care among first responders: "Removing the darkness." *Journal of the American Psychiatric Nurses Association, 26*, 43–54.

Kupferschmid, B., Rowsey, P., & Riviera, M. (2020). Characterization of spatial learning and sickness responses in aging rats following recurrent lipopolysaccharide administration. *Biological Research for Nursing, 22*, 92–102.

Pu, L., Moyle, W., & Jones, C. (2020). How people with dementia perceive a therapeutic robot called PARO in relation to their pain and mood: a qualitative study. *Journal of Clinical Nursing, 29*, 437–446.

**Schnall, R., Musgrove, K., & Batey, D. (2020). Symptom profile and technology use of persons living with HIV who access services at a community-based organization in the Deep South. *The Journal of the Association of Nurses in AIDS Care, 31*, 42–50.

Silva, M. C. (1995). *Ethical guidelines in the conduct, dissemination, and implementation of nursing research*. Washington, DC: American Nurses Association.

Stievano, A., & Tschudin, V. (2019). The ICN code of ethics for nurses: A time for revision. *International Nursing Review, 66*, 154–166.

Strandås, M., Wackerhausen, S., & Bondas, T. (2019). The nurse-patient relationship in the New Public Management era, in public home care: A focused ethnography. *Journal of Advanced Nursing, 75*, 400–411.

Suchting, R., Colpo, G., Rocha, N., & Ahn, H. (2020). The effect of transcranial direct current stimulation on inflammation in older adults with knee osteoarthritis: A Bayesian residual change analysis. *Biological Research for Nursing, 22*, 57–63.

Ungpakorn, R., & Rae, B. (2020). Health-related street outreach: Exploring the perceptions of homeless people with experience of sleeping rough. *Journal of Advanced Nursing, 76*, 253–263.

*A link to this open-access article is provided in the Internet Resources section on thePoint° website.

**This journal article is available on thePoint° for this chapter.

5 · Identifying Research Problems, Research Questions, and Hypotheses

Learning Objectives

On completing this chapter, you will be able to:

- Describe the process of developing and refining a research problem
- Distinguish the functions and forms of purpose statements and research questions for quantitative and qualitative studies
- Describe the purpose and characteristics of research hypotheses
- Critically appraise statements of purpose, research questions, and hypotheses in research reports with respect to their placement, clarity, wording, and relevance to nursing
- Define new terms in the chapter

Key Terms

- Directional hypothesis
- Hypothesis
- Nondirectional hypothesis
- Null hypothesis
- Problem statement
- Research hypothesis
- Research problem
- Research question
- Statement of purpose

OVERVIEW OF RESEARCH PROBLEMS

Studies begin in much the same fashion as an evidence-based practice (EBP) effort—as problems that need to be solved or questions that need to be answered. This chapter discusses research problems and research questions. We begin by clarifying some terms.

Basic Terminology

Researchers begin with a *topic* on which to focus. Claustrophobia during magnetic resonance imaging (MRI) tests and pain management for sickle cell disease are examples of research topics. Within broad topic areas are many possible research problems. In this section, we illustrate various terms using the topic *side effects of chemotherapy*.

A **research problem** is an enigmatic or troubling condition. The purpose of research is to "solve" the problem—or to contribute to its solution—by gathering relevant data.

TABLE 5.1 Terms Relating to Research Problems With Examples

Term	Example
Topic	Side effects of chemotherapy
Research problem (problem statement)	Nausea and vomiting are common side effects among patients on chemotherapy, and interventions to date have been only moderately successful in reducing these effects. New interventions that can reduce these side effects need to be identified.
Statement of purpose	The purpose of the study is to compare the effectiveness of patient-controlled versus nurse-administered antiemetic therapy for controlling nausea and vomiting in patients on chemotherapy.
Research question	What is the relative effectiveness of patient-controlled antiemetic therapy versus nurse-controlled antiemetic therapy with regard to (1) medication consumption and (2) control of nausea and vomiting in patients on chemotherapy?
Hypotheses	Patients receiving antiemetic therapy by a patient-controlled pump will (1) be less nauseous, (2) vomit less, and (3) consume less medication than patients receiving nurse-administered therapy.

A **problem statement** articulates the problem and offers an *argument* explaining the need for a study. Table 5.1 presents a simplified problem statement related to the topic of side effects of chemotherapy.

Many reports provide a **statement of purpose** (or *purpose statement*), which summarizes an overall goal. **Research questions** are the specific queries researchers want to answer. Researchers who make specific predictions about the answers to research questions pose **hypotheses** that are then tested. These terms are not always consistently defined in research textbooks. Table 5.1 illustrates the interrelationships among terms as we define them.

Research Problems and Paradigms

Some research problems are better suited to qualitative versus quantitative inquiry. Quantitative studies usually involve concepts that are well developed and for which methods of measurement have been (or can be) developed. For example, a quantitative study might be undertaken to assess whether people with chronic illness are more depressed than people without a chronic illness. There are good measures of depression that would yield quantitative data about the level of depression in those with and without a chronic illness.

Qualitative studies are undertaken because a researcher wants to develop a rich, context-bound understanding of a poorly understood phenomenon. Qualitative methods would not be well suited to comparing levels of depression among those with and without chronic illness, but they would be ideal for exploring the *meaning* or *experience* of depression among chronically ill people. In appraising a research report, one consideration is whether the research problem is suitable for the chosen paradigm.

Sources of Research Problems

Where do ideas for research problems come from? At the most basic level, research topics originate with researchers' interests. Because research is a time-consuming enterprise, curiosity about a topic that is appealing is essential to a project's success.

Research reports rarely indicate the origin of researchers' inspiration for a study, but a variety of sources can fuel their curiosity, such as their clinical experience or readings in the nursing literature. Also, topics are sometimes suggested by global social or political issues of relevance to the health care community (e.g., health disparities). Theories from nursing and other disciplines sometimes generate a research problem. Additionally, researchers who have developed a *program of research* may get inspiration for "next steps" from their own work or from discussions of their findings with others.

> **Example of a problem source for a quantitative study** • • • • • • • • • • • • • • • • • •
> Beck, one of this book's authors, has developed a strong research program on postpartum depression (PPD). Beck was approached by Dr. Carol Lammi-Keefe, a professor in nutritional sciences and a PhD student (Michelle Judge), who had been researching the effect of DHA (docosahexaenoic acid; a fat found in cold-water fish) on fetal brain development. The literature suggested that DHA might play a role in reducing the severity of PPD and so these researchers collaborated in a project to test the effect of dietary supplements of DHA during pregnancy on the incidence and severity of PPD. The researchers found that women in the DHA experimental group had fewer symptoms of postpartum depression compared to women who did not receive the DHA intervention (Judge et al., 2014).

Development and Refinement of Research Problems

Developing a research problem is a creative process. Researchers often begin with interests in a broad topic area and then develop a more specific researchable problem. For example, suppose a clinical nursing instructor wonders about secondary traumatic stress (the stress resulting from helping traumatized or suffering patients) in nursing students. The nurse has read that registered nurses report high levels of secondary traumatic stress and wonders if nursing students are also susceptible. This broad interest in secondary traumatic stress in students may lead to more specific musings, such as whether the students' type of nursing program is relevant to their secondary traumatic stress. The nurse also observes nursing students who have clinical rotations on her unit and may notice that students struggle caring for certain types of patients. These reflections may lead the nurse to have a discussion with colleagues, which may result in several research questions, such as the following:

- What is the experience of secondary traumatic stress like among nursing students?
- What is the frequency and intensity of secondary traumatic stress symptoms in nursing students?
- Do baccalaureate and associate degree nursing students differ in their level of secondary traumatic stress symptoms?
- What patient characteristics or clinical situations are most likely to provoke secondary traumatic stress in students?

These questions stem from the same broad problem, yet some suggest a qualitative approach and others suggest a quantitative one. Symptoms of secondary traumatic stress (Q2), type of nursing program (Q3), and patient characteristics (Q4) are all attributes that can be measured and suggest a quantitative inquiry. A qualitative researcher would be more interested in understanding the *essence* of students' stressful experiences or the *process* by which the stress was alleviated (Q1). These aspects of the problem would be difficult to measure. Researchers choose a problem to study based on its inherent interest to them and its fit with a paradigm of preference.

COMMUNICATING RESEARCH PROBLEMS AND QUESTIONS

Every study should have a problem statement that articulates clearly what is problematic and what must be solved. Most research reports also present either a statement of purpose, research questions, or hypotheses, and often, combinations of these three elements are included.

> **Box 5.1 Draft Problem Statement on Humor and Stress**
>
> A diagnosis of cancer is associated with high levels of stress. Sizeable numbers of patients who receive a cancer diagnosis describe feelings of uncertainty, fear, anger, and loss of control. Interpersonal relationships, psychological functioning, and role performance have all been found to suffer following cancer diagnosis and treatment.
>
> A variety of alternative/complementary therapies have been developed in efforts to decrease the harmful effects of cancer-related stress on psychological and physiological functioning, and resources devoted to these therapies have increased in recent years. However, many of these therapies have not been carefully evaluated to assess their efficacy, safety, or cost-effectiveness. For example, the use of humor has been recommended as a therapeutic device to improve quality of life, decrease stress, and perhaps improve immune functioning, but the evidence to justify its advocacy is scant.

Many students do not really understand problem statements and may have trouble identifying them in a research article. A problem statement is presented early in the report, whereas research questions, purpose statements, or hypotheses appear later in the introduction.

Problem Statements

A good problem statement is a declaration of what it is that is problematic, what it is that "needs fixing," or what it is that is poorly understood. Problem statements, especially for quantitative studies, usually have most of the following six components:

1. *Problem identification*: What is wrong with the current situation?
2. *Background*: What is the nature of the problem, or the context of the situation, that readers need to understand?
3. *Scope of the problem*: How big a problem is it? How many people are affected?
4. *Consequences of the problem*: What is the cost of *not* fixing the problem?
5. *Knowledge gaps*: What information about the problem is lacking?
6. *Proposed solution*: How will the new study contribute to the solution of the problem?

Let us suppose that our topic was humor as a complementary therapy for reducing stress in hospitalized patients with cancer. One research question (discussed later in this section) might be, "What is the effect of nurses' use of humor on stress and natural killer cell activity in hospitalized cancer patients?" Box 5.1 presents a rough draft of a problem statement for such a study. This problem statement is a reasonable draft, but it can be improved.

Box 5.2 illustrates how the problem statement was strengthened by adding information about scope, long-term consequences, and possible solutions. This second draft builds a more compelling *argument* for new research: Millions of people are affected by cancer, and the disease has adverse consequences not only for patients and their families but also for society. The revised problem statement also suggests a possible solution that is the basis for the new study.

 HOW-TO-TELL TIP How can you tell a problem statement? Problem statements are rarely explicitly labeled. The first sentence of a research report is often the starting point of a problem statement. The problem statement is usually interwoven with findings from the research literature, which provide supporting evidence and suggest gaps in knowledge. In many articles, it is difficult to disentangle the problem statement from the literature review, unless there is a subsection specifically labeled "Literature Review" or something similar.

Box 5.2 Some Possible Improvements to Problem Statement on Humor and Stress

Each year, over 1 million people are diagnosed with cancer, which remains one of the top causes of death among both men and women (reference citations).* Numerous studies have documented that a diagnosis of cancer is associated with high levels of stress. Sizeable numbers of patients who receive a cancer diagnosis describe feelings of uncertainty, fear, anger, and loss of control (citations). Interpersonal relationships, psychological functioning, and role performance have all been found to suffer following cancer diagnosis and treatment (citations). These stressful outcomes can, in turn, adversely affect health, long-term prognosis, and medical costs among cancer survivors (citations).

A variety of alternative/complementary therapies have been developed in efforts to decrease the harmful effects of cancer-related stress on psychological and physiological functioning, and resources devoted to these therapies (money and staff) have increased in recent years (citations). However, many of these therapies have not been carefully evaluated to assess their efficacy, safety, or cost-effectiveness. For example, the use of humor has been recommended as a therapeutic device to improve quality of life, decrease stress, and perhaps improve immune functioning (citations), but the evidence to justify its advocacy is scant. Preliminary findings from a recent small-scale endocrinology study with a healthy sample exposed to a humorous intervention (citation), however, holds promise for further inquiry with immuno-compromised populations.

*Reference citations would be inserted to support the statements.

Problem statements for a qualitative study similarly express the nature of the problem, its context, its scope, and information needed to address it. Qualitative studies embedded in a research tradition often incorporate terms and concepts that foreshadow the tradition in their problem statements. For example, a problem statement for a phenomenological study might note the need to learn more about people's experiences or meanings they attribute to those experiences.

Statements of Purpose

Many researchers articulate their research goal as a statement of purpose. The purpose statement establishes the general direction of the inquiry and captures the study's substance. It is usually easy to identify a purpose statement because the word *purpose* is explicitly stated: "The purpose of this study was . . ."—although sometimes the words *aim, goal,* or *objective* are used instead, as in "The aim of this study was . . . ."

In a quantitative study, a statement of purpose identifies the key study variables and their possible interrelationships as well as the population of interest (i.e., all the PICO elements).

Example of a statement of purpose from a quantitative study • • • • • • • • • • •
Lee and colleagues (2020) studied the relationship between implantable cardioverter defibrillator (ICD) shocks and psychological distress. One of the stated purposes was to "compare ICD-related concerns, perceived control, anxiety, and depressive symptoms between patients who received shocks and patients who did not" (p. 67).

This purpose statement indicates that the population (P) of interest is patients with an ICD. The key study variables were the patients' status as having or not having ICD shocks (I and C components—the independent variable), and the patients' concerns, perceived control, anxiety, and depressive symptoms (the Os or dependent variables).

In qualitative studies, the statement of purpose indicates the nature of the inquiry; the key concept or phenomenon; and the group, community, or setting under study.

Example of a statement of purpose from a qualitative study • • • • • • • • • • • • •
"The primary objective of the present study was to explore cancer patients' experiences of participating in a 12-month individualized comprehensive lifestyle intervention study focusing on physical activity, diet, smoking cessation, and stress management while undergoing . . . chemotherapy" (Mikkelsen et al., 2020).

This statement indicates that the population under study was cancer patients undergoing chemotherapy, and the central phenomenon was the patients' experiences during their participation in a 12-month lifestyle intervention.

Researchers often communicate information about their approach through their choice of verbs. A study whose purpose is to *explore, investigate,* or *describe* some phenomenon is likely to be an investigation of a little-researched topic, often involving a qualitative approach such as phenomenology or ethnography. A statement of purpose for a qualitative study—especially a grounded theory study—may also use verbs such as *understand, discover,* or *generate*. Statements of purpose in qualitative studies also may "encode" the tradition of inquiry through certain terms or "buzz words" associated with those traditions, as follows:

- *Grounded theory*: processes; social structures; social interactions
- *Phenomenological studies*: experience; lived experience; meaning; essence
- *Ethnographic studies*: culture; roles; lifeways; cultural behavior

Quantitative researchers also use verbs to communicate the nature of the inquiry. A statement indicating that the study purpose is to *test* or *evaluate* something (e.g., an intervention) suggests an experimental design, for example. A study whose purpose is to *examine* or *explore* the relationship between two variables is more likely to involve a nonexperimental design. Sometimes the verb is ambiguous: If a purpose statement states that the researcher's intent is to *compare* two things, the comparison could involve alternative treatments (using an experimental design) or two preexisting groups such as smokers and nonsmokers (using a nonexperimental design). In any event, verbs such as *test, evaluate,* and *compare* suggest quantifiable variables and designs with scientific controls.

The verbs in a purpose statement should signal objectivity. A statement of purpose indicating that the study goal was to *prove, demonstrate,* or *show* something suggests a bias.

Research Questions

Research questions are, in some cases, direct rewordings of statements of purpose, phrased interrogatively rather than declaratively, as in the following example:

- *Purpose*: The purpose of this study is to assess the relationship between the functional dependence level of renal transplant recipients and their rate of recovery.
- *Question*: Is the functional dependence level (I) of renal transplant recipients (P) related to their rate of recovery (O)?

Some research articles omit a statement of purpose and state only research questions—or vice versa. Some researchers use research questions to add greater specificity to a global purpose statement.

Research Questions in Quantitative Studies

In Chapter 1, we discussed questions to guide an EBP inquiry. The EBP question templates in Table 1.3 could yield questions to guide a research project as well, but *researchers* tend to conceptualize their questions in terms of their *variables*. Take, for example, the first question in Table 1.3: "In (population), what is the effect of (intervention) on (outcome)? A researcher would be more likely to think of the question in these terms: "In (population), what is the effect of (independent variable) on (dependent variable)?" Thinking in terms of variables helps to guide researchers' decisions about how to operationalize them. Thus, in quantitative studies, research questions identify the population (P) under study, the key study variables (I, C, and O components), and relationships among the variables.

Most research questions concern relationships among variables, and thus, many quantitative research questions could be articulated using a general question template: "In (population), what is the relationship between (independent variable or IV) and (dependent variable or DV)?" Examples of variations include the following:

- *Therapy/intervention*: In (population), what is the effect of (IV: intervention vs. an alternative) on (DV)?
- *Prognosis*: In (population), does (IV: a disease or illness vs. its absence) affect or increase the risk of (DV)?
- *Etiology/harm*: In (population), does (IV: exposure vs. nonexposure) cause or increase the risk of (DV)?

Not all research questions are about relationships—some are descriptive. As examples, here are two descriptive questions that could be answered in a quantitative study on nurses' use of humor:

- What is the frequency with which nurses use humor as a complementary therapy with hospitalized cancer patients?
- What are the characteristics of nurses who use humor as a complementary therapy with hospitalized cancer patients?

Answers to such questions might be useful in developing effective strategies for reducing stress in patients with cancer.

Example of a research question from a quantitative study • • • • • • • • • • • • • •
Higbee and colleagues (2020) undertook a study that addressed the following question: Is there a relationship between energy drink consumption and sleep quality, sleep quantity, and perceived stress in nurses working in a clinical setting?

In this example, the question asks about the relationship between an independent variable (consumption [I] vs. nonconsumption [C] of energy drinks) and three dependent variables (sleep quality, sleep quantity, and perceived stress—the Os) in a population of nurses working in a clinical setting (P).

Research Questions in Qualitative Studies

Research questions in qualitative studies stipulate the phenomenon and population of interest. Grounded theory researchers are likely to ask *process* questions, phenomenologists tend to ask *meaning* and *experience* questions, and ethnographers generally ask *descriptive* questions about cultures. The terms associated with the various traditions, discussed previously in connection with purpose statements, are likely to be incorporated into the research questions.

Example of a research question from a phenomenological study • • • • • • • • •
"What is the lived experience of adult Haitian immigrants in the United States who are self-managing their type 2 diabetes?" (Magny-Normilus et al., 2020).

Not all qualitative studies are rooted in a specific research tradition. Many researchers use constructivist approaches to describe or explore phenomena without focusing on cultures, meaning, or social processes.

Example of a research question from a descriptive qualitative study •••••••
In their descriptive qualitative study, Watermeyer and colleagues (2020) asked, "What are the barriers and facilitators to care experienced by people living with types 1 and 2 diabetes and healthcare professionals at a healthcare site in Johannesburg, South Africa?" (p. 241).

In qualitative studies, research questions sometimes evolve during the study. Researchers begin with a *focus* that defines the broad boundaries of the inquiry, but the boundaries are not cast in stone. Constructivists are often sufficiently flexible that the question can be modified as new information makes it relevant to do so.

 TIP Researchers most often state their purpose or research questions at the end of the introduction or immediately after the review of the literature. Sometimes, a separate section of a research article is devoted to formal statements about the research problem formally and might be labeled "Purpose," "Statement of Purpose," "Research Questions," or, in quantitative studies, "Hypotheses."

RESEARCH HYPOTHESES

A hypothesis is a prediction, usually involving a predicted relationship between two or more variables. Qualitative researchers do not have formal hypotheses because qualitative researchers want the inquiry to be guided by participants' viewpoints rather than by their own hunches. Thus, our discussion focuses on hypotheses in quantitative research.

Function of Hypotheses in Quantitative Research

Many research questions ask about relationships between variables, and hypotheses are predicted answers to these questions. For instance, the research question might ask: Does sexual abuse in childhood affect the development of irritable bowel syndrome in women? The researcher might predict the following: Women (P) who suffered sexual abuse in childhood (I) have a higher incidence of irritable bowel syndrome (O) than women who were not abused (C).

Hypotheses sometimes emerge from a theory. Scientists reason from theories to hypotheses and test those hypotheses in the real world (see Chapter 7). Even in the absence of a theory, hypotheses offer direction and suggest explanations. For example, suppose we hypothesized that the incidence of desaturation in low-birth-weight infants undergoing intubation and ventilation would be lower using the closed tracheal suction system (CTSS) than using partially ventilated endotracheal suction (PVETS). Our hypothesis might be based on prior studies or clinical observations.

Now let us suppose the hypothesis is not confirmed in a study; that is, we find that rates of desaturation are similar for both the PVETS and CTSS methods. *The failure of data to support a prediction forces researchers to analyze theory or previous research critically, to scrutinize study limitations, and to explore alternative explanations for the findings.* The use of hypotheses tends to promote critical thinking. Now, suppose we conducted the study guided only by the question, Is there a relationship between suction method and rates of desaturation? Without a hypothesis, the researcher is seemingly prepared to accept any results. The problem is that it is almost always possible to explain something superficially after the fact, no matter what the findings are. Hypotheses reduce the possibility that spurious results will be misconstrued.

TIP Some quantitative research articles explicitly state the hypotheses that guided the study, but many do not. The absence of a stated hypothesis often means that the researchers failed to disclose their hunches.

Characteristics of Testable Hypotheses

Research hypotheses usually state the expected relationship between the independent variable (the presumed cause or influence) and the dependent variable (the presumed outcome or effect) within a population.

Example of a research hypothesis •
Brenner and coresearchers (2020) hypothesized that patients diagnosed with peripheral artery disease who participated in a 12-week low-intensity walking intervention, compared to patients who did not participate, would have improved autonomic function.

In this example, the population is patients with peripheral artery disease. The independent variable is participation versus nonparticipation in the walking intervention, and the outcome variable is autonomic function. The hypothesis predicts that, in the population, participation in the program is related to subsequent autonomic function.

Hypotheses that do not make a relational statement are difficult to test. Take the following example: *Pregnant women who receive prenatal instruction about postpartum experiences are unlikely to experience postpartum depression.* This statement expresses no anticipated relationship and cannot be tested using standard statistical procedures. In our example, how would we decide whether to accept or reject the hypothesis?

We could, however, modify the hypothesis as follows: Pregnant women who receive prenatal instruction are less likely than those who do not to experience postpartum depression. Here, the outcome variable (O) is postpartum depression, and the independent variable is receipt (I) versus nonreceipt (C) of prenatal instruction. The relational aspect of the prediction is embodied in the phrase *less . . . than*. If a hypothesis lacks a phrase such as *more than*, *less than*, *different from*, *related to*, or something similar, it is not testable. To test the revised hypothesis, we could ask two groups of women with different prenatal instruction experiences to respond to questions on depression and then compare the groups' responses.

 TIP Hypotheses are typically fairly easy to identify because researchers make statements such as, "The study tested the hypothesis that . . ." or, "It was predicted that . . . ."

Wording of Hypotheses

Hypotheses can be stated in various ways, as in the following example:

1. Older patients are more likely to fall than younger patients.
2. There is a relationship between a patient's age and the likelihood of falling.
3. The risk of falling increases with the age of the patient.
4. Older patients differ from younger ones with respect to their risk of falling.

In each example, the hypothesis states the population (patients), the independent variable (age), the outcome variable (falling), and an anticipated relationship between them.

Hypotheses can be either directional or nondirectional. A **directional hypothesis** specifies the expected direction of the relationship between variables. In the four versions of the hypothesis, versions 1 and 3 are directional because they predict that older patients are more likely to fall than younger ones. A **nondirectional hypothesis** does not stipulate the direction of the relationship (versions 2 and 4). These versions predict that a patient's age and falling are related but do not specify whether *older* or *younger* patients are predicted to be at greater risk.

 TIP Hypotheses can be either *simple hypotheses* (with a single independent variable and dependent variable) or *complex* (multiple independent or dependent variables). We discuss simple versus complex hypotheses in the supplement to this chapter on thePoint°. We also briefly describe moderator and mediating variables in the supplement.

Another distinction is between research and null hypotheses. **Research hypotheses** are statements of expected relationships between variables. All the hypotheses presented thus far are research hypotheses that indicate actual expectations.

Statistical inference operates on a logic that may be confusing. This logic requires that hypotheses be expressed as an expected *absence* of a relationship. **Null hypotheses** state that there is no relationship between the independent and dependent variables. The null form of the first hypothesis in our example would be "Older patients and younger patients are equally likely to fall." The null hypothesis can be compared with the assumption of innocence in many systems of criminal justice: The variables are assumed to be "innocent" of a relationship until they can be shown "guilty" through statistical tests.

Research articles typically state research rather than null hypotheses. In statistical testing, underlying null hypotheses are assumed, without being stated.

 TIP If a researcher uses statistical tests (which is true in most quantitative studies), it means that there are underlying hypotheses—regardless of whether the researcher explicitly stated them—because statistical tests are designed to test hypotheses.

Hypothesis Testing and Proof

Hypotheses are formally tested through statistical analysis. Researchers use statistics to test whether their hypotheses have a high probability of being correct (i.e., has a probability < .05). Statistical analysis does not offer proof, it only supports inferences that a hypothesis is *probably* correct (or not). Hypotheses are never *proved* or *disproved*; rather, they are *supported* or *rejected*. Hypotheses come to be increasingly supported with evidence from multiple studies.

To illustrate why this is so, suppose we hypothesized that height and weight are related. We predict that, on average, tall people weigh more than short people. Suppose we happened by chance to get a sample of short, heavy people and tall, thin people. Our results might indicate that there is no relationship between a person's height and weight. But we would not be justified in concluding that the study *proved* or *demonstrated* that height and weight are unrelated.

This example illustrates the difficulty of using observations from a sample to generalize to a population. Issues other than sampling, such as measurement flaws and the effects of confounding variables, prevent researchers from concluding that hypotheses are proved.

CRITICAL APPRAISAL OF RESEARCH PROBLEMS, RESEARCH QUESTIONS, AND HYPOTHESES

The problem statement, purpose, research questions, and hypotheses set the stage for describing what was done and what was learned. You should not have to dig too deeply to figure out the research problem or discover the questions.

> **Box 5.3 Guidelines for Critically Appraising Research Problems, Research Questions, and Hypotheses**
>
> 1. What was the research problem? Was the problem statement easy to locate and was it clearly stated? Did the problem statement build a coherent and persuasive argument for the new study?
> 2. Does the problem have significance for nursing?
> 3. Was there a good fit between the research problem and the paradigm (and tradition) within which the research was conducted?
> 4. Did the report formally present a statement of purpose, research question, and/or hypotheses? Was this information communicated clearly and concisely, and was it placed in a logical and useful location?
> 5. Were purpose statements or research questions worded appropriately (e.g., were key concepts/variables identified and the population specified?)
> 6. If there were no formal hypotheses, was their absence justified? Were statistical tests used in analyzing the data despite the absence of stated hypotheses?
> 7. Were hypotheses (if any) properly worded—did they state a predicted relationship between two or more variables? Were they presented as research or as null hypotheses?

A critical appraisal of the research problem involves multiple dimensions. Substantively, you need to consider whether the problem has significance for nursing. Studies that build on existing evidence in a meaningful way can make contributions to evidence-based nursing practice. Also, research problems stemming from research priorities (see Chapter 1) have a high likelihood of yielding important evidence for nurses.

Another dimension in appraising the research problem concerns methodologic issues—in particular, whether the research problem is compatible with the chosen research paradigm and its associated methods. You should also evaluate whether the statement of purpose or research questions lend themselves to research inquiry.

If an article describing a quantitative study does not state hypotheses, you should consider whether their absence is justified. If there are hypotheses, you should evaluate whether the hypotheses are sensible and consistent with existing evidence or relevant theory. Also, hypotheses are valid guideposts in scientific inquiry only if they are testable. To be testable, hypotheses must predict a relationship between two or more measurable variables.

Specific guidelines for appraising research problems, research questions, and hypotheses are presented in Box 5.3.

RESEARCH EXAMPLES WITH CRITICAL THINKING EXERCISES

This section describes how the research problem and research questions were communicated in two nursing studies, one quantitative and one qualitative. Read the summaries and then answer the critical thinking questions that follow, referring to the full research report if necessary. Answers to Exercises 1 and 2 are available to instructors on thePoint° website. The critical thinking questions for Exercises 3 and 4 are based on the studies that appear in their entirety in Appendices A and B of this book. Our comments for these exercises are in the Student Resources section on thePoint°.

EXAMPLE 1: QUANTITATIVE RESEARCH

Study: Efficacy of osteoporosis prevention smartphone app (Ryan et al., 2020)

Problem Statement (excerpt): "Osteoporosis is a condition that compromises the density and microarchitecture of bone. Decreases in the amount and strength of bone can result in fractures . . . Osteoporotic fractures occur in 50% of all White women, and its prevalence is rapidly increasing among Latina and Black women . . . Although it is recommended that all women should engage in behaviors that promote or maintain healthy bones . . . , fewer than 20% of healthy middle-aged women regularly follow these recommendations . . . Interventions that enhance long-term maintenance of osteoporosis health promotion behaviors have not been identified" (p. 31). (Citations were omitted to streamline the presentation.)

Statement of Purpose: "The goal of this health promotion study was to test the efficacy of an intervention designed to enhance knowledge and beliefs, engagement in self-regulation processes, and social facilitation using an app that dynamically and automatically prepared information and activities matched to each individual" (p. 32).

Hypothesis: "We hypothesized that active use of the app over the 12-month study period would result in better distal outcomes [bone mineral density and trabecular bone scores] than use of a more traditional e-book app" (p. 32).

Study Methods: The Striving to be Strong study was a clinical trial in which 290 healthy women between 40 and 60 years of age were randomly assigned to one of three groups: (1) the "Striving" app—a dynamically tailored, person-centered app; (2) "Boning up," a standardized osteoporosis-education e-book; and (3) a wait-list group in which participants were offered a choice of apps in the final 3 months of the 12-month study. Bone mineral density (BMD) and trabecular bone scores (TBS) were measured at the outset of the study and 12 months later.

Key Findings: Overall, there were smaller-than-expected decreases in BMD over time, but no differences among the groups. TBS improved across all three groups. The researchers speculated that several factors could have contributed to the absence of differences among the groups.

Critical Thinking Exercises

1. Answer the relevant questions from Box 5.3 regarding this study.
2. Also consider the following targeted questions:
   a. Where in the research report do you think the researchers presented the hypotheses? Where in the report would the results of the hypothesis tests be placed?
   b. Was the stated hypothesis directional or nondirectional?
   c. Was the researchers' hypothesis supported in the statistical analysis?

EXAMPLE 2: QUALITATIVE RESEARCH

Study: Caregivers experiences in symptom management for their children who require medical technology at home (Spratling & Lee, 2020)

Problem Statement (excerpt): "Children who require medical technology have complex chronic conditions and are part of the estimated 11 million children (15%) with special health care needs in the United States. With the number of children with chronic illnesses and the advances in technology in home care, there are growing numbers of children who require medical technology at home to support them in their daily lives . . . Despite diligence in care by caregivers, children who require medical technology have frequent ED [emergency department] visits and hospitalizations due to commonly experienced symptoms and used technologies . . . Little is known about how caregivers of children who require technology manage daily care challenges at home and why these children are so often hospitalized" (p. 2). (Citations were omitted to streamline the presentation.)

Statement of Purpose: "The purpose of this study is to explore the daily care experiences of caregivers of children who require medical technology at home. Specific aims were to gain an understanding of their perceptions of (a) how caregivers manage symptoms for their children . . . (b) why the caregivers seek ED and hospital care, and (c) what the caregivers need to manage their children's symptoms at home" (p. 2).

Research Question: "What are the education, skills, and support caregivers report needing to effectively manage their child's symptoms and prevent avoidable ED visits and hospitalization?" (p. 2)

Method: The researchers recruited a sample of nine primary caregivers of children who required medical technology from an outpatient pulmonary clinic in a pediatric hospital system. In-depth interviews were audiorecorded and transcribed for analysis. Caregivers were asked several broad questions, such as "How have you managed symptoms at home?" and "What services would help you to better manage your child's care?"

Key Findings: The researchers identified three themes in their data: "Knowing my child's normal and having confidence with daily caregiving," "This is much different from my child's normal . . . this is an emergency," and "We cannot sleep and we are exhausted."

Critical Thinking Exercises

1. Answer the relevant questions from Box 5.3 regarding this study.
2. Also consider the following targeted questions:
   a. Where in the research report do you think the researchers presented the statement of purpose and research questions?
   b. Does it appear that this study was conducted within one of the three main qualitative traditions? If so, which one?
3. If the results of this study are trustworthy, what are some of the uses to which the findings might be put in clinical practice?

EXAMPLE 3: QUANTITATIVE RESEARCH IN APPENDIX A

1. Read the abstract and the introduction of Swenson and colleagues' study ("Parents' use of praise and criticism in a sample of young children seeking mental health services") in Appendix A of this book and then answer the relevant questions in Box 5.3.
2. Also consider the following question: What might a hypothesis for this study be? State it as a research hypothesis and as a null hypothesis.

EXAMPLE 4: QUALITATIVE RESEARCH IN APPENDIX B

1. Read the abstract and introduction from Beck and Watson's study ("Posttraumatic growth after birth trauma") in Appendix B of this book and then answer the relevant questions in Box 5.3.
2. Also consider the following question: Do you think that Beck and Watson provided a sufficient rationale for the significance of their research problem?

WANT TO KNOW MORE?

A wide variety of resources to enhance your learning and understanding of this chapter is available on thePoint°.

- Chapter Supplement on Complex Relationships and Hypotheses
- Answers to the Critical Thinking Exercises for Examples 3 and 4
- Internet Resources with useful websites for Chapter 5
- A Wolters Kluwer journal article on a topic related to this chapter

Additional study aids, including eight journal articles and related questions, are also available in *Study Guide for Essentials of Nursing Research, 10e*.

Summary Points

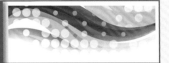

- A **research problem** is a perplexing or troubling situation that a researcher wants to address through disciplined inquiry.

- Researchers usually identify a broad *topic*, narrow the scope of the problem, and then identify research questions consistent with a paradigm of choice.

- Researchers communicate their aims in research articles as problem statements, statements of purpose, research questions, or hypotheses.

- A **problem statement** articulates the problem and an *argument* that explains the need for a study. Problem statements typically include several components: problem identification; background, scope, and consequences of the problem; knowledge gaps; and possible solutions to the problem.

- A **statement of purpose**, which summarizes the overall study goal, identifies the key concepts (variables) and the study group or population. Purpose statements often communicate, through the choice of verbs and other key terms, aspects of the study design, or the research tradition.

- **Research questions** are the specific queries researchers want to answer in addressing the research problem.

- A **hypothesis** states predicted relationships between two or more variables—that is, the anticipated association between independent and dependent variables.

- **Directional hypotheses** predict the direction of a relationship; **nondirectional hypotheses** predict the existence of relationships, not their direction.

- **Research hypotheses** predict the existence of relationships; **null hypotheses**, which express the absence of relationships, are the hypotheses subjected to statistical testing.

- Hypotheses are never proved or disproved—they are accepted or rejected, supported or not supported by the data.

REFERENCES FOR CHAPTER 5

Brenner, I., Brown, C., Hains, S., Trammer, J., Zelt, D., & Brown, P. (2020). Low-intensity exercise training increases heart rate variability in patients with peripheral artery disease. *Biological Research for Nursing, 22,* 24–33.

Higbee, M., Chilton, J., El-Saidi, M., Duke, G., & Haas, B. (2020). Nurses consuming energy drinks report poorer sleep and higher stress. *Western Journal of Nursing Research, 42,* 24–31.

Judge, M., Beck, C. T., Durham, H., McKelvey, M., & Lammi-Keefe, C. (2014). Pilot trial evaluating maternal docosahexaenoic acid consumption during pregnancy: Decreased postpartum depressive symptomatology. *International Journal of Nursing Sciences, 1,* 339–345.

Lee, K., Kim, J., Kang, K., Miller, J., McEvedy, S., Hwang, S., & Moser, D. (2020). Implantable cardioverter defibrillator shocks and psychological distress: Examining the mediating roles of implantable cardioverter defibrillator-related concerns and perceived control. *Journal of Cardiovascular Nursing, 35,* 66–73.

Magny-Normilus, C., Mawn, B., & Dalton, J. (2020). Self-management of type 2 diabetes in adult Haitian immigrants: A qualitative study. *Journal of Transcultural Nursing, 31,* 51–58.

Mikkelsen, H., Vassbakk-Brovold, K., Antonsen, A., Berntsen, S., Kersten, C., & Fegran, L. (2020). Cancer patients' long-term experiences of participating in a comprehensive lifestyle intervention study while receiving chemotherapy. *Cancer Nursing, 43,* 60–68.

**Ryan, P., Brown, R., Csuka, M., & Papanek, P. (2020). Efficacy of osteoporosis prevention smartphone app. *Nursing Research, 69,* 31–41.

Spratling, R., & Lee, J. (2020). Caregivers experiences in symptom management for their children who require medical technology at home. *Journal for Specialists in Pediatric Nursing, 25,* e12275.

Watermeyer, J., Hume, V., Seabi, T., & Pauly, B. (2020). "It's got its own life, and you can't contain it": A qualitative study of patient and health professional experiences of diabetes care. *Journal of Clinical Nursing, 29,* 240–250.

**This journal article is available on thePoint® for this chapter.

6 Finding and Reviewing Research Evidence in the Literature

Learning Objectives

On completing this chapter, you will be able to:

- Understand the steps involved in doing a literature review
- Identify bibliographic aids for retrieving research reports, and locate references for a research topic
- Understand the process of screening, abstracting, appraising, and organizing research evidence
- Evaluate the style, content, and organization of a literature review
- Define new terms in the chapter

Key Terms

- Bibliographic database
- CINAHL
- Google Scholar
- Keyword
- Literature review
- MEDLINE
- MeSH
- Primary source
- PubMed
- Secondary source

A **literature review** is a written summary of the state of evidence on a research problem. It is useful for consumers of nursing research to acquire skills for reading, appraising, and preparing written evidence summaries.

BASIC ISSUES RELATING TO LITERATURE REVIEWS

Before discussing the activities involved in undertaking a research-based literature review, we briefly discuss some general issues. The first concerns the purposes of doing a literature review.

Purposes of Research Literature Reviews

The primary purpose of literature reviews is to summarize evidence on a topic—to sum up what is known and what is not known. Literature reviews are sometimes stand-alone reports intended to communicate the state of evidence to others, but reviews are also used to lay the foundation for new studies and to help researchers interpret their findings.

 TIP Sometimes, stand-alone reviews are called *integrative reviews*, a term that most often is used when a literature review integrates evidence from both qualitative and quantitative studies. Whittemore and Knafl (2005) and de Souza et al. (2010) offer further guidance.

In qualitative research, opinions about doing an upfront literature review vary. Grounded theory researchers typically begin to collect data before examining the literature. As a theory takes shape, researchers turn to the literature, seeking to relate prior findings to the theory. Phenomenologists and ethnographers often undertake a literature search at the outset of a study.

Regardless of when they perform the review, researchers usually include a brief summary of relevant literature in the introductions of their reports. The literature review summarizes current evidence on a topic and illuminates the significance of the new study. Literature reviews are often intertwined with the problem statement as part of the argument for the new study.

Types of Information to Seek for a Research Review

Findings from prior studies are the "data" for a research review. If you are preparing a literature review, you should rely mostly on **primary sources**, which are descriptions of studies written by the researchers who conducted them. **Secondary sources** are descriptions of studies prepared by someone else. Literature reviews are secondary sources. Recent reviews are a good place to start because they offer overviews and valuable bibliographies. If you are doing your own literature review, however, secondary sources should not be considered substitutes for primary sources because secondary sources lack details and may not be completely objective.

 TIP For an evidence-based practice (EBP) project, a recent, high-quality systematic review may provide the needed information about the evidence base, although it is usually a good idea to search for studies published after the review. We provide more explicit guidance on searching for evidence for an EBP query in the supplement to this chapter on thePoint® website.

A literature search may yield nonresearch references, such as case reports or clinical opinions. Such materials may broaden understanding of a problem or demonstrate a need for research. These writings have limited utility in research reviews; however, they do not address the central question: What is the current state of *evidence* on this research problem?

Major Steps and Strategies in Doing a Literature Review

Conducting a literature review is a little bit like doing a study: A reviewer starts with a question and then must gather, analyze, and interpret the information. Figure 6.1 depicts the literature review process and shows that there are potential feedback loops, with opportunities to go back to earlier steps in search of more information.

Reviews should be unbiased, thorough, and up-to-date. Decision rules for including a study should be explicit—a good review should be reproducible. This means that another diligent reviewer would be able to apply the same decision rules and come to similar conclusions about the state of evidence on the topic.

 TIP Locating all relevant information on a research question is like being a detective. The literature retrieval tools we discuss in this chapter are helpful, but there inevitably needs to be some digging for, and sifting of, the clues to evidence on a topic. Be prepared for sleuthing!

Doing a literature review is in some ways similar to undertaking a qualitative study. It is useful to have a flexible approach to "data collection" and to think creatively about opportunities for new sources of information.

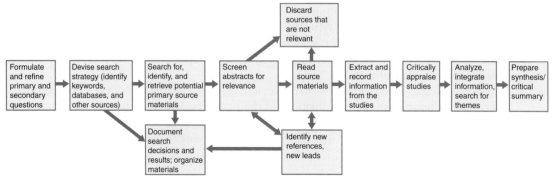

Figure 6.1   Flow of tasks in a literature review.

LOCATING RELEVANT LITERATURE FOR A RESEARCH REVIEW

An early step in a literature review is devising a strategy to locate relevant studies. The ability to locate evidence on a topic is an important skill that requires adaptability—rapid technological changes mean that new methods of searching the literature are introduced continuously. We urge you to consult with librarians or faculty at your institution for updated suggestions.

Developing a Search Strategy

A particular productive approach to locating studies is to search for evidence in bibliographic databases, which we discuss next. Reviewers also use the *ancestry approach* ("footnote chasing"), in which citations from relevant studies are used to track down earlier research on which the studies are based (the "ancestors"). A third strategy, the *descendancy approach*, involves finding a pivotal early study and searching forward to find more recent studies ("descendants") that cited the key study.

 TIP   You may be tempted to begin a literature search through an Internet search engine, such as Yahoo, Google, or Bing. Such a search is likely to yield a lot of "hits" on your topic but is unlikely to give you full bibliographic information on *research* literature on your topic.

Decisions must also be made about limiting the search. For example, reviewers may restrict their search to reports written in one language. You may also want to limit your search to studies conducted within a certain time frame (e.g., within the past 10 years).

Searching Bibliographic Databases

Bibliographic databases are accessed by computer. Most databases can be accessed through user-friendly software with menu-driven systems and on-screen support so that minimal instruction is needed to retrieve articles. Your university or hospital library probably has subscriptions to these services.

Getting Started With an Electronic Search

Before searching a bibliographic database, you should become familiar with the features of the software through which it is accessed. The software has options for restricting or expanding your search, for combining two searches, for saving your search, and so on. Most programs have tutorials, and most also have Help buttons.

An early task in an electronic search is identifying keywords to launch the search (an *author search* for prominent researchers in a field also can be done). A **keyword** is a word or phrase that captures key concepts in your review question. For quantitative studies, the keywords are usually the independent or dependent variables and perhaps the population. For qualitative studies, the keywords are the central phenomenon and the population. If you use the question templates for asking clinical questions in Table 1.3, the words you enter in the blanks are likely to be good keywords.

 TIP If you want to identify all research reports on a topic, you need to be flexible and to think broadly about keywords. For example, if you are interested in anorexia, you might look up *anorexia, eating disorders,* and *weight loss* and perhaps *appetite, eating behavior, food habits, bulimia,* and *body weight changes.*

There are various approaches for a bibliographic search. All citations in a database are coded so they can be retrieved, and coders use database-specific systems of categorizing entries. The indexing systems have specific *subject headings* (subject codes).

You can undertake a *subject search* by entering a keyword into the search field. You do not have to worry about knowing the subject codes because most software has mapping capabilities. *Mapping* is a feature that allows you to search for topics using your own keywords rather than the exact subject heading used in the database. The software translates ("maps") your keywords into the most plausible subject heading and then retrieves citation records that have been coded with that subject heading.

When you enter a keyword into the search field, the program likely will launch both a subject search and a textword search. A *textword search* looks for your keyword in the text fields of the records—in the title and the abstract. Thus, if you searched for *cancer* in the MEDLINE database (described in a subsequent section), the search would retrieve citations coded for the MEDLINE subject code of *neoplasms* as well as any entries in which the phrase *cancer* appeared in text fields even if it had not been coded for the *neoplasm* subject heading.

Some features of an electronic search are similar across databases, such as the use of *Boolean operators* to expand or delimit a search. Three widely used Boolean operators are AND, OR, and NOT (in all caps). The operator *AND* delimits a search. If we searched for *pain AND children,* the software would retrieve only records that have both terms. The operator *OR* expands the search: *pain OR children* could be used in a search to retrieve records with either term. Finally, *NOT* narrows a search: *pain NOT children* would retrieve all records with pain that did not include the term *children.*

Truncation symbols are another useful tool. A *truncation symbol* (often an asterisk, *) expands a search term to include all forms of a root. For example, a search for *child** would instruct the computer to search for any word that begins with "child" such as children, childhood, or childbearing. For each database, it is important to learn what the special symbols are and how they work. The use of special symbols, while useful, may turn off a software's mapping feature.

One way to force a textword search in some databases is to use quotation marks around a phrase to retrieve citations in which the exact phrase appears in text fields. In other words, searches for *lung cancer* and "lung cancer" might yield different results. A thorough search strategy might entail doing a search with and without quotation marks.

Two especially useful electronic databases for nurses are CINAHL (**C**umulative **I**ndex to **N**ursing and **A**llied **H**ealth **L**iterature) and MEDLINE (**Med**ical **L**iterature On-**L**ine), which we discuss in the next sections. We also briefly discuss Google Scholar. Other useful bibliographic databases for nurses include the Cochrane Database of Systematic Reviews, Web of Knowledge, Scopus, and EMBASE (the Excerpta Medica database). The Web of Science database is useful for a descendancy search strategy because of its strong citation indexes.

 TIP If your goal is to conduct a *systematic* review, you will need to establish an explicit formal plan about your search strategy and keywords, as discussed in Chapter 17.

The CINAHL Database

CINAHL is an important electronic database for nurses. It covers references to thousands of nursing and allied health journals as well as to books and dissertations. CINAHL contains more than 6 million records.

CINAHL provides information for locating references (i.e., the author, title, journal, year of publication, volume, and page numbers) and abstracts for most citations. We illustrate features of CINAHL but note that some features may be different at your institution and changes are introduced regularly.

A "basic search" in CINAHL involves entering keywords in the search field (more options for expanding and limiting the search are available in the "Advanced Search" mode). You can restrict your search to records with certain features (e.g., only ones with abstracts), to specific publication dates (e.g., only those after 2010), and to those with certain attributes (e.g., those published in English or those from specific countries).

To illustrate with a concrete example, suppose we were interested in research on nurses' pain management for children. We entered the following terms in the search field and placed only one limit on the search—only records with abstracts:

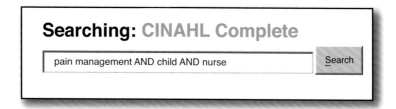

By clicking the Search button, we got 160 "hits" (citations). Note that we used one Boolean operator. The use of "AND" ensured that the retrieved records had to include all three keywords.

By clicking the Search button, all of the identified references would be displayed on the monitor, and we could view and print full information for ones that seemed promising. An example of a CINAHL record entry for a report identified through this search is presented in Figure 6.2. The title of the article and author information is displayed, followed by source information. The source indicates the following:

- Name of the journal (*Pain Management Nursing*)
- Year of publication (2015)
- Volume (16)
- Issue (1)
- Page numbers (40–50)

The abstract for the study is then presented; based on the abstract, we would decide whether this reference was pertinent to our inquiry. Note that there is also a sidebar link in each record, labeled *Find Similar Results*, that can be used to identify other relevant references.

The MEDLINE Database

The **MEDLINE** database, developed by the U.S. National Library of Medicine, is the premier source for bibliographic coverage of the biomedical literature. MEDLINE covers about 5,250 medical, nursing, and health journals and has more than 26 million records. MEDLINE can be accessed for free on the Internet at the **PubMed** website. PubMed is a lifelong resource regardless of your institution's access to bibliographic databases.

MEDLINE uses a controlled vocabulary called **MeSH** (Medical Subject Headings) to code and index articles. MeSH terminology provides a consistent way to retrieve information

Title:	**Nurses'** Provision of Parental Guidance Regarding School-Aged **Children's** Postoperative **Pain Management:** A Descriptive Correlational Study
Authors:	He, Hong-Gu; Klainin-Yobas, Piyanee; Ang, Emily Neo Kim; Sinnappan, Rajammal; Pölkki, Tarja; Wang, Wenru
Affiliation:	Alice Lee Centre for Nursing Studies Department, Yong Loo Lin School of Medicine, National University of Singapore, Singapore; Clinical and Oncology Nursing, National University Hospital, Singapore; Division of Nursing, KK Women's and Children's Hospital, Singapore; Institute of Health Sciences, University of Oulu, Oulu, Finland
Source:	Pain Management Nursing (PAIN MANAGE NURS), Feb2015; 16(1): 40-50. (11p)
Publication Type:	Journal Article - research
Language:	English
Major Subjects:	Postoperative Pain – Prevention and Control – In Infancy and Childhood Parental Role Nurse Attitudes – Evaluation Parents – Education Pediatric Nursing
Minor Subjects:	Human; Multiple Linear Regression; Descriptive Research; Descriptive Statistics; Correlational Studies; Convenience Sample; T-Tests; Hospitals – Singapore; Singapore; Age Factors; Educational Status; Questionnaires; Adult; Child
Abstract:	Involving parents in children's pain management is essential to achieve optimal outcomes. Parents need to be equipped with sufficient knowledge and information. Only a limited number of studies have explored nurses' provision of parental guidance regarding the use of nonpharmacologic methods in children's pain management. This study aimed to examine nurses' perceptions of providing preparatory information and nonpharmacologic methods to parents, and how their demographics and perceived knowledge adequacy of these methods influence this guidance. A descriptive correlational study using questionnaire surveys was conducted to collect data from a convenience sample of 134 registered nurses working in seven pediatric wards of two public hospitals in Singapore. Descriptive statistics, independent-samples t test, and multiple linear regression were used to analyze the data. Most nurses provided various types of cognitive information to parents related to their children's surgery, whereas information about children's feelings was less often provided. Most nurses provided guidance to parents on positioning, breathing technique, comforting/reassurance, helping with activities of daily living, relaxation, and creating a comfortable environment. Nurses' provision of parental guidance on preparatory information and nonpharmacologic methods was significantly different between subgroups of age, education, parent or not, and perceived knowledge adequacy of nonpharmacologic methods. Nurses' perceived knowledge adequacy was the main factor influencing their provision of parental guidance. More attention should be paid to nurses who are younger, have less working experience, and are not parents. There is a need to educate nurses about nonpharmacologic pain relief methods to optimize their provision of parental guidance.
Journal Subset:	Blind Peer Reviewed; Core Nursing; Editorial Board Reviewed; Expert Peer Reviewed; Nursing; Peer Reviewed; USA
Special Interest:	Pain and Pain Management; Pediatric Care; Perioperative Care
ISSN:	1524-9042
MEDLINE info:	*NLM UID*: 100890606
Entry Date:	20150115
Revision Date:	20150710
DOI:	http://dx.doi.org.libraryproxy.griffith.edu.au/10.1016/j.pmn.2014.03.002
Accession No:	103873708

Figure 6.2 Example of a record from a CINAHL search. (Abstract reprinted with permission from He, H. G., Klainin-Yobas, P., Ang, E., Sinnappan, R., Pölkki, T., & Wang, W. [2015]. Nurses' provision of parental guidance regarding school-aged children's postoperative pain management: A descriptive correlational study. *Pain Management Nursing, 16,* 40–50.)

that may use different terminology for the same concepts. Once you have begun a search, a field on the right side of the screen labeled "Search Details" lets you see how the search terms you entered mapped onto MeSH terms, which might lead you to pursue other leads.

When we did a PubMed search of MEDLINE analogous to the one we described earlier for CINAHL, using the same keywords and restrictions, 450 records were retrieved. The list of records in the PubMed and CINAHL searches overlapped considerably, but new references were found in each search. Both searches, however, retrieved the study by

Pain Manag Nurs. 2015 Feb;16(1):40-50. doi: 10.1016/j.pmn.2014.03.002. Epub 2014 Jun 21.

Nurses' provision of parental guidance regarding school-aged children's postoperative pain management: a descriptive correlational study.

He HG[1], Klainin-Yobas P[2], Ang EN[3], Sinnappan R[4], Pölkki T[5], Wang W[2].

Author information: 1 Alice Lee Centre for Nursing Studies Department, Yong Loo Lin School of Medicine, National University of Singapore, Singapore. Electronic address: nurhhg@nus.edu.sg. 2 Alice Lee Centre for Nursing Studies Department, Yong Loo Lin School of Medicine, National University of Singapore, Singapore. 3 Clinical and Oncology Nursing, National University Hospital, Singapore. 4 Division of Nursing, KK Women's and Children's Hospital, Singapore. 5 Institute of Health Sciences, University of Oulu, Oulu, Finland.

Abstract:
Involving parents in children's pain management is essential to achieve optimal outcomes. Parents need to be equipped with sufficient knowledge and information. Only a limited number of studies have explored nurses' provision of parental guidance regarding the use of nonpharmacologic methods in children's pain management. This study aimed to examine nurses' perceptions of providing preparatory information and nonpharmacologic methods to parents, and how their demographics and perceived knowledge adequacy of these methods influence this guidance. A descriptive correlational study using questionnaire surveys was conducted to collect data from a convenience sample of 134 registered nurses working in seven pediatric wards of two public hospitals in Singapore. Descriptive statistics, independent-samples t test, and multiple linear regression were used to analyze the data. Most nurses provided various types of cognitive information to parents related to their children's surgery, whereas information about children's feelings was less often provided. Most nurses provided guidance to parents on positioning, breathing technique, comforting/reassurance, helping with activities of daily living, relaxation, and creating a comfortable environment. Nurses' provision of parental guidance on preparatory information and nonpharmacologic methods was significantly different between subgroups of age, education, parent or not, and perceived knowledge adequacy of nonpharmacologic methods. Nurses' perceived knowledge adequacy was the main factor influencing their provision of parental guidance. More attention should be paid to nurses who are younger, have less working experience, and are not parents. There is a need to educate nurses about nonpharmacologic pain relief methods to optimize their provision of parental guidance.

PMID: 24957816   DOI: 10.1016/j.pmn.2014.03.002

MeSH Terms

- Child
- Female
- Humans
- Male
- Nursing Education Research
- Nursing Staff, Hospital/statistics & numerical data*
- Pain Management/nursing*
- Pain, Postoperative/prevention & control*
- Parent-Child Relations
- Parents/education*
- Postoperative Care/nursing*
- Professional-Family Relations*
- Singapore

Figure 6.3   Example of record from PubMed search. (Abstract reprinted with permission from He, H. G., Klainin-Yobas, P., Ang, E., Sinnappan, R., Pölkki, T., & Wang, W. [2015]. Nurses' provision of parental guidance regarding school-aged children's postoperative pain management: A descriptive correlational study. *Pain Management Nursing, 16*, 40–50.)

He et al.—the CINAHL record in Figure 6.2. Figure 6.3, the PubMed record for this study, provides similar information, but it also lists the MeSH terms that were indexed for this study at the bottom. In PubMed, after identifying a relevant study, you could review the list of "similar articles" that appears beneath the abstract to locate additional studies.

 TIP   Note that in both the CINAHL and PubMed records, the authors' names are hyperlinks that can be clicked on to retrieve other articles written by these authors.

Google Scholar

Google Scholar (GS) is a bibliographic search engine that was launched in 2004. Google Scholar includes articles in journals from scholarly publishers in all disciplines as well as books, technical reports, and other documents. GS is accessible free of charge over the Internet. Like other bibliographic search engines, GS allows users to search by topic, by a title, and by author, and uses Boolean operators and other search conventions. Because of its expanded coverage of material, GS can provide greater access to free full-text publications.

In the field of medicine, GS has generated controversy, with some arguing that it is of similar utility and quality to popular medical databases and others urging caution in depending primarily on GS. The capabilities and features of Google Scholar may improve in the years ahead, but at the moment, it is risky to depend on GS exclusively. We note that a Google Scholar search with the same search terms used in CINAHL and PubMed did not retrieve the Pérez-Ros et al. study.

Example of a bibliographic search •
In their literature review on the effects of movement-based mind–body interventions such as yoga and tai chi for patients with back pain, Park and colleagues (2020) searched six electronic databases, including MEDLINE and CINAHL. A total of 625 studies were initially identified, of which 149 full-text articles were screened and 32 were included in the review.

Screening, Documentation, and Abstracting

After searching for and retrieving references, several important steps remain before a synthesis can begin.

Screening and Gathering References

References that have been identified in the search need to be screened for relevance. You can usually surmise relevance by reading the abstract. When you find a relevant article, you should obtain a full copy rather than relying on information in the abstract only.

 TIP The *open-access journal* movement is gaining momentum in health care publishing. Open-access journals provide articles free of charge online. When an article is not available online or through your library resources, you may be able to access it by communicating with the lead author, either directly through an email or through scholarly collaboration networks such as *Research Gate* (www.researchgate.net).

Documentation in Literature Retrieval

Search strategies are often complex, so it is wise to document your search actions and results. You should make note of databases searched, keywords used, limits instituted, and any other information that would help you keep track of what you did. Part of your strategy can be documented by printing your search history from the electronic databases. Documentation will promote efficiency by preventing unintended duplication and will also help you to assess what else needs to be tried.

Extracting and Recording Information

Once you have retrieved useful articles, you need a strategy to organize the information in the articles. For simple reviews, it may be sufficient to make notes about key features of the retrieved studies and to base your review on these notes. When a literature review involves a large number of studies, a formal system of recording information from each study may be needed. One mechanism that we recommend for complex reviews is to *code* the characteristics of each study and then record codes in matrices, a system that we describe in detail elsewhere (Polit & Beck, 2021). Another approach is to use a form that allows you to record systematically important features of the study (e.g., number of study participants, type of design, main findings, and so on).

CRITICAL APPRAISAL OF THE EVIDENCE

In drawing conclusions about a body of evidence, reviewers must make judgments about the worth of the studies. Thus, an important part of doing a literature review is evaluating the body of completed research and integrating the evidence across studies.

Appraising Studies for a Review

In reviewing the literature, you would not undertake a comprehensive critique of every study, but you would need to assess the quality of each study so that you could draw conclusions about the overall body of evidence and about gaps in the evidence. Appraisals for a literature review tend to focus on study methods, and so the guidelines in Tables 3.1 and 3.2 might be useful.

In literature reviews, methodological features of the studies under review need to be assessed with an eye to answering a broad question: To what extent do the findings reflect the *truth* (the true state of affairs) or, conversely, to what extent do flaws undermine the believability of the evidence? The "truth" is most likely to be discovered when researchers use powerful designs, good sampling plans, high-quality data collection procedures, and appropriate analyses.

Analyzing and Synthesizing Evidence

Once relevant studies have been retrieved and appraised, the information has to be analyzed and synthesized. We find the analogy between doing a literature review and doing a qualitative study useful: In both, the focus is on the identification of important *themes*.

A thematic analysis essentially involves detecting patterns and regularities—as well as inconsistencies. Several different types of theme can be identified for a literature review, three of which are as follows:

- *Substantive themes*: What is the pattern of evidence—what findings predominate? How much evidence is there? How consistent is the body of evidence? What gaps are there in the evidence?
- *Methodologic themes*: What methods have been used to address the question? What are major methodologic deficiencies and strengths?
- *Generalizability/transferability themes*: To what population does the evidence apply? Do the findings vary for different types of people (e.g., men vs. women) or setting (e.g., urban vs. rural)?

In preparing a review, you would need to determine which themes are most relevant for the purpose at hand. Substantive themes usually are of greatest interest.

PREPARING A WRITTEN LITERATURE REVIEW

Writing a literature review can be challenging, especially when voluminous information and thematic analyses must be condensed into a few pages. We offer some suggestions, but we note that skills in writing literature reviews develop over time.

Organizing a Written Review

Organization is crucial in preparing a written review. When literature on a topic is extensive, it is useful to summarize the retrieved information in a table. The table could include columns with headings such as Author and Year, Sample, Design, and Key Findings. Such a table provides a quick overview that allows you to make sense of a mass of information.

Most writers find an outline helpful. Unless the review is simple, it is important to have an organizational plan so that the review has a meaningful and understandable flow. Although the specifics of the organization differ from topic to topic, the goal is to structure the review to lead logically to a conclusion about the state of evidence on the topic. After finalizing an organizing structure, you should review your notes or protocols to decide where a particular reference fits in the outline. If some references do not seem to fit anywhere, they may need to be omitted. Remember that the number of references is less important than their relevance.

Writing a Literature Review

It is beyond the scope of this textbook to offer detailed guidance on writing research reviews, but we offer a few comments on their content and style. Additional assistance is provided in books such as those by Fink (2020) and Garrard (2017).

Content of the Written Literature Review

A written research review should provide readers with an objective synthesis of current evidence on a topic. Although key studies may be described in detail, it is not necessary to provide particulars for every reference. Studies with similar findings often can be summarized together—for example, Several studies have found . . . (Forbes, 2020; Lowe, 2019; Rivera, 2021).

Findings should be summarized in your own words. The review should demonstrate that you have considered the cumulative worth of the body of research. Stringing together quotes from articles fails to show that previous research has been assimilated and understood.

The review should be as unbiased as possible. The review should not omit a study because its findings contradict those of other studies or conflict with your ideas. Inconsistent results should be analyzed objectively.

A literature review typically concludes with a summary of current evidence on the topic. When the literature review is conducted for a new study, the summary should demonstrate the need for the research.

As you read this book, you will become increasingly proficient in critically evaluating the research literature. We hope you will understand the mechanics of doing a research review once you have completed this chapter, but we do not expect that you will be in a position to write a state-of-the-art review until you have acquired more skills in research methods.

Style of a Research Review

Students preparing research reviews often have trouble writing in an acceptable style. Remember that hypotheses cannot be proved or disproved by statistical testing, and no question can be definitely answered in a single study. The problem is partly semantic: Hypotheses are not proved or verified, they are *supported* by research findings.

 TIP Phrases indicating the tentativeness of research results, such as the following, are appropriate:
- Several studies have *found* . . .
- Findings thus far *suggest* . . .
- The results *are consistent* with the conclusion that . . .
- There *appears* to be evidence that . . .

Also, a literature review should include opinions sparingly and should explicitly reference the source. Reviewers' own opinions do not belong in a review, with the exception of assessments of study quality.

Box 6.1 Guidelines for Critically Appraising Literature Reviews

1. Does the review seem thorough and up-to-date? Did it include major studies on the topic? Did it include recent research?
2. Did the review rely mainly on research reports, using primary sources?
3. Did the review critically appraise and compare key studies? Did it identify important gaps in the literature?
4. Was the review well organized? Is the development of ideas clear?
5. Did the review use appropriate language, suggesting the tentativeness of prior findings? Is the review objective?
6. If the review was in the introduction for a new study, did the review support the need for the study?
7. If the review was designed to summarize evidence for clinical practice, did it draw appropriate conclusions about practice implications?

CRITICAL APPRAISAL OF RESEARCH LITERATURE REVIEWS

Some nurses never prepare a written research review, and perhaps you will never be required to do one. Most nurses, however, do *read* research reviews (including the literature review sections of research reports), and they should be prepared to evaluate such reviews critically.

It is often difficult to appraise a research review if you are not familiar with the topic. You may not be able to judge whether the review includes all relevant literature and is an adequate summary of knowledge on that topic. Some aspects of a research review, however, are amenable to evaluation by readers who are not experts on the topic. A few suggestions for appraising research reviews are presented in Box 6.1. Additional appraisal questions relevant for systematic reviews are presented in Chapter 17.

In assessing a literature review, the overarching question is whether it summarizes the current state of research evidence. If the review is written as part of an original research report, an equally important question is whether the review lays a solid foundation for the new study.

 TIP   Literature reviews in the introductions of research articles are almost always very brief and are unlikely to present a thorough critique of existing evidence. Gaps in what has been studied, however, should be identified.

RESEARCH EXAMPLES WITH CRITICAL THINKING EXERCISES

The best way to learn about the style, content, and organization of a research literature review is to read reviews that appear in the nursing literature. We present an excerpt from a review for a quantitative study. The excerpt is followed by some questions to guide critical thinking—you can refer to the entire report if needed. Answers to the questions for Exercise 1 are available to instructors on thePoint®. The critical thinking questions for Exercises 2 and 3 are based on the studies that appear in their entirety in Appendices A and B of this book. Our comments for these exercises are in the Student Resources section on thePoint®.

EXAMPLE 1: EXAMPLE OF A LITERATURE REVIEW FROM A QUANTITATIVE STUDY

Study: Predictors of parental presence in the neonatal intensive care unit (Zauche et al., 2020)

Statement of Purpose: The purpose of this study was to identify sociodemographic, clinical, environmental, and maternal psychological factors that predict parent presence in the NICU.

Literature Review*: "Advances in medical care have led to a remarkable improvement in the survival of preterm infants over the past few decades.[1,2] Infants are admitted to the neonatal intensive care unit (NICU), where they often have lengthy hospital stays and are physically separated from their parents. This separation, along with the medical condition of the preterm infant, limits early parent–infant interactions, which increase preterm infants' risk for social isolation and impaired attachment.[3] Extensive evidence from animal models demonstrates that delayed attachment due to early, prolonged maternal separation has lasting effects on neurodevelopment, self-regulation, and emotional and behavioral health.[4-7] Absent or reduced early parent–infant interactions in the NICU may contribute to the known disparities in the socioemotional and neurodevelopmental outcomes between preterm and term-born children.[8-10]

Preterm birth confers both biological and environmental risks on an infant's developmental trajectory.[11-13] Although biological risks are not easily modified, parent involvement in the NICU, which is modifiable, is thought to be a significant mediating factor between the infant's perinatal risk and developmental outcomes.[3,14] Evidence supports the benefits of parental involvement through breastfeeding, kangaroo care, touch and massage, and maternal voice on the clinical status of preterm infants.[15-20] These modalities have been demonstrated to lessen physical responses to painful procedures, decrease levels of cortisol, improve sleep, increase weight gain, provide exposure to positive sensory stimuli, and increase the concentration of hormones that promote bonding and synaptic plasticity.[16,21] Therefore, parent involvement may have a critical role in enhancing the neurobehavioral and neurodevelopmental outcomes of preterm infants.

Involvement in the NICU necessitates the presence of a parent. However, previous studies have suggested that parent visitation patterns vary significantly.[22-26] While few studies have examined the relationship between the frequency or duration of parent visits and infant outcomes, higher visitation frequency has been associated with shorter NICU length of stay, lower rates of behavioral problems at school entry, and decreased levels of parent stress and depression.[14,26] With a growing consensus that parental presence has the potential to improve outcomes, recent efforts to encourage parental presence and to support parents as caregivers of their infant have been implemented in many NICUs throughout the country. Examples of such efforts include revising visitation protocols to allow 24-hour access to parents and transitioning from traditional open-bay units to single-family rooms, which offer a more private environment and recliners or beds for parents to sleep in overnight.[13,27] In addition, programs in which parents serve as the primary caregivers in the NICU while nurses provide support and education, such as in the Family Integrated Care program, have been developed.[21] These efforts are contributing to a necessary shift in which parents are not seen as 'visitors' but rather essential providers in their infant's care.

Few studies have described predictors of parental presence in the NICU and most of the studies conducted were published more than a decade ago. These studies consistently found that infants with siblings were visited less frequently than infants who were their parents' first child.[22-25,28,29] Increased length of hospitalization was also associated with decreased parental presence, but the infant's medical condition and maternal health had no effect on parental presence.[3,22,23,25,28,29] Findings from these studies are inconsistent for the effect of gestational age, birth weight, maternal marital status, and maternal age on visitation frequency.[23-25,28,30] Understanding factors that contribute to parental presence may help identify infants at risk for low parental presence and thus at a higher risk for delayed attachment and poor outcomes (pp. 251–252)."

---

*References within this literature review are not provided.

Critical Thinking Exercises

1. Answer the relevant questions from Box 6.1 regarding this literature review.
2. Also consider the following targeted questions, which may further sharpen your critical thinking skills and assist you in understanding this study:
   a. In performing the literature review, what keywords might the researchers have used to search for prior studies?
   b. Using the keywords, perform a search of a bibliographic database to see if you can find a recent relevant study to augment the review.

EXAMPLE 2: QUANTITATIVE RESEARCH IN APPENDIX A

1. Read the introduction to Swenson and colleagues' study ("Parents' use of praise and criticism in a sample of young children seeking mental health services") in Appendix A of this book and then answer the relevant questions in Box 6.1.
2. Also consider the following targeted questions:
   a. In performing the literature review, what keywords might have been used to search for prior studies?
   b. Using the keywords, perform a search of a bibliographic database to see if you can find a recent relevant study to augment the review.

EXAMPLE 3: QUALITATIVE RESEARCH IN APPENDIX B

1. Read the abstract and introduction from Beck and Watson's study ("Posttraumatic growth after birth trauma") in Appendix B of this book and then answer the relevant questions in Box 6.1.
2. Also consider the following targeted questions:
   a. What was the central phenomenon in this study? Was that phenomenon adequately covered in the literature review?
   b. In performing their literature review, what keywords might Beck and Watson have used to search for prior studies?

WANT TO KNOW MORE?

A wide variety of resources to enhance your learning and understanding of this chapter is available on thePoint.

- Interactive Critical Thinking Activity
- Chapter Supplement on Finding Evidence for a Clinical Query in PubMed
- Answers to the Critical Thinking Exercises for Examples 2 and 3
- Internet Resources with useful websites for Chapter 6
- A Wolters Kluwer journal article on a topic related to this chapter

Additional study aids, including eight journal articles and related questions, are also available in *Study Guide for Essentials of Nursing Research, 10e.*

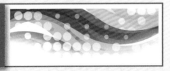

Summary Points

- A research **literature review** is a written summary of the state of evidence on a research problem.

- The major steps in preparing a written research review include formulating a question, devising a search strategy, searching and retrieving relevant sources, abstracting and encoding information, appraising studies, analyzing and integrating the information, and preparing a written synthesis.

- Research reviews rely primarily on findings in research reports. Information in nonresearch references (e.g., opinion articles, case reports) may broaden understanding of a problem but has limited utility in summarizing evidence.

- A **primary source** is the original description of a study prepared by the researcher who conducted it; a **secondary source** is a description of a study by another person. Literature reviews should rely mostly on primary source material.

- Strategies for finding studies on a topic not only include electronic searches of **bibliographic databases** but also include the *ancestry approach* (tracking down earlier studies cited in a reference list) and the *descendancy approach* (using a pivotal study to search forward to subsequent studies that cited it.)

- The bibliographic databases that are especially useful for nurses are **CINAHL** and **MEDLINE**. **Google Scholar** and **PubMed** (for the MEDLINE database) are free bibliographic resources.

- In searching a bibliographic database, users can do a **keyword** search that looks for terms in *text fields* of a database record (or that *maps* keywords onto the database's subject codes), or they can search according to the *subject heading* codes themselves.

- References identified in the search must be retrieved and screened for relevance; then, pertinent information can be extracted and encoded for subsequent analysis. Studies must also be appraised for the quality of the evidence.

- The analysis of information from a literature search essentially involves the identification of important *themes*—regularities and patterns in the information.

- In preparing a written review, it is important to organize materials coherently. Preparation of an outline is recommended. The reviewers' role is to point out what has been studied, how adequate and dependable the studies are, and what gaps exist in the body of research.

REFERENCES FOR CHAPTER 6

*de Souza, M., da Silva, M., & de Carvalho, R. (2010). Integrative review: What is it? How to do it? *Einstein (Sao Paulo)*, *8*, 102–106.

Fink, A. (2020). *Conducting research literature reviews: From the Internet to paper* (5th ed.). Thousand Oaks, CA: Sage.

Garrard, J. (2017). *Health sciences literature review made easy: The matrix method* (5th ed.). Burlington, MA: Jones & Bartlett Learning.

He, H. G., Klainin-Yobas, P., Ang, E., Sinnappan, R., Polkki, T., & Wang, W. (2015). Nurses' provision of parental guidance regarding school-aged children's postoperative pain management: A descriptive correlational study. *Pain Management Nursing*, *16*, 40–50.

Park, J., Krause-Parello, C., & Barnes, C. (2020). A narrative review of movement-based mind-body interventions: Effects of yoga, tai chi, and qigong for back pain patients. *Holistic Nursing Practice*, *34*, 3–23.

Polit, D., & Beck, C. (2021). *Nursing research: Generating and assessing evidence for nursing practice* (11th ed.) Philadelphia, PA: Lippincott Williams & Wilkins.

Whittemore, R., & Knafl, K. (2005). The integrative review: Updated methodology. *Journal of Advanced Nursing*, *52*, 546–553.

**Zauche, L., Zauche, M., Dunlop, A., & Williams, B. (2020). Predictors of parental presence in the neonatal intensive care unit. *Advances in Neonatal Care*, *20*, 251–259.

*A link to this open-access article is provided in the Internet Resources section on thePoint® website.

**This journal article is available on thePoint® for this chapter.

7 Understanding Theoretical and Conceptual Frameworks

Learning Objectives

On completing this chapter, you will be able to:

- Identify major characteristics of theories, conceptual models, and frameworks
- Identify several conceptual models or theories frequently used by nurse researchers
- Describe how theory and research are linked in quantitative and qualitative studies
- Appraise the appropriateness of a conceptual/theoretical framework—or its absence—in a study
- Define new terms in the chapter

Key Terms

- Conceptual framework
- Conceptual map
- Conceptual model
- Descriptive theory
- Framework
- Middle-range theory
- Model
- Schematic model
- Theoretical framework
- Theory

High-quality studies typically achieve a high level of *conceptual integration*. This happens when the research questions fit the chosen methods, when the questions are consistent with existing evidence, and when there is a conceptual rationale for expected outcomes—including a rationale for any hypotheses or interventions. For example, suppose a research team hypothesized that a nurse-led smoking cessation intervention would reduce smoking among patients with cardiovascular disease. Why would they make this prediction—what is the "theory" about how the intervention might change people's behavior? Do the researchers predict that the intervention will change patients' knowledge? their attitudes? their motivation? The researchers' theoretical expectations about how the intervention would "work" should drive the design of the intervention and the study.

Studies are not developed in a vacuum—researchers have an underlying conceptualization of people's behaviors and characteristics. In some studies, the conceptualization is fuzzy or unstated, but in good research, it is made explicit. This chapter discusses theoretical and conceptual contexts for nursing research problems.

THEORIES, MODELS, AND FRAMEWORKS

Many terms are used in connection with conceptual contexts for research, such as theories, models, frameworks, schemes, and maps. We offer guidance in distinguishing these terms.

Theories

In nursing education, the term *theory* is used to refer to content covered in classrooms, as opposed to actual nursing practice. In both lay and scientific language, *theory* connotes an *abstraction*.

Theory is often defined as an abstract generalization that explains how phenomena are interrelated. As classically defined, theories consist of two or more concepts and a set of propositions that form a logically interrelated system, providing a mechanism for deducing hypotheses. To illustrate, consider *reinforcement theory*, which posits that behavior that is reinforced (i.e., rewarded) tends to be repeated and learned. The proposition lends itself to hypothesis generation. For example, we could deduce from the theory that hyperactive children who are rewarded when they engage in quiet play will exhibit less acting-out behavior than unrewarded children. This prediction, as well as others based on reinforcement theory, could be tested in a study.

The term *theory* is also used less restrictively to refer to a broad characterization of a phenomenon. A **descriptive theory** accounts for and thoroughly describes a phenomenon. Descriptive theories are inductive, observation-based abstractions that describe or classify characteristics of individuals, groups, or situations by summarizing their commonalities. Such theories play an important role in qualitative studies.

Theories can help to make research findings interpretable. Theories may guide researchers' understanding not only of the "what" of natural phenomena but also of the "why" of their occurrence. Theories can also help to stimulate research by providing direction and impetus.

Theories vary in their level of generality. *Grand theories* (or *macrotheories*) claim to explain large segments of human experience. In nursing, there are grand theories that offer explanations of the whole of nursing and that characterize the nature and mission of nursing practice, as distinct from other disciplines. An example of a nursing theory that has been described as a grand theory is Parse's Humanbecoming Paradigm (Parse, 2014). Theories of relevance to researchers are often less abstract than grand theories. **Middle-range theories** attempt to explain such phenomena as stress, comfort, and health promotion. Middle-range theories, compared to grand theories, are more specific and more amenable to empirical testing.

Models

A **conceptual model** deals with abstractions (concepts) that are assembled because of their relevance to a common theme. Conceptual models provide a conceptual perspective on interrelated phenomena, but they are more loosely structured than theories and do not link concepts in a logical deductive system. A conceptual model broadly presents an understanding of a phenomenon and reflects the assumptions of the model's designer. Conceptual models can serve as springboards for generating hypotheses.

Some writers use the term **model** to designate a method of representing phenomena with a minimal use of words. Two types of models used in research contexts are schematic models and statistical models. *Statistical models*, not discussed here, are equations that mathematically express relationships among a set of variables and are tested statistically.

Schematic models (or **conceptual maps**) visually represent relationships among phenomena and are used in both qualitative and quantitative research. Concepts and linkages between them are depicted graphically through boxes, arrows, or other symbols. As an example of a schematic model, Figure 7.1 shows *Pender's Health Promotion Model*, which is a model for explaining and predicting the health-promotion component of lifestyle (Murdaugh et al., 2019). Schematic models are appealing as visual summaries of complex ideas.

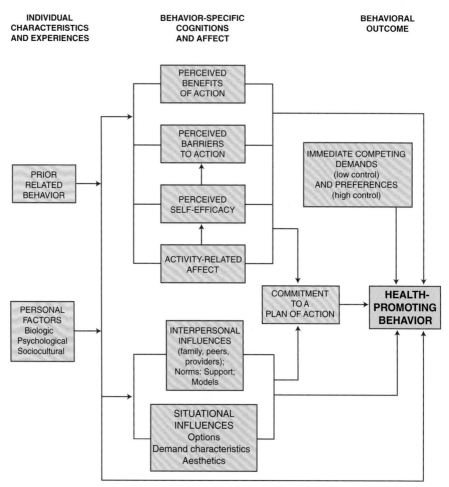

INDIVIDUAL CHARACTERISTICS AND EXPERIENCES	BEHAVIOR-SPECIFIC COGNITIONS AND AFFECT	BEHAVIORAL OUTCOME

Figure 7.1   Pender's Health Promotion Model. (Reprinted with permission from www.nursing.umich.edu/faculty/pender/chart.gif. Retrieved https://nolapender.weebly.com/critical-elements.html.)

Frameworks

A **framework** is the conceptual underpinning of a study. Not every study is based on a theory or model, but every study has a framework. In a study based on a theory, the framework is called the **theoretical framework**; in a study that has its roots in a conceptual model, the framework may be called the **conceptual framework**. However, the terms *conceptual framework*, *conceptual model*, and *theoretical framework* are often used interchangeably.

A study's framework is often implicit (i.e., not formally stated). Worldviews shape how concepts are defined, but researchers often fail to clarify the conceptual foundations of their concepts. Researchers who clarify conceptual definitions of key variables provide important information about the study's framework.

In recent years, *concept analysis* has become an important enterprise among students and nurse scholars. Several methods have been proposed for undertaking a concept analysis and clarifying conceptual definitions (e.g., Walker & Avant, 2018). Efforts to analyze concepts of relevance to nursing should facilitate greater conceptual clarity among nurse researchers.

Example of developing a conceptual definition •
Streck and colleagues (2020) used Walker and Avant's (2018) eight-step concept analysis approach to conceptually define *family caregiver-receiver mutuality*. They performed a literature search that yielded 168 relevant articles. They proposed the following definition: "Family caregiver-receiver mutuality is a phenomenon of shared experience and reciprocity resulting in strengthened caregiver-receiver relationships" (p. E71).

The Nature of Theories and Conceptual Models

Theories, conceptual frameworks, and models are not *discovered*; they are created. Theory building depends not only on observable evidence but also on a theorist's ingenuity in pulling evidence together and making sense of it. Because theories are not just "out there" waiting to be discovered, it follows that theories are tentative. A theory cannot be proved—a theory represents a theorist's best efforts to describe and explain phenomena. Through research, theories evolve and are sometimes discarded. This may happen if new evidence undermines a previously accepted theory. Or, a new theory might integrate new observations with an existing theory to yield a more parsimonious explanation of a phenomenon.

Theory and research have a reciprocal relationship. Theories are built inductively from observations, and research is an excellent source for those observations. The theory, in turn, must be tested by subjecting deductions from it (hypotheses) to systematic inquiry. Thus, research plays a dual and continuing role in theory building and testing.

CONCEPTUAL MODELS AND THEORIES USED IN NURSING RESEARCH

Nurse researchers have used both nursing and nonnursing frameworks as conceptual contexts for their studies. This section briefly discusses several frameworks that have been found useful by nurse researchers.

 TIP Links to websites devoted to several theories mentioned in this chapter are provided in the Internet Resources on thePoint®.

Conceptual Models of Nursing

Several nurses have formulated conceptual models representing explanations of what the nursing discipline is and what the nursing process entails. As Fawcett and DeSanto-Madeya (2013) have noted, four concepts are central to models of nursing: *human beings*, *environment*, *health*, and *nursing*. The various conceptual models define these concepts differently, link them in diverse ways, and emphasize different relationships among them. Moreover, the models emphasize different processes as being central to nursing.

The conceptual models were not developed primarily as a base for nursing research. Indeed, most models have had more impact on nursing education and clinical practice than on research. Nevertheless, some nurse researchers have turned to these conceptual frameworks for inspiration in formulating research questions and hypotheses.

 TIP The supplement to Chapter 7 on thePoint® website includes a table of several prominent conceptual models in nursing. The table describes the model's key features and identifies a study that claimed the model as its framework.

Let us consider one conceptual model of nursing that has received research attention, **Roy's Adaptation Model**. In this model, humans are viewed as biopsychosocial adaptive systems who cope with environmental change through the process of adaptation (Roy & Andrews, 2009). Within the human system, there are four subsystems: physiologic/physical, self-concept/group identity, role function, and interdependence. These subsystems constitute adaptive modes that provide mechanisms for coping with environmental stimuli and change. Health is viewed as both a state and a process of becoming integrated and whole that reflects the mutuality of persons and environment. The goal of nursing, according to this model, is to promote client adaptation. Nursing interventions usually take the form of increasing, decreasing, modifying, removing, or maintaining internal and external stimuli that affect adaptation. Roy's Adaptation Model has been the basis for several middle-range theories and dozens of studies.

Example using Roy's Adaptation model •
Lok and colleagues (2020) studied the effects of an intervention (Cognitive Stimulation Therapy based on Roy's Adaptation Model) on the coping and adaptation skills and quality of life of patients with Alzheimer's disease.

Middle-Range Theories Developed by Nurses

In addition to conceptual models that describe and characterize the nursing process, nurses have developed middle-range theories and models that focus on more specific phenomena of interest to nurses. Examples of middle-range theories that have been used in research include Beck's (2015) Theory of Traumatic Childbirth, Kolcaba's (2003) Comfort Theory, Murdaugh et al. (2019) Pender's Health Promotion Model, and Mishel's (1990) Uncertainty in Illness Theory. The latter two are briefly described here.

Nola Pender's **Health Promotion Model (HPM)** focuses on explaining health-promoting behaviors, using a wellness orientation (Murdaugh et al., 2019). According to the model (see Fig. 7.1), *health promotion* entails activities directed toward developing resources that maintain or enhance a person's well-being. The model embodies several propositions that can be used to develop interventions and to understand health behaviors. For example, one HPM proposition is that people engage in behaviors from which they anticipate deriving valued benefits, and another is that perceived competence (or *self-efficacy*) relating to a given behavior increases the likelihood of performing it.

Example using the Health Promotion Model •
Seo and Ha (2019), using the Health Promotion Model, studied factors that influence physical activity (as a health-promoting action) differentially for male and female college students in Korea.

Mishel's **Uncertainty in Illness Theory** (Mishel, 1990) focuses on the concept of uncertainty—a person's inability to determine the meaning of illness-related events. According to this theory, people develop subjective appraisals to assist them in interpreting the experience of illness and treatment. Uncertainty occurs when people are unable to recognize and categorize stimuli. Uncertainty results in the inability to obtain a clear conception of the situation, but a situation appraised as uncertain will mobilize individuals to use their resources to adapt to the situation. Mishel's conceptualization of uncertainty and her Uncertainty in Illness Scale have been used in many nursing studies.

Example using Uncertainty in Illness Theory •••••••••••••••••••••••
Adarve and Osorio (2019) sought to understand the frequency of uncertainty, and sociodemographic and clinical predictors of uncertainty, in patients scheduled to undergo hematopoietic stem cell transplantation.

Other Models Used by Nurse Researchers

Many concepts in which nurse researchers are interested are not unique to nursing, and so their studies are sometimes linked to frameworks that are not models from nursing. Several alternative models have gained prominence in the development of nursing interventions to promote health-enhancing behaviors and life choices. Four nonnursing theories have frequently been used in nursing studies: Social Cognitive Theory, the Transtheoretical (Stages of Change) Model, the Health Belief Model, and the Theory of Planned Behavior.

Social Cognitive Theory (Bandura, 2001), which is sometimes called *self-efficacy theory*, offers an explanation of human behavior using the concepts of self-efficacy, outcome expectations, and incentives. Self-efficacy concerns people's belief in their own ability to carry out certain behaviors (e.g., smoking cessation). Self-efficacy expectations determine the behaviors people choose to perform, their degree of perseverance, and the quality of the performance. For example, Frensham and colleagues (2020) tested the effectiveness of an online health promotion intervention that had been developed on the basis on Social Cognitive Theory. This study is described in greater detail at the end of the chapter.

 TIP Self-efficacy is a key construct in several models. Self-efficacy has repeatedly been found to affect people's behaviors *and* to be amenable to change. Self-efficacy enhancement is often a goal in interventions designed to change people's health-related behavior.

In the **Transtheoretical Model** (Prochaska et al., 2002), the core construct is *stages of change*, which conceptualizes a continuum of motivational readiness to change problem behavior. The five stages of change are precontemplation, contemplation, preparation, action, and maintenance. Studies have found that successful self-changers use different processes at each stage, thus suggesting the desirability of interventions that are individualized to the person's stage of readiness for change. For example, Temuchin and Nahcivan (2020) tested the effects of a nurse navigation program that was guided by the Transtheoretical Model on colorectal cancer screening behaviors in adults aged 50 to 70 years old.

Becker's **Health Belief Model** (HBM) (1974) is a framework for explaining people's health-related behavior, such as compliance with a medical regimen. According to the model, health-related behavior is influenced by a person's perception of a threat posed by a health problem as well as by the value associated with actions aimed at reducing the threat (Becker, 1976). Nurse researchers have used the HBM extensively. For example, Wang and colleagues (2020) tested the effects of a comprehensive reminder system based on the HBM for patients who had had a stroke.

The **Theory of Planned Behavior** (TPB; Ajzen, 2005), which is an extension of another theory called the Theory of Reasoned Action, offers a framework for understanding people's behavior and its psychological determinants. According to the theory, behavior that is volitional is determined by people's *intention* to perform that behavior. Intentions, in turn, are affected by attitudes toward the behavior, subjective norms (i.e., perceived social pressure to perform or not perform the behavior), and perceived behavioral control (i.e., anticipated ease or difficulty of engaging in the behavior). Tseng and colleagues (2020) used the TPB as a framework for their study of safe sexual behavior intention among female youth aged 15 to 24 years old.

USING A THEORY OR FRAMEWORK IN RESEARCH

The ways in which theory is used by qualitative and quantitative researchers is elaborated on in this section. The term *theory* is used in its broadest sense to include conceptual models, formal theories, and frameworks.

Theories and Qualitative Research

Theory is almost always present in studies that are embedded in a qualitative research tradition such as ethnography or phenomenology. However, different traditions involve theory in different ways.

Sandelowski (1993) distinguished between *substantive theory* (conceptualizations of a specific phenomenon) and theory reflecting a conceptualization of human inquiry. Some qualitative researchers insist on an atheoretical stance vis-à-vis the phenomenon of interest, with the goal of suspending prior conceptualizations (substantive theories) that might bias their inquiry. For example, phenomenologists are committed to theoretical naiveté and try to hold preconceived views of the phenomenon in check. Nevertheless, phenomenologists are guided by a framework that focuses their inquiry on certain aspects of a person's lifeworld—i.e., lived experiences.

Ethnographers bring a cultural perspective to their studies, and this perspective shapes their fieldwork. Cultural theories include *ideational theories*, which suggest that cultural conditions stem from mental activity and ideas, and *materialistic theories*, which view material conditions (e.g., resources, production) as the source of cultural developments (Fetterman, 2010).

The theoretical underpinning of grounded theory is a melding of sociologic formulations, the most prominent of which is *symbolic interaction*. Three underlying premises include (1) humans act toward things based on the meanings that the things have for them; (2) the meaning of things is derived from the human interactions; and (3) meanings are handled in, and modified through, an interpretive process (Blumer, 1986).

Example of a grounded theory study •
Xavier and colleagues (2020) did a grounded theory study within a symbolic interaction framework to explore the stages through which family caregivers assign meanings about children's chronic disease diagnosis.

Despite this theoretical perspective, grounded theory researchers, like phenomenologists, try to hold prior substantive theory about the phenomenon in abeyance until their own substantive theory emerges. The goal of grounded theory is to develop a conceptually dense understanding of a phenomenon that is *grounded* in actual observations. Grounded theory researchers, who focus on social or psychological processes, often develop conceptual maps to illustrate how a process works or unfolds. Figure 7.2 illustrates such a conceptual map for a study of the process of self-management by young adolescents and young adults after a stem cell transplant (Morrison et al., 2018).

In recent years, some qualitative nurse researchers have used *critical theory* as a framework in their research. Critical theory is a paradigm that involves a critique of society and societal structures, as we discuss in Chapter 10.

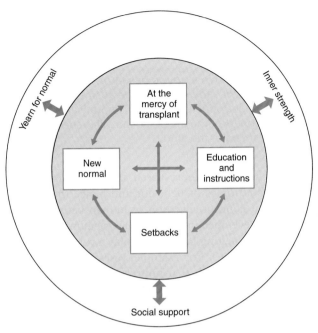

Figure 7.2 A grounded theory of the self-management process of adolescents and young adults after a stem cell transplant. Process starts with "At the mercy of transplant" and proceeds through the cycle. Adolescents/young adults may skip setbacks and proceed to new normal, or they may revert back to another stage and repeat the cycle. "Yearn for normal," Inner strength," and "Social support" influence and are influenced by the context of Social Cognitive Theory and self-management. (Adapted with permission from Morrison C., Martsolf D., Borich A., Coleman K., Ramirez P., Wehrkamp N., . . . Pai, A. [2018]. Follow the yellow brick road: Self-management by adolescents and young adults after a stem cell transplant. *Cancer Nursing, 41,* 347–358.)

Qualitative researchers sometimes use conceptual models of nursing or other theories as interpretive frameworks. For example, a number of qualitative nurse researchers acknowledge that the philosophic roots of their studies lie in conceptual models of nursing such as those developed by Roy (Roy & Andrews, 2009), Rogers (1994), or Newman (1997).

 TIP Systematic reviews of qualitative studies on a specific topic can lead to substantive theory development. In metasyntheses, qualitative studies are combined to identify their essential elements that are then used for theory building.

Theories in Quantitative Research

Quantitative researchers link research to theory or models in various ways. The classic approach is to test hypotheses deduced from an existing theory. For example, a nurse might read about Pender's Health Promotion Model (see Fig. 7.1) and might reason as follows: If the HPM is valid, then I would expect that patients with osteoporosis who perceive the benefit of a calcium-enriched diet would be more likely to alter their eating patterns than those who perceive no benefits. This hypothesis could be tested through statistical analysis of data on patients' perceptions in relation to their eating habits. Repeated acceptance of hypotheses derived from a theory lends support to the theory.

 TIP When a quantitative study is based on a theory or model, the research article typically states this fact early—often in the abstract or the title. Some reports also have a subsection of the introduction called "Theoretical Framework." The report usually includes a brief overview of the theory so that all readers can understand, in a broad way, the conceptual context of the study.

Some researchers test theory-based interventions. Theories have implications for modifying people's attitudes or behavior and hence their health outcomes. Interventions based on an explicit conceptualization of human behavior have a better chance of being effective than ones developed in a conceptual vacuum. Interventions rarely affect outcomes directly—there are mediating factors that play a role in the pathway between the intervention and desired outcomes. For example, researchers developing interventions based on Social Cognitive Theory posit that improvements to a person's self-efficacy will result in positive changes in health behaviors or health outcomes.

Many researchers who cite a theory or model as their framework are not directly *testing* the theory but using the theory to provide an *organizing structure*. In such an approach, researchers *assume* that the model they adopt is valid and then use its constructs to provide an interpretive context.

CRITICAL APPRAISAL OF FRAMEWORKS IN RESEARCH REPORTS

It is often challenging to critically appraise the theoretical context of a research report—or its absence—but we offer a few suggestions.

In a qualitative study in which a grounded theory is developed, you may not be given enough information to refute the proposed theory because only evidence supporting the theory is presented. You can, however, assess whether conceptualizations are insightful and whether the evidence is convincing. In a phenomenological study you should look for a discussion of the study's philosophical underpinnings, that is, the philosophy of phenomenology.

For quantitative studies, the first task is to see whether the study has an explicit conceptual framework. If there is no mention of a theory, model, or framework (and often there is not), you should consider whether this absence diminishes the value of the study. Research often benefits from an explicit conceptual context, but some studies are so pragmatic that the lack of a theory has no effect on its utility. If, however, the study involves the test of a hypothesis or a complex intervention, the absence of a formal framework suggests conceptual fuzziness.

If the study does have an explicit framework, you can reflect on its appropriateness. You may not be able to challenge the researcher's use of a particular theory, but you can assess whether the link between the problem and the theory is genuine. Did the researcher present a convincing rationale for the framework used? In quantitative studies, did the hypotheses *flow* from the theory? Did the researcher interpret the findings within the context of the framework? If the answer to such questions is no, you may have grounds for criticizing the study's framework, even though you may not be able to suggest ways to improve the conceptual basis of the study. Some suggestions for evaluating the conceptual basis of a quantitative study are offered in Box 7.1.

> ### Box 7.1 Guidelines for Critically Appraising Theoretical/Conceptual Frameworks in a Research Report
>
> 1. Did the report describe an explicit theoretical or conceptual framework for the study? If not, does the absence of a framework detract from the study's conceptual integration?
> 2. Did the report adequately describe the major features of the theory or model so that readers could understand the conceptual basis of the study?
> 3. Is the theory or model appropriate for the research problem? Does the purported link between the problem and the framework seem contrived?
> 4. Was the theory or model used for generating hypotheses, or is it used as an organizational or interpretive framework? Do the hypotheses (if any) naturally flow from the framework?
> 5. Were concepts defined in a way that is consistent with the theory? If there was an intervention, were intervention components consistent with the theory?
> 6. Did the framework guide the study methods? For example, was the appropriate research tradition used if the study was qualitative? If quantitative, do the operational definitions correspond to the conceptual definitions?
> 7. Did the researcher tie the study findings back to the framework at the end of the report? Were the findings interpreted within the context of the framework?

 TIP Some studies claim theoretical linkages that are contrived. This is most likely to occur when researchers first formulate the research problem and then later find a theoretical context to fit it. An after-the-fact linkage of theory to a research question is often artificial. If a research problem is truly linked to a conceptual framework, then the design of the study, the measurement of key constructs, and the analysis and interpretation of data will *flow* from that conceptualization.

RESEARCH EXAMPLES WITH CRITICAL THINKING EXERCISES

This section presents an example of a study that described its theoretical links. Read the summary and then answer the critical thinking questions, referring to the full research report if necessary. Answers to the questions for Exercise 1 are available to instructors on thePoint®. The critical thinking questions for Exercises 2 and 3 are based on the studies that appear in their entirety in Appendices A and B of this book. Our comments for these exercises are in the Student Resources section on thePoint®.

EXAMPLE 1: SOCIAL COGNITIVE THEORY IN A QUANTITATIVE STUDY

Study: Predicting engagement with online walking promotion among metropolitan and rural cancer survivors (Frensham et al., 2020)

Statement of Purpose: The purpose of the study was to evaluate the effectiveness of a 12-week online intervention (Steps Toward Improving Diet and Exercise or STRIDE) that was designed to promote walking and other health-promoting behaviors among cancer survivors living in rural and urban areas of Australia.

Theoretical Framework: The intervention was developed in accordance with Social Cognitive Theory (SCT). As noted by the authors, SCT informed the development of STRIDE in that it "posits that physical activity interventions are most effective when they consider intrapersonal mediators (including goal setting, self-monitoring, and self-efficacy), social mediators (family and peer support), and environmental mediators (access to facilities and opportunities)" (p. 53). The researchers also noted that STRIDE "resonates" with another theory that has been used by many nurse researchers, Self-Determination Theory.

Method: In the trial, 91 cancer survivors who were insufficiently active were assigned to either the intervention or to a control group. Control group members were offered a pedometer but did not have access to the online STRIDE program. Outcomes, which included walking activity, motivation, and self-efficacy, were measured at baseline, 12 weeks later (postintervention), and at a 3-month follow-up.

Key Findings: The researchers observed an increase in steps per day at 12 weeks in both groups, with a larger increase in the intervention group than control group (a 32% vs. 13% increase). The increases were not sustained at the 3-month point. However, both groups remained above their baseline step levels at follow-up. Changes in self-efficacy were predictive of changes in the number of steps "in line with the theoretical basis of the STRIDE intervention" (p. 58).

Critical Thinking Exercises

1. Answer the relevant questions from Box 7.1 regarding this study.
2. Also consider the following targeted question: Is there another model or theory that was described in this chapter that could have been used to study the effect of this intervention?
3. If the results of this study are valid and generalizable, what might be some of the uses to which the findings could be put in clinical practice?

EXAMPLE 2: QUANTITATIVE RESEARCH IN APPENDIX A

1. Read the introduction of Swenson and colleagues' study ("Parents' use of praise and criticism in a sample of young children seeking mental health services") in Appendix A of this book and then answer relevant questions from Box 7.1.
2. Also consider the following question: Would any of the other theories or models described in this chapter have provided an appropriate conceptual context for this study?

EXAMPLE 3: QUALITATIVE RESEARCH IN APPENDIX B

1. Read the introduction of Beck and Watson's study ("Posttraumatic growth after birth trauma") in Appendix B of this book and then answer relevant questions from Box 7.1.
2. Also consider the following targeted questions:
    a. Do you think that a schematic model would have helped to summarize the findings in this report?
    b. Did Beck and Watson present convincing evidence to support their use of the philosophy of phenomenology?

WANT TO KNOW MORE?

A wide variety of resources to enhance your learning and understanding of this chapter is available on thePoint.

- Chapter Supplement on Prominent Conceptual Models of Nursing Used by Nurse Researchers
- Answers to the Critical Thinking Exercises for Examples 2 and 3
- Internet Resources with useful websites for Chapter 7
- A Wolters Kluwer journal article on a topic related to this chapter

Additional study aids, including eight journal articles and related questions, are also available in *Study Guide for Essentials of Nursing Research, 10e.*

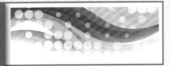

Summary Points

- High-quality research requires *conceptual integration*, one aspect of which is having a defensible theoretical rationale for the study.

- As classically defined, a **theory** consists of two or more concepts and propositions that form a logically interrelated system, providing a mechanism for deducing hypotheses. **Descriptive theory** thoroughly describes a phenomenon.

- *Grand theories* (or *macrotheories*) attempt to describe or explain large segments of the human experience. **Middle-range theories** are specific to certain phenomena; examples include Pender's Health Promotion Model and Mishel's Uncertainty in Illness Theory.

- Concepts are also the basic elements in **conceptual models**, but concepts are not linked in a logically ordered, deductive system.

- In research, the goals of theories and models are to make findings meaningful, to integrate knowledge into coherent systems, to stimulate new research, and to explain phenomena and relationships among them.

- **Schematic models** (or **conceptual maps**) are graphic representations of phenomena and their interrelationships using symbols or diagrams and a minimal use of words.

- A **framework** is the conceptual underpinning of a study, including an overall rationale and conceptual definitions of key concepts. In qualitative studies, the framework often springs from distinct research traditions.

- Several conceptual models of nursing have been used in nursing research. The concepts central to models of nursing are *human beings*, *environment*, *health*, and *nursing*. An example of a model of nursing used by nurse researchers is Roy's Adaptation Model. Nonnursing models are also used by nurse researchers (e.g., Bandura's Social Cognitive Theory).

- In some qualitative research traditions (e.g., phenomenology), the researcher strives to suspend previously held *substantive theories* of the specific phenomena under study, but each tradition has rich theoretical underpinnings.

- Some qualitative researchers seek to develop *grounded theories*, data-driven explanations to account for phenomena under study through inductive processes.

- In the classical use of theory, researchers test hypotheses deduced from an existing theory. An emerging trend is the testing of theory-based interventions.

- In both qualitative and quantitative studies, researchers sometimes use a theory or model as an organizing framework or as an interpretive tool.

REFERENCES FOR CHAPTER 7

Adarve, S., & Osorio, J. (2019). Factors associated with uncertainty in patients scheduled to undergo hematopoietic stem cell transplantation. *Cancer Nursing*, Advance online publication. doi:10.1097/NCC.0000000000000773.

Ajzen, I. (2005). *Attitudes, personality and behavior* (2nd ed.). Milton Keynes, United Kingdom: Open University Press/McGraw Hill.

Bandura, A. (2001). Social cognitive theory: An agentic perspective. *Annual Review of Psychology*, *52*, 1–26.

*Beck, C. T. (2015). Middle-range theory of traumatic childbirth: The ever-widening ripple effect. *Global Qualitative Nursing Research*, *2*, 1–13.

Becker, M. (1976). *Health Belief Model and personal health behavior*. Thorofare, NJ: Slack.

Blumer, H. (1986). *Symbolic interactionism: Perspective and method*. Berkeley, CA: University of California Press.

Fawcett, J., & DeSanto-Madeya, S. (2013). *Contemporary nursing knowledge: Analysis and evaluation of nursing models and theories* (3rd ed.). Philadelphia, PA: F.A. Davis.

Fetterman, D. M. (2010). *Ethnography: Step by step* (3rd ed.). Newbury Park, CA: Sage.

**Frensham, L., Parfitt, G., & Dollman, J. (2020). Predicting engagement with online walking promotion among metropolitan and rural cancer survivors. *Cancer Nursing*, *43*, 52–59.

Kolcaba, K. (2003). *Comfort theory and practice: A vision for holistic health care and research*. New York, NY: Springer Publishing.

Lok, N., Buldukoglu, K., & Barcin, E. (2020). Effects of the cognitive stimulation therapy based on Roy's adaptation model on Alzheimer's patients' cognitive functions, coping-adaptation skills, and quality of life: A randomized controlled trial. *Perspectives in Psychiatric Care*, *56*, 581–592.

Mishel, M. H. (1990). Reconceptualization of the Uncertainty in Illness Theory. *Image—The Journal of Nursing Scholarship*, *22*(4), 256–262.

Morrison, C., Martsolf, D., Borich, A., Coleman, K., Ramirez, P., Wehrkamp, N., . . . Pai, A. (2018). Follow the yellow brick road: Self-management by adolescents and young adults after a stem cell transplant. *Cancer Nursing*, *41*, 347–358.

Murdaugh, C., Parsons, M. A., & Pender, N. J., (2019). *Health promotion in nursing practice* (8th ed.). Upper Saddle River, NJ: Pearson.

Newman, M. (1997). Evolution of the theory of health as expanding consciousness. *Nursing Science Quarterly*, *10*, 22–25.

Parse, R. R. (2014). *The Humanbecoming Paradigm: A transformational worldview*. Pittsburgh, PA: Discovery International Publication.

Prochaska, J. O., Redding, C. A., & Evers, K. E. (2002). The Transtheoretical Model and stages of changes. In K. Glanz, B. K. Rimer, & F. M. Lewis (Eds). *Health behavior and health education: Theory, research, and practice* (3rd ed., pp. 99–120). San Francisco, CA: Jossey-Bass.

Rogers, M. E. (1994). The science of unitary human beings: Current perspectives. *Nursing Science Quarterly*, *7*, 33–35.

Roy, C., & Andrews, H. (2009). *The Roy Adaptation Model* (3rd ed.). Upper Saddle River, NJ: Prentice Hall.

Sandelowski, M. (1993). Theory unmasked: The uses and guises of theory in qualitative research. *Research in Nursing & Health*, *16*, 213–218.

*Seo, Y., & Ha, Y. (2019). Gender differences in predictors of physical activity among Korean college students based on the Health Promotion Model. *Asian/Pacific Island Nursing Journal*, *4*, 1–10.

Streck, B., Wardell, D., & LoBiondo Wood, G. (2020). Family caregiver-receiver mutuality: A concept analysis. *ANS. Advances in Nursing Science*, *43*, E71–E79.

Temucin, E., & Nahcivan, O. (2020). The effects of the Nurse Navigation Program in promoting colorectal cancer screening behaviors: A randomized controlled trial. *Journal of Cancer Education*, *35*, 112–124.

Tseng, Y. H., Cheng, C. P., Kuo, S. H., Hou, W. L., Chan, T. F., & Chou, F. H. (2020). Safe sexual behaviors intention among female youth: The construction on extended Theory of Planned Behavior. *Journal of Advanced Nursing*, *76*, 814–823.

Walker, L., & Avant, K. (2018). *Strategies for theory construction in nursing* (6th ed.). Upper Saddle River, NJ: Prentice-Hall.

Wang, M., Shen, M., Wan, L., Mo, M., Wu, Z., Li, L., & Neidlinger, S. (2020). Effects of a comprehensive reminder system based on the Health Belief Model for patients who have had a stroke on health behaviors, blood pressure, disability, and recurrence from baseline to 6 months: A randomized controlled trial. *The Journal of Cardiovascular Nursing*, *35*, 156–164.

*Xavier, D., Gomes, G., & Cezar-Vaz, M. (2020). Meanings assigned by families about children's chronic disease diagnosis. *Revista Brasileira de Enfermagem*, *73*, e20180742.

*A link to this open-access article is provided in the Internet Resources section on thePoint° website.

**This journal article is available on thePoint° for this chapter.

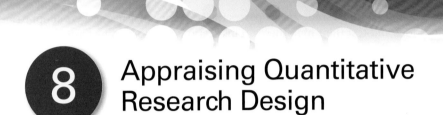

8 Appraising Quantitative Research Design

Learning Objectives

On completing this chapter, you will be able to:

- Discuss key research design decisions for a quantitative study
- Discuss the concept of causality and identify criteria for causal relationships
- Describe and identify experimental, quasi-experimental, and nonexperimental designs
- Distinguish between cross-sectional and longitudinal designs
- Identify and evaluate alternative methods of controlling confounding variables
- Understand various threats to the validity of quantitative studies
- Evaluate a quantitative study in terms of its research design and methods of controlling confounding variables
- Define new terms in the chapter

Key Terms

- Attrition
- Baseline data
- Blinding
- Case-control design
- Cause
- Cohort design
- Construct validity
- Control (comparison) group
- Correlation
- Correlational research
- Crossover design
- Cross-sectional design
- Descriptive research
- Effect
- Experiment
- Experimental group
- External validity
- History threat
- Homogeneity
- Internal validity
- Intervention
- Longitudinal design
- Matching
- Maturation threat
- Mortality threat
- Nonequivalent control group design
- Nonexperimental study
- Placebo
- Posttest data
- Pretest–posttest design
- Prospective design
- Quasi-experiment
- Randomization (random assignment)
- Randomized controlled trial (RCT)
- Research design
- Retrospective design
- Selection threat (self-selection)
- Statistical conclusion validity
- Statistical power
- Threats to validity
- Time-series design
- Validity

For quantitative studies, no aspect of a study's methods has a bigger impact on the validity of the results than the research design—particularly if the inquiry is *cause-probing*. This chapter has information about how you can draw conclusions about key aspects of evidence quality in a quantitative study.

OVERVIEW OF RESEARCH DESIGN ISSUES

The **research design** of a study encompasses the strategies that researchers adopt to answer their questions and test their hypotheses. This section describes some basic design issues.

Key Research Design Features

Table 8.1 describes seven key features that are typically addressed in the design of a quantitative study. Design decisions that researchers must make include the following:

- *Will there be an intervention?* A basic design issue is whether researchers will introduce an intervention and test its effects—the distinction between experimental and nonexperimental research.
- *What types of comparisons will be made?* Quantitative researchers often make comparisons to provide an interpretive context. Sometimes, the *same* people are compared at different points in time (e.g., preoperatively vs. postoperatively), but often, different people are compared (e.g., those getting vs. not getting an intervention).
- *How will confounding variables be controlled?* In quantitative research, efforts are often made to control factors extraneous to the research question.
- *Will* **blinding** *be used?* Researchers must decide if information about the study (e.g., who is getting an intervention) will be withheld from data collectors, study participants, or others to minimize the risk of *expectation bias*—i.e., the risk that such knowledge could influence study outcomes.

TABLE 8.1 **Key Design Features**

Feature	Key Questions	Design Options
Intervention	Will there be an intervention?	Experimental (RCT), quasi-experimental, nonexperimental/observational design
Comparisons	What type of comparisons will be made to illuminate relationships?	Same participants at different times or conditions OR different participants
Control over confounding variables	How will confounding variables be controlled? Which confounding variables will be controlled?	Randomization, crossover, homogeneity, matching, statistical control
Blinding	From whom will critical information be withheld to avoid bias?	Blinding of participants, interventionists, other staff, data collectors
Time frames	How often will data be collected? When, relative to other events, will data be collected?	Cross-sectional, longitudinal design
Relative timing	When will information on independent and dependent variables be collected— looking backward or forward?	Retrospective (case control), prospective (cohort) design
Location	Where will the study take place?	Setting selection; single site versus multisite

- *How often will data be collected?* Data sometimes are collected from participants at a single point in time (*cross-sectionally*), but other studies involve multiple points of data collection (*longitudinally*).
- *When will "effects" be measured, relative to potential causes?* Some studies collect information about outcomes and then look back *retrospectively* for potential causes. Other studies begin with a potential cause and then see what outcomes ensue, in a *prospective* fashion.
- *Where will the study take place?* Data for quantitative studies are collected in various settings, such as in hospitals or people's homes. Researchers must also decide how many sites will be involved in the study—a decision that could affect the generalizability of the results.

Many design decisions are independent of the others. For example, both experimental and nonexperimental studies can compare different people or the same people at different times.

 TIP Information about a study's research design usually appears early in the method section of a research article.

Causality

Many research questions are about *causes* and *effects*. For example, does turning patients cause reductions in pressure ulcers? Does exercise cause improvements in heart function? Causality is a hotly debated issue, but we all understand the general concept of a **cause**. For example, we understand that failure to sleep *causes* fatigue and that high caloric intake *causes* weight gain. Most phenomena are multiply determined. Weight gain, for example, can reflect high caloric intake *or* other factors. Causes are seldom *deterministic*—they only increase the likelihood that an effect will occur. For example, smoking is a cause of lung cancer, but not everyone who smokes develops lung cancer, and not everyone with lung cancer smoked.

While it might be easy to grasp what researchers mean when they talk about a *cause*, what exactly is an **effect**? One way to understand an effect is by conceptualizing a counterfactual (Shadish et al., 2002). A *counterfactual* is what would happen to people if they were exposed to a causal influence and were simultaneously *not* exposed to it. An effect represents the difference between what actually did happen with the exposure and what would have happened without it. A counterfactual clearly can never be realized, but it is a good model to keep in mind in thinking about research design.

Three criteria for establishing causal relationships are attributed to John Stuart Mill.

1. *Temporal*: A cause must precede an effect in time. If we test the hypothesis that smoking causes lung cancer, we need to show that cancer occurred *after* smoking began.
2. *Relationship*: There must be an association between the presumed cause and the effect. In our example, we have to demonstrate an association between smoking and cancer—that is, that a higher percentage of smokers than nonsmokers get lung cancer.
3. *Confounders*: The relationship cannot be explained as being *caused by a third variable*. Suppose that smokers tended to live predominantly in urban environments. There would then be a possibility that the relationship between smoking and lung cancer reflects an underlying causal connection between the environment and lung cancer.

Other criteria for causality have been proposed. One important criterion in health research is *biological plausibility*—evidence from basic physiological studies that a causal pathway is credible. Researchers investigating casual relationships must provide persuasive evidence regarding these criteria through their research design.

TABLE 8.2 **Hierarchy of Designs for Different Cause-Probing Research Questions**

Type of Question	Hierarchy of Designs
Therapy/Intervention	RCT/Experimental > Quasi-experimental > Cohort > Case control > Descriptive correlational
Prognosis	Cohort > Case control > Descriptive correlational
Etiology (causation)/ prevention of harm	RCT/Experimental > Quasi-experimental > Cohort > Case control > Descriptive correlational

Research Questions and Research Design

Different quantitative designs are appropriate for different types of question. In this chapter, we focus primarily on designs for Therapy, Prognosis, Etiology/Harm, and Description questions; Meaning questions require a qualitative approach and are discussed in Chapter 10.

Except for Description, questions that call for a quantitative approach usually concern causal relationships:

- Does a telephone counseling intervention (I) for patients with prostate cancer (P) *cause* improvements in their psychological distress (O)? (Therapy question)
- Do birth weights under 1,500 g (I) *cause* developmental delays (O) in children (P)? (Prognosis question)
- Does salt (I) *cause* high blood pressure (O) in adults (P)? (Etiology/Harm question)

Some designs are better at revealing cause-and-effect relationships than others. In particular, experimental designs (**randomized controlled trials** or **RCTs**) are the best possible designs for illuminating causal relationships—but using such designs is not always possible. Table 8.2 summarizes a "hierarchy" of designs for answering different types of causal questions and augments the evidence hierarchy presented in Figure 1.2 (Chapter 1).

EXPERIMENTAL, QUASI-EXPERIMENTAL, AND NONEXPERIMENTAL DESIGNS

This section describes designs that differ with regard to whether or not there is an intervention.

Experimental Design: Randomized Controlled Trials

Early scientists learned that complexities occurring in nature can make it difficult to understand relationships through pure observation. This problem was addressed by isolating phenomena and controlling the conditions under which they occurred. These experimental procedures have been adopted by researchers interested in human physiology and behavior.

Characteristics of True Experiments

A true **experiment** is characterized by the following properties:

- *Intervention*—The experimenter *does* something to some participants by manipulating the independent variable.
- *Control*—The experimenter introduces controls into the study, including devising an approximation to a counterfactual—usually a *control group* that does not receive the intervention.
- *Randomization*—The experimenter assigns participants to a control or experimental condition on a random basis.

By introducing an **intervention**, experimenters consciously vary the independent variable and then observe its effect on the outcome. To illustrate, suppose we were investigating the effect of gentle massage (I), compared to no massage (C), on pain (O) in nursing home residents (P). One experimental design for this question is a **pretest–posttest design**, which involves observing the outcome (pain levels) before and after the intervention. Participants in the experimental group receive a gentle massage, whereas those in the control group do not. This design permits us to see whether changes in pain were *caused* by the massage because only some people received it, providing an important comparison. In this example, we met the first criterion of a true experiment by varying massage receipt, the independent variable.

This example also meets the second requirement for experiments, use of a control group. Inferences about causality require a comparison, but not all comparisons yield equally persuasive evidence. For example, if we were to supplement the diet of premature babies (P) with special nutrients (I) for 2 weeks, their weight (O) at the end of 2 weeks would tell us nothing about the intervention's effectiveness. At a minimum, we would need to compare posttreatment weight with pretreatment weight to see if weight had increased. But suppose we find an average weight gain of 1 pound. Does this finding support an inference of a causal connection between the nutritional intervention (the independent variable) and weight gain (the outcome)? No, because infants normally gain weight as they mature. Without a control group—a group that does not receive the supplements (C)—it is impossible to separate the effects of maturation from those of the treatment. The term **control group** refers to a group of participants whose performance on an outcome is used to evaluate the performance of the **experimental group** (the group getting the intervention) on the same outcome.

Experimental designs also involve placing participants in groups at random. Through **randomization** (also called **random assignment**), every participant has an equal chance of being included in any group. If people are randomly assigned, there is no systematic bias in the groups with regard to attributes that may affect the outcome. *Randomly assigned groups are expected to be comparable, on average, with respect to an infinite number of biological, psychological, and social traits at the outset of the study*. Group differences on outcomes observed *after* randomization can therefore be inferred as being caused by the intervention.

Random assignment can be accomplished by flipping a coin or pulling names from a hat. Researchers typically use computers to perform the randomization.

 TIP   There is a lot of confusion about random assignment versus random sampling. Random assignment is a *signature* of an experimental design (RCT). If subjects are not randomly assigned to treatment groups, then the design is not a true experiment. Random *sampling*, by contrast, refers to a method of selecting people for a study, as we discuss in Chapter 9. Random sampling is *not* a signature of an experimental design. In fact, random sampling is seldom used in RCTs.

Experimental Designs

The most basic experimental design involves randomizing people to different groups and then measuring outcomes. This design is sometimes called a *posttest-only design*. A more widely used design is the pretest–posttest design, which involves collecting **baseline** (pretest) **data** on the dependent variable before the intervention and **posttest** (outcome) **data** after it.

Example of a pretest–posttest design •••••••••••••••••••••••••••••••••
Huang and colleagues (2020) tested the effectiveness of a tailored rehabilitation education program to improve the health literacy and health status of patients with breast cancer. A total of 99 women were randomized to the intervention or a control group. Data on health literacy, upper extremity function, and overall health were gathered 1 day before the intervention and 1 month later.

TIP   Experimental designs can be depicted graphically using symbols to represent design features. Many such diagrams are shown in the chapter supplement on thePoint˙.

The people who are randomly assigned to different conditions usually are different people. For example, if we were testing the effect of music on agitation (O) in patients with dementia (P), we could give some patients music (I) and others no music (C). A **crossover design**, by contrast, involves exposing people to more than one treatment. Such studies are true experiments only if people are randomly assigned to different orderings of treatment. For example, if a crossover design were used to compare the effects of music on patients with dementia, some would be randomly assigned to receive music first followed by a period of no music, and others would receive no music first. In such a study, the three conditions for an experiment have been met: There is intervention, randomization, and control—with *participants serving as their own control group.*

A crossover design has the advantage of ensuring the highest possible equivalence among the people exposed to different conditions. Such designs are sometimes inappropriate, however, because of possible *carryover effects*. When participants are exposed to two different treatments, they may be influenced in the second condition by their experience in the first. However, when carryover effects are implausible, as when intervention effects are immediate and short-lived, a crossover design is powerful.

> **Example of a crossover design** •
> Kudo and Sasaki (2020) used a crossover design to test the effects of a hand massage with a warm hand bath on sleep outcomes in elderly women with sleep disturbances. Participants were randomly assigned to be either in the intervention or control (no massage) group first.

Experimental and Control Conditions

To give an intervention a fair test, researchers need to design one of sufficient intensity and duration that effects on the outcome might reasonably be expected. Researchers describe the intervention in formal *protocols* that stipulate exactly what the treatment is.

Researchers have choices about what to use as the control condition, and the decision affects the interpretation of the findings. Among the possibilities for the control condition are the following:

- "Usual care"—standard or normal procedures
- An alternative treatment (e.g., music vs. massage)
- A **placebo** or pseudointervention presumed to have no therapeutic value
- An *attention control condition* (the control group gets attention but not the intervention's active ingredients)
- *Delayed treatment,* i.e., control group members are *wait-listed* and exposed to the intervention after outcomes are assessed

> **Example of a wait-listed control group** •
> Chiang and colleagues (2020) tested the effectiveness of a mental health promotion mind-training program on improving the subjective well-being of institutionalized older people. Participants living on different floors of a geriatric institution were randomly assigned to either receive the intervention immediately or to receive it after the first group completed the 6-week program.

Ethically, the delayed treatment design is attractive but is not always feasible. Testing two alternative interventions is also appealing ethically and clinically, but a risk is that the results will be inconclusive if differential effects of two good treatments cannot be detected. However, there is growing interest in such *comparative effectiveness research*, which we discuss at greater length in subsequent chapters.

Researchers must also consider possibilities for blinding. Many nursing interventions do not lend themselves easily to blinding. For example, if the intervention were a smoking cessation program, participants would know whether they were receiving the intervention, and the intervener would know who was in the program. It is usually possible and desirable, however, to blind the participants' group status from the people collecting outcome data.

Example of an RCT with blinding •
Yeh and an interdisciplinary team (2020) described a protocol for an RCT to test the effects of auricular point acupressure (APA) to manage low back pain in older adults. Participants will be randomized to the APA condition, a sham treatment group, or an educational control group. Those in the first two groups will be blinded to their treatment group, as will the interventionists. The technician collecting biomarker data and the data analysts will also be blinded.

 TIP The term *double blind* is widely used when more than one group is blinded (e.g., participants and interventionists). However, this term is falling into disfavor because of its ambiguity, in favor of clear specifications about exactly who was blinded and who was not.

Advantages and Disadvantages of Experiments

RCTs are the "gold standard" for Therapy questions because they yield the most persuasive evidence about the effects of an intervention. Through randomization to groups, researchers come as close as possible to attaining an ideal counterfactual.

The great strength of experiments lies in the confidence with which causal relationships can be inferred. Through the controls imposed by intervening, comparing, and—especially—randomizing, alternative explanations can often be ruled out. For this reason, meta-analyses of RCTs, which integrate evidence from multiple experimental studies, are at the pinnacle of evidence hierarchies for cause-and-effect questions (Fig. 1.2, Chapter 1).

Despite the advantages of experiments, they have limitations. First, many interesting variables simply are not amenable to intervention. A large number of human traits, such as disease or health habits, cannot be randomly conferred. That is why RCTs are not at the top of the hierarchy for Prognosis questions (Table 8.2), which concern the consequences of health problems. For example, infants could not be randomly assigned to having or not having cystic fibrosis to see if this disease causes poor psychosocial adjustment.

Second, many variables could technically—but not ethically—be experimentally varied. For example, there have been no RCTs to study the effect of cigarette smoking on lung cancer. Such a study would require people to be assigned randomly to a smoking group (people forced to smoke) or a nonsmoking group (people prohibited from smoking). Thus, although RCTs are technically at the top of the evidence hierarchy for Etiology/Harm questions (Table 8.2), many etiology questions cannot be answered using an experimental design.

Sometimes, RCTs are not feasible because of practical issues. It may, for instance, be impossible to secure administrative approval to randomize people to groups. In summary, experimental designs have some limitations that restrict their use for some real-world problems; nevertheless, RCTs have a clear superiority to other designs for testing causal hypotheses.

 HOW-TO-TELL TIP   How can you tell if a study is experimental? Researchers usually indicate in the method section of their reports that they used an experimental or randomized design (RCT). If such terms are missing, you can conclude that a study is experimental if the article says that the study purpose was to *test the effects of* an intervention AND if participants were put into groups at random.

Quasi-Experiments

Quasi-experiments (called *trials without randomization* in the medical literature) also involve an intervention; however, quasi-experimental designs lack randomization, the signature of a true experiment. Some quasi-experiments even lack a control group. The signature of a quasi-experimental design is the testing of an intervention in the absence of randomization.

Quasi-Experimental Designs

A frequently used quasi-experimental design is the **nonequivalent control group** pretest–posttest design, which involves comparing two or more groups of people before and after implementing an intervention. For example, suppose we wished to study the effect of a chair yoga intervention (I) for older people (P) on quality of life (O). The intervention is being offered to everyone at a community senior center, and randomization is not possible. For comparative purposes, we collect outcome data at a different senior center that is not instituting the intervention (C). Data on quality of life (QOL) are collected from both groups at baseline and 10 weeks later.

This quasi-experimental design is identical to a pretest–posttest experimental design, *except* people were not randomized to groups. The quasi-experimental design is weaker because, without randomization, *it cannot be assumed that the experimental and comparison groups are equivalent at the outset.* The design is, nevertheless, strong because the baseline data allow us to see whether elders in the two senior centers had similar QOL scores, on average, before the intervention. If the groups are comparable at baseline, we could be relatively confident inferring that posttest differences in QOL were the result of the yoga intervention. If QOL scores are different initially, however, postintervention differences are hard to interpret. Note that in quasi-experiments, the term **comparison group** is often used in lieu of *control group* to refer to the group against which outcomes in the treatment group are evaluated.

Now suppose we had been unable to collect baseline data. Such a design (*nonequivalent control group posttest-only*) has a flaw that is hard to remedy. We no longer have information about initial equivalence. If QOL in the experimental group is higher than that in the control group at the posttest, can we conclude that the intervention *caused* improved QOL? There could be other explanations for the differences. In particular, the QOL of people in the two centers might have differed initially. The hallmark of strong quasi-experiments is the effort to introduce control mechanisms, such as baseline measurements.

Example of a nonequivalent control group design •
Tsai and colleagues (2020) used a nonequivalent control group pretest–posttest design to test the effects of a smartphone-based videoconferencing program for nursing home residents in terms of depression, loneliness, and QOL. Residents of five nursing homes received the intervention, and those in two nursing homes comprised the control group. Outcomes were measured at baseline and at several points post intervention.

Some quasi-experiments have neither randomization nor a comparison group. Suppose a hospital implemented rapid response teams (RRTs) in its acute care units and wanted to learn the effects on patient outcomes (e.g., mortality). For the purposes of this example, assume no other hospital would be a good comparison, and so the only possible comparison is a before–after contrast. If RRTs were implemented in January, we could compare the mortality rate, for example, during the 3 months before RRTs with the mortality rate in the subsequent 3-month period.

This *one-group pretest–posttest design* seems logical, but it has weaknesses. What if one of the 3-month periods is atypical, apart from the RRTs? What about the effect of other changes instituted during the same period? What about the effects of external factors, such as seasonal morbidity? The design in question offers no way to control these factors.

However, the design could be modified so that some alternative explanations for changes in mortality could be ruled out. For example, **time-series designs** involve collecting data over an extended time period and introducing the treatment during that period. Our study could be designed with four observations before the RRTs are introduced (e.g., four quarters of mortality data for the prior year) and four observations after it (mortality for the next four quarters). Although a time-series design does not eliminate all interpretive problems, the extended time perspective strengthens the ability to attribute improvements to the intervention.

Example of a time-series design •
Loresto and colleagues (2020) used a time-series design to test the effect of regular audits of the Fall Champion team on patient fall rates on a medical oncology unit. Monthly data on fall rates on the unit were gathered from January 2017 (9 months before Fall Champion audits were instituted) to June 2018.

Advantages and Disadvantages of Quasi-Experiments

One strength of quasi-experiments is their practicality. Nursing research often occurs in natural settings, where it is difficult to deliver an innovative treatment randomly to some people but not to others. Strong quasi-experimental designs introduce some research control when full experimental rigor is not possible.

Another issue is that people are not always willing to be randomized. Quasi-experimental designs, because they do not involve random assignment, are likely to be acceptable to more people. This, in turn, has implications for the generalizability of the results—but the problem is that the results are less conclusive.

The major disadvantage of quasi-experiments is that causal inferences cannot be made as readily as with RCTs. Alternative explanations for results abound with quasi-experiments. For example, suppose we administered a special diet to a group of frail nursing home residents to assess its impact on weight gain. If we use a nonequivalent control group and then observe a weight gain, we must ask: Is it *plausible* that some other factor caused the gain? Is it *plausible* that pretreatment differences in weight or diet between the groups resulted in differential gain? Is it *plausible* that there was an average weight gain simply because the most frail died or were transferred to a hospital? If the answer to any of these *rival hypotheses* is yes, then inferences about the causal effect of the intervention are weakened. With quasi-experiments, there is almost always at least one plausible rival explanation.

 HOW-TO-TELL TIP   How can you tell if a study is quasi-experimental? Researchers do not always identify their designs as quasi-experimental. If a study involves the testing of an intervention and if the report does not explicitly mention random assignment, it is probably safe to conclude that the design is quasi-experimental.

Nonexperimental Studies

Many cause-probing questions cannot be addressed with an RCT or quasi-experiment. For example, take this Prognosis question: Do birth weights under 1,500 g *cause* developmental delays in children? Clearly, we cannot manipulate birth weight, the independent variable. When researchers do not intervene by controlling the independent variable, the study is **nonexperimental**, or, in the medical literature, *observational*.

There are various reasons for doing a nonexperimental study. In some situations, the independent variable inherently cannot be manipulated (Prognosis questions), and in others, it would be unethical to manipulate the independent variable (some Etiology questions). Experimental designs are also not appropriate for Description questions.

Types of Nonexperimental/Observational Studies

When researchers study the effect of a cause they cannot manipulate, they undertake **correlational research** to examine relationships between variables. A **correlation** is an association between two variables, that is, a tendency for variation in one variable (e.g., weight) to be related to variation in another (e.g., height). Correlations can be detected through statistical analysis.

It is risky to infer causal relationships in correlational research. In RCTs, investigators predict that deliberate variation of the independent variable will result in a change to the outcome variable. In correlational research, investigators do not control the independent variable, which often has already occurred. A famous research dictum is relevant: *Correlation does not prove causation.* The mere existence of a relationship between variables is not enough to conclude that one variable caused the other, even if the relationship is strong.

Correlational studies are weaker than RCTs for cause-probing questions, but different designs offer varying degrees of supportive evidence. The strongest design for Prognosis questions, and for Etiology questions when randomization is impossible, is a cohort design (Table 8.2). Observational studies with a **cohort design** (sometimes called a **prospective design**) start with a presumed cause and then go forward to the presumed effect. For example, in prospective lung cancer studies, researchers start with a cohort of adults (P) that includes smokers (I) and nonsmokers (C) and then compare subsequent lung cancer incidence (O) in the two groups.

> **Example of a cohort (prospective) design** ●
> Osis and Diccini (2020) conducted a prospective study of risk factors associated with pressure injury in patients with traumatic brain injury. They found, for example, that a moderate or severe brain injury classification was a risk factor for subsequent pressure injury. They also found that the presence of a pressure injury was associated with mortality within 30 days of hospitalization.

 TIP RCTs are inherently prospective because the researcher institutes the intervention and subsequently examines its effect.

In correlational studies with a **retrospective design**, an effect (outcome) observed in the present is linked to a potential cause occurring in the past. For example, in retrospective lung cancer research, researchers begin with some people who have lung cancer and others who do not and then look for differences in antecedent behaviors or conditions, such as smoking habits. This type of study uses a **case-control design**—*cases* with a certain condition such as lung cancer are compared to *controls* without it. In designing a case-control study, researchers try to identify controls who are as similar as possible to cases with regard to confounding variables (e.g., age, gender). The difficulty, however, is that the two groups are almost never comparable with respect to *all* factors influencing the outcome.

Example of a case-control design ••••••••••••••••••••••••••••••••
Weaver and colleagues (2020) conducted an exploratory study of gene expression in patients with irritable bowel syndrome (IBS). Part of their study involved comparing gene expression and perceived stress in 27 participants with IBS with that of 43 healthy controls.

Prospective studies are more costly, but stronger, than retrospective studies. For one thing, any ambiguity about the temporal sequence of phenomena is resolved in prospective research (i.e., smoking is known to precede the lung cancer). In addition, samples are more likely to be representative of smokers and nonsmokers.

A second broad class of nonexperimental studies is **descriptive research**. The purpose of descriptive studies is to observe, describe, and document aspects of a situation. For example, an investigator may wish to discover the percentage of teenagers who smoke—i.e., the *prevalence* of certain behaviors. Sometimes a study design is *descriptive correlational*, meaning that researchers seek to describe relationships among variables, without inferring causal connections. For example, researchers might be interested in describing the relationship between fatigue and psychological distress in HIV patients. In such situations, a descriptive nonexperimental design is appropriate.

Example of a descriptive correlational study ••••••••••••••••••••••••
Kim (2020) conducted a descriptive correlational study of nurses from 27 Korean hospitals to examine relationships among stress, emotional labor strategies (e.g., regulation and suppression of felt emotions), and burnout.

 TIP For Description questions, the strongest design is a nonexperimental study that relies on random sampling of participants. Random sampling is discussed in Chapter 9.

Advantages and Disadvantages of Nonexperimental Research

The major disadvantage of nonexperimental studies is that they yield weak evidence for causal inferences. This is not a problem when the aim is description, but correlational studies are often undertaken to explore causes. Yet, correlational studies are susceptible to faulty interpretation because groups being compared have formed through **self-selection**. A researcher doing a correlational study cannot assume that any groups being compared were similar before the occurrence of the independent variable.

As an example of such interpretive problems, suppose we studied differences in depression (O) of patients with cancer (P) who do (I) or do not (C) have good social support. Suppose we found a correlation—i.e., that patients without social support were more depressed than patients with social support. We could interpret this to mean that patients' emotional state is influenced by the adequacy of their social support, as diagrammed in Figure 8.1A. There are, however, alternative interpretations. Maybe a third variable influences *both* social support and depression, such as whether the patients are married. Having a spouse may influence patients' depression *and* the quality of their social support (Fig. 8.1B). A third possibility is reversed causality (Fig. 8.1C). Depressed cancer patients may find it more difficult to elicit social support than patients who are cheerful. In this interpretation, the person's depression causes the amount of received social support, not the other way around. The point is that correlational results should be interpreted cautiously.

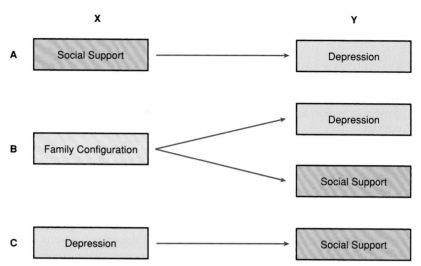

Figure 8.1 Alternative explanations for correlation between depression and social support in cancer patients.

TIP Be prepared to think critically when a researcher claims to be studying the "effects" of one variable on another in a nonexperimental study. For example, if a report title were "The Effects of Eating Disorders on Depression," the study would be nonexperimental (i.e., participants were not randomly assigned to an eating disorder). In such a situation, you might ask, Did the eating disorder have an effect on depression—or did depression have an effect on eating patterns? or Did a third variable (e.g., childhood abuse) have an effect on both?

Nevertheless, nonexperimental studies play a big role in nursing because many important problems are not amenable to intervention. An example is whether smoking causes lung cancer. Despite the absence of any RCTs with humans, few people doubt that this causal connection exists. There is ample evidence of a relationship between smoking and lung cancer and, through prospective studies, that smoking precedes lung cancer. In numerous replications, researchers have been able to control for, and thus rule out, other possible "causes" of lung cancer.

Correlational research offers an efficient way to collect large amounts of data about a problem. For example, it would be possible to collect information about people's health problems and their diet. Researchers could then examine which problems correlate with which dietary patterns. By doing this, many relationships could be discovered in a short time. By contrast, an experimenter looks at only a few variables at a time. For example, one RCT might manipulate cholesterol, whereas another might manipulate protein. Nonexperimental work is often necessary before interventions can be justified.

THE TIME DIMENSION IN RESEARCH DESIGN

Research designs incorporate decisions about when and how often data will be collected. A major distinction is between cross-sectional and longitudinal designs.

Cross-Sectional Designs

In **cross-sectional designs**, data are collected at one point in time. For example, a researcher might study whether psychological symptoms in menopausal women are correlated contemporaneously with physiological symptoms. Retrospective studies are usually cross-sectional: Data on the independent and outcome variables are collected concurrently (e.g., participants' lung cancer status and smoking habits), but the independent variable usually involves events or behaviors occurring in the past.

Cross-sectional designs can be used to study time-related phenomena, but they are less persuasive than longitudinal designs. Suppose we were studying changes in children's health promotion activities between ages 8 and 10 years. One way to investigate this would be to interview children at age 8 years and then 2 years later at age 10 years—a longitudinal design. Or, we could question two groups of children, ages 8 and 10 years, at one point in time and then compare responses—a cross-sectional design. If 10-year-olds engaged in more health-promoting activities than 8-year-olds, it might be inferred that children made healthier choices as they aged. To make this inference, we have to assume that the older children would have responded as the younger ones did had they been questioned 2 years earlier or, conversely, that 8-year-olds would report more health-promoting activities if they were questioned again 2 years later.

Cross-sectional designs are economical, but they pose problems for inferring changes over time. The amount of social and technological change that characterizes our society makes it questionable to assume that differences in the behaviors or characteristics of different age groups are the result of the passage through time rather than cohort differences.

Example of a cross-sectional study •
McAlpine and colleagues (2020) conducted a cross-sectional study that examined factors associated with the use of micronutrient supplements by pregnant women. They found that nulliparous women were more likely to use supplements than multiparous women.

Longitudinal Designs

Longitudinal designs involve collecting data multiple times over an extended period. Such designs are useful for studying changes over time and for establishing the sequencing of phenomena, which is a criterion for inferring causality.

In nursing research, longitudinal studies are often *follow-up studies* of a clinical population, undertaken to assess the subsequent status of people with a specified condition or who received an intervention. For example, patients who received a smoking cessation intervention could be followed up to assess its long-term effectiveness. As a nonexperimental example, samples of premature infants could be followed up to assess subsequent motor development.

Example of a longitudinal study •
Kuo and colleagues (2020) studied the association between rest–activity rhythms and survival in older adults with lung cancer. Data were first collected within 2 weeks of hospitalization, before treatment. Participants were then followed up at 1.5, 3, 6, and 12 months after treatment initiation.

In longitudinal studies, researchers must decide the number of data collection points and the time intervals between them. When change is rapid, numerous data collection points at relatively short intervals may be required to understand transitions. By convention, however, the term *longitudinal* implies multiple data collection points over an extended period of time.

A challenge in longitudinal studies is the loss of participants (**attrition**) over time. Attrition is problematic because those who drop out of a study usually differ in important ways from those who continue to participate, resulting in potential biases and problems with generalizability.

TIP Not all longitudinal studies are prospective because sometimes, the independent variable occurred even before the initial wave of data collection. And not all prospective studies are longitudinal in the classic sense. For example, an experimental study that collects data at 1, 2, and 4 hours after an intervention would be prospective but not longitudinal (i.e., data are not collected over a long time period).

TECHNIQUES OF RESEARCH CONTROL

A major goal of research design in quantitative studies is to maximize researchers' control over confounding variables. Two broad categories of confounders need to be controlled—those that are intrinsic to study participants and those that are situational factors.

Controlling the Study Context

External factors, such as the research context, can affect outcomes. In well-controlled quantitative research, steps are taken to achieve *constancy of conditions* so that researchers can be confident that outcomes reflect the effect of the independent variable and not the study context.

Researchers cannot totally control study contexts, but some opportunities exist. For example, blinding is a way to control bias. By keeping data collectors and others unaware of group allocation, researchers minimize the risk that other people involved in the study will influence the results.

Most quantitative studies also standardize communications to participants. Formal scripts are often prepared to inform participants about the study purpose and methods. In intervention studies, researchers develop formal intervention protocols. Careful researchers pay attention to *intervention fidelity*—that is, they monitor whether an intervention is faithfully delivered in accordance with its plan and that the intended treatment was actually received.

Example of attention to intervention fidelity ••••••••••••••••••••••••
McGuire and coresearchers (2019) described their extensive efforts to ensure intervention fidelity in a multicomponent behavioral change trial for heart failure patients. For example, intervention agents received detailed scripts to use in coaching sessions, and intervention delivery was monitored in several ways (e.g., via video recordings).

Controlling Participant Factors

Outcomes of interest to nurse researchers are affected by dozens of attributes, and most are irrelevant to the research question. For example, suppose we were investigating the effects of a physical fitness program on the physical functioning of nursing home residents. In this study, variables such as the participants' age, gender, and smoking history would be confounding variables; each is likely to be related to the outcome variable (physical functioning), independent of the program. In other words, the effects that these variables have on the outcome are extraneous to the study. In this section, we review strategies researchers can use to control confounding variables.

Randomization

Randomization is the most effective way to control participants' characteristics. A critical advantage of randomization, compared with other control strategies, is that it controls *all* possible sources of extraneous variation, without any conscious decision about which variables should be controlled. In our example of a physical fitness intervention, random assignment of elders to an intervention or control group would yield groups presumably comparable in terms of age, gender, smoking history, and dozens of other characteristics that could affect the outcome. Randomization to different treatment orderings in a crossover design is especially powerful: Participants serve as their own controls, thereby controlling all confounding characteristics.

Homogeneity

When randomization is not feasible, other methods of controlling extraneous characteristics can be used. One alternative is **homogeneity**, in which only people who are similar with respect to confounding variables are included in the study. In the physical fitness example, if gender were a confounding variable, we could recruit only men (or women) as participants. If age was considered a confounder, participation could be limited to a specified age range. Using a homogeneous sample is easy, but a consequence is limits to generalizability.

Example of control through homogeneity •
Bang and colleagues (2018) used a nonequivalent control group design to test the effects of a health promotion program on the psychological health of elementary school children in Korea. Several variables were controlled through homogeneity, including the children's age (all in grades 4 to 6), socioeconomic background (all children were considered "vulnerable"), and all were getting social services in community centers.

Matching

A third method of controlling confounding variables is **matching**, which involves consciously forming comparable groups. For example, suppose we began with a group of nursing home residents who agreed to participate in the physical fitness program. A comparison group of nonparticipating residents could be created by matching participants on the basis of important confounding variables (e.g., age and gender). This procedure results in groups known to be similar on specific confounding variables. Matching is often used to form comparable groups in case-control designs.

Matching has some drawbacks, however. To match effectively, researchers must know what the relevant confounders are. Also, after two or three variables, it becomes difficult to match. Suppose we wanted to control age, gender, and length of nursing home stay. In this situation, if a program participant were an 85-year-old woman whose length of stay was 5 years, we would have to seek another woman with these characteristics as a comparison group counterpart. With more than three variables, matching may not be possible. Thus, matching is a control method used primarily when more powerful procedures are not feasible.

Example of control through matching •
Telli and Gürkan (2019) studied the effects of a mastectomy on women's sexual and dyadic adjustment. A sample of 88 women who underwent mastectomy surgery were compared to 88 women without a mastectomy. The two groups were matched for age and levels of education.

Statistical Control

Researchers can also control confounding variables statistically. Methods of statistical control are complex, and so a detailed description of powerful statistical control mechanisms, such as *analysis of covariance*, will not be attempted. You should recognize, however, that nurse researchers are increasingly using powerful statistical techniques to control confounding variables. A brief description of statistical control methods is presented in Chapter 13.

Evaluation of Control Methods

Random assignment is the most effective approach to controlling confounding variables because randomization tends to control individual variation on all possible confounders. Crossover designs are especially powerful, but they cannot be used in many situations because of the risk of carryover effects. The alternatives described here share two disadvantages. First, researchers must decide in advance which variables to control. To select homogeneous samples, match, or use statistical control, researchers must identify which variables to control. Second, these methods control only the specified characteristics, leaving others uncontrolled.

Although randomization is an excellent tool, it is not always feasible. It is better to use matching or statistical control than to ignore the problem of confounding variables.

CHARACTERISTICS OF GOOD DESIGN

An important question in critically appraising a quantitative study is whether the research design yielded valid evidence. Four key questions regarding research design, particularly in cause-probing studies, are as follows:

1. What is the strength of evidence that a relationship between variables really exists?
2. If a relationship exists, what is the strength of evidence that the independent variable (e.g., an intervention), rather than other factors, *caused* the outcome?
3. What is the strength of evidence that observed relationships are generalizable across people, settings, and time?
4. What are the theoretical constructs underlying the study variables, and are those constructs adequately captured?

These questions, respectively, correspond to four aspects of a study's **validity**: (1) statistical conclusion validity, (2) internal validity, (3) external validity, and (4) construct validity (Shadish et al., 2002).

Statistical Conclusion Validity

A criterion for establishing causality is a demonstrated relationship between the independent and dependent variable. Statistical tests are used to support inferences about whether such a relationship exists. Several threats can undermine a study's **statistical conclusion validity**.

Statistical power, the capacity to detect true relationships, affects statistical conclusion validity. The most straightforward way to achieve adequate statistical power is to use a sufficiently large sample. With small samples, the analyses may fail to show that the independent variable and the outcome are related—*even when they are*. Power and sample size are discussed in Chapter 9.

Researchers can also enhance power by strengthening differences on the independent variable (i.e., making the *cause* powerful) so as to maximize differences on the outcome (the effect). If the groups or treatments are not very different, the statistical analysis might not be sufficiently sensitive to detect effects that actually exist. Intervention fidelity can enhance the power of an intervention.

Thus, if you are appraising a study in which outcomes for the groups being compared were not significantly different, one possibility is that the study had low statistical conclusion validity. The report might give clues about this possibility (e.g., too small a sample or substantial attrition) that should be taken into consideration in interpreting what the results mean.

Internal Validity

Internal validity is the extent to which it can be inferred that the independent variable is causing the outcome. RCTs tend to have high internal validity because randomization enables researchers to rule out competing explanations for group differences in outcomes. With quasi-experiments and correlational studies, there are rival explanations, which are sometimes called **threats to internal validity**. Evidence hierarchies rank study designs mainly in terms of internal validity.

Threats to Internal Validity

Temporal Ambiguity

In a causal relationship, the cause precedes the effect. In RCTs, researchers create the independent variable and then observe the outcome, so establishing a temporal sequence is never a problem. In correlational studies, however—especially ones using a cross-sectional design—it may be unclear whether the independent variable preceded the dependent variable, or vice versa, as illustrated in Figure 8.1.

Selection

The **selection threat (self-selection)** reflects biases stemming from preexisting differences between groups. When people are not assigned randomly to groups, the groups being compared may not be equivalent; group differences in the outcome may be caused by extraneous factors rather than by the independent variable. Selection bias is the most challenging threat to the internal validity of studies not using an experimental design, but it can be partially addressed using control strategies described in the previous section.

History

The **history threat** is the occurrence of events concurrent with the independent variable that can affect the outcome. For example, suppose we were studying the effectiveness of a community program to encourage flu shots among the elderly. Now suppose a story about a flu epidemic was aired in the national media at about the same time. Our outcome variable, number of flu shots administered, is now influenced by at least two forces, and it would be hard to disentangle the two effects. In RCTs, history is not typically a threat because external events are as likely to affect one randomized group as another. The designs most likely to be affected by the history threat are one-group pretest–posttest designs and time-series designs.

Maturation

The **maturation threat** arises from processes occurring as a result of time (e.g., growth, fatigue) rather than the independent variable. For example, if we were studying the effect of an intervention for developmentally delayed children, our design would have to deal with the fact that progress would occur without an intervention. *Maturation* does not refer only to developmental changes but to any change that occurs as a function of time. Phenomena such as wound healing or postoperative recovery occur with little intervention, and so maturation may be a rival explanation for favorable posttreatment outcomes if the design does not include a comparison group. One-group pretest–posttest designs are especially vulnerable to the maturation threat.

Mortality/Attrition

Mortality is the threat that arises from attrition in groups being compared. If different kinds of people remain in the study in one group versus another, then these differences, rather than the independent variable, could account for group differences in outcomes. The most severely ill patients might drop out of an experimental condition because it is too demanding, for example. Attrition bias essentially is a selection bias that occurs after the study unfolds: Groups initially equivalent can lose comparability because of attrition, and differential group composition, rather than the independent variable, could be the "cause" of any group differences on outcomes.

TIP If attrition is random (i.e., those dropping out of a study are similar to those remaining in it), then there would not be bias. However, attrition is rarely random. In general, the higher the rate of attrition, the greater the risk of bias. Biases are usually of concern if the rate exceeds 10% to 15%.

Internal Validity and Research Design

Quasi-experimental and correlational studies are especially susceptible to internal validity threats, which compete with the independent variable as a cause of the outcome. *The aim of a good quantitative research design is to rule out these competing explanations.* The control mechanisms previously described are strategies for improving internal validity—and thus for strengthening the quality of evidence that studies yield.

An experimental design often, but not always, eliminates competing explanations. Attrition is a particularly salient threat. Because researchers do different things with the groups, members may drop out of the study for different reasons. This is particularly likely to happen if the intervention is stressful or time-consuming or if the control condition is boring or disappointing. Participants remaining in a study may differ from those who left, nullifying the initial equivalence of the groups.

You should carefully consider possible rival explanations for study results, especially in non-RCT studies. When researchers do not have control over critical confounding variables, caution in drawing conclusions about causal relationships is appropriate.

External Validity

External validity concerns inferences about whether relationships observed for study participants might hold true for different people and settings. External validity is critical to evidence-based practice (EBP) because it is important to generalize evidence from controlled research settings to real-world practice settings.

External validity questions can take several different forms. For example, we may ask whether relationships observed with a study sample can be generalized to a larger population—for example, whether results about rates of postpartum depression in Boston can be generalized to mothers in northeastern United States. Thus, one aspect of a study's external validity concerns sampling. If the sample is representative of the population, generalizing results to the population is safer (Chapter 9).

Other external validity questions are about generalizing to different types of people, settings, or situations. For example, can findings about a pain reduction treatment in Norway be generalized to people in the United States? New studies are often needed to answer questions about generalizability. *Replication* is an important concept. Multisite studies are powerful because generalizability of the results can be enhanced if the results have been replicated in several sites—particularly if the sites differ on important dimensions (e.g., size). In studies with a diverse sample of participants, researchers can assess whether results are replicated for various subgroups—for example, whether an intervention benefits older and younger people. Systematic reviews represent a crucial aid to external validity precisely because they explore consistency in results based on replications across time, space, people, and settings.

The demands for internal and external validity may conflict. If a researcher exercises tight control to maximize internal validity, the setting may become too artificial to generalize to more natural environments. We discuss this issue in Chapter 18.

Construct Validity

Research involves constructs. Researchers conduct a study with specific exemplars of treatments, outcomes, settings, and people, but these are all stand-ins for broad constructs.

Construct validity involves inferences from the particulars of the study to the higher order constructs they are intended to represent. If studies contain construct errors, the evidence could be misleading. One aspect of construct validity concerns the degree to which an intervention is a good representation of the construct that was theorized as having the potential to cause beneficial outcomes. Lack of blinding can be a threat to construct validity: Is it the intervention, or *awareness* of the intervention, that resulted in benefits? Another issue is whether the measures used to represent the research variables are good operationalizations of constructs. This aspect of construct validity is discussed in Chapter 9.

CRITICAL APPRAISAL OF QUANTITATIVE RESEARCH DESIGNS

A key evaluative question is whether the research design enabled researchers to get good answers to the research question. This question has both substantive and methodological facets.

Substantively, the issue is whether the design matches the aims of the research. If the research purpose is descriptive or exploratory, an experimental design is not appropriate. If the researcher is searching to understand the full nature of a phenomenon about which little is known, a structured design that allows little flexibility might block insights (flexible designs are discussed in Chapter 10). We have discussed research control as a bias-reducing strategy, but too much control can introduce bias—for example, when a researcher tightly controls how a phenomenon under study can be manifested and so obscures its true nature.

Methodologically, the main design issue in quantitative studies is whether the research design provides the most valid, unbiased, and interpretable evidence possible. Indeed, there usually is no other aspect of a quantitative study that affects the quality of evidence as much as research design. Box 8.1 provides questions to assist you in appraising research designs.

Box 8.1 Guidelines for Critically Appraising Research Design in a Quantitative Study

1. Was the design experimental, quasi-experimental, or nonexperimental? What specific design was used? Was this a cause-probing study? Given the type of question (Therapy, Prognosis, etc.), was the most rigorous possible design used?
2. What type of comparison was called for in the research design? Was the comparison strategy effective in illuminating key relationships?
3. If the study involved an intervention, were the intervention and control conditions adequately described? Was blinding used, and if so, who was blinded? If not, is there a good rationale for failure to use blinding?
4. If the study was nonexperimental, why did the researcher opt not to intervene? If the study was cause-probing, which criteria for inferring causality were potentially compromised? Was a retrospective or prospective design used, and was such a design appropriate?
5. Was the study longitudinal or cross-sectional? Were the number and timing of data collection points appropriate?
6. What did the researcher do to control confounding participant characteristics, and were the procedures effective? What are the threats to the study's internal validity? Did the design enable the researcher to draw causal inferences about the relationship between the independent variable and the outcome?
7. What are the major limitations of the design used? Were these limitations acknowledged by the researcher and taken into account in interpreting results? What can be said about the study's external validity?

RESEARCH EXAMPLES WITH CRITICAL THINKING EXERCISES

This section presents examples of studies with different research designs. Read these summaries and then answer the critical thinking questions, referring to the full research report if necessary. Answers to the questions for Exercise 1 are available to instructors on thePoint®. The critical thinking questions for Exercises 2 and 3 are based on studies that appear in their entirety in Appendices C and A, respectively, of this book. Our comments for these questions are in the Student Resources section on thePoint®.

EXAMPLE 1: EXAMPLE OF A QUASI-EXPERIMENT

Study: Effects of a coping-oriented supportive programme for people with spinal cord injury during inpatient rehabilitation: A quasi-experimental study (Li et al., 2020).

Statement of Purpose: The purpose of the study was to evaluate the effectiveness of a coping-oriented supportive program in improving people's psychosocial outcomes following a spinal cord injury. It was hypothesized that participation in the program would contribute to greater improvement in coping ability and self-efficacy.

Treatment Groups: The program was a psychosocial intervention for people with spinal cord injury (SCI) undergoing inpatient rehabilitation. The program consisted of eight weekly group sessions lasting 1 to 1.5 hours that provided guidance on problem solving, adaptive coping, and communication skills. The program was delivered by registered nurses in two similar rehabilitation hospitals. One ward in each hospital was selected, at random, to receive the intervention. Patients from two different wards in the same hospitals received an attention control treatment involving eight brief educational sessions (e.g., self-care information, bowel and bladder training).

Method: To estimate their sample size needs, the researchers undertook a power analysis (see Chapter 9) that suggested that a sample of 50 patients per group would be needed to achieve statistical conclusion validity. A total of 99 patients (50 in the intervention group and 49 in the comparison group) participated in the research. Patient-reported assessment data for the primary outcomes and several secondary outcomes (e.g., anxiety, depression) were gathered at baseline, immediately after the intervention, and at two follow-ups. At the final 12-week follow-up, data were collected from 43 patients in the intervention group and 41 patients in the control group.

Key Findings: The intervention and comparison group members were similar demographically and clinically on most baseline traits, but people in the comparison group were less likely to be married and less likely to use analgesic or psychotropic medication than those in the intervention group. The analysis of program effects revealed statistically significant improvements for those in the intervention group, compared to those in the comparison group, with respect to coping, self-efficacy, depression, anxiety, and life satisfaction.

Critical Thinking Exercises

1. Answers the relevant questions from Box 8.1 regarding this study.
2. Also consider the following targeted question: What can be inferred about the statistical conclusion validity of the study?

EXAMPLE 2: RANDOMIZED CONTROLLED TRIAL IN APPENDIX C

1. Read the method section from Wilson and colleagues' study ("A randomized controlled trial of an individualized preoperative education intervention . . . ") in Appendix C of this book and then answer the questions in Box 8.1.
2. Also consider the following targeted question: Could a crossover design have been used in this study?

EXAMPLE 3: NONEXPERIMENTAL STUDY IN APPENDIX A

1. Read the method section from Swenson and colleagues' study ("Parents' use of praise and criticism in a sample of young children seeking mental health services") in Appendix A of this book and then answer the questions in Box 8.1.
2. Suggest modifications to the design of this study that might improve its external validity.

WANT TO KNOW MORE?

A wide variety of resources to enhance your learning and understanding of this chapter is available on thePoint®.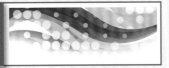

- Chapter Supplement on Selected Experimental and Quasi-Experimental Designs: Diagrams, Uses, and Drawbacks
- Answers to the Critical Thinking Exercises for Examples 2 and 3
- Internet Resources with useful websites for Chapter 8
- A Wolters Kluwer journal article on a topic related to this chapter

Additional study aids, including eight journal articles and related questions, are also available in *Study Guide for Essentials of Nursing Research, 10e.*

Summary Points

- A **research design** is the overall plan for answering research questions. In quantitative studies, the design designates whether there is an intervention, the nature of any comparisons, methods for controlling confounding variables, whether there will be blinding, and the timing and location of data collection.

- Therapy, Prognosis, and Etiology questions are cause-probing; the challenge of research design is to facilitate causal inferences.

- Key criteria for inferring causality include the following: (1) a **cause** (the independent variable) must precede an **effect** (the outcome), (2) there must be a detectable relationship between a cause and an effect, and (3) the relationship between the two does not reflect the influence of a third (confounding) variable.

- A *counterfactual* is what would have happened to the same people simultaneously exposed *and* not exposed to a causal factor. The *effect* is the difference between the two. A good research design for cause-probing questions entails finding a good approximation to the idealized counterfactual.

- **Experiments** (or **randomized controlled trials [RCTs]**) involve an **intervention** (the researcher manipulates the independent variable by introducing an intervention), control (including the use of a **control group** that does not receive the intervention), and **randomization/random assignment** (with participants allocated to experimental and control conditions at random to achieve group comparability at the outset).

- RCTs are considered the gold standard for Therapy questions because they come closer than any other design to meeting the criteria for inferring causal relationships.

- In **pretest–posttest designs**, data are collected both before the intervention (at **baseline**) and after it.

- In **crossover designs**, people are exposed to more than one condition in random order and serve as their own controls. Crossover designs are inappropriate if there is a risk of *carryover effects*.

- Possible control group conditions include standard treatment ("usual care"), an alternative treatment, a **placebo** (a pseudointervention), an *attention control* condition, or a *wait-list* (*delayed treatment*) condition.

- **Quasi-experiments** (*trials without randomization*) involve an intervention but lack a comparison group or randomization. Strong quasi-experimental designs introduce features to compensate for these missing components.

- The **nonequivalent control group,** pretest–posttest **design** involves a **comparison group** that was not created through randomization and the collection of pretreatment data from both groups to assess initial group equivalence.

- In a **time-series design**, outcome data are collected over a period of time before and after the intervention, usually for a single group.

- **Nonexperimental** (*observational*) **studies** include **descriptive research**—studies that summarize the status of phenomena—and **correlational studies** that examine relationships among variables but do not involve an intervention.

- In **prospective (cohort) designs**, researchers begin with a possible cause and then subsequently collect data about outcomes.

- **Retrospective designs (case-control designs)** involve collecting data about an outcome in the present and then looking back in time for possible causes.

- Making causal inferences in correlational studies is risky; a basic research dictum is that *correlation does not prove causation*.

- **Cross-sectional designs** involve the collection of data at one time period, whereas **longitudinal designs** involve data collection at two or more times over an extended period. In nursing, longitudinal studies often are *follow-up studies* of clinical populations.

- Longitudinal studies are typically expensive, time-consuming, and subject to the risk of **attrition** (loss of participants over time), but they yield valuable information about time-related phenomena.

- Quantitative researchers strive to control external factors that could affect study outcomes and participant characteristics that are extraneous to the research question.

- Researchers delineate the intervention in formal *protocols* that stipulate exactly what the treatment is. Careful researchers attend to *intervention fidelity*—whether the intervention was properly implemented as planned and actually received.

- Techniques for controlling participant characteristics include **homogeneity** (restricting the sample to reduce variability on confounding variables), **matching** (deliberately making groups comparable on some extraneous variables), statistical procedures, and randomization—the most effective method because it controls all possible confounding variables without researchers having to identify them.

- Study **validity** concerns the extent to which appropriate inferences can be made. **Threats to validity** are reasons that an inference could be wrong. A key function of quantitative research design is to rule out validity threats.

- **Statistical conclusion validity** concerns the strength of evidence that a relationship exists between two variables. One threat to statistical conclusion validity is low **statistical power** (the ability to detect true relationships among variables).

- **Internal validity** concerns inferences that outcomes were caused by the independent variable, rather than by extraneous factors. Threats to internal validity include temporal ambiguity (uncertainty about whether the presumed cause preceded the outcome), **selection** (pre-existing group differences), **history** (external events that could affect outcomes), **maturation** (changes due to the passage of time), and **mortality** (effects attributable to attrition).

- **External validity** concerns inferences about generalizability—whether findings hold true over variations in people, conditions, and settings.

REFERENCES FOR CHAPTER 8

*Bang, K., Kim, S., Song, M., Kang, K., & Jeong, Y. (2018). The effects of a health promotion program using urban forests and nursing student mentors on the perceived and psychological health of elementary school children in vulnerable populations. *International Journal of Environmental Research and Public Health, 15,* 1977.

Chiang, Y., Lee, C., & Hsueh, S. (2020). Happiness or hopelessness in late life: A cluster RCT of the 3L-Mind-Training programme among the institutionalized older people. *Journal of Advanced Nursing, 76,* 312–323.

**Huang, S., Kuo, S., Tsai, P., Tsai, C., Chen, S., Lin, C., . . . Hou, W. (2020). Effectiveness of tailored rehabilitation education in improving the health literacy and health status of postoperative patients with breast cancer. *Cancer Nursing, 43,* E38–E46.

Kim, J. (2020). Emotional labor strategies, stress, and burnout among hospital nurses. *Journal of Nursing Scholarship, 52,* 105–112.

Kudo, Y., & Sasaki, M. (2020). Effect of a hand massage with a warm hand bath on sleep and relaxation in elderly women with disturbance of sleep: A crossover trial. *Japanese Journal of Nursing Science, 17,* e12327.

Kuo, L., Chang, W., Huang, H., & Lin, C. (2020). Association of time-varying rest-activity rhythms with survival in older adults with lung cancer. *Cancer Nursing, 43,* 45–51.

Li, Y., Chien, W., & Bressington, D. (2020). Effects of a coping-oriented supportive programme for people with spinal cord injury during inpatient rehabilitation: A quasi-experimental study. *Spinal Cord, 58,* 58–69.

Loresto, F., Jr., Grant, C., Solberg, J., & Eron, K. (2020). Assessing the effect of unit champion-initiated audits on fall rates: Improving awareness. *Journal of Nursing Care Quality, 35,* 227–232.

McAlpine, J., Vanderlelie, J., Vincze, L., & Perkins, A. (2020). Use of micronutrient supplements in pregnant women of southeast Queensland. *The Australia & New Zealand Journal of Obstetrics & Gynaecology,* Advance online publication. doi:10.1111/ajo.13109.

McGuire, R., Duncan, K., & Pozehl, B. (2019). Incorporating intervention fidelity components into randomized controlled trials promoting exercise adherence in heart failure patients. *Research in Nursing & Health, 42,* 306–316.

Osis, S., & Diccini, S. (2020). Incidence and risk factors associated with pressure injury in patients with traumatic brain injury. *International Journal of Nursing Practice, 26,* e12821.

Shadish, W. R., Cook, T. D., & Campbell, D. T. (2002). *Experimental and quasi-experimental designs for generalized causal inference.* Boston, MA: Houghton Mifflin.

*Telli, S., & Gürkan, A. (2019). Examination of sexual quality of life and dyadic adjustment among women with mastectomy. *European Journal of Breast Health, 16,* 48–54.

*Tsai, H., Cheng, C., Shieh, W., & Chang, Y. (2020). Effects of a smartphone-based videoconferencing program for older nursing home residents on depression, loneliness, and quality of life: A quasi-experimental study. *BMC Geriatrics, 20,* 27.

Weaver, K., Melkus, G., Fletcher, J., & Henderson, W. (2020). Relevance and subtype in patients with IBS: An exploratory study of gene expression. *Biological Research for Nursing, 22,* 13–23.

*Yeh, C., Li, C., Glick, R., Schlenk, E., Albers, K., Suen, L., . . . Christo, P. (2020). A prospective randomized controlled study of auricular acupressure to manage chronic lower back pain in older adults: Study protocol. *Trials, 21,* 99.

*A link to this open-access article is provided in the Internet Resources section on thePoint° website.

**This journal article is available on thePoint° for this chapter.

9 Appraising Sampling and Data Collection in Quantitative Studies

Learning Objectives

On completing this chapter, you will be able to:

- Distinguish nonprobability and probability samples and compare their advantages and disadvantages
- Identify and describe several sampling designs in quantitative studies
- Evaluate the appropriateness of the sampling method and sample size used in a study
- Discuss dimensions along which data collection approaches vary
- Identify phenomena that lend themselves to self-reports, observation, and physiological measurement
- Describe various approaches to collecting self-report data (e.g., interviews, questionnaires, composite scales)
- Describe methods of collecting and recording observational data
- Describe the major features and advantages of biomarkers
- Critically appraise researchers' decisions about a data collection plan
- Describe approaches for assessing the reliability and validity of measures
- Define new terms in the chapter

Key Terms

- Biophysiological measure
- Biomarker
- Category system
- Checklist
- Closed-ended question
- Consecutive sampling
- Construct validity
- Content validity
- Convenience sampling
- Criterion validity
- Eligibility criteria
- Face validity
- Internal consistency
- Interrater reliability
- Interview schedule
- Likert scale
- Measurement
- Measurement property
- Nonprobability sampling
- Observational methods
- Open-ended question
- Patient-reported outcome (PRO)
- Population
- Power analysis
- Probability sampling
- Psychometric assessment
- Purposive sampling
- Questionnaire
- Quota sampling
- Rating scale
- Reliability
- Response options
- Response rate
- Response set bias
- Sample
- Sample size
- Sampling bias
- Sampling plan
- Scale
- Self-reports
- Simple random sampling
- Strata
- Stratified random sampling
- Summated rating scale
- Test–retest reliability
- Validity

This chapter covers two important research topics—how quantitative researchers select study participants and how they collect data from them.

SAMPLING IN QUANTITATIVE RESEARCH

Researchers answer research questions using data from a sample of participants. In testing the effects of an intervention for pregnant women, nurse researchers reach conclusions without testing it with all pregnant women. Quantitative researchers develop a **sampling plan** that specifies in advance how—and how many—participants will be selected.

Basic Sampling Concepts

Let us begin by considering some terms associated with sampling.

Populations

A **population** ("P" in PICO questions) is the entire group of interest. For instance, if a researcher were studying American nurses with doctoral degrees, the population could be defined as all registered nurses (RNs) in the United States with a doctoral-level degree. Other populations might be all patients who had cardiac surgery in St. Peter's Hospital in 2021 or all Australian children younger than age 10 years with cystic fibrosis. Populations are not restricted to people. A population might be all patient records in Memorial Hospital. A population is an entire aggregate of elements.

Researchers specify population characteristics through **eligibility criteria**. For example, consider the population of American nursing students. Does the population include part-time students? Are RNs returning to school for a bachelor's degree included? Researchers establish criteria to determine whether a person qualifies as a member of the population (*inclusion* criteria) or should be excluded (*exclusion* criteria). For example, patients who are severely ill might be excluded.

> **Example of inclusion and exclusion criteria** •
> Becker and coresearchers (2020) analyzed the effects of an intervention to improve cognitive abilities in patients with multiple sclerosis (MS). To be eligible for the study, patients had to have a physician diagnosis of MS for at least 6 months, have self-reported cognitive problems, and be between 18 and 60 years of age. Those with an exacerbation in the previous 3 months were excluded.

Quantitative researchers sample from an accessible population in the hope of generalizing to a target population. The *target population* is the entire population of interest. The *accessible population* is the portion of the target population that is accessible to the researcher. For example, a researcher's target population might be all diabetic patients in the United States, but, in reality, the population that is accessible might be diabetic patients in a particular city.

Samples and Sampling

Sampling involves selecting cases to represent the population—a **sample** is a subset of population elements. In nursing research, the *elements* (basic units) are usually humans. Researchers work with samples rather than populations for practical reasons.

Information from samples can, however, lead to faulty conclusions. In quantitative studies, a criterion for judging a sample is its representativeness. A *representative sample* is one whose characteristics closely approximate those of the population. Some sampling plans are more likely to yield biased samples than others. **Sampling bias** is the systematic overrepresentation or underrepresentation of a population segment on a characteristic relevant to the research question (e.g., too few or too many men in the sample).

Strata

Populations consist of subpopulations, or **strata**. Strata are mutually exclusive segments of a population based on a specific characteristic. For instance, a population consisting of all RNs in the United States could be divided into two strata based on attainment or nonattainment of a bachelor's degree. Strata can be designated in sample selection to enhance the sample's representativeness—elements in each stratum can be sampled in the correct proportions.

 TIP The sampling plan is usually discussed in a report's method section, sometimes in a subsection labeled "Sample" or "Study participants." Sample characteristics (e.g., average age) are often described in the results section.

Sampling Designs in Quantitative Studies

The two broad classes of sampling designs in quantitative research are probability sampling and nonprobability sampling.

Nonprobability Sampling

In **nonprobability sampling**, researchers select elements by nonrandom methods in which every element does not have a chance to be included. Nonprobability sampling is less likely than probability sampling to produce representative samples—and yet, *most* research samples in nursing and other disciplines are nonprobability samples.

Convenience sampling entails selecting the most conveniently available people as participants. A nurse who distributes questionnaires about vitamin use to college students leaving the library is sampling by convenience, for example. The problem with convenience sampling is that people who are readily available might be atypical of the population. The price of convenience is the risk of bias. Convenience sampling is the weakest form of sampling, but it is also the most commonly used method.

Example of a convenience sample •
Zhang and colleagues (2020) studied self-management among elderly patients with hypertension in China. A convenience sample of 301 patients was recruited in two tertiary Chinese hospitals.

In **quota sampling**, researchers identify population strata and figure out how many people are needed from each stratum. By using information about the population, researchers can ensure that diverse segments are represented in the sample. For example, if the population is known to have 48% males, 48% females, and 4% other gender, then the sample should have similar percentages. Procedurally, quota sampling is similar to convenience sampling: Participants are a convenience sample from each stratum. Because of this fact, quota sampling shares some weaknesses of convenience sampling. Nevertheless, quota sampling is a big improvement over convenience sampling and does not require sophisticated skills or a lot of effort. Surprisingly, few researchers use this strategy.

Example of a quota sample •
Cheung and colleagues (2018) studied anticipatory grief in spousal and adult children caregivers of community-dwelling people with dementia. They recruited 108 caregivers and used quota sampling to ensure that half of the sample members were spousal caregivers and the other half were adult children caregivers.

Consecutive sampling is a nonprobability sampling method that involves recruiting *all* people from an accessible population over a specific time interval or for a specified sample size. For example, in a study of ventilator-associated pneumonia in intensive care unit (ICU) patients, a consecutive sample might consist of all eligible patients who were admitted to an ICU over a 6-month period. Or it might be the first 250 eligible patients admitted to the ICU, if 250 were the targeted sample size. Consecutive sampling is often the best possible choice when there is "rolling enrollment" into an accessible population.

Example of a consecutive sample •
Lee and colleagues (2020) studied the relationship between self-leadership skills and the performance and maintenance of an exercise program regimen among patients with colorectal cancer. A total of 350 consecutive eligible patients who had follow-up visits in clinics were recruited.

Purposive sampling involves using researchers' knowledge about the population to handpick sample members. Researchers might decide purposely to select people judged to be knowledgeable about the issues under study. This method can lead to bias but can be a useful approach when researchers want a sample of experts.

Example of purposive sampling •
Phillips and colleagues (2020) invited two panels of experts to review a draft of an instrument the researchers were developing to assess the connectedness of health care providers of adolescents and young adults (AYAs) with cancer. Purposive samples of five AYAs and six clinical experts were selected.

 HOW-TO-TELL TIP   How can you tell what type of sampling design was used in a quantitative study? If the report does not explicitly mention or describe the sampling design, it is usually safe to assume that a convenience sample was used.

Probability Sampling

Probability sampling involves random selection of elements from a population. With random sampling, each element in the population has an equal, independent chance of being selected. Random selection should not be (although it often is) confused with random assignment, which is a signature of a randomized controlled trial (RCT; see Chapter 8). Random *assignment* to different treatment conditions has no bearing on how participants in the RCT were selected.

The most basic probability sampling is **simple random sampling**. Researchers using simple random sampling often establish a *sampling frame*—a list of population elements. If nursing students at the University of Connecticut were the population, a student roster would be the sampling frame. Elements in a sampling frame are numbered and then a table of random numbers or an online randomizer is used to draw a random sample of the desired size. Samples selected randomly are unlikely to be biased. There is no *guarantee* of a representative sample, but random selection guarantees that differences between the sample and the population are purely a function of chance. The probability of selecting a markedly atypical sample through random sampling is low and decreases as sample size increases.

Example of a simple random sample •
Hughes and colleagues (2020) did a study of 2,000 randomly selected patients who presented with pain as a symptom in a large inner-city emergency department (ED). The researchers examined whether the length of time to the first administration of analgesic medication was related to the patients' length of stay in the ED.

In **stratified random sampling**, the population is first divided into two or more strata, from which elements are randomly selected. As with quota sampling, the aim of stratified sampling is to enhance representativeness.

Example of stratified random sampling •
Gathara and colleagues (2020) studied missed nursing care on newborn units in six hospitals in Nairobi, Kenya. The researchers made direct observations of nursing care for 216 newborns. In each hospital, they randomly sampled 12 shifts, stratified by day/night shift and weekday/weekend shift for the observations.

 TIP   Many large national studies use *multistage sampling*, in which large units are first randomly sampled (e.g., census tracts, hospitals), then smaller units are selected (e.g., individual people). Another type of sampling used by some researchers is *systematic sampling*, which involves the selection of every *k*th person on a list, such as every 10th person. If the first person is chosen at random, systematic sampling is essentially the same as simple random sampling.

Evaluation of Nonprobability and Probability Sampling

Probability sampling is the only viable method of obtaining representative samples. If all elements in a population have an equal chance of being selected, then the resulting sample is likely to do a good job of representing the population. Probability sampling also allows researchers to estimate the magnitude of *sampling error*, which is the difference between population values (e.g., the average age of the population) and sample values (e.g., the average age of the sample).

Nonprobability samples are rarely representative of the population—some segment of the population is likely to be underrepresented. When there is sampling bias, there is a chance that the results could be misleading. Why, then, are nonprobability samples used in most studies? Clearly, the advantage lies in their ease and expediency. Quantitative researchers using nonprobability samples must be cautious about the inferences drawn from the data, and consumers should be alert to possible sampling biases.

 TIP   The quality of the sampling plan is of particular importance when the focus of the research is to obtain descriptive information about prevalence or average values for a population. For quantitative studies whose purpose is primarily description, data from a probability sample would be high on an evidence hierarchy for individual studies.

Sample Size in Quantitative Studies

Sample size—the number of study participants—is a major concern in quantitative research. There is no simple formula to determine how large a sample should be, but larger is usually better than smaller. When researchers calculate a percentage or an average using sample data, the purpose is to estimate a population value, and larger samples have less sampling error.

Researchers can estimate how large their samples should be for testing hypotheses through **power analysis**. An example can illustrate basic principles of power analysis. Suppose we were testing effectiveness of an intervention to help people quit smoking; smokers would be randomized to an intervention group or a control group. How many people should be in the sample? When using power analysis, researchers must estimate how large the group difference will be on a key outcome (e.g., daily number of cigarettes smoked). The estimate is often based on prior research. When differences are expected to be sizeable, a large sample is not needed to reveal group differences statistically; but when small differences are predicted, large samples are necessary. In our example, if a small-to-moderate group difference in postintervention smoking were expected, the sample size needed to test group differences in smoking, with standard statistical criteria, would be about 250 smokers (125 per group).

The risk of "getting it wrong" (i.e., failing to achieve statistical conclusion validity) increases when samples are too small: Researchers risk gathering data that will not support their hypotheses *even when those hypotheses are correct*. Large samples are no assurance of accuracy, though: With nonprobability sampling, even a large sample can harbor bias. A famous illustration of this point is the 1936 U.S. presidential poll conducted by the magazine *Literary Digest*, which predicted that Alfred Landon would defeat Franklin Roosevelt by a landslide. A sample of about 2.5 million people were polled, but biases arose because the sample was drawn from telephone directories and auto registrations during a Depression year when only the well-to-do (who favored Landon) had a car or telephone.

A large sample cannot correct for a faulty sampling design; nevertheless, a large nonprobability sample is better than a small one. When appraising quantitative studies, you must assess both the sample size and the sample selection method to judge how good the sample was.

 TIP The sampling plan is often one of the weakest aspects of quantitative studies. Most nursing studies use samples of convenience, and many are based on small samples that risk disappointing results.

Critical Appraisal of Sampling Plans

In coming to conclusions about the quality of evidence that a study yields, the sampling plan merits special scrutiny. If the sample is seriously biased or too small, the findings may be misleading or just plain wrong.

In appraising the description of a sampling plan, you should consider whether the researcher has adequately explained the sampling strategy. Ideally, research reports should describe the following:

- The type of sampling approach used (e.g., convenience, consecutive, random)
- The population and eligibility criteria for sample selection
- The sample size, with a rationale
- A description of the sample's main characteristics (e.g., age, gender, clinical status, and so on)

A second issue is whether the researcher made good sampling decisions. We have stressed that a key criterion for assessing a sampling plan in quantitative research is whether the sample is representative of the population. You will never know for sure, of course, but if the sampling strategy is weak or if the sample size is small, there is reason to suspect some bias.

Even with a rigorous sampling plan, the sample may be biased if not all people invited to participate in a study agree to do so. If certain subgroups in the population decline to participate, then a biased sample can result, even when probability sampling is used. Research reports ideally should provide information about **response rates** (i.e., the number of people actually participating in a study relative to the number of people sampled) and

---

Box 9.1 Guidelines for Critically Appraising Quantitative Sampling Plans

1. Was the population identified? Were eligibility criteria specified?
2. What type of sampling design was used? Was the sampling plan one that could be expected to yield a representative sample?
3. How many participants were in the sample? Was the sample size affected by high rates of refusals or attrition? Was the sample size large enough to support statistical conclusion validity? Was the sample size justified on the basis of a power analysis or other rationale?
4. Were key characteristics of the sample described (e.g., mean age, percentage of female)?
5. To whom can the study results reasonably be generalized?

---

about possible *nonresponse bias*—differences between participants and those who declined to participate (also sometimes referred to as *response bias*).

Your job as reviewer is to come to conclusions about the reasonableness of generalizing the findings from the researcher's sample to the accessible population and a broader target population. If the sampling plan is flawed, it is risky to generalize the findings at all without replicating the study with another sample. Replication is, in any event, always desirable.

Box 9.1 presents some guiding questions for appraising the sampling plan of a quantitative research report.

DATA COLLECTION IN QUANTITATIVE RESEARCH

Phenomena in which researchers are interested must be translated into data that can be analyzed. This section discusses the challenging task of collecting quantitative research data.

Overview of Data Collection and Data Sources

Data collection methods vary along several dimensions. One issue is whether the researcher collects original data or uses existing data. Existing *records*, for example, are an important data source for nurse researchers. A wealth of clinical data gathered for nonresearch purposes can be fruitfully analyzed to answer research questions.

Example of a study using records •
Davis and coresearchers (2020) studied sociodemographic factors and referral triggers for inclusion in perinatal and neonatal palliative and supportive care programs. Data were collected from the medical records of 135 women enrolled in a newly developed program.

Researchers usually collect new data and must decide the type of data to gather. Three types have been frequently used by nurse researchers: self-reports, observations, and biomarkers. **Self-report** data—also called **patient-reported outcome (PRO)** data—are participants' responses to researchers' questions, such as in an interview. In nursing studies, self-reports are the most common data collection approach. Direct **observation** of people's behaviors and characteristics can be used for certain questions. Nurses also use **biomarkers** (biophysiological measures) to assess important clinical variables.

Regardless of type of data collected in a study, data collection methods vary along several dimensions, including degree of structure, quantifiability, and objectivity. Data for quantitative studies tend to be quantifiable and structured, with the same information gathered from all participants in a comparable, prespecified way. Quantitative researchers generally strive for methods that are as objective as possible.

Self-Reports/Patient-Reported Outcomes

Structured self-report methods are used when researchers know in advance exactly what they need to know and can frame appropriate questions to obtain the desired information. Structured self-report data are collected with a formal, written document—an *instrument*. The instrument is known as an **interview schedule** when the questions are asked orally face-to-face or by telephone and as a **questionnaire** when respondents complete the instrument themselves.

Question Form and Wording

In a totally structured instrument, participants are asked to respond to the same questions in the same order. **Closed-ended questions** are ones in which the **response options** are prespecified. The options may range from a simple yes or no to complex expressions of opinion. Such questions ensure comparability of responses and facilitate analysis. Some examples of closed-ended questions are presented in Table 9.1.

Some structured instruments also include **open-ended questions**, which allow participants to respond to questions in their own words (e.g., Why did you stop smoking?). When open-ended questions are included in questionnaires, respondents must write out their responses. In interviews, the interviewer records responses verbatim.

If participants are verbally expressive and cooperative, open-ended questions provide richer information than closed-ended questions. However, responses to closed-ended questions are easier to analyze, and people may be unwilling to compose lengthy written responses to open-ended questions in questionnaires. A major drawback of closed-ended questions is that researchers might fail to include important responses, and some respondents may object to choosing from alternatives that do not reflect their opinions precisely.

In drafting questions for a structured instrument, researchers must carefully monitor the wording of each question for clarity, absence of bias, and (in questionnaires) reading level. Questions must be sequenced in a psychologically meaningful order that encourages cooperation and candor. Developing, pretesting, and refining a self-report instrument can take months.

TABLE 9.1 Examples of Closed-Ended Questions

Question Type	Example
1. Dichotomous question	Have you ever been pregnant? 1. Yes 2. No
2. Multiple-choice question	How important is it to you to avoid a pregnancy at this time? 1. Extremely important 2. Very important 3. Somewhat important 4. Not important
3. Forced-choice question	Which statement most closely represents your point of view? 1. What happens to me is my own doing. 2. Sometimes I feel I don't have enough control over my life.
4. Rating question	On a scale from 0 to 10, where 0 means "extremely dissatisfied" and 10 means "extremely satisfied," how satisfied were you with the nursing care you received during your hospitalization?

Interviews Versus Questionnaires

Researchers using structured self-reports must decide whether to use interviews or self-administered questionnaires. Questionnaires have the following advantages:

- Questionnaires are less costly and are advantageous for geographically dispersed samples. Internet questionnaires are especially economical and are an increasingly important means of gathering self-report data, although response rates to Internet questionnaires tend to be low.
- Questionnaires offer the possibility of anonymity, which may be crucial in obtaining information about certain opinions or traits.

Example of Internet questionnaires •
Wahlström, Harder, and colleagues (2020) sent a web-based questionnaire to school nurses in Sweden to investigate the nurses' self-assessed cultural competence in health visits with children of foreign origin. Responses were received from 816 nurses.

The strengths of interviews outweigh those of questionnaires. Among the advantages are the following:

- Response rates tend to be high in face-to-face interviews. Respondents are less likely to refuse to talk to an interviewer than to ignore a questionnaire. Low response rates can lead to bias because respondents are rarely a random subset of the original sample. In the web-based survey of school nurses (Wahlström, Harder, et al., 2020), 816 nurses completed the questionnaire out of 3,331 nurses to whom it was sent, a response rate of 24%.
- Some people cannot fill out a questionnaire (e.g., young children). Interviews are feasible with most people.

Some advantages of face-to-face interviews also apply to telephone interviews. Long or complex instruments are not well suited to telephone administration, but for relatively brief instruments, telephone interviews combine relatively low costs with high response rates.

Example of telephone interviews •
Craswell and Dwyer (2019) collected data regarding people's reasons for choosing or refusing care from a nurse practitioner by means of telephone calls to randomly selected Australian households (both landlines and mobile phones). Up to five callbacks were made if the phone was not answered.

Summated Rating Scales

Psychosocial scales are often incorporated into self-report instruments. A **scale** is a device that assigns a numeric score to people along a continuum, like a scale for measuring weight. Psychosocial scales are used to measure attitudes, perceptions, and psychological traits such as anxiety or depression.

One technique is the **Likert scale**, which traditionally consists of several declarative statements (*items*) that express a viewpoint on a topic. Respondents are asked to indicate how much they agree or disagree with the statement. Table 9.2 presents a six-item Likert scale for measuring attitudes toward condom use. In this example, agreement with positively worded statements is assigned a higher score. The first statement is positively worded; agreement indicates a favorable attitude toward condom use. Because there are five response alternatives, a score of 5 would be given for *strongly agree*, 4 for *agree*, and so on. Responses of two

TABLE 9.2 Example of a Likert Scale to Measure Attitudes Toward Using Condoms

Direction of Scoring*	Item	Responses†					Score	
		SA	A	?	D	SD	Person 1 (✓)	Person 2 (X)
+	1. Using a condom shows you care about your partner.		✓			X	4	1
−	2. My partner would be angry if I talked about using condoms.			X		✓	5	3
−	3. I wouldn't enjoy sex as much if my partner and I used condoms.			X	✓		4	2
+	4. Condoms are a good protection against AIDS and other sexually transmitted diseases.				✓	X	3	2
+	5. My partner would respect me if I insisted on using condoms.	✓				X	5	1
−	6. I would be too embarrassed to ask my partner about using a condom.			X		✓	5	2
	Total score						26	11

*Researchers would not indicate the direction of scoring on a Likert scale administered to participants. The scoring direction is indicated in this table for illustrative purposes only.
†SA, strongly agree; A, agree; ?, uncertain; D, disagree; SD, strongly disagree.

hypothetical participants are shown by a check or an X, and their item scores are shown in the right-hand columns. Person 1, who agreed with the first statement, has a score of 4, whereas person 2, who strongly disagreed, got a score of 1. The second statement is negatively worded, and so scoring is reversed—a score of 1 is assigned for *strongly agree*, and so forth. *Item reversals* ensure that a high score consistently reflects positive attitudes toward condom use.

A person's total score is the sum of item scores—hence, such scales are often called **summated rating scales** or *composite scales*. In our example, person 1 has a more positive attitude toward condoms (total score = 26) than person 2 (total score = 11). Summing item scores makes it possible to finely discriminate among people with different opinions. Composite scales are often composed of two or more *subscales* that measure different aspects of a construct. Developing high-quality scales requires a lot of skill and effort.

 TIP Summated rating scales can be used to measure a wide array of attributes. The bipolar scale is not always on an agree/disagree continuum—it might be always/never, likely/unlikely, and so on.

Example of a summated rating scale •
Fortney and colleagues (2020) studied neonatal nurses' perceptions of infant well-being in relation to their own self-reported distress, using scales created by the study team. For example, one scale measured perceived infant suffering with item response options on a 5-point scale ranging from 0 = "Not at all" to 4 = "Very much." Perceived infant quality of life was measured with a scale that had item response options ranging from 0 = "Poor" to 4 = "Excellent."

Scales permit researchers to efficiently quantify subtle gradations in the intensity of individual characteristics. Scales can be administered either verbally or in writing and so can be used with most people. Scales are susceptible to several common problems, however, referred to as **response set biases**, which include the following:

- *Social desirability response set bias*—a tendency to misrepresent oneself by giving answers that are consistent with prevailing social views
- *Extreme response set bias*—a tendency to consistently select extreme alternatives (e.g., strongly agree), leading to distortions if the extreme responses reflect a personality trait and not intense feelings about the phenomenon under study
- *Acquiescence response set bias*—a tendency of some people to agree with statements regardless of their content (*yea-sayers*). The opposite tendency for other people to disagree with statements independently of the question content (*naysayers*) is less common.

Researchers can reduce these biases by developing sensitively worded questions, creating a nonjudgmental atmosphere, and guaranteeing the confidentiality of responses.

 TIP   Other self-report approaches include vignettes, visual analog scales, and Q-sorts. *Vignettes* are brief descriptions of situations to which respondents are asked to react. *Visual analog scales* are used to measure subjective experiences (e.g., fatigue) on a bipolar continuum. *Q sorts* present participants with a set of cards on which statements are written. Participants are asked to sort the cards along a specified dimension, such as most helpful/least helpful. These three approaches are described in the chapter supplement on thePoint® website.

Evaluation of Self-Report Methods

If researchers want to know how people feel or what they believe, the most direct approach is to ask them. Self-reports frequently yield information that would be difficult or impossible to gather by other means. Behaviors can be *observed* but only if people are willing to engage in them publicly—and engage in them at the time of data collection.

Nevertheless, self-reports have some weaknesses. The most serious issue concerns the validity and accuracy of self-reports: How can we be sure that participants feel or act the way they say they do? Investigators usually have no choice but to assume that most respondents have been frank. Yet, we all have a tendency to present ourselves in the best light, and this may conflict with the truth. When reading research reports, you should be alert to potential biases in self-reported data.

Observational Methods

For some research questions, direct observation of people's behavior is an alternative to self-reports, especially in clinical settings. **Observational methods** can be used to gather such information as patients' conditions (e.g., their sleep–wake state), verbal communication (e.g., exchange of information at discharge), nonverbal communication (e.g., body language), activities (e.g., geriatric patients' self-grooming activities), and environmental conditions (e.g., noise levels).

In studies that use observation, researchers have flexibility on several dimensions. For example, the focus of the observation can be on broadly defined events (e.g., patient mood swings) or on small, specific behaviors (e.g., facial expressions). Observations can be made through the human senses and then recorded manually, but they can also be done with equipment such as video recorders.

TIP Researchers often use structured observations when participants cannot be asked questions or cannot be expected to provide reliable answers. Many observational instruments are designed to capture the behaviors of infants, children, or people whose communication skills are impaired.

Structured observation involves the use of formal instruments and protocols that dictate what to observe, how long to observe it, and how to record the data. Structured observation is not intended to capture a broad slice of life but rather to document specific behaviors, actions, and events. Structured observation requires the formulation of a system for accurately categorizing, recording, and encoding the observations.

Methods of Structured Observation

The most common approach to making structured observations is to use a category system for classifying observed phenomena. A **category system** represents a method of recording in a systematic fashion the behaviors and events of interest that transpire within a setting.

Some category systems require that *all* observed behaviors in a specified domain (e.g., body positions) be classified. A contrasting technique is a system in which only particular types of behavior (which may or may not occur) are categorized. For example, if we were studying children's aggressive behavior, we might develop such categories as "strikes another child" or "throws objects." In this category system, many behaviors—all that are nonaggressive—would not be classified; some children may exhibit *no* aggressive actions.

> **Example of nonexhaustive categories for observation** •
> Abraham and colleagues (2019) used an experimental design to test the effectiveness of an intervention to prevent the use of physical restraints in nursing homes. The use of physical restraints was measured using an observational checklist that listed various types of physical restraint (e.g., use of a belt in a chair, restrictive bed rails). Observers, who were blinded to treatment group, made observations twice a day.

Category systems must have careful, explicit definitions of the behaviors and characteristics to be observed. Each category must be explained, and observers must be given clearcut criteria for assessing the occurrence of the phenomenon.

Category systems are the basis for constructing a **checklist**—the instrument observers use to record observations. The checklist is usually formatted with a list of behaviors from the category system on the left and space for tallying the frequency or duration on the right. Observers using an exhaustive category system must place *all* observed behaviors in one category for each "unit" of behavior (e.g., a time interval). With nonexhaustive category systems, categories of behaviors that may or may not be manifested are listed. The observer watches for instances of these behaviors and records their occurrence.

Another approach to structured observations is to use a **rating scale**, an instrument that requires observers to rate phenomena along a continuum. The observer may be required to make ratings at intervals throughout the observation or to summarize an entire episode after observation is completed.

> **Example of observational ratings** •
> Rasheed and coresearchers (2019) compared the utility of two observational scales to measure patient agitation. The scale that they found to have better properties was the Richmond Agitation-Sedation Scale, which requires ratings on a 10-point scale, from +4 (combative) to −5 (unarousable).

Observational Sampling

Researchers must decide when, and for how long, structured observations will be undertaken. Observational sampling methods are a means of obtaining representative examples of the behaviors being observed. One system is *time sampling*, which involves selecting time periods during which observations will occur. Time frames may be selected systematically (e.g., for 30 seconds at 5-minute intervals) or at random.

With *event sampling*, researchers select integral events to observe. Event sampling requires researchers to either know when events will occur (e.g., nursing shift changes) or wait for their occurrence. Event sampling is a good choice when events of interest are infrequent and may be missed if time sampling is used. When behaviors and events are frequent, however, time sampling enhances the representativeness of the observed behaviors.

Example of observational sampling •
Park and colleagues (2020) studied preterm infants' sleep–wake state trajectories in relation to feeding progression during the infants' hospitalization. For 3 weeks, observations of sleep–wake behaviors were made during 2-hour interfeeding periods twice a day—nighttime and daytime. During the observations, sleep and wake states were recorded every 10 seconds.

Evaluation of Observational Methods

Certain research questions are better suited to observation than to self-reports, such as when people cannot describe their own behaviors. This may be the case when people are unaware of their behavior (e.g., stress-induced behavior), when behaviors are emotionally laden (e.g., grieving), or when people are not capable of reporting their actions (e.g., young children). Observational methods have an intrinsic appeal for directly capturing behaviors. Nurses are often in a position to watch people's behaviors and may, by training, be especially sensitive observers.

Shortcomings of observational methods include possible *reactivity* (behavioral distortions resulting from being observed) when the observer is conspicuous and the vulnerability of observations to bias. For example, the observer's values and prejudices may lead to faulty inference. Observational biases probably cannot be eliminated, but they can be minimized by training and monitoring observers.

Biomarkers

Nurse researchers have used biomarkers (**biophysiological measures**) for a wide variety of purposes. Examples include studies of basic biophysiological processes, explorations of the ways in which nursing actions and interventions affect physiological outcomes, product assessments, studies to evaluate the accuracy of biophysiological information gathered by nurses, and studies of the correlates of physiological functioning in patients with health problems.

Both *in vivo* and *in vitro* measurements are used in research. *In vivo* measurements are those performed directly within or on living organisms, such as blood pressure and body temperature measurement. Technological advances continue to improve the ability to measure biophysiological phenomena accurately and conveniently. With *in vitro* measures, data are gathered from participants by extracting biophysiological material from them and subjecting it to laboratory analysis. *In vitro* measures include chemical measures (e.g., hormone levels), microbiological measures (e.g., bacterial counts and identification), and cytological or histological measures (e.g., tissue biopsies). Recently, there has been a growing interest among nurse researchers about microbiomes, especially gut microbiomes. Nurse researchers also use *anthropomorphic measures*, such as the body mass index and waist circumference.

Example of a study with in vivo and in vitro measures • • • • • • • • • • • • • • • • • •
Wahlström, Rosenqvist, and colleagues (2020) studied the effectiveness of a self-management therapeutic yoga program for patients with paroxysmal atrial fibrillation. The researchers measured heart rate, blood pressure, and N-terminal pro b-type natriuretic peptide at baseline and 12 weeks after the start of the intervention.

Biomarkers are relatively accurate and precise, especially compared to psychological measures, such as self-report measures of anxiety or pain. Biophysiological measures are also objective. Two nurses reading from the same spirometer output are likely to record identical tidal volume measurements, and two spirometers are likely to produce the same readouts. Patients cannot easily distort measurements of biophysiological functioning. Finally, biophysiological instruments provide valid measures of targeted variables: Thermometers can be relied on to measure temperature and not blood volume, and so forth. For nonbiophysiological measures, there are often concerns about whether an instrument is really measuring the target concept.

Data Quality in Quantitative Research

In developing a data collection plan, researchers must strive for the highest possible quality data. One aspect of data quality concerns the procedures used to collect the data. For example, the people who collect and record the data must be properly trained to ensure that procedures are diligently followed. Another aspect concerns the circumstances of data collection. For example, it is important to ensure privacy and to create an atmosphere that encourages participant candor.

A crucial issue for data quality concerns the adequacy of the *measures* used to operationalize constructs. **Measurement** involves assigning numbers to represent the amount of an attribute present in a person or object. When a new measure of a construct (e.g., anxiety) is developed, rules for assigning numerical values (*scores*) need to be established. Then, the rules must be evaluated to see if they are good rules—they must yield numbers that accurately correspond to different amounts of the targeted trait.

Measures that are not perfectly accurate yield measurements that contain some error. Many factors contribute to *measurement error*, including personal states (e.g., fatigue), response set biases, and situational factors (e.g., temperature). In self-report measures, measurement errors can result from question wording.

Careful researchers select measures that are known to be psychometrically sound. *Psychometrics* is the branch of psychology concerned with the theory and methods of measurements of psychosocial phenomena, such as depression, pain, or anxiety. When a new measure is developed, the developers undertake a **psychometric assessment**, which involves an evaluation of the measure's **measurement properties**.

Psychometricians (and most nurse researchers) have traditionally focused on two measurement properties when assessing the quality of a measure: reliability and validity. In recent years, measurement experts in medicine have advocated attending to additional measurement properties that concern the measurement of change (Polit & Yang, 2016). Here, we describe the two properties that you are most likely to encounter in reading articles in the nursing literature. Methods used to assess these properties are briefly described in the chapter on statistical analysis (see Chapter 13).

Reliability

Reliability, broadly speaking, is the extent to which scores are free from measurement error. Reliability can also be defined as the extent to which scores for people *who have not changed* are the same for repeated measurements. In other words, reliability concerns consistency—the *absence* of variation—in measuring a stable attribute. In all types of assessments, reliability involves a *replication* to evaluate the extent to which scores for a stable trait are the same.

In **test–retest reliability**, replication takes the form of administering a measure to the same people on two occasions (e.g., 1 week apart). The assumption is that for traits that have not changed, any differences in people's scores on the two testings are the result of measurement error. When score differences across waves are small, reliability is high. Except for highly volatile constructs (e.g., mood), test–retest reliability can be assessed for most measures, including biophysiological ones.

When measurements involve people who make scoring judgments, a key source of measurement error stems from the person making the measurements. This is the situation for observational measures (e.g., ratings of agitation) and for some biophysiological measurements (e.g., skinfold measurement). In such situations, it is important to evaluate how reliably the measurements reflect attributes of the person being rated rather than attributes of the raters. The most typical approach is to undertake an **interrater** (or *interobserver*) **reliability** assessment, which involves having two or more observers independently applying the measure with the same people to see if the scores are consistent across raters.

Another aspect of reliability is **internal consistency**. In responding to a self-report item, people are influenced not only by the underlying construct but also by idiosyncratic reactions to item wording. By combining multiple items with various wordings, item irrelevancies are expected to cancel each other out. An instrument is said to be internally consistent to the extent that its items measure the same trait. For internal consistency, replication involves people's responses to multiple items during a single administration. Whereas other reliability estimates assess a measure's degree of consistency across time or raters, internal consistency captures consistency across items.

As we explain in Chapter 13, assessments of reliability yield coefficients that summarize how reliable a measure is. *Reliability coefficients* range in value from .00 to 1.00, with higher values being desirable. Coefficients of .80 or higher usually are considered acceptable. Researchers should select instruments with demonstrated reliability and should document this in their reports. Researchers undertaking a study often compute internal consistency reliability coefficients with their own data.

> **Example of internal consistency reliability** •
> Oh and Cho (2020) studied changes in fatigue and psychological outcomes after chemotherapy in women with breast cancer. They chose an existing measure of fatigue that had high internal consistency (.93). In their own sample of 50 women, internal consistency was .89.

Validity

Validity in a measurement context is the degree to which an instrument is measuring the construct it purports to measure. When researchers develop a scale to measure *resilience*, they need to be sure that the resulting scores validly reflect this construct and not something else, such as self-efficacy or perseverance. Assessing the validity of abstract constructs requires a careful conceptualization of the construct—as well as a conceptualization of what the construct is *not*. Like reliability, measurement validity has different aspects: face validity, content validity, criterion validity, and construct validity.

Face validity refers to whether the instrument *looks* like it is measuring the target construct. Although face validity is not considered good evidence of validity, it is helpful for a measure to have face validity. If patients' resistance to being measured reflects the view that the scale is not relevant to their problems or situations, then face validity is an issue.

Content validity may be defined as the extent to which an instrument's content adequately captures the construct—that is, whether a composite instrument (e.g., a multi-item scale) has an appropriate sample of items for the construct being measured. Content validity is assessed by having a panel of experts rate the scale items for relevance to the construct and comment on the need for revisions.

Criterion validity is the extent to which the scores on a measure are a good reflection of a "gold standard"—i.e., a criterion considered an ideal measure of the construct. Not all measures can be validated using a criterion approach because there is not always a "gold standard" criterion. As an example, scores on a self-report scale to measure stress could be compared to wake-up salivary free cortisol levels (a *concurrent* criterion). Screening scales are often tested against some future criterion—namely, the occurrence of the phenomenon for which a screening tool is sought (e.g., a patient fall). This is called *predictive validity*.

For many abstract, unobservable human attributes (constructs), no gold standard criterion exists, and so other validation avenues must be pursued. **Construct validity** is the degree to which evidence about a measure's scores in relation to other variables supports the inference that the construct has been well represented. Construct validity typically involves hypothesis testing, which follow a similar path: Hypotheses are developed about a relationship between scores on the focal measure and values on other constructs, data are collected to test the hypotheses, and then validity conclusions are reached based on the results of the hypothesis tests.

One approach to construct validity is called *known-groups validity*, which tests hypotheses about a measure's ability to discriminate between two or more groups known (or expected) to differ with regard to the construct of interest. For instance, in validating a measure of anxiety about the labor experience, the scores of primiparas and multiparas could be contrasted. Evidence suggests that, on average, women who have never given birth experience more anxiety than women who already have children; one might question the validity of the instrument if such differences did not emerge.

Example of known-groups validity •
Pados and colleagues (2019) evaluated the validity of the Neonatal Assessment Tool—a parent-report assessment measure. As hypothesized, infants with feeding problems scored significantly higher on the scale measuring problematic feeding symptoms than infants without feeding problems.

 TIP   Another aspect of construct validity is called cross-cultural validity, which is relevant for measures that have been translated or adapted for use with a different cultural group than that for the original instrument. *Cross-cultural validity* is the degree to which the components (e.g., items) of a translated or culturally adapted measure perform adequately and equivalently relative to their performance on the original instrument.

An instrument does not possess or lack validity; it is a question of degree. An instrument's validity is not proved, demonstrated, or verified but rather is supported to a greater or lesser extent by evidence. Researchers strive to select measures for which good validity information is available.

Critical Appraisal of Data Collection Methods

The goal of a data collection plan is to produce data that are of excellent quality. Decisions that researchers make about their data collection methods and procedures can affect data quality and hence the quality of the study.

Box 9.2 Guidelines for Critically Appraising Quantitative Data Collection Plans

1. Did the researchers use the best method of capturing study phenomena (i.e., self-reports, observation, biomarkers)?
2. If self-report methods were used, did the researchers make good decisions about the specific methods used to solicit information (e.g., in-person interviews, Internet questionnaires, and so on)? Were composite scales used? If not, should they have been?
3. If observational methods were used, did the report adequately describe what the observations entailed and how observations were sampled? Were risks of observational bias addressed? Were biomarkers used in the study, and was this appropriate?
4. Did the report provide adequate information about data collection procedures (e.g., the training of the data collectors)?
5. Did the report offer evidence of the reliability of measures? Did the evidence come from the research sample itself, or was it based on other studies? If reliability was reported, which estimation method was used? Was the reliability sufficiently high?
6. Did the report offer evidence of the validity of the measures? If validity information was reported, which validity approach was used?
7. If there was no reliability or validity information, what conclusion can you reach about the quality of the data in the study?

It may, however, be difficult to critically appraise data collection methods in studies reported in journals because researchers' descriptions are seldom detailed. However, researchers do have a responsibility to communicate basic information about their approach so that readers can assess the quality of evidence that the study yields.

Information about data quality (reliability and validity of the measures) should be provided in quantitative research reports. Ideally—especially for composite scales—the report should provide internal consistency coefficients based on data from the study itself, not just from previous research. Interrater or interobserver reliability is especially crucial for assessing data quality in studies that use observational methods. The values of the reliability coefficients should be sufficiently high to support confidence in the findings.

Validity is more difficult to document than reliability. At a minimum, researchers should defend their choice of existing measures based on validity information from the developers, and they should cite the relevant publication. Guidelines for appraising data collection methods are presented in Box 9.2.

RESEARCH EXAMPLES WITH CRITICAL THINKING EXERCISES

In this section, we describe the sampling and data collection plan of a quantitative nursing study. Read the summary and then answer the critical thinking questions that follow, referring to the full research report if necessary. Answers to the questions for Exercise 1 are available to instructors on thePoint˙. The critical thinking questions for Exercise 2 are based on the study that appears in its entirety in Appendix A of this book. Our comments for these exercises are in the Student Resources section on thePoint˙.

EXAMPLE 1: SAMPLING AND DATA COLLECTION IN A QUANTITATIVE STUDY

Study: Integration of different sensory interventions from mother's breast milk for preterm infant pain during peripheral venipuncture procedures (Wu et al., 2020)

Statement of Purpose: The purpose of the study was to compare the effects of integrating mother's breast milk with three different combinations of sensory stimuli on preterm infant pain during peripheral venipuncture procedures.

Design and Treatment Conditions: The researchers used a randomized design with four treatment conditions: (1) usual care (the control group), (2) breast milk odor or taste, (3) breast milk odor or taste + mothers' heartbeat sounds, and (4) breast milk odor or taste + heartbeat sounds + nonnutritive sucking. For those in the three intervention groups, breast milk odor was placed around the infants' nose, and 2 mL of breast milk was provided 2 minutes before the venipuncture.

Sampling: The inclusion criteria for infants in the study were gestational age of 28 to 37 weeks, postnatal age of 3 to 28 days, scheduled to receive a venipuncture, no opioids within 24 hours prior to venipuncture, and in stable condition (based on an illness severity or Apgar score). Infants were excluded if they had a condition that might influence their response to pain. A total of 225 preterm infants were sampled by convenience and screened for eligibility in a medical center in Taiwan; 198 met the inclusion criteria, but not all parents consented to have their infants participate in the study. A final sample of 140 infants was randomly assigned to one of the four treatment conditions by a statistician. The researchers had undertaken a power analysis that estimated that a sample of 127 infants would meet standard criteria for statistical conclusion validity. There was no attrition from the study.

Data Collection: Information about the infants' baseline characteristics (e.g., birth weight, Apgar scores) was obtained from medical charts. Infant pain was measured with a scale (the Premature Infant Pain Profile-Revised, PIPP-R) that combined physiological information (heart rate and oxygen saturation) with information gathered through observations of the infants' behavior as captured on videotapes (e.g., brow bulge, eye squeeze). A trained research assistant who scored the observational items was blinded to group assignment. Infant pain was measured at 1-minute intervals during the videotaped venipuncture procedures, which were divided into phases (baseline, disinfection, puncture, and recovery). Interrater reliability in scoring the PIPP-R was high.

Key Findings: The four groups of infants were comparable in terms of such characteristics as gestational age, birth weight, Apgar scores, and baseline pain scores. Infants who received treatment no. 4 had significantly lower increases in pain scores compared to those in the control group across all postbaseline phases. Those receiving treatments no. 2 or no. 3 had significant reductions in pain during the disinfecting and recovery phases compared to controls.

Critical Thinking Exercises

1. Answer the relevant questions from Box 9.1 regarding this study.
2. Answer the relevant questions from Box 9.2 regarding this study.
3. Are there variables in this study that could have been measured through self-report but were not?
4. If the results of this study are valid and reliable, what might be some of the uses to which the findings could be put in clinical practice?

EXAMPLE 2: SAMPLING AND DATA COLLECTION IN THE STUDY IN APPENDIX A

Read the method section of Swenson and colleagues' study ("Parents' use of praise and criticism in a sample of young children seeking mental health services") in Appendix A of this book.

1. Answer the relevant questions from Box 9.1 regarding this study.
2. Answer the relevant questions from Box 9.2 regarding this study.

WANT TO KNOW MORE?

A wide variety of resources to enhance your learning and understanding of this chapter is available on thePoint®.

- Chapter Supplement on Vignettes, Q Sorts, and Visual Analog Scales
- Answers to the Critical Thinking Exercises for Example 2
- Internet Resources with useful websites for Chapter 9
- A Wolters Kluwer journal article on a topic related to this chapter

Additional study aids, including eight journal articles and related questions, are also available in *Study Guide for Essentials of Nursing Research, 10e.*

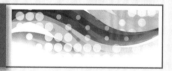

Summary Points

- **Sampling** is the process of selecting elements from a **population**, which is an entire aggregate. An *element* is the basic unit of a population—usually humans in nursing research.

- **Eligibility criteria** (including both *inclusion criteria* and *exclusion criteria*) are used to define population characteristics.

- A key criterion in assessing a sample in a quantitative study is its *representativeness*—the extent to which the sample is similar to the population and avoids bias. **Sampling bias** is the systematic overrepresentation or underrepresentation of some segment of the population.

- **Nonprobability sampling** (in which elements are selected by nonrandom methods) includes convenience, quota, consecutive, and purposive sampling. Nonprobability sampling is convenient and economical; a major disadvantage is its potential for bias.

- **Convenience sampling** uses the most readily available or convenient people.

- **Quota sampling** divides the population into homogeneous **strata** (subpopulations) to ensure representation of the subgroups in the sample; within each stratum, people are sampled by convenience.

- **Consecutive sampling** involves taking *all* of the people from an accessible population who meet the eligibility criteria over a specific time interval or for a specified sample size.

- In **purposive sampling**, participants are handpicked to be included in the sample based on the researcher's knowledge about the population.

- **Probability sampling** designs, which involve the random selection of elements from the population, yield more representative samples than nonprobability designs and permit estimates of the magnitude of *sampling error*.

- **Simple random sampling** involves the random selection of elements from a *sampling frame* that enumerates all the elements; **stratified random sampling** divides the population into homogeneous subgroups from which elements are selected at random.

- In quantitative studies, researchers can use a **power analysis** to estimate **sample size** needs. Large samples are preferable because they enhance statistical conclusion validity and tend to be more representative, but large samples do not *guarantee* representativeness.

- The three principal data collection methods for nurse researchers are self-reports, observations, and biomarkers.

- **Self-reports**, which are also called **patient-reported outcomes** or PROs, involve directly questioning study participants and are the most widely used method of collecting data for nursing studies.

- Structured self-reports for quantitative studies involve a formal **instrument**—a **questionnaire** or **interview schedule**—that may contain **open-ended questions** (which permit respondents to respond in their own words) and multiple **closed-ended questions** (which offer respondents **response options** from which to choose).

- Questionnaires are less costly than interviews and offer the possibility of anonymity, but interviews yield higher response rates and are suitable for a wider variety of people.

- Social psychological **scales** are self-report instruments for measuring such characteristics as attitudes and psychological attributes. **Summated rating scales** such as **Likert scales** present respondents with a series of *items*; each item is scored on a continuum (e.g., from strongly agree to strongly disagree) and then summed into a composite score.

- Scales are versatile and powerful but are susceptible to **response set biases**—the tendency of some people to respond to items in characteristic ways, independently of item content.

- **Observational methods** are techniques for acquiring data through the direct observation of phenomena.

- Structured observations dictate what the observer should observe; they often involve **checklists**—instruments based on **category systems** for recording the appearance, frequency, or duration of behaviors or events. Observers may also use **rating scales** to rate phenomena along a dimension of interest (e.g., lethargic/energetic).

- Structured observations often involve a sampling plan (such as *time sampling* or *event sampling*) for selecting the behaviors, events, and conditions to be observed. When observers are conspicuous, *reactivity* (behavioral distortions) can affect data quality.

- Data may also be derived from biophysiological measures (**biomarkers**), which include *in vivo* measurements (those performed within or on living organisms) and *in vitro* measurements (those performed outside the organism's body, such as blood tests). Biomarkers have the advantage of being objective, accurate, and precise.

- In quantitative studies, variables are measured. **Measurement** involves assigning numbers to represent the amount of an attribute present in a person, using a set of rules; researchers strive to use measures that have good rules that minimize *measurement error*.

- *Measures* (and the quality of the data that the measures yield) can be evaluated in a **psychometric assessment** in terms of several **measurement properties**, most often reliability and validity.

- **Reliability** is the extent to which scores for people *who have not changed* are the same for repeated measurements. A reliable measure minimizes measurement error.

- Methods of assessing reliability include **test–retest reliability** (administering a measure twice in a short period to see if the measure yields consistent scores), **interrater reliability** (assessing whether two raters or observers independently assign similar scores), and **internal consistency** (assessing whether there is consistency across items in a composite scale in measuring a trait).

- Reliability is assessed statistically by computing coefficients that range from .00 to 1.00; higher values indicate greater reliability.

- **Validity** is the degree to which an instrument measures what it is supposed to measure.

- Aspects of validity include **face validity** (the extent to which a measure looks like it is measuring the target construct), **content validity** (in composite scales, the extent to which an instrument's content adequately captures the construct), **criterion validity** (the extent to which scores on a measure are a good reflection of a "gold standard"), and **construct validity** (the extent to which an instrument adequately measures the targeted construct, as assessed mainly by testing hypotheses).

- A measure's validity is not proved or established but rather is supported to a greater or lesser extent by evidence.

REFERENCES FOR CHAPTER 9

Abraham, J., Kupfer, R., Behncke, A., Berger-Höger, B., Icks, A., Haastert, B., . . . Möhler, R. (2019). Implementation of a multicomponent intervention to prevent physical restraints in nursing homes (IMPRINT): A pragmatic cluster randomized controlled trial. *International Journal of Nursing Studies*, 96, 27–34.

Becker, H., Stuifbergen, A., Zhang, W., & Sales, A. (2020). Moderator effects in intervention studies. *Nursing Research*, 69, 62–68.

*Cheung, D., Ho, K., Cheung, T., Lam, S., & Tse, M. (2018). Anticipatory grief of spousal and adult children caregivers of people with dementia. *BMC Palliative Care*, 17, 124.

Craswell, A., & Dwyer, T. (2019). Reasons for choosing or refusing care from a nurse practitioner: Results from a national population-based survey. *Journal of Advanced Nursing*, 75, 3668–3676.

Davis, S., Harmon, C., Baker Urquhart, B., Moore, B., & Sprague, R. (2020). Women and infants in the Deep South receiving perinatal and neonatal palliative and supportive care services. *Advances in Neonatal Care*, 20, 216–222.

**Fortney, C., Pratt, M., Dunnells, Z., Rausch, J., Clark, O., Baughcum, A., & Gerhardt, C. (2020). Perceived infant well-being and self-reported distress in neonatal nurses. *Nursing Research*, 69, 127–132.

*Gathara, D., Serem, G., Murphy, G., Obengo, A., Tallam, E., Jackson, D., . . . English, M. (2020). Missed nursing care in newborn units: A cross-sectional direct observational study. *BMJ Quality & Safety*, 29, 19–30.

Hughes, J., Brown, N., Chiu, J., Allwood, B., & Chu, K. (2020). The relationship between time to analgesic administration and emergency department length of stay: A retrospective review. *Journal of Advanced Nursing*, 76, 183–190.

Lee, M., Park, S., & Choi, G. (2020). Association of self-leadership and planning with performing an exercise in patients with colorectal cancer: Cross-sectional study. *Cancer Nursing*, 43, E1–E9.

Oh, P., & Cho, J. (2020). Changes in fatigue, psychological distress, and quality of life after chemotherapy in women with breast cancer: A prospective study. *Cancer Nursing*, 43, E54–E60.

*Pados, B., Thoyre, S., & Galer, K. (2019). Neonatal Eating Assessment Tool—Mixed breastfeeding and bottle-feeding (NeoEAT—mixed feeding): Factor analysis and psychometric properties. *Maternal Health, Neonatology, and Perinatology*, 5, 12.

Park, J., Silva, S., Thoyre, S., & Brandon, D. (2020). Sleep-wake states and feeding progression in preterm infants. *Nursing Research*, 69, 22–30.

Phillips, C., Haase, J., & Bakoyannis, G. (2020). Development and psychometric evaluation of the Connectedness with Health Care Providers Scale for adolescents and young adults with cancer. *Journal of Adolescent and Young Adult Oncology*, 9, 271–277.

Polit, D. F., & Yang, F. M. (2016). *Measurement and the measurement of change: A primer for health professionals*. Philadelphia, PA: Lippincott.

Rasheed, A., Amirah, M., Abdallah, M., Parameaswari, P. J., Issa, M., & Alharthy, A. (2019). Ramsay Sedation Scale and Richmond Agitation Sedation Scale: A cross-sectional study. *Dimensions of Critical Care Nursing*, 38, 90–95.

Wahlström, E., Harder, M., Granlund, M., Holmström, I., Larm, P., & Golsäter, M. (2020). School nurses' self-assessed cultural competence when encountering children of foreign origin: A cross-sectional study. *Nursing & Health Sciences*, 22, 226–234.

Wahlström, M., Rosenqvist, M., Medin, J., Walfridsson, U., & Rydell-Karlsson, M. (2020). MediYoga as a part of a self-management programme among patients with paroxysmal atrial fibrillation—A randomised study. *European Journal of Cardiovascular Nursing*, 19, 74–82.

Wu, H., Yin, T., Hsieh, K., Lan, H., Feng, R., Chang, Y., & Liaw, J. (2020). Integration of different sensory interventions from mother's breast milk for preterm infant pain during peripheral venipuncture procedures: A prospective randomized controlled trial. *Journal of Nursing Scholarship*, 52, 75–84.

Zhang, X., Qiu, C., Zheng, Y., Zang, X., & Zhao, Y. (2020). Self-management among elderly patients with hypertension and its association with individual and social environmental factors in China. *The Journal of Cardiovascular Nursing*, 35, 45–53.

*A link to this open-access article is provided in the Internet Resources section on thePoint® website.

**This journal article is available on thePoint® for this chapter.

10 Appraising Qualitative Designs and Approaches

Learning Objectives

On completing this chapter, you will be able to:

- Discuss the rationale for an emergent design in qualitative research and describe qualitative design features
- Identify the major research traditions for qualitative research and describe the domain of inquiry of each
- Describe the main features and methods associated with ethnographic, phenomenological, and grounded theory studies
- Describe key features of case studies, narrative analyses, and descriptive qualitative studies
- Discuss the goals and features of research with ideological perspectives
- Define new terms in the chapter

Key Terms

- Basic social process (BSP)
- Bracketing
- Case study
- Constant comparison
- Constructivist grounded theory
- Core variable
- Critical ethnography
- Critical theory
- Descriptive phenomenology
- Descriptive qualitative study
- Emergent design
- Ethnonursing research
- Feminist research
- Grounded theory
- Hermeneutics
- Interpretive phenomenology
- Narrative analysis
- Participant observation
- Participatory action research (PAR)
- Reflexive journal

THE DESIGN OF QUALITATIVE STUDIES

Quantitative researchers develop a research design before collecting their data and rarely depart from that design once the study is underway: They design and *then* they do. In qualitative research, by contrast, the study design often evolves during the project: Qualitative researchers design *as* they do. Qualitative studies use an **emergent design** that evolves as researchers make ongoing decisions about their data needs based on what they have already learned. An emergent design supports the researchers' desire to have the inquiry reflect the realities and viewpoints of those under study—realities and viewpoints that are not known at the outset.

Characteristics of Qualitative Research Design

Qualitative inquiry has been guided by different disciplines with distinct methods and approaches. Some characteristics of qualitative research design are broadly applicable, however. In general, qualitative design

- Is flexible, capable of adjusting to what is learned during data collection
- Benefits from ongoing data analysis to guide subsequent strategies
- Often involves triangulating various data sources
- Tends to be holistic, aimed at understanding the whole
- Requires researchers to become intensely involved and reflexive

Although design decisions are not finalized beforehand, qualitative researchers typically do advance planning that supports their flexibility. For example, qualitative researchers make advance decisions with regard to the study site, a broad data collection strategy, and the equipment they will need in the field. Qualitative researchers plan for a variety of circumstances, but decisions about how to deal with them are resolved when the social context is better understood.

Qualitative Design Features

Some of the design features discussed in Chapter 8 apply to qualitative studies. To contrast qualitative and quantitative research design, we consider the elements identified in Table 8.1.

Intervention, Control, and Blinding

Qualitative research is almost always nonexperimental—although a qualitative component may be embedded in an experiment (see Chapter 12). Qualitative researchers do not conceptualize their studies as having independent and dependent variables and rarely control the people or environment under study. Blinding is rarely used by qualitative researchers. The goal is to develop a rich understanding of a phenomenon as it exists and as it is constructed by individuals within their own context.

Comparisons

Qualitative researchers typically do not plan to make group comparisons because the intent is to thoroughly describe or explain a phenomenon. Yet, patterns emerging in the data sometimes suggest illuminating comparisons. Indeed, as Morse (2004) noted in an editorial in *Qualitative Health Research*, "All description requires comparisons" (p. 1323). In analyzing qualitative data and in determining whether categories are saturated, there is a need to compare "this" to "that."

Example of qualitative comparisons •
Ventura and colleagues (2020) explored the decision-making process of patients with an insertable cardiac monitor. They found that patients who perceived their experience as life-threatening trusted their health care provider and assented to the insertion. Those who perceived symptoms as episodic used other strategies to resolve symptoms before making the decision.

Research Settings

Qualitative researchers usually collect their data in naturalistic settings. And, whereas quantitative researchers usually strive to collect data in one type of setting to maintain constancy of conditions (e.g., conducting all interviews in participants' homes), qualitative researchers may deliberately study phenomena in various natural contexts, especially in ethnographic research.

Time Frames

Qualitative research, like quantitative research, can be either cross-sectional, with one data collection point, or longitudinal, with multiple data collection points designed to observe the evolution of a phenomenon.

Example of a longitudinal qualitative study •
Dale and an interprofessional team (2020) conducted a longitudinal qualitative study to understand the transition experience of adolescents receiving long-term home mechanical ventilation to adult health care services.

Causality and Qualitative Research

In evidence hierarchies that rank evidence in terms of support of causal inferences (e.g., the one in Figure 1.2), qualitative research is often near the base, which has led some to criticize evidence-based initiatives. The issue of causality, which has been controversial throughout the history of science, is especially contentious in qualitative research.

Some believe that causality is an inappropriate construct within the naturalistic paradigm. For example, Lincoln and Guba (1985) devoted an entire chapter of their book to a critique of causality and argued that it should be replaced with a concept that they called *mutual shaping*. According to their view, "Everything influences everything else, in the here and now." (p. 151).

Others, however, believe that qualitative methods are especially well suited to understanding causal relationships. For example, Maxwell (2012) argued that qualitative research is important for causal explanations, noting that they "depend on the in-depth understanding of meanings, contexts, and processes that qualitative research can provide" (p. 655).

In attempting to not only describe but also explain phenomena, qualitative researchers who undertake in-depth studies will inevitably reveal patterns and processes suggesting causal interpretations. These interpretations can be (and often are) subjected to more systematic testing using more controlled methods of inquiry.

QUALITATIVE RESEARCH TRADITIONS

There is a wide variety of qualitative approaches. One classification system involves categorizing qualitative research according to disciplinary traditions. These traditions vary in their conceptualization of the types of questions that are important to ask and in the methods considered appropriate for answering them. This section describes traditions that have been prominent in nursing research.

Ethnography

Ethnography, the research tradition of anthropologists, involves the description and interpretation of a culture and cultural behavior. *Culture* refers to the way a group of people live—the patterns of human activity and the values and norms that give activity significance. Ethnographies typically involve extensive *fieldwork*, which is the process by which the ethnographer comes to understand a culture. Because culture is, in itself, not visible or tangible, it must be inferred from the words, actions, and products of members of a group.

Ethnographic research sometimes concerns broadly defined cultures (e.g., the Maori culture of New Zealand) in a *macroethnography*. However, ethnographers sometimes focus on more narrowly defined cultures in a *focused ethnography*. Focused ethnographies are studies of small units in a group or culture (e.g., the culture of an intensive care unit). An underlying assumption of the ethnographer is that every human group eventually evolves a culture that guides the members' view of the world and the way they structure their experiences.

> **Example of a focused ethnography** •
> Josi and Bianchi (2019) used a focused ethnographic approach to study the professional roles of advanced practice nurses, registered nurses (RNs), and medical practice assistants in new care models in Swiss primary care.

Ethnographers seek to learn from (rather than to study) members of a cultural group—to understand their world view. Ethnographers distinguish "emic" and "etic" perspectives. An *emic perspective* refers to the way the members of the culture regard their world—the insiders' view. The emic is the local concepts or means of expression used by members of the group under study to characterize their experiences. The *etic perspective*, by contrast, is the outsiders' interpretation of the culture's experiences—the words and concepts they use to refer to the same phenomena. Ethnographers strive to acquire an emic perspective of a culture and to reveal *tacit knowledge*—information about the culture that is so deeply embedded in cultural experiences that members do not talk about it or may not even be consciously aware of it.

Three broad types of information are usually sought by ethnographers: cultural behavior (what members of the culture do), cultural artifacts (what members make and use), and cultural speech (what they say). Ethnographers rely on a wide variety of data sources, including observations, in-depth interviews, records, and other types of physical evidence (e.g., photographs, diaries). Ethnographers typically use a strategy called **participant observation** in which they make observations of the culture under study while participating in its activities. Ethnographers also enlist *key informants* to help them understand and interpret the events and activities being observed.

Ethnographic research is time-consuming—months and even years of fieldwork may be required to learn about a culture. Ethnography requires a certain level of intimacy with members of the cultural group, and such intimacy can be developed only over time and by working with those members as active participants.

The products of ethnographies are rich, holistic descriptions and interpretations of the culture under study. Among health care researchers, ethnography provides access to the health beliefs and health practices of a culture. Ethnographic inquiry can thus help to foster understanding of behaviors affecting health and illness. Leininger (1985) coined the phrase **ethnonursing research**, which she defined as "the study and analysis of the local or indigenous people's viewpoints, beliefs, and practices about nursing care behavior and processes of designated cultures" (p. 38).

> **Example of an ethnonursing study** •
> Carron and coresearchers (2020) conducted an ethnonursing study to understand and describe cultural experiences, patterns, and practices of American Indian women with polycystic ovary syndrome.

Ethnographers are often, but not always, "outsiders" to the culture under study. A type of ethnography that involves the scrutiny of groups or cultures to which researchers themselves belong is called *autoethnography* or *insider research*. Autoethnography has several advantages, including ease of recruitment and the ability to get candid data based on preestablished trust. The drawback is that an "insider" may have biases about certain issues or may be so entrenched in the culture that valuable data get overlooked.

Phenomenology

Phenomenology is an approach to understanding people's everyday life experiences. Phenomenological researchers ask: What is the *essence* of this phenomenon as experienced by people and what does it *mean?* Phenomenologists assume there is an *essence*—an essential structure—that can be understood, much as ethnographers assume that cultures exist. Essence is what makes a phenomenon what it is, and without which it would not be what it is. Phenomenologists investigate subjective phenomena in the belief that critical truths about reality are grounded in people's lived experiences. The topics appropriate to phenomenology are ones that are fundamental to the life experiences of humans, such as the meaning of suffering or the grief of losing a child to cancer.

In phenomenological studies, the main data source is in-depth conversations. Through these conversations, researchers strive to gain entrance into the informants' world and to have access to their experiences as lived. Phenomenological studies usually involve a small number of participants—often fewer than 15. For some phenomenological researchers, the inquiry includes gathering not only information from informants but also efforts to experience the phenomenon, through participation, observation, and reflection. Phenomenologists share their insights in rich, vivid reports that describe key *themes*. The results section in a phenomenological report should help readers "see" something in a different way that enriches their understanding of experiences.

Phenomenology has two main variants: descriptive phenomenology and interpretive phenomenology (hermeneutics).

Descriptive Phenomenology

Descriptive phenomenology was developed first by Husserl, who was primarily interested in the question: *What do we know as persons?* Descriptive phenomenologists insist on the careful portrayal of ordinary conscious experience of everyday life—a depiction of "things" as people experience them to understand the *essence* of the experience. These "things" include hearing, seeing, believing, feeling, remembering, deciding, and evaluating.

Descriptive phenomenological studies often involve the following four steps: bracketing, intuiting, analyzing, and describing. **Bracketing** refers to the process of identifying and holding in abeyance preconceived beliefs and opinions about the phenomenon under study. Researchers strive to bracket out presuppositions in an effort to confront the data in pure form. Phenomenological researchers (and other qualitative researchers) often maintain a **reflexive journal** in their efforts to bracket.

Intuiting, the second step in descriptive phenomenology, occurs when researchers remain open to the meanings attributed to the phenomenon by those who have experienced it. Phenomenological researchers then proceed to an analysis (i.e., extracting significant statements, categorizing, and making sense of essential meanings). Finally, the descriptive phase occurs when researchers come to understand and define the phenomenon.

Example of a descriptive phenomenological study •
Walker and co-investigators (2020) used a descriptive phenomenological approach in their study of the lived experience of persons with malignant pleural mesothelioma. The researchers discovered three themes in data from in-depth interviews with seven patients: uncertainty and worry about the future, value in relationships, and adapting to a new norm.

Interpretive Phenomenology

Heidegger, a student of Husserl, is the founder of **interpretive phenomenology** or hermeneutics. Heidegger stressed interpreting—not just describing—human experience. He believed that lived experience is inherently an interpretive process and argued that **hermeneutics** ("understanding") is a basic characteristic of human existence. (The term *hermeneutics* refers to the art and philosophy of interpreting the meaning of an object such as a *text* or work of art.) The goals of interpretive phenomenological research are to enter another's world and to discover the understandings found there.

Gadamer, another interpretive phenomenologist, described the interpretive process as a circular relationship—the *hermeneutic circle*—where one understands the whole of a text (e.g., an interview transcript) in terms of its parts and the parts in terms of the whole. Researchers continually question the meanings of the text.

Heidegger believed it is impossible to bracket one's being-in-the-world, so bracketing does not occur in interpretive phenomenology. Hermeneutics presupposes prior understanding on the part of the researcher. Interpretive phenomenologists ideally approach each interview text with openness—they must be open to hearing what it is the text is saying.

Interpretive phenomenologists, like descriptive phenomenologists, rely primarily on in-depth interviews with individuals who have experienced the phenomenon of interest, but they may go beyond a traditional approach to gathering and analyzing data. For example, interpretive phenomenologists sometimes augment their understandings of the phenomenon through an analysis of relevant supplementary texts, such as novels, poetry, or other artistic expressions.

Example of a hermeneutic study •
Solberg and Nåden (2020) used Gadamer's hermeneutic approach in their study of the meaning of dignity among patients with substance use disorders. They asked: What is dignity for the patient? and What could enhance the experience of dignity in encounters with home-based health care staff?

 HOW-TO-TELL TIP How can you tell if a phenomenological study is descriptive or interpretive? Phenomenologists often use terms that can help you make this determination. In a descriptive phenomenological study such terms may be *bracketing*, *description*, or *essence*. The names Colaizzi, van Kaam, or Giorgi may be mentioned in the method section. In an interpretive phenomenological study, key terms can include *being-in-the-world*, *hermeneutics*, and *understanding*. The names van Manen or Benner may appear in the method section, as we discuss in Chapter 15 on qualitative data analysis.

Grounded Theory

Grounded theory research has contributed to the development of many middle-range theories of phenomena relevant to nurses. Grounded theory was developed in the 1960s by two sociologists, Glaser and Strauss (1967), whose theoretical roots were in *symbolic interaction*, which focuses on the manner in which people make sense of social interactions.

Grounded theory tries to account for people's actions from the perspective of those involved. Grounded theory researchers seek to identify a main concern or problem and then to understand the behavior designed to resolve it—the **core variable**. One type of core variable is a **basic social process (BSP)**. Grounded theory researchers generate conceptual categories and integrate them into a substantive theory, grounded in the data.

Grounded Theory Methods

Grounded theory methods constitute an entire approach to the conduct of field research. A study that truly follows Glaser and Strauss's precepts does not begin with a focused research problem. The problem and the process used to resolve it emerge from the data and are discovered during the study. In grounded theory research, data collection, data analysis, and sampling of participants occur simultaneously. The grounded theory process is recursive: Researchers collect data, categorize them, describe the emerging central phenomenon, and then recycle earlier steps.

A procedure called **constant comparison** is used to develop and refine theoretically relevant concepts and categories. Categories elicited from the data are constantly compared with data obtained earlier so that commonalities and variations can be detected. As data collection proceeds, the inquiry becomes increasingly focused on the emerging theory.

In-depth interviews and participant observation are common data sources in grounded theory studies, but existing documents and other data may also be used. Typically, a grounded theory study involves interviews with a sample of about 20 to 30 people.

Alternate Views of Grounded Theory

In 1990, Strauss and Corbin published a controversial book, *Basics of Qualitative Research: Grounded Theory Procedures and Techniques*. The book's stated purpose was to provide beginning grounded theory researchers with basic procedures for building a grounded theory. The book is currently in its fourth edition (Corbin & Strauss, 2015).

Glaser, however, disagreed with some procedures advocated by Strauss (his original co-author) and Corbin (a nurse researcher). Glaser (1992) believed that Strauss and Corbin (1990) developed a method that is not grounded theory but rather what he called "full conceptual description." According to Glaser, the purpose of grounded theory is to generate concepts and theories that explain and account for variation in behavior in the substantive area under study. *Conceptual description*, by contrast, is aimed at describing the full range of behavior of what is occurring in the substantive area.

Nurse researchers have conducted grounded theory studies using both the original Glaser and Strauss (1967) and the Corbin and Strauss (2015) approaches. They also use an approach called **constructivist grounded theory** (Charmaz, 2014). Charmaz (2014) regards Glaser and Strauss's grounded theory as having positivist roots. In Charmaz's approach, the developed grounded theory is seen as an interpretation. The data collected and analyzed are acknowledged to be constructed from shared experiences and relationships between the researcher and the participants. Data and analyses are viewed as social constructions.

Example of a grounded theory study •
Tafjord (2020) used constructivist grounded theory methods to explore nurses' recognition of *insufficient competence* in their direct involvement with the adolescent children of patients with cancer. Data were gathered in in-depth interviews with 12 nurses.

OTHER TYPES OF QUALITATIVE RESEARCH

Qualitative studies often can be characterized and described in terms of the disciplinary research traditions discussed in the previous section. However, several other important types of qualitative research that are not associated with a particular discipline also deserve mention.

Case Studies

Case studies are in-depth investigations of a single entity or small number of entities. The entity may be an individual, family, institution, or other social unit. Case study researchers attempt to understand issues that are important to the circumstances of the focal entity.

In most studies, whether qualitative or quantitative, certain phenomena or variables are the core of the inquiry. In a case study, the *case* itself is at "center stage." The focus of case studies is typically on understanding *why* a person thinks, behaves, or develops in a particular manner rather than on *what* his or her status or actions are. Probing research of this type may require study over a considerable period. Data are often collected not only about the person's present state but also about past experiences relevant to the problem being examined.

The greatest strength of case studies is the depth that is possible when a small number of entities are being investigated. Case study researchers can gain an intimate knowledge of a person's feelings, actions, and intentions. Yet, this same strength is a potential weakness: Researchers' familiarity with the case may make objectivity more difficult. Another limitation concerns generalizability: If researchers discover important relationships, it is difficult to know whether the same relationships would occur with others. However, case studies can play a role in challenging generalizations from other types of research.

Example of a case study •
Geryk and colleagues (2019) explored the processes used by older individuals to self-manage their health during the first month after a hospital discharge. The researchers used a multiple case study approach that involved interviews, observations, and diaries from three women who were 75 years old or older and had been recently discharged.

Narrative Analyses

Narrative analysis focuses on *story* as the object of inquiry to understand how individuals make sense of events in their lives. A basic premise of narrative research is that people most effectively make sense of their world—and communicate these meanings—by narrating stories. Individuals construct stories when they wish to understand specific events and situations that require linking an inner world of needs to an external world of observable actions. Analyzing stories opens up *forms* of telling about experience and is more than just content. Narrative analysts ask, *Why did the story get told that way?* A number of structural approaches can be used to analyze stories, including ones based in literary analysis and linguistics.

Example of a narrative analysis •
Meraz (2020) conducted a narrative analysis to understand the medication decision-making process and experiences of older adults with heart failure. The personal narratives of 11 adults with heart failure were gathered and analyzed using narrative analysis. Meraz learned that the participants made intentional decisions to take particular medications differently than prescribed.

Descriptive Qualitative Studies

Many qualitative studies claim no particular disciplinary or methodological roots. The researchers may simply indicate that they have conducted a qualitative study, a naturalistic inquiry, or a *content analysis* or *thematic analysis* of qualitative data (i.e., an analysis of themes and patterns that emerge in the narrative content). Thus, some qualitative studies do not have a formal name or do not fit into the typology we have presented in this chapter. We refer to these as **descriptive qualitative studies**.

Descriptive qualitative studies tend to be eclectic in their methods and are based on the general premises of constructivist inquiry. The chapter supplement on thePoint® website presents information on descriptive qualitative studies.

 TIP The supplement to this chapter also describes a qualitative approach that nurse researcher Sally Thorne (2013) called *interpretive description* and briefly describes historical nursing research.

Example of a descriptive qualitative study •
Fowler (2020) undertook a descriptive qualitative study to explore critical care nurses' perceptions of hope-inspiring strategies. In the analysis of in-depth interviews with 14 critical care nurses, Fowler found that hope was described as something "to hang on to" and to move forward toward and that hope was inspired through communication.

Research With Ideological Perspectives

Some qualitative researchers conduct inquiries within an ideological framework, typically to draw attention to social problems or the needs of certain groups and to bring about change. These approaches represent important investigative avenues.

Critical Theory

Critical theory originated with a group of Marxist-oriented German scholars in the 1920s. Essentially, a critical researcher is concerned with a critique of society and with envisioning new possibilities. Critical research is action oriented. Its aim is to make people aware of contradictions and disparities in social practices and to inspire them to make changes. Critical theory calls for inquiries that foster enlightened self-knowledge and sociopolitical action.

Critical researchers often triangulate methods and emphasize multiple perspectives (e.g., alternative racial or social class perspectives) on problems. Critical researchers typically interact with participants in ways that emphasize participants' expertise.

Critical theory has been applied in several disciplines but has played an especially important role in ethnography. **Critical ethnography** focuses on raising consciousness in the hope of effecting social change. Critical ethnographers attempt to increase the political dimensions of cultural research and undermine oppressive systems.

Example of a critical ethnography •
Bidabadi and colleagues (2019) undertook a critical ethnography designed to uncover the cultural factors that impeded maintaining patients' dignity in the cardiac surgery intensive care unit. Data were collected in 30 interviews, 200 hours of participant observation, and document assessments. The researchers found that the prevailing atmosphere in the unit culture was reductionist and paternalistic.

Feminist Research

Feminist research is similar to critical theory research, but the focus is on gender domination and discrimination within patriarchal societies. Similar to critical researchers, feminist researchers seek to establish collaborative and nonexploitative relationships with their informants and to conduct research that is transformative. Feminist investigators seek to understand how gender and a gendered social order have shaped women's lives. The aim is to facilitate change in ways relevant to ending women's unequal social position.

Feminist research methods typically include in-depth, interactive, and collaborative individual or group interviews that offer the possibility of reciprocally educational encounters. Feminists usually seek to negotiate the meanings of the results with those participating in the study and to be self-reflective about what they themselves are learning.

Example of feminist research •
Van Daalen-Smith and colleagues (2020) used a feminist lens (based on Feminist Standpoint Theory) in their study of Canadian women's experiences of psychiatric hospitalization. Overarching themes were docility making, harm, betrayal, indifference, and resistance.

Participatory Action Research

Participatory action research (PAR) is based on the view that the production of knowledge can be used to exert power. PAR researchers typically work with groups or communities that are vulnerable to the control or oppression of a dominant group.

The PAR tradition has as its starting point a concern for the powerlessness of the group under study. In PAR, researchers and participants collaborate in defining the problem, selecting research methods, analyzing the data, and deciding how the findings will be used. The aim of PAR is to produce not only knowledge but also action, empowerment, and consciousness raising.

In PAR, the research methods are designed to facilitate processes of collaboration that can motivate and generate community solidarity. Thus, "data-gathering" strategies are not only the traditional methods of interview and observation but may include storytelling, sociodrama, photography, and other activities designed to encourage people to find creative ways to explore their lives, tell their stories, and recognize their own strengths.

Example of participatory action research •
Peake and coresearchers (2020) used PAR in an effort to develop culturally appropriate health resources for Australian aboriginal communities.

CRITICAL APPRAISAL OF QUALITATIVE DESIGNS

Evaluating a qualitative design is often difficult. Qualitative researchers do not always describe design decisions or the process by which such decisions were made. Researchers often do, however, indicate whether the study was conducted within a specific qualitative tradition. This information can be used to come to some conclusions about the study design. For example, if a report indicated that the researcher conducted 2 months of fieldwork for an ethnographic study, you might suspect that insufficient time had been spent in the field to obtain an emic perspective of the culture under study. Ethnographic studies may also be critiqued if their only source of information was from interviews, rather than from a broader range of data sources, particularly observations.

In a grounded theory study, look for evidence about when the data were collected and analyzed. If the researcher collected all the data before analyzing any of it, you might question whether the constant comparative method was used correctly.

In appraising a phenomenological study, you should first determine if the study is descriptive or interpretive. This will help you to assess how closely the researcher kept to the

> ### Box 10.1 Guidelines for Critically Appraising Qualitative Designs
>
> 1. Was the research tradition for the qualitative study identified? If none was identified, can one be inferred?
> 2. Is the research question congruent with a specific research tradition? Are the data sources and research methods congruent with the research tradition?
> 3. How well was the research design described? Are design decisions explained and justified? Does it appear that the design emerged during data collection, allowing researchers to capitalize on early information?
> 4. Did the design lend itself to a thorough, in-depth examination of the focal phenomenon? Was there evidence of reflexivity? What design elements might have strengthened the study (e.g., a longitudinal perspective rather than a cross-sectional one)?
> 5. Was the study undertaken with an ideological perspective? If so, is there evidence that ideological goals were achieved (e.g., Was there full collaboration between researchers and participants? Did the research have the power to be transformative?)?

basic tenets of that qualitative research tradition. For example, in a descriptive phenomenological study, did the researcher bracket? When appraising a phenomenological study, you should also look at its power in capturing the meaning of the phenomena being studied.

No matter what qualitative design is identified in a study, look to see if the researchers stayed true to a single qualitative tradition throughout the study or if they mixed qualitative traditions. For example, did the researcher state that grounded theory was used but then present results that described *themes* instead of a substantive theory?

The guidelines in Box 10.1 are designed to assist you in appraising the design of qualitative studies.

RESEARCH EXAMPLES WITH CRITICAL THINKING EXERCISES

This section presents examples of qualitative studies. Read about the studies and then answer the critical thinking questions, referring to the full research report if necessary. Answers to the questions for Exercise 1 are available to instructors on the Point®. The critical thinking questions for Exercise 2 are based on the phenomenological study that appears in its entirety in Appendix B of this book. Our comments for this exercise are in the Student Resources section on the Point®.

EXAMPLE 1: AN ETHNOGRAPHIC STUDY

Study: Health care experiences of Korean women divers (Jeju haenyeos) (Kim & Kim, 2018)

Statement of Purpose: Jeju haenyeos are female divers who collect seafood while holding their breath, without equipment. They work in groups and have developed a unique culture. The study sought to explore the health beliefs and experiences of the Jeju haenyeos and how they manage and maintain their health in their daily work lives.

Setting: The research was conducted in the eastern part of Jeju in South Korea.

Method: An ethnographic approach was used, with fieldwork conducted over a 4-month period. The researchers received permission from the Jeju haeyeos' association chairperson to observe the participants at work. A 73-year-old diver who had started working at the age of 5 years served as a key informant.

She provided access to other divers and rich information about the divers' health management. She allowed the researchers to stay in her home for 3 days so she could observe the divers' daily lives and interactions. Observations were also made in the fitting rooms before dives and at a seawall where the diving occurred. The researchers conducted individual face-to-face interviews with 14 other divers. On average, the divers in the study had been working for 55 years.

Key Findings: The main theme of the divers' health management approach was "a life of listening to the body and mind, controlling greed, and adjusting work for safe diving" (p. 756). The study revealed that the divers led communal lives centered on their work and promoted safety by working collectively. The researchers found, however, that the Jeju haenyeos used a range of preventive drugs before work to relieve their minds and bodies. They also used other drugs and lacked understanding of how the diverse drugs potentially interact.

Critical Thinking Exercises

1. Answer the relevant questions from Box 10.1 regarding this study.
2. Also consider the following targeted questions:
   a. Comment on the amount of time spent in the field in this study (4 months).
   b. Could this study have been undertaken as a phenomenological inquiry? A grounded theory study?
3. If the results of this study are trustworthy, what are some of the uses to which the findings might be put in clinical practice?

EXAMPLE 2: PHENOMENOLOGICAL STUDY IN APPENDIX B

1. Read the method section from Beck and Watson's study ("Posttraumatic growth after birth trauma") in Appendix B of this book and then answer the relevant questions in Box 10.1.
2. Also consider the following targeted questions:
   a. Was this study a descriptive or interpretive phenomenology?
   b. Could this study have been conducted as a grounded theory study? As an ethnographic study? Why or why not?
   c. Could this study have been conducted as a feminist inquiry? If yes, what might Beck and Watson have done differently?

WANT TO KNOW MORE?

A wide variety of resources to enhance your learning and understanding of this chapter is available on thePoint.

- Chapter Supplement on Qualitative Description, Interpretive Description, and Historical Research
- Answer to the Critical Thinking Exercise for Example 2
- Internet Resources with useful websites for Chapter 10
- A Wolters Kluwer journal article on a topic related to this chapter

Additional study aids, including eight journal articles and related questions, are also available in *Study Guide for Essentials of Nursing Research, 10e*.

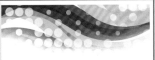

Summary Points

- Qualitative research involves an **emergent design** that develops in the field as the study unfolds. Qualitative studies can be either cross-sectional or longitudinal.

- Ethnography focuses on the culture of a group of people and relies on extensive fieldwork that usually includes **participant observation** and in-depth interviews with *key informants*. Ethnographers strive to acquire an *emic* (insider's) *perspective* of a culture rather than an *etic* (outsider's) *perspective*.

- Nurses sometimes refer to their ethnographic studies as **ethnonursing research.**

- Phenomenologists seek to discover the *essence* and *meaning* of a phenomenon as it is experienced by people, mainly through in-depth interviews with people who have had the relevant experience.

- In **descriptive phenomenology**, which seeks to describe lived experiences, researchers strive to **bracket** out preconceived views and to *intuit* the essence of the phenomenon by remaining open to meanings attributed to it by those who have experienced it.

- **Interpretive phenomenology (hermeneutics)** focuses on interpreting the meaning of experiences rather than just describing them.

- **Grounded theory** researchers try to account for people's actions by focusing on the main concern that their behavior is designed to resolve. The manner in which people resolve this main concern is the **core variable**. A prominent type of core variable is called a **basic social process (BSP)** that explains the processes of resolving the problem.

- Grounded theory uses **constant comparison**: Categories elicited from the data are constantly compared with data obtained earlier.

- Grounded theory researchers opt to follow either the original approach of Glaser and Strauss (1967) or to use procedures adapted by Strauss and Corbin (2015). Glaser (1997) argued that the latter approach does not result in *grounded theories* but rather in *conceptual descriptions*. More recently, Charmaz's (2014) **constructivist grounded theory** has emerged, emphasizing interpretive aspects in which the grounded theory is constructed from relationships between the researcher and participants.

- **Case studies** are intensive investigations of a single entity or a small number of entities, such as individuals, groups, families, or communities.

- **Narrative analysis** focuses on *story* in studies in which the purpose is to determine how individuals make sense of events in their lives.

- **Descriptive qualitative studies** are not embedded in a disciplinary tradition. Such studies may be referred to as qualitative studies, naturalistic inquiries, or as qualitative content analyses.

- Research is sometimes conducted within an ideological perspective. **Critical theory** is concerned with a critique of existing social structures; critical researchers conduct studies in collaboration with participants in an effort to foster self-knowledge and transformation. **Critical ethnography** uses the principles of critical theory in the study of cultures.

- **Feminist research**, like critical research, aims at being transformative, but the focus is on how gender domination and discrimination shape women's lives.

- **Participatory action research (PAR)** produces knowledge through close collaboration with groups that are vulnerable to oppression by a dominant culture; in PAR, a goal is to develop processes that can motivate people and generate community solidarity.

REFERENCES FOR CHAPTER 10

Bidabadi, F., Yazdannik, A., & Zargham-Boroujeni, A. (2019). Patient's dignity in intensive care unit: A critical ethnography. *Nursing Ethics, 26,* 738–752.

Carron, R., Kooienga, S., Gilman-Kehrer, E., & Alvero, R. (2020). Cultural experiences, patterns, and practices of American Indian women with polycystic ovary syndrome: An ethnonursing study. *Journal of Transcultural Nursing, 31,* 162–170.

Charmaz, K. (2014). *Constructing grounded theory* (2nd ed.). Thousand Oaks, CA: Sage.

Corbin, J., & Strauss, A. (2015). *Basics of qualitative research: Techniques and procedures for developing grounded theory* (4th ed.). Thousand Oaks, CA: Sage.

Dale, C., Carbone, S., Amin, R., Amaria, K., Varadi, K., Goldstein, R., & Rose, L. (2020). A transition program to adult health services for teenagers receiving long-term home mechanical ventilation: A longitudinal qualitative study. *Pediatric Pulmonology, 55,* 771–779.

Fowler, S. (2020). Critical-care nurses' perceptions of hope: Original qualitative research. *Dimensions of Critical Care Nursing, 39,* 110–115.

Geryk, T., Jacelon, C., LeBlanc, R., & Choi, J. (2019). Self-management after hospitalisation. *International Journal of Older People Nursing, 14,* e12257.

Glaser, B. G. (1992). *Emergence versus forcing: Basics of grounded theory analysis.* Mill Valley, CA: Sociology Press.

Glaser, B. G., & Strauss, A. L. (1967). *The discovery of grounded theory: Strategies for qualitative research.* Chicago, CA: Aldine.

*Josi, R., & Bianchi, M. (2019). Advanced practice nurses, registered nurses and medical practice assistants in new care models in Swiss primary care: A focused ethnography of their professional roles. *BMJ Open, 9,* e033929.

Kim, J. I., & Kim, M. (2018). Health care experiences of Korean women divers (Jeju haenyeos). *Qualitative Health Research, 28,* 756–765.

Leininger, M. M. (Ed.). (1985). *Qualitative research methods in nursing.* New York, NY: Grune and Stratton.

Lincoln, Y. S., & Guba, E. G. (1985). *Naturalistic inquiry.* Newbury Park, CA: Sage.

Maxwell, J. (2012). The importance of qualitative research for causal explanation in education. *Qualitative Inquiry, 18,* 655–661.

Meraz, R. (2020). Medication nonadherence or self-care? Understanding the medication decision-making process and experiences of older adults with heart failure. *Journal of Cardiovascular Nursing, 35,* 26–34.

Morse, J. M. (2004). Qualitative comparison: Appropriateness, equivalence, and fit. *Qualitative Health Research, 14,* 1323–1325.

Peake, R., Jackson, D., Lea, J., & Usher, K. (2020). Meaningful engagement with aboriginal communities using participatory action research to develop culturally appropriate health resources. *Journal of Transcultural Nursing.* Advance online publication. doi:10.1177/1043659619899999

Solberg, H., & Nåden, D. (2020). It is just that people treat you like a human being: The meaning of dignity for patients with substance use disorders. *Journal of Clinical Nursing, 29,* 480–491.

Strauss, A., & Corbin, J. (1990). *Basics of qualitative research: Grounded theory procedures and techniques.* Newbury Park, CA: Sage.

**Tafjord, T. (2020). Recognition of insufficient competence—Nurses' experiences in direct involvement with adolescent children of cancer patients. *Cancer Nursing, 43,* 32–44.

Thorne, S. (2013). Interpretive description. In C. T. Beck (Ed.), *Routledge international handbook of qualitative nursing research* (pp. 295–306). New York, NY: Routledge.

van Daalen-Smith, C., Adam, S., Hassim, F., & Santerre, F. (2020). A world of indifference: Canadian women's experiences of psychiatric hospitalization. *Issues in Mental Health Nursing, 41,* 315–327.

Ventura, A., Horne, C., Crane, P., Mendes, M., & Sears, S. (2020). Exploring the experiences of individuals with an insertable cardiac monitor: Making the decision for device insertion. *Heart & Lung, 49,* 86–91.

Walker, S., Crist, J., Shea, K., Holland, S., & Cacchione, P. (2020). The lived experience of persons with malignant pleural mesothelioma in the United States. *Cancer Nursing.* Advance online publication. doi:10.1097/NCC.0000000000000770

*A link to this open-access article is provided in the Internet Resources section on thePoint® website.

**This journal article is available on thePoint® for this chapter.

Appraising Sampling and Data Collection in Qualitative Studies

Learning Objectives

On completing this chapter, you will be able to:

- Describe the logic of sampling for qualitative studies
- Identify and describe several types of sampling approaches in qualitative studies
- Evaluate the appropriateness of the sampling method and sample size used in a qualitative study
- Identify and describe methods of collecting unstructured self-report data
- Identify and describe methods of collecting and recording unstructured observational data
- Critically appraise a qualitative researcher's decisions regarding the data collection plan
- Define new terms in the chapter

Key Terms

- Data saturation
- Diary
- Field notes
- Focus group interview
- Key informant
- Log
- Maximum variation sampling
- Participant observation
- Photo elicitation
- Photovoice
- Purposive (purposeful) sampling
- Semi-structured interview
- Snowball sampling
- Theoretical sampling
- Topic guide
- Unstructured interview

This chapter covers two important aspects of qualitative studies—sampling (selecting informative study participants) and data collection (gathering the right types and amount of information to address the research question).

SAMPLING IN QUALITATIVE RESEARCH

Qualitative studies typically rely on small nonprobability samples. Qualitative researchers are as concerned as quantitative researchers with the quality of their samples, but they use different considerations in selecting study participants.

The Logic of Qualitative Sampling

Quantitative researchers measure attributes and identify relationships in a population; they desire a representative sample so that findings can be generalized. The aim of most qualitative studies is to discover *meaning* and to uncover multiple realities, not to generalize to a population.

Qualitative researchers ask such sampling questions as, Who would be an *information-rich* data source for my study? Whom should I talk to, or what should I observe, to maximize my understanding of the phenomenon? A first step in qualitative sampling is selecting settings with potential for information richness.

As the study progresses, new sampling questions emerge, such as, Whom can I talk to or observe who would confirm, challenge, or enrich my understandings? As with the overall design, sampling design in qualitative studies tends to be an emergent one that capitalizes on early information to guide subsequent action.

TIP Like quantitative researchers, qualitative researchers identify eligibility criteria for their studies. Although they do not specify an explicit population to whom results could be generalized, they do establish the kinds of people who are eligible to participate in their research.

Types of Qualitative Sampling

Qualitative researchers avoid random samples because they are not the best method of selecting people who are knowledgeable, articulate, reflective, and willing to talk at length with researchers. Qualitative researchers use various nonprobability sampling designs.

Convenience and Snowball Sampling

Qualitative researchers often begin with a *volunteer* (convenience) *sample*. Volunteer samples are often used when researchers want participants to come forward and identify themselves. For example, if we wanted to study the experiences of people with frequent nightmares, we might recruit them by placing a notice on the Internet on a relevant website. We would be less interested in obtaining a representative sample of people with nightmares, than in recruiting a group with diverse nightmare experiences.

Sampling by convenience is efficient but is not a preferred approach. The aim in qualitative studies is to extract the greatest possible information from a small number of people, and a convenience sample may not provide the most information-rich sources. However, convenience sample may be an economical way to begin the sampling process.

Example of a convenience sample •
Childers and Aleshire (2020) explored the use of essential oils by health care professionals for health maintenance. They used a convenience sample of 10 participants who worked at a residential care facility.

Qualitative researchers also use **snowball sampling** (or *network sampling*), asking early informants to make referrals. A weakness of this approach is that the eventual sample might be restricted to a small network of acquaintances. Also, the quality of the referrals may be affected by whether the referring sample member trusted the researcher and truly wanted to cooperate.

Example of a snowball sample •
In their descriptive qualitative study, Link and coresearchers (2020) explored the burden of farmer suicide on surviving family members. Study participants were recruited using snowball sampling, based on Link's connections to farming communities.

Purposive Sampling

Qualitative sampling may begin with volunteer informants and may be supplemented with new participants through snowballing. Many qualitative studies, however, evolve to a **purposive** (or **purposeful**) **sampling** strategy in which researchers deliberately choose the cases or types of cases that will best contribute to the study.

Dozens of purposive sampling strategies have been identified (Patton, 2015), only some of which are mentioned here. Researchers do not necessarily refer to their sampling plans with Patton's labels; his classification shows the diverse strategies qualitative researchers have adopted to meet the conceptual needs of their research:

- **Maximum variation sampling** involves deliberately selecting cases with a range of variation on dimensions of interest.
- *Extreme (deviant) case sampling* provides opportunities for learning from the most unusual and extreme informants (e.g., outstanding successes and notable failures).
- *Typical case sampling* involves the selection of participants who illustrate or highlight what is typical or average.
- *Criterion sampling* involves studying cases who meet a predetermined criterion of importance.

Maximum variation sampling is often the sampling mode of choice in qualitative research because it is useful in illuminating the scope of a phenomenon and in identifying important patterns that cut across variations. Other strategies can also be used advantageously, however, depending on the nature of the research question.

Example of maximum variation sampling •••••••••••••••••••••••••••
Nilsson and coresearchers (2020) explored the ways in which young survivors of childhood cancer that had a risk of infertility understood their ability to have children. Maximum variation sampling was used to recruit people who differed in terms of diagnosis, age, time since diagnosis, gender, and relationship status.

Sampling confirming and disconfirming cases is another purposive strategy used toward the end of data collection. As researchers analyze their data, emerging conceptualizations sometimes need to be checked. *Confirming cases* are additional cases that fit researchers' conceptualizations and strengthen credibility. *Disconfirming cases* are new cases that do not fit and serve to challenge researchers' interpretations. These "negative" cases may offer insights about how the original conceptualization needs to be revised.

 TIP   Some qualitative researchers call their sample *purposive* simply because they "purposely" selected people who experienced the phenomenon of interest. Exposure to the phenomenon is, however, an eligibility criterion. If the researcher then recruits *any* person with the desired experience, the sample is selected by convenience, not purposively. Purposive sampling implies an intent to choose *particular* exemplars or *types* of people who can best enhance the researcher's understanding of the phenomenon.

Theoretical Sampling

Theoretical sampling is used in grounded theory studies. Theoretical sampling involves decisions about where to find data to develop an emerging theory. The basic question in theoretical sampling is What types of people should the researcher turn to next to further the theoretical development of the emerging conceptualization?

Example of a theoretical sampling •••••••••••••••••••••••••••••••
Andrews and colleagues (2020) used theoretical sampling in their grounded theory study of self-care and self-compassion in nursing. Purposive sampling was used at the initial state of recruitment, but theoretical sampling was used as the study progressed: " . . . it became apparent from the data that it would be useful to sample nurse leaders and newly qualified nurses to expand some of the emerging categories and to follow-up leads within the data" (p. 3).

Sample Size in Qualitative Research

Sample size in qualitative research is usually based on informational needs. **Data saturation** involves sampling until no new information is obtained and redundancy is achieved. The number of participants needed to reach saturation depends on various factors. For example, the broader the scope of the research question, the more participants will likely be needed. Data quality can affect sample size: If participants are insightful and can communicate effectively, saturation can be achieved with a relatively small sample. Also, a larger sample is likely to be needed with maximum variation sampling than with typical case sampling.

Example of data saturation •
Wang and colleagues (2020) studied the views of Chinese patients with cancer regarding disclosure of their cancer diagnosis to their minor children. A total of 18 patients were interviewed. The researchers noted that "[d]ata were saturated after 15 interviews, but 3 more interviews were conducted to ensure full data saturation" (p. 4).

 TIP Sample size adequacy in a qualitative study is difficult to evaluate because the main criterion is information redundancy, which consumers cannot judge. Some (but not all) reports explicitly mention that saturation was achieved.

Sampling in the Three Main Qualitative Traditions

There are similarities among the main qualitative traditions with regard to sampling: Small samples and nonrandom methods are used, and final sampling decisions usually take place during data collection. However, there are some differences as well.

Sampling in Ethnography

Ethnographers often begin with a "big net" approach—they mingle and converse with many members of the culture. However, they usually rely heavily on a smaller number of **key informants**, who are knowledgeable about the culture and serve as the researcher's main link to the "inside." Ethnographers may use an initial framework to develop a pool of potential key informants. For example, an ethnographer might decide to recruit different types of key informants based on their *roles* (e.g., nurses, advocates). Once potential key informants are identified, key considerations for final selection are their level of knowledge about the culture and willingness to collaborate with the ethnographer in revealing and interpreting the culture.

Sampling in ethnography typically involves sampling *things* as well as people. For example, ethnographers make decisions about observing *events* and *activities*, about examining *records* and *artifacts*, and about exploring *places* that provide clues about the culture. Key informants often help ethnographers decide what to sample.

Example of an ethnographic sample •
In their ethnographic study of the cultural features of waiting in an emergency department in Iran, Hassankhani and colleagues (2019) conducted 34 informal interviews during the course of their participant observation. Then, 13 in-depth interviews were conducted to explore cultural meanings "from culturally sensitive informants (2 patients, 4 relatives, 4 nurses, and 3 physicians)" (p. 2).

Sampling in Phenomenological Studies

Phenomenologists tend to rely on very small samples of participants—typically 15 or fewer. Two principles guide the selection of a sample for a phenomenological study:

(1) All participants must have experienced the phenomenon and (2) they must be able to articulate what it is like to have lived that experience. Phenomenological researchers often want to explore diversity of individual experiences, and so, they may specifically look for people with demographic or other differences who have shared a common experience.

> **Example of a sample in a phenomenological study** •
> In their phenomenological study of health-related adherence of patients who had had a myocardial infarction (MI), Hanna and colleagues (2020) recruited a purposive sample of 22 post-MI patients from a cardiac rehabilitation unit and from two communities in Northern Israel. One was an Arab community, and the other was a Kibbutz. The researchers noted that participants "were chosen from different cultures to obtain a diversity of experiences" (p. 3).

Interpretive phenomenologists may, in addition to sampling people, sample artistic or literary sources. Experiential descriptions of a phenomenon may be selected from literature, such as poetry, novels, or autobiographies. These sources can help increase phenomenologists' insights into the phenomena under study.

Sampling in Grounded Theory Studies

Grounded theory research is typically done with samples of about 20 to 30 people, using theoretical sampling. The goal in a grounded theory study is to select informants who can best contribute to the evolving theory. Sampling, data collection, data analysis, and theory construction occur concurrently, and so, study participants are selected serially and contingently (i.e., contingent on the emerging conceptualization). Sampling might evolve as follows:

1. The researcher begins with a general notion of where and with whom to start. The first few cases may be sampled by convenience.
2. Maximum variation sampling might be used next to gain insights into the range and complexity of the phenomenon.
3. The sample is continually adjusted: Emerging conceptualizations inform the theoretical sampling process.
4. Sampling continues until saturation is achieved.
5. Final sampling may include a search for confirming and disconfirming cases to test, refine, and strengthen the theory.

Critically Appraising Qualitative Sampling Plans

Qualitative sampling plans can be evaluated in terms of their adequacy and appropriateness (Morse, 1991). *Adequacy* refers to the sufficiency and quality of the data the sample yielded. An adequate sample provides data without "thin" spots. When researchers have truly obtained saturation, informational adequacy has been achieved, and the resulting description or theory is richly textured and complete.

Appropriateness concerns the methods used to select a sample. An appropriate sample results from the selection of participants who can best supply information that meets the study's conceptual requirements. The sampling strategy must yield a full understanding of the phenomenon of interest. A sampling approach that excludes negative cases or that fails to include people with unusual experiences may not fully address the study's information needs.

Another important issue concerns the potential for transferability of the findings. The transferability of study findings is a function of the similarity between the study sample and other people to whom the findings might be applied. Thus, in appraising a report, you should assess whether the researcher provided an adequately *thick description* of the sample

---

Box 11.1 Guidelines for Critically Appraising Qualitative Sampling Plans

1. Was the setting appropriate for addressing the research question, and was it adequately described?
2. What type of sampling strategy was used?
3. Were the eligibility criteria for the study specified? How were participants recruited into the study?
4. Given the information needs of the study—and, if applicable, its qualitative tradition—was the sampling approach effective?
5. Was the sample size adequate and appropriate? Did the researcher indicate that saturation had been achieved? Do the findings suggest a richly textured and comprehensive set of data without any apparent "holes" or thin areas?
6. Were key characteristics of the sample described (e.g., age, gender)? Was a rich description of participants and context provided, allowing for an assessment of the transferability of the findings?

---

and the study context so that someone interested in transferring the findings could make an informed decision. Further guidance in critically appraising qualitative sampling is presented in Box 11.1.

 TIP The issue of transferability within the context of broader models of generalizability is discussed in the supplement to this chapter on the book's website.

DATA COLLECTION IN QUALITATIVE STUDIES

In-depth interviews are the most common method of collecting qualitative data. Observation is used in some qualitative studies as well. Physiological data are rarely collected in a constructivist inquiry. Table 11.1 compares the types of data and aspects of data

TABLE 11.1 **Comparison of Data Collection in Three Qualitative Traditions**

Issue	Ethnography	Phenomenology	Grounded Theory
Types of data	Primarily observation and interviews plus artifacts, documents, photographs, social network diagrams	Primarily in-depth interviews, sometimes diaries, other written materials, observations	Primarily individual interviews, sometimes group interviews, observation, diaries, documents
Unit of data collection	Cultural systems	Individuals	Individuals
Data collection points	Cross-sectional or longitudinal	Mainly cross-sectional	Cross-sectional or longitudinal
Length of time for data collection	Typically long, several months or years	Typically moderate	Typically moderate
Data recording	Field notes/logs, interview notes or recordings	Interview notes or recordings	Interview notes or recordings, memos, observational notes
Salient field issues	Gaining entrée, determining a role, learning how to participate, encouraging candor, loss of objectivity, premature exit, reflexivity	Bracketing one's views, building rapport, encouraging candor, listening while preparing what to ask next, keeping "on track," handling emotionality	Building rapport, encouraging candor, listening while preparing what to ask next, keeping "on track," handling emotionality

collection used by researchers in the three main qualitative traditions. Ethnographers typically collect a wide array of data, with observation and interviews being the primary methods. Ethnographers also gather or examine products of the culture under study, such as documents, artifacts, photographs, and so on. Phenomenologists and grounded theory researchers rely primarily on in-depth interviews, although observation sometimes plays a role.

Qualitative Self-Report Techniques

Qualitative researchers do not have a set of questions that must be asked in a specific order and worded in a given way. Instead, they start with general questions and allow respondents to tell their narratives in a naturalistic fashion. Qualitative interviews tend to be conversational. Interviewers encourage respondents to define the important dimensions of a phenomenon and to elaborate on what is relevant to them.

Types of Qualitative Self-Reports

Researchers use completely **unstructured interviews** when they have no preconceived view of the information to be gathered. Researchers begin by asking a *grand tour question* such as "What happened when you first learned that you had AIDS?" Subsequent questions are guided by initial responses. Ethnographic and phenomenological studies often gather data through unstructured interviews.

Semi-structured (or *focused*) **interviews** are used when researchers have a list of topics or broad questions that must be covered in an interview. Interviewers use a written **topic guide** to ensure that all question areas are addressed. The interviewer's function is to encourage participants to talk freely about all the topics on the guide.

Example of a semi-structured interview •
Barsuk and colleagues (2020) studied the perceptions of patients, caregivers, and clinicians regarding the existing self-care training for ventricular assist devices. Topic guides were developed, informed by a formal theory of heart failure self-care. Three interviewers—all of whom had previous interview experience—practiced the questions together before conducting interviews.

Focus group interviews involve groups of about 5 to 10 people whose opinions and experiences are solicited simultaneously. The interviewer (or *moderator*) guides the discussion using a topic guide. A group format is efficient and can generate a lot of dialogue, but not everyone is comfortable sharing their views or experiences in front of a group.

Example of focus group interviews •
Kim and colleagues (2020) explored the self-management needs of breast cancer survivors after treatment. A total of 20 women participated in three separate focus groups. Each session took place in a quiet seminar room in a hospital in South Korea. All sessions, which lasted about 2 hours, were audiorecorded, and notes were taken by an assistant moderator.

Personal **diaries** are a standard data source in historical research. It is also possible to generate new data for a study by asking participants to maintain a diary over a specified period. Diaries can be useful in providing an intimate description of a person's everyday life. The diaries may be completely unstructured; for example, individuals who had an organ transplantation could be asked to spend 15 minutes a day jotting down their thoughts. Frequently, however, people are asked to make diary entries regarding some specific aspect of their lives.

Example of diaries •••
Alsaigh and Coyne (2019) undertook a hermeneutic study to understand the meaning of mothers' experiences of caring for children who were receiving growth hormone treatment. In-depth interviews were conducted with 16 mothers, 8 of whom maintained and shared diaries about their experiences. Quotes from the diary entries were included in the report.

Photo elicitation involves an interview guided by photographic images. This procedure, most often used in ethnographies and participatory action research, can help to promote a collaborative discussion. The photographs sometimes are ones that researchers have made of the participants' world, but photo elicitation can also be used with photos in participants' homes. Researchers have also used the technique of asking participants to take photographs themselves and then interpret them, a method sometimes called **photovoice**.

Example of a photovoice study ••••••••••••••••••••••••••••••••••••
Duck and colleagues (2020) studied adults' and children's perceptions regarding barriers and facilitators of school-aged children's physical activity in a low-income urban neighborhood. Photovoice was used to prompt discussions that took place in focus group sessions.

Gathering Qualitative Self-Report Data

Researchers gather narrative self-report data to develop a construction of a phenomenon that is consistent with that of participants. This goal requires researchers to overcome communication barriers and to enhance the flow of information. Although qualitative interviews are conversational, the conversations are purposeful ones that require preparation. For example, the wording of questions should reflect the participants' worldview and language. In addition to being good questioners, researchers must be good listeners. Only by attending carefully to what respondents are saying can in-depth interviewers develop useful follow-up questions.

Unstructured interviews are typically long, sometimes lasting an hour or more, and so, an important issue is how to record such abundant information. Some researchers take notes during the interview, but this is risky in terms of data accuracy. Most researchers record the interviews for later transcription. Although some respondents are self-conscious when their conversation is recorded, they typically forget about the presence of recording equipment (often a cell phone) after a few minutes.

 TIP Although qualitative self-report data are often gathered in face-to-face interviews, they can also be collected in writing. Internet "interviews" are also possible.

Evaluation of Qualitative Self-Report Methods

In-depth interviews are a flexible approach to gathering data and, in many research contexts, offer distinct advantages. In clinical situations, for example, it is often appropriate to let people talk freely about their problems and concerns, allowing them to take the initiative in directing the flow of conversation. Unstructured self-reports may allow investigators to ascertain what the basic issues or problems are, how sensitive or controversial the topic is, how individuals conceptualize and talk about the problems, and what range of opinions or behaviors exist relevant to the topic. In-depth interviews may also help elucidate the underlying meaning of a relationship repeatedly observed in more structured research. On the other hand, qualitative methods are very time-consuming and demanding of researchers' skills in gathering, analyzing, and interpreting the resulting data.

Qualitative Observational Methods

Qualitative researchers sometimes collect loosely structured observational data, often as a supplement to self-report data. The aim of qualitative observation is to understand the behaviors and experiences of people as they occur in naturalistic settings. Skillful observation permits researchers to see the world as participants see it, to develop a rich understanding of the focal phenomenon, and to grasp subtleties of cultural variation.

Unstructured observational data are often gathered through **participant observation**. Participant observers take part in the functioning of the group under study and strive to observe, ask questions, and record information within the contexts and structures that are relevant to group members. Participant observation is characterized by prolonged periods of social interaction between researchers and participants. By assuming a participating role, observers often have insights that would have eluded more passive or concealed observers.

 TIP Not all qualitative observational research is *participant* observation (i.e., with observations occurring from *within* the group). Some unstructured observations involve watching and recording behaviors without the observers' active participation in activities. Be on the alert for the misuse of the term "participant observation." Some researchers use the term inappropriately to refer to all unstructured observations conducted in the field.

The Observer-Participant Role in Participant Observation

In participant observation, the role that observers play in the group is important because their social position determines what they are likely to see. The extent of the observers' actual participation in a group is best thought of as a continuum. At one extreme is complete immersion in the setting, with researchers assuming full participant status; at the other extreme is complete separation, with researchers as onlookers. Researchers may in some cases assume a fixed position on this continuum throughout the study, but often researchers' role evolves toward increasing participation over the course of the fieldwork.

Observers must overcome two major hurdles in assuming a satisfactory role in the group. The first is to gain entrée into the group under study; the second is to establish rapport and trust within that group. Without gaining entrée, the study cannot proceed; but without the group's trust, the researcher will be restricted to "front stage" knowledge—information distorted by the group's protective facades. The goal of participant observers is to "get backstage"—to learn the true realities of the group's experiences. On the other hand, being a fully participating member does not *necessarily* offer the best perspective for studying a phenomenon—just as being an actor in a play does not offer the most advantageous view of the performance.

Gathering Participant Observation Data

Participant observers typically place few restrictions on the nature of the data collected, but they often have a broad plan for types of information desired. Among the aspects of an observed activity likely to be considered relevant are the following:

1. *The physical setting—Where questions.* What are the main features of the setting?
2. *The participants—Who questions.* Who is present and what are their characteristics?

3. *Activities—What questions*. What is going on? What are participants doing?
4. *Frequency and duration—When questions*. When did the activity begin and end? Is the activity a recurring one?
5. *Process—How questions*. How is the activity organized? How does it unfold?
6. *Outcomes—Why questions*. Why is the activity happening? What did not happen (especially if it ought to have happened) and why?

Participant observers must decide how to sample events and select observational locations. They often use a variety of positioning approaches—staying in a single location to observe activities in that location (*single positioning*), moving around to observe behaviors from different locations (*multiple positioning*), or following a person around (*mobile positioning*).

Direct observation is usually supplemented with information from interviews. For example, key informants may be asked to describe what went on in a meeting the observer was unable to attend or to describe an event that occurred before the study began. In such cases, the informant functions as the observer's observer.

Recording Observations

The most common forms of record keeping for participant observation are logs and field notes, but photographs and video recordings may also be used. A **log** (or *field diary*) is a daily record of events and conversations. **Field notes** are broader and more interpretive. Field notes represent the observer's efforts to record information and to synthesize and understand the data.

Field notes serve multiple purposes. *Descriptive notes* are objective descriptions of events and conversations that were observed. *Reflective notes* document researchers' personal experiences, reflections, and progress in the field. For example, some notes document the observers' interpretations; others are reminders about how future observations should be made. Observers often record personal notes, which are comments about their own feelings during the research process.

The success of participant observation depends on the quality of the logs and field notes. It is essential to record observations as quickly as possible, but participant observers cannot usually record information by openly carrying a clipboard or a recording device because this would undermine their role as ordinary participants. Observers must develop skills in making detailed mental notes that can later be written or recorded.

Evaluation of Unstructured Observational Methods

Qualitative observational methods—especially participant observation—can provide a deeper understanding of human behaviors and social situations than is possible with structured methods. Participant observation offers opportunities to delve deeply into a situation and illuminate its complexities. Participant observation can answer questions about phenomena that are difficult for insiders themselves to explain because these phenomena are taken for granted.

Like all research methods, however, participant observation faces potential problems. Observers may lose objectivity in sampling, viewing, and interpreting observations. Once they begin to participate in a group's activities, emotional involvement might become a concern. Researchers in their member role may develop a myopic view on issues of importance to the group. Finally, the success of participant observation depends on the observer's observational and interpersonal skills—skills that may be difficult to cultivate.

Example of participant observation •

Anderson and colleagues (2020) conducted an ethnographic study to explore the relationship between nursing identity and advanced nursing practice (ANP) in two general practice sites. In addition to conducting interviews with ANPs and other nurses, the researchers used participant observation in their study. The ANPs were observed in team meetings, during supervision, and during formal and informal interactions. The fieldwork took place at different times of the day, different days of the week, and in different settings and contexts. A total of 127 hours of participant observation was undertaken.

Critical Appraisal of Unstructured Data Collection

It is often difficult to critically appraise the decisions that researchers made in collecting qualitative data because details about those decisions are seldom spelled out. In particular, there is often scant information about participant observation. It is not uncommon for a report to simply say that the researcher undertook participant observation, without descriptions of how much time was spent in the field, what exactly was observed, how observations were recorded, and what level of participation was involved. Thus, one aspect of an appraisal is likely to involve an evaluation of how much information the article provided about the data collection methods. Even though space constraints in journals make it impossible for researchers to fully elaborate their methods, researchers have a responsibility to communicate basic information about their approach so that readers can assess the quality of evidence that the study yields. Researchers should provide examples of questions asked and types of observations made.

Triangulation of methods provides important opportunities for qualitative researchers to enhance the integrity of their data. Thus, an important issue to consider in evaluating unstructured data is whether the types and amount of data collected are sufficiently rich to support an in-depth, holistic understanding of the phenomena under study. Box 11.2 provides guidelines for appraising the collection of unstructured data.

Box 11.2 Guidelines for Critically Appraising Data Collection Methods in Qualitative Studies

1. Given the research question and the characteristics of study participants, did the researcher use the best method of capturing study phenomena (i.e., self-reports, observation)? Should supplementary methods have been used to enrich the data available for analysis?
2. If self-report methods were used, did the researcher make good decisions about the specific method used to solicit information (e.g., unstructured interviews, focus group interviews, and so on)?
3. If a topic guide was used, did the report present examples of specific questions? Did the wording of questions encourage rich responses?
4. Were interviews recorded and transcribed? If interviews were not recorded, what steps were taken to ensure data accuracy?
5. If observational methods were used, did the report adequately describe what the observations entailed? What did the researcher actually observe, in what types of setting did the observations occur, and how often and over how long a period were observations made?
6. What role did the researcher assume in terms of being an observer and a participant? Was this role appropriate?
7. How were observational data recorded? Did the recording method maximize data quality?

RESEARCH EXAMPLES WITH CRITICAL THINKING EXERCISES

In this section, we describe the sampling plan and data collection strategies used in a qualitative nursing study. Read the summary and then answer the critical thinking questions that follow, referring to the full research report if necessary. Answers to the questions for Exercise 1 are available to instructors on thePoint®. The critical thinking questions for Exercise 2 are based on the study that appears in its entirety in Appendix B of this book. Our comments for this exercise are in the Student Resources section on thePoint®.

EXAMPLE 1: SAMPLING AND DATA COLLECTION IN A QUALITATIVE STUDY

Study: The experience of the self in Canadian youth living with anxiety: A qualitative study (Woodgate et al., 2020)

Statement of Purpose: The purpose of this study was to explore the experience of the sense of self among Canadian youth who live with anxiety.

Design: The researchers stated that they used a hermeneutic approach in their study. They noted that this approach "afforded the opportunity to understand how living with anxiety shaped youth's sense of self from their frames of reference and experiences of reality" (p. 4).

Sampling Strategy: Youth with a primary diagnosis of an anxiety disorder (e.g., social anxiety disorder, generalized anxiety disorder) were invited to participate. They were recruited from a hospital-based program that deals in the treatment of anxiety and from youth centers, schools, and via social media. Parents of the youth completed a diagnostic interview to assess the presence of their children's anxiety disorders. The researchers used maximum variation sampling to recruit a diverse sample of youth. Recruitment stopped when data saturation was achieved. The sample included 58 youth who were aged 10 to 22 years at the time of the study. The mean age was 14.5 years; 44 participants identified as female and 14 as male.

Data Collection: In-depth face-to-face interviews were conducted with study participants, typically in their own homes. Participants were interviewed a second time, which allowed "for follow-up questions that add to topics and themes discovered in the initial interview" (p. 4). The interviews, which were digitally recorded, lasted between 30 minutes and 3 hours. Here is an example of a question from the first interview: "What worries do you have when you are feeling really nervous or scared?" Field notes that detailed the interview context were recorded after each interview. Ecomaps (graphic portrayals of people and objects that play a role in the youth's lives) were used to supplement the data during the first interview. Before the initial interview, the youth were given instructions and were asked to draw an ecomap that was used as a point of discussion in the interview. At the completion of the first interview, the youth were given a digital camera and asked to take pictures over the next few weeks of things that portrayed their experience of living with anxiety. Photovoice discussions were incorporated into the second interview.

Key Findings: The six core themes identified by analyzing the data included *the self as fractured, being there for oneself, discovery of the self, masking the self, trust in the self,* and *transcendental self.* "A fractured sense of self underlined their experience, setting up for a great deal of self-scrutiny and a lack of self-compassion" (p. 1). The study also revealed that the youth were interested in self-discovery.

Critical Thinking Exercises

1. Answer the relevant questions from Box 11.1 and Box 11.2 regarding this study.
2. Comment on the researchers' overall data collection plan in terms of the amount of information gathered.
3. If the results of this study are valid and trustworthy, what might be some of the uses to which the findings could be put in clinical practice?

EXAMPLE 2: SAMPLING AND DATA COLLECTION IN THE STUDY IN APPENDIX B

1. Read the method section from Beck and Watson's study ("Posttraumatic growth after birth trauma") in Appendix B of this book and then answer the relevant questions in Box 11.1 and 11.2.
2. Also consider the following targeted questions, which may further sharpen your critical thinking skills and assist you in assessing aspects of the study's merit:
   a. Comment on the characteristics of the participants, given the purpose of the study.
   b. Do you think that Beck and Watson should have limited their sample to women from one country only? Provide a rationale for your answer.
   c. Did Beck and Watson's study involve a "grand tour" question?

WANT TO KNOW MORE?

A wide variety of resources to enhance your learning and understanding of this chapter is available on the Point.

- Chapter Supplement on Transferability and Generalizability
- Answer to the Critical Thinking Exercise for Example 2
- Internet Resources with useful websites for Chapter 11
- A Wolters Kluwer journal article on a topic related to this chapter

Additional study aids, including eight journal articles and related questions, are also available in *Study Guide for Essentials of Nursing Research, 10e.*

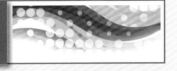
Summary Points

- Qualitative researchers typically select articulate and reflective informants with relevant experiences in an emergent way, capitalizing on early learning to guide subsequent sampling decisions.

- Qualitative researchers may start with convenience or **snowball sampling** but usually rely eventually on **purposive sampling** to guide them in selecting data sources that maximize information richness.

- One purposive strategy is **maximum variation sampling**, which entails purposely selecting cases that are diverse on key traits. Another important strategy is *sampling confirming and disconfirming cases*—i.e., selecting cases that enrich and challenge the researchers' conceptualizations.

- Samples in qualitative studies are typically small and based on information needs. A guiding principle is **data saturation**, which involves sampling to the point at which no new information is obtained and redundancy is achieved.

● Ethnographers make numerous sampling decisions, including not only *whom* to sample but also *what* to sample (e.g., activities, events, documents, artifacts); decision making is often aided by **key informants** who serve as guides and interpreters of the culture.

● Phenomenologists typically work with a small sample of people (usually 15 or fewer) who meet the criterion of having lived the experience under study.

● Grounded theory researchers typically use **theoretical sampling** in which sampling decisions are guided in an ongoing fashion by the emerging theory. Samples of about 20 to 30 people are typical.

● In-depth interviews are the most widely used method of collecting data for qualitative studies. Self-reports in qualitative studies include completely **unstructured interviews**, which are conversational discussions on the topic of interest; **semi-structured** (or *focused*) **interviews**, using a broad **topic guide**; **focus group interviews**, which involve discussions with small groups; **diaries**, in which respondents are asked to maintain daily records about some aspects of their lives; and **photo elicitation** interviews, which are guided and stimulated by photographic images, sometimes using photos that participants themselves take (**photovoice**).

● In qualitative research, self-reports are often supplemented by direct observations in naturalistic settings. One type of unstructured observation is **participant observation**, in which the researcher gains entrée into a social group and participates to varying degrees in its functioning while making in-depth observations of activities and events. **Logs** of daily events and **field notes** of the experiences and interpretations are the major data collection documents.

REFERENCES FOR CHAPTER 11

Alsaigh, R., & Coyne, I. (2019). Mothers' experiences of caring for children receiving growth hormone treatment. *Journal of Pediatric Nursing, 49*, e63–e73.

Anderson, H., Birks, Y., & Adamson, J. (2020). Exploring the relationship between nursing identity and advanced nursing practice: An ethnographic study. *Journal of Clinical Nursing, 29*, 1195–1208.

Andrews, H., Tierney, S., & Seers, K. (2020). Needing permission: The experience of self-care and self-compassion in nursing: A constructivist grounded theory study. *International Journal of Nursing Studies, 101*, 103436.

**Barsuk, J., Cohen, E., Harap, R., Grady, K., Wilcox, J., Shanklin, K., . . . Cameron, K. (2020). Patient, caregiver, and clinician perceptions of ventricular assist device self-care education inform the development of a simulation-based mastery learning curriculum. *The Journal of Cardiovascular Nursing, 35*, 54–65.

Childers, P., & Aleshire, M. (2020). Use of essential oils by health care professionals for health maintenance. *Holistic Nursing Practice, 34*, 91–102.

Duck, A., Robinson, J., & Stewart, M. (2020). Adults' and children's perceptions of barriers and facilitators of school-aged children's physical activity in an inner-city urban area. *Journal for Specialists in Pediatric Nursing, 25*, e12278.

Hanna, A., Yael, E-M., Hadassa, L., Iris, E., Eugenia, N., Lior, G., . . . Liora, P. (2020). "It's up to me with a little support"—Adherence after myocardial infarction: A qualitative study. *International Journal of Nursing Studies, 101*, 103416.

Hassankhani, H., Soheili, A., Vahdati, S., Mozaffari, F., Wold, L., & Wiseman, T. (2019). "Me first, others later": A focused ethnography of ongoing cultural features of waiting in an Iranian emergency department. *International Emergency Nursing, 47*, 100804.

Kim, S., Park, S., Kim, S., Hur, M., Lee, B., & Han, M. (2020). Self-management needs of breast cancer survivors after treatment: Results from a focus group interview. *Cancer Nursing, 43*, 78–85.

Link, K., Garrett-Wright, D., & Jones, M. (2020). The burden of farmer suicide on surviving family members: A qualitative study. *Issues in Mental Health Nursing, 41*, 66–72.

Morse, J. M. (1991). Strategies for sampling. In J. M. Morse (Ed.), *Qualitative nursing research: A contemporary dialogue* (pp. 127–145). Newbury Park, CA: Sage.

Nilsson, J., Röing, M., Malmros, J., & Winterling, J. (2020). Ways of understanding the ability to have children among young adult survivors of childhood cancer—A phenomenographic study. *European Journal of Oncology Nursing, 44*, 101710.

Patton, M. Q. (2015). *Qualitative research & evaluation methods* (4th ed.). Thousand Oaks, CA: Sage.

Wang, Q., Arber, A., Shen, A., & Qiang, W. (2020). Perspectives of Chinese cancer patients toward disclosure of cancer diagnosis to their minor children. *Cancer Nursing, 43*, 2–11.

*Woodgate, R., Tailor, K., Tennent, P., Wener, P., & Altman, G. (2020). The experience of the self in Canadian youth living with anxiety: A qualitative study. *PLoS One, 15*, e0228193.

*A link to this open-access article is provided in the Internet Resources section on thePoint® website.

**This journal article is available on thePoint® for this chapter.

12

Understanding Mixed Methods Research, Quality Improvement, and Other Special Types of Research

Learning Objectives

On completing this chapter, you will be able to:

- Understand the advantages of mixed methods research and describe specific applications
- Describe strategies and designs for conducting mixed methods research
- Distinguish research and quality improvement (QI), and describe QI strategies
- Identify the purposes and some of the distinguishing features of specific types of research (e.g., clinical trials, evaluations, outcomes research, surveys)
- Define new terms in the chapter

Key Terms

- Clinical trial
- Comparative effectiveness research (CER)
- Concurrent design
- Convergent design
- Delphi survey
- Economic (cost) analysis
- Evaluation research
- Explanatory design
- Exploratory design
- Health services research
- Improvement science
- Intervention research
- Intervention theory
- Methodological study
- Mixed methods research
- Nursing sensitive outcome
- Outcomes research
- Patient-centered outcomes research
- Plan-Do-Study-Act (PDSA)
- Pragmatism
- Process analysis
- Quality improvement (QI)
- Root cause analysis (RCA)
- Secondary analysis
- Sequential design
- Survey

In this final chapter on research designs, we explain several special types of research. We begin by discussing mixed methods research that combines qualitative and quantitative approaches.

MIXED METHODS RESEARCH

A growing trend in nursing research is the planned collection and integration of qualitative and quantitative data within a single study or coordinated clusters of studies. This section discusses the rationale for such **mixed methods research** and presents a few applications.

Rationale for Mixed Method Research

The dichotomy between quantitative and qualitative data represents a key methodological distinction. It is now widely believed, however, that many areas of inquiry can be enriched by integrating qualitative and quantitative data. The advantages of a mixed methods (MM) design include the following:

- *Complementarity.* Qualitative and quantitative data are complementary. By using MM, researchers can avoid the limitations of a single approach.
- *Practicality.* Given the complexity of phenomena, it is practical to use whatever methodological tools are best suited to addressing pressing research questions.
- *Enhanced validity.* When a hypothesis or model is supported by multiple and complementary types of data, researchers can be more confident about their inferences.

Perhaps the strongest argument for MM research, however, is that some questions *require* MM. The paradigm called **pragmatism** is often associated with MM research—a paradigm that some consider offers an "umbrella worldview" for a study (Creswell & Plano Clark, 2018, p. 69). Pragmatist researchers consider that it is the research question that should drive the research design. They reject a forced choice between the traditional positivist and constructivist modes of inquiry.

Purposes and Applications of Mixed Methods Research

In MM research, there are inevitably at least two research questions, each of which requires a different approach. For example, MM researchers may ask both exploratory (qualitative) and confirmatory (quantitative) questions. In an MM study, researchers can examine causal *effects* in a quantitative component but can shed light on causal *mechanisms* in a qualitative component. In addition to mono-method questions, MM studies ideally ask a specific MM question relating to the integration of qualitative and quantitative data and that makes explicit what will be answered through such integration.

Creswell and Plano Clark (2018) identified seven broad types of research situations that are especially well suited to MM research. Here are a few examples:

1. Neither a qualitative nor a quantitative approach, by itself, is adequate in addressing the complexity of the research problem.
2. The findings from one approach can be greatly enhanced with a second source of data that has explanatory power.
3. Quantitative results from an intervention study require qualitative data to help to explain and interpret the results.
4. A program (or formal instrument) needs to be developed and evaluated.

As this list suggests, MM research can be used in various situations. Some major applications include the following:

- *Hypothesis generation.* In-depth qualitative studies are often fertile with insights about constructs and relationships among them. These insights then can be tested with larger samples in quantitative studies.
- *Explication.* Qualitative data are sometimes used to explicate the *meaning* of quantitative relationships. Quantitative methods can demonstrate that variables are systematically related but may fail to explain *why* they are related.
- *Instrument development.* Nurse researchers sometimes gather qualitative data as the basis for generating construct-valid questions for quantitative scales that are then subjected to rigorous testing.
- *Intervention development.* Qualitative research also plays an important role in the development of nursing interventions that are then rigorously tested for efficacy.

Example of MM in intervention development research • • • • • • • • • • • • • • • •
Redeker and an interdisciplinary team (2018) published a protocol for an MM study of sleep in children from disadvantaged urban areas. They launched a community-engaged study to understand the perspectives of key stakeholders (e.g., parents, pediatric health care providers) about children's sleep habits and difficulties. The team collected in-depth data through interviews with stakeholders and 9 days of objective sleep data (wrist actigraphy) from 32 infants and toddlers (Caldwell et al., 2020). Data from the study will be used to develop a contextually relevant program to promote sleep health.

Mixed Method Designs and Strategies

In designing MM studies, researchers make many important decisions. We briefly describe a few.

Design Decisions and Notation

Two decisions in MM design concern sequencing and prioritization. There are three options for sequencing components of an MM study: Qualitative data are collected first, quantitative data are collected first, or both types are collected simultaneously. When the data are collected at the same time, the approach is **concurrent**. The design is **sequential** when the two types of data are collected in phases. In well-conceived sequential designs, the analysis and interpretation in one phase informs the collection of data in the second.

In terms of prioritization, researchers decide which approach—qualitative or quantitative—to emphasize. One option is to give the two components (*strands*) equal, or roughly equal, weight. Usually, however, one approach is given priority. The distinction is sometimes referred to as *equal status* versus *dominant status*.

Janice Morse (1991), a prominent nurse researcher, contributed to MM research by proposing a notation system for sequencing and prioritization. In this system, priority is designated by upper- and lowercase letters: QUAL/quan designates an MM study in which the dominant approach is qualitative, whereas QUAN/qual designates the reverse. If neither approach is dominant (i.e., both are equal), the notation is QUAL/QUAN. Sequencing is indicated by the symbols + or →. The arrow designates a sequential approach. For example, QUAN → qual is the notation for a primarily quantitative MM study in which qualitative data are collected in phase 2. When both approaches occur concurrently, a plus sign is used (e.g., QUAL + quan).

Specific Mixed Methods Designs

Numerous design typologies have been proposed by different MM methodologists. We illustrate a few core designs described by Creswell and Plano Clark (2018).

The purpose of the **convergent design** is to obtain different, but complementary, data about the central phenomenon under study. The goal of this design is to converge on "the truth" about a problem or phenomenon by allowing the limitations of one approach to be offset by the strengths of the other. In this design, qualitative and quantitative data are collected simultaneously, with equal priority (QUAL + QUAN).

Example of a convergent design •
Kalanlar and Kuru Alici (2020) used a convergent design to study the effect of care burden on formal caregivers' quality of work life. Structured questionnaires were used to obtain quantitative data about the key constructs. In-depth interviews were also undertaken with some caregivers, who were asked such questions as, "What are the most challenging situations while giving care?" and "How does your care burden affect your home life?"

Explanatory designs are sequential designs with quantitative data collected in the first phase, followed by qualitative data collected in the second phase. Either the qualitative or the quantitative strand can be given a stronger priority: The design can be either QUAN → qual or quan → QUAL. In explanatory designs, qualitative data from the second phase are used to build on or explain the quantitative data from the initial phase. This design is especially suitable when results are complex and tricky to interpret.

Example of an explanatory design ••••••••••••••••••••••••••••••••••
Dove-Medows and colleagues (2020) used an MM design to study pregnant African American women's perceptions of stressful environments and psychological distress as influences on birth outcomes. A sample of 38 women completed structured questionnaires that measured their views on neighborhood disorder, experiences of racial discrimination, and depression and emotional well-being. Then, about 5 weeks later, 7 women participated in in-depth interviews. The researchers found that the in-depth interviews provided data about the women's experiences that brought into focus the depth of the women's perceptions.

Exploratory designs are sequential MM designs, with qualitative data being collected first. The design has as its central premise the need for initial in-depth exploration of a phenomenon, often to better understand contextual or cultural issues relevant to a phenomenon. Its intent is use rich contextualized information to inform the development of a quantitative feature, such as a new measure, survey, intervention, or digital tool such as a website or app. The overall design of the previously described MM project by Redeker and colleagues (2018) would be considered exploratory; the first phase primarily involved the collection of qualitative data from a range of stakeholders concerning the sleep problems of children who are economically disadvantaged (Caldwell et al., 2020).

 TIP In an earlier edition of their MM textbook, Creswell and Plano Clark (2018) described a design called the *embedded design*. An embedded design is one in which a second type of data is totally subservient to the other type of data. Creswell and Plano Clark now see embedding as an analytic strategy rather than as a design type.

Sampling and Data Collection in Mixed Methods Research

Sampling and data collection in MM studies are often a blend of approaches described in earlier chapters. A few special issues for an MM study merit brief discussion.

MM researchers can combine sampling designs in various ways. The quantitative component is likely to rely on a sampling strategy that enhances the researcher's ability to generalize from the sample to a population. For the qualitative component, MM researchers usually adopt purposive sampling methods to select people who are good informants about the phenomenon of interest. Sample sizes are also likely to be different in the qualitative and quantitative strands, with larger samples for the quantitative component. A unique sampling issue in MM studies concerns whether the same people will be in both the strands. The best strategy depends on the study purpose and research design, but using overlapping samples can be advantageous. Indeed, a popular strategy is a *nested* approach in which a subset of participants from the quantitative strand is included in the qualitative strand.

Example of nested sampling •••••••••••••••••••••••••••••••••••••••
Makic and colleagues (2020) undertook an MM study to characterize the fatigue experiences and self-management behaviors of people living with HIV. A sample of 55 people living with HIV completed daily surveys on their smartphones. A nested sample of 25 participants also completed in-depth interviews about their experiences.

In terms of data collection, all of the data collection methods discussed previously can be creatively combined and triangulated in an MM study. Thus, possible sources of data include group and individual interviews, psychosocial scales, observations, biophysiological measures, records, diaries, and so on. MM studies can involve *intramethod mixing* (e.g., structured and unstructured self-reports) and *intermethod mixing* (e.g., biophyisiological measures and unstructured observation). A fundamental issue concerns the methods' complementarity—that is, having the limitations of one method be balanced and offset by the strengths of the other.

 TIP   One challenge in doing MM research concerns how best to analyze the qualitative and quantitative data. The benefits of MM research require an effort to merge results from the two strands and to develop interpretations and recommendations based on integrated understandings.

QUALITY IMPROVEMENT

Quality improvement (QI) involves assessments of a problem in patient care with the aim of improving clinical care and patient outcomes within a health care organization. A decade ago, there was a lot of discussion in nursing journals about the differences and similarities among QI, research, and evidence-based practice projects. All three have a lot in common, notably the use of systematic methods of solving health problems with an overall aim of fostering improvements in health care.

Shirey and colleagues (2011) created a comparison chart describing the similarities and differences of the three types of efforts on over 20 dimensions. On some dimensions, the differences noted in the chart continue to be relevant. For example, one issue is whether approval from an ethics committee is needed. Most QI efforts are not subject to the regulations protecting human subjects in research, and patient informed consent is typically not obtained.

On other dimensions, however, differences between QI and research are becoming less clear-cut. For example, one dimension on the comparison chart was "expectations for knowledge dissemination." A decade ago, publication in a professional journal was considered by many a criterion for classifying something as "research" rather than QI, but this is no longer the case. Many QI projects are described in professional journals, and several journals are now devoted specifically to improvement activities.

A related dimension on which QI, evidence-based practice, and research were compared by Shirey and colleagues (2011) was the generalizability of the knowledge gained from the project. Their chart stated that knowledge from QI is not generalizable—it is specific to the organization in which the QI is undertaken. However, the growing interest in health care improvement has led to efforts to inspire more systematic, rigorous, theoretical, and replicable improvement activity—in short, to develop **improvement science** (Marshall et al., 2015). Increasingly, improvement researchers are developing their own base of QI evidence.

Features of Quality Improvement and Improvement Science

QI projects typically have as their primary goal the swift attainment of positive change in a health care service. QI projects are practical and typically focus on a specific problem identified in a local context. QI can also involve an ongoing process in which interprofessional teams collaborate to improve systems and processes, with the goals of reducing waste, increasing efficiency, and improving satisfaction. The ongoing nature of such efforts is integral to a quality management philosophy called *continuous quality improvement* (CQI). CQI encourages members of health care teams to continuously ask such questions as, "How are we doing?" and "Can we do this better?"

Several features characterize many QI projects. For example, the intervention or protocol for an improvement project can change as it is being evaluated to incorporate new ideas and insights—unlike what occurs in a research study. Another feature is that QI projects are designed to achieve an improvement that is sustainable. Typically, QI projects are interprofessional, involving a team with diverse perspectives on a problem.

Marshall and colleagues (2015) are among a growing group of advocates promoting improvement science as a distinct discipline. They have argued that improvement science "aims to generate local wisdom and generalisable or transferable knowledge with robust, well established research methods applied in highly pragmatic ways" (p. 419). They and other commentators have noted that QI projects are often methodologically weak and called for the adoption of a more scientific approach to health care improvement.

 TIP Nurses are being encouraged to not only participate in QI efforts but also to play a lead role. As Johnson (2012) observed, "Who better to lead the effort to improve health care delivery and outcomes than the professionals delivering the majority of health care . . . ?" (p. 113).

Efforts to improve quality and safety in health care organizations have involved a wide variety of strategies to effecting positive change. QI interventions include (1) provider education (teaching health care teams how best to manage particular situations), (2) provider reminders (providing decision support materials to prompt health care professionals to undertake some action), (3) patient education (increasing patient's understanding of a prevention or treatment strategy), (4) patient reminders (reminding patients to keep appointments or adhere to regimens), and (5) structural changes (creating care coordination or case management systems).

Example of reminders and education in a QI project •
Bauer and colleagues (2020) gathered data from parents in an effort to identify barriers to their immunizing their young children against influenza. Based on the feedback they received, the team developed a QI program that included reminder phone calls, parent education, and proactive appointment scheduling.

Quality Improvement Planning Tools

During the planning of QI initiatives, a major issue is the identification of a problem on which to focus. This is likely to involve discussions with key stakeholders, brainstorming, a review of institutional trends, a search for relevant evidence, and the creation of flowcharts and process maps.

Once a problem or process has been selected for improvement, the QI team usually tries to investigate the *causes* of the problem. It is difficult to develop solutions to institutional problems without understanding the underlying factors contributing to them. QI teams often undertake what is called a **root cause analysis (RCA)**, which involves efforts to identify underlying process deficiencies (Haxby & Shuldham, 2018).

One tool for identifying the root cause of a problem is a process called the *5 Whys*. The process begins by identifying the specific problem and then asking why the problem happens. If the answer fails to get to the underlying cause, "Why" is asked again. Here is an example (Chambers et al., 2014):

Problem: Patient falls while toileting.

1. Why do patients fall while toileting? → *Because nurses do not stay in the bathroom with their patients.*
2. Why don't nurses stay in the bathroom with patients? → *Because patients don't understand that a nurse should stay with them.*

3. Why don't patients understand why a nurse should stay? → *Because they don't know that they might be unstable and that nurses can prevent them from falling if they stay in the room.*
4. Why don't patients know this? → *Because nurses have not explained this safety precaution to them.*
5. Why don't nurses explain this safety precaution to them? → *Because current training and practice does not address this strategy.*

QI teams use such tools to determine the causes of undesirable outcomes and to understand why current practices deviate from best practices. Then, the team can consider specific aspects of a problem that will be addressed.

Quality Improvement Approaches

QI projects typically are based on one of several broad models to guide processes and activities. For example, health care institutions have used the *lean approach* (also called the *Toyota Production System*) in efforts to achieve improved quality and efficiency at lower costs. A major feature of lean is that it strives to eliminate three types of waste: (1) unnecessary actions, (2) unevenness and variability in product or in flow of information, and (3) unreasonableness of a process for a person's capability. The goal of a lean process is to eliminate non–value-added steps, to identify what "value" means to customers (patients), and to serve customers' needs.

The most widely used QI model in health care is **Plan-Do-Study-Act (PDSA)**, which is sometimes called *Plan-Do-Check-Act* (PDCA). The PDSA cycle was originally introduced as a framework for CQI in business and manufacturing. Typically, PDSA relies on multiple *rapid cycles* of investigating and acting on a problem. The idea underpinning rapid cycle improvement is to first try an improvement strategy on a small scale to see how well it works and then modify it and try it again until there is confidence in the effectiveness of the change.

PDSA allows the QI team to test improvement strategies in a controlled manner, to measure results of these strategies, and to drive further improvements. The PDSA/PDCA process involves the following:

1. **Plan:** The QI team initially works on developing explicit strategies or interventions to address the problem identified before the project gets underway. During this phase, the team also develops a plan for data collection and identifies measures that will be used to assess improvement. Baseline (pre-QI intervention) data typically are collected during this phase.
2. **Do:** The team then implements the QI intervention and collects data on key outcomes to assess whether improvement occurred. In a PDSA cycle, each improvement is tested on a fairly small scale.
3. **Study/Check:** Data from the trial run are analyzed to see if a positive change occurred.
4. **Act:** If the QI project resulted in improved outcomes, the team considers how best to sustain (and perhaps disseminate) the practice change. If no improvements were observed, or were modest, the team would work through the PDSA/PSCA cycle again, starting with decisions on what changes to make next.

Many QI projects use simple research designs. Conducting projects within real-world health care settings makes it challenging to use powerful designs, but those who promote a more rigorous approach are urging QI teams to consider designs that offer better internal validity. Randomized controlled trials (RCTs) are rare in the field of QI, but they do exist. RCTs are especially suitable when an improvement intervention is being considered for widespread use based on early evidence.

Most QI teams adopt quasi-experimental designs to test the effectiveness of changes to systems or processes of care. Before–after designs, which measure changes to key outcomes after implementing a QI intervention, are especially common, but they are notably weak designs. Time series–type designs are especially useful for sorting out the effects of seasonal or cyclical trends from QI intervention effects.

Example of a quality improvement project •
An interprofessional team (Griffith et al., 2020) conducted a QI project to address communication problems between (1) patients with left ventricular assist devices (VADs) having an emergency and (2) VAD-trained personnel. The team undertook an RCA analysis and then used the PDSA model to implement processes to reduce waiting time between a patient call and response by appropriate personnel. A pretest–posttest design was used to assess changes.

 TIP Many QI projects use MM designs that involve collecting both qualitative and quantitative data. Qualitative methods are especially well suited during the planning phase and during the "Act" phase when the QI team must consider what to do next.

OTHER SPECIAL TYPES OF RESEARCH

The remainder of this chapter briefly describes types of research that vary by study purpose rather than by research design or tradition.

Intervention Research

In Chapter 8, we discussed RCTs and other designs for testing the effects of interventions. In actuality, intervention research is often more complex than a simple experimental–control group comparison of outcomes—indeed, intervention research often relies on MM to develop, refine, test, and understand the intervention and its effects.

Different disciplines have developed their own approaches and terminology in connection with intervention efforts. *Clinical trials* are associated with medical research, *evaluation research* is linked to the fields of education and public policy, and nurses are developing their own tradition of intervention research. We briefly describe these three approaches.

Clinical Trials

Clinical trials test clinical interventions. Clinical trials that are undertaken to evaluate an innovative therapy or drug are often designed in a series of phases:

- *Phase I* of the trial is designed to establish safety, tolerance, and dose with a simple design (e.g., one-group pretest–posttest). The focus is on developing the best treatment.
- *Phase II* is a pilot test of treatment effectiveness. Researchers see if the intervention is feasible and holds promise. This phase is designed as a small-scale experiment or quasi-experiment.
- *Phase III* is a full experimental test of the intervention—an RCT with random assignment to treatment conditions. The objective is to develop evidence about the treatment's *efficacy*—i.e., whether the intervention is more efficacious than usual care or an alternative. When the term *clinical trial* is used, it often is referring to a phase III trial.
- *Phase IV* of clinical trials involves studies of the *effectiveness* of an intervention in the general population. The emphasis in effectiveness studies is on the external validity of an intervention that has demonstrated efficacy under controlled (but artificial) conditions.

Evaluation Research

Evaluation research focuses on developing useful information about a program or policy—information that decision makers need on whether to adopt, modify, or abandon the program.

Evaluations are undertaken to answer various questions. Questions about program effectiveness rely on experimental or quasi-experimental designs, but other questions do not. Many evaluations are MM studies with distinct components.

For example, a **process analysis** is often undertaken to obtain descriptive information about the process by which a program gets implemented and how it actually functions. A process analysis addresses such questions as the following: What exactly *is* the treatment, and how does it differ from traditional practices? What are the barriers to successful program implementation? How do staff and clients feel about the intervention? Qualitative data play a big role in process analyses.

Evaluations may also include an **economic** (or **cost**) **analysis** to assess whether program benefits outweigh its monetary costs. Administrators make decisions about resource allocation for health services not only on the basis of whether something "works" but also based on economic viability. Cost analyses are often done when researchers are also evaluating program efficacy.

Example of an economic analysis ••••••••••••••••••••••••••••••••••••
Mitchell and colleagues (2019) assessed the cost-effectiveness of switching from saline to 0.1% chlorhexidine for meatal cleaning prior to urinary catheter insertion. They estimated that making the switch would save nearly 400,000 Australian dollars per 100,000 catheterizations.

 TIP Some nurse researchers have begun to undertake a *realist evaluation*, which is a theory-driven approach to evaluating programs—especially complex programs or interventions. The realist approach acknowledges that interventions are not always effective for everyone because people are diverse and embedded in complicated social and cultural contexts. In a realist evaluation, the focus is on understanding why certain groups benefitted from an intervention, whereas others did not benefit.

Nursing Intervention Research

Both clinical trials and evaluations involve *interventions*. However, the term **intervention research** is increasingly being used by nurse researchers to describe an approach characterized by a distinctive *process* of planning, developing, and testing interventions—especially *complex interventions*. Proponents of the process are critical of the simplistic, atheoretical approach that is often used to design and evaluate interventions. The recommended process involves an in-depth understanding of the problem and the target population; careful, collaborative planning with a diverse team; and the development or adoption of a theory to guide the inquiry.

Similar to clinical trials, nursing intervention research that involves the development of a complex intervention typically involves several phases: (1) basic developmental research, (2) pilot research, (3) evaluation of intervention efficacy, and (4) implementation research.

Conceptualization, a major focus of the development phase, is supported through collaborative discussions, consultations with experts, critical literature reviews, and in-depth qualitative research to understand the problem. The construct validity of the intervention is enhanced through efforts to develop an **intervention theory** that clearly articulates what must be done to achieve desired outcomes. The intervention design, which emerges from the intervention theory, specifies what the clinical inputs should be. During the developmental phase, key *stakeholders*—people who have a stake in the intervention—are often identified and "brought on board." Stakeholders include potential beneficiaries of the intervention and their families, advocates and community leaders, and health care staff.

The second phase of nursing intervention research is a pilot test of the intervention. The central activities during the pilot test are to secure preliminary evidence of the intervention's benefits, to assess the feasibility of a rigorous test, and to refine the intervention theory and intervention protocols. The feasibility assessment should involve an analysis of factors that affected implementation during the pilot (e.g., recruitment, retention, and adherence problems). Qualitative research can be used to gain insight into how the intervention should be refined.

As in a classic clinical trial, the third phase involves a full experimental test of the intervention. The final phase focuses on implementation and effectiveness in real-world clinical settings.

> **Example of nursing intervention research** •
> Kinser and colleagues (2020) developed and are pilot testing a self-management intervention entitled "Mindful Moms," which is designed to foster pregnant women's ability to address depressive symptoms and enhance resilience. The 12-week intervention has three components: (1) a nurse–participant partnership to foster awareness of depressive symptoms; (2) mindful physical activity through prenatal yoga classes; and (3) self-directed, home-based mindful physical activity.

Comparative Effectiveness Research

Comparative effectiveness research (CER) involves direct comparisons of two or more health interventions. Like realist approaches, CER seeks insights into which intervention works best for which patients. CER has emerged as a major force in health research. Disappointment with some of the methods favored for evidence-based practice—especially the strong reliance on tightly controlled RCTs with placebo comparators—has led to the development of new ideas, new models, and new methods of research that fall within the umbrella of CER.

The impetus for CER in the United States crystalized when the Institute of Medicine published a report (2009) that proposed priorities for CER. CER was defined as follows: "Comparative effectiveness research (CER) is the generation and synthesis of evidence that compares the benefits and harms of alternative methods to prevent, diagnose, treat, and monitor a clinical condition or to improve the delivery of care. The purpose of CER is to assist consumers, clinicians, purchasers, and policy makers to make informed decisions that will improve health care at both the individual and population level" (p. 41).

Another major stimulus for CER in the United States was the creation in 2010 of the independent nonprofit organization, the *Patient-Centered Outcomes Research Institute* (PCORI). PCORI specifically sponsors CER—in fact, CER is sometimes referred to as **patient-centered outcomes research**. PCORI funds research that is designed to help patients select the health care options that best meet their needs. CER studies often incorporate outcomes that are especially important to patients and their caregivers. The standard outcomes used in medical research (e.g., blood pressure, mortality) are increasingly being supplemented by outcomes in which patients have a strong interest, such as functional limitations, quality of life, and experiences with care.

Designs for CER vary widely. Some studies are RCTs involving a comparison of two or more active (nonplacebo) treatments. Some CER projects, however, are observational studies using data from large databases, such as patient registries. CER is described at greater length in Chapter 18.

Example of comparative effectiveness research •
In 2017, PCORI awarded $14 million to an interprofessional team led by a nurse re-searcher (Huong Nguyen) for a 15-site project called "A non-inferiority comparative effectiveness trial of home-based palliative care in older adults (HomePal)." The project, which will compare home-based palliative care with in-person or video consultation, is expected to be completed in 2024 (see https://www.pcori.org/research-results/2017/comparing-home-based-palliative-care-person-or-video-consultation).

Health Services and Outcomes Research

Health services research is the broad interdisciplinary field that studies how organizational structures and processes, health technologies, social factors, and personal behaviors affect access to health care, the cost and quality of health care, and, ultimately, people's health and well-being. **Outcomes research**, a subset of health services research, comprises efforts to understand the end results of particular health care practices and to assess the effectiveness of health care services. Outcomes research represents a response to the increasing demand from policy makers and the public to justify care practices in terms of improved patient outcomes and costs.

Many nursing studies evaluate patient outcomes, but efforts to appraise the quality and impact of nursing care—as distinct from care provided by the overall health care system—are less common. A major obstacle is attribution—that is, linking patient outcomes to specific nursing actions, distinct from those of other members of the health care team. It is also often difficult to ascertain a causal connection between outcomes and health care interventions because factors outside the health care system (e.g., patient characteristics) affect outcomes in complex ways.

Donabedian (1987), whose pioneering efforts created a framework for outcomes research, emphasized three factors in appraising quality in health care services: structure, process, and outcomes. The *structure* of care refers to broad organizational and administrative features. Nursing skill mix, for example, is a structural variable that has been found to be related to patient outcomes. *Processes* involve aspects of clinical management and decision making. *Outcomes* refer to specific clinical end results of patient care. Much progress has been made in identifying **nursing sensitive outcomes**—patient outcomes that improve if there is greater quantity or quality of nurses' care.

Several modifications to Donabedian's (1987) framework for appraising health care quality have been proposed, the most noteworthy of which is the Quality Health Outcomes Model developed by the American Academy of Nursing (Mitchell et al., 1998). This model is more dynamic than Donabedian's original framework and takes client characteristics (e.g., illness severity) and system characteristics into account.

Outcomes research usually concentrates on studying linkages within such models rather than on testing the overall model. Some studies have examined the effect of health care structures on health care processes or outcomes, for example. Outcomes research in nursing often has focused on the process–patient–outcomes nexus. Examples of nursing process variables include nursing actions, nurses' problem solving and decision making, clinical competence and leadership, and specific activities or interventions (e.g., communication, touch).

Example of outcomes research •
Magnowski and Cleveland (2020) used the Donabedian (1987) framework in their study of two different types of nursing shift assignments (milieu nurse–client vs. individual nurse–client shift assignments—a structural feature) on monthly restraint rates in an inpatient child/adolescent psychiatric unit.

Survey Research

A **survey** obtains quantitative information about the prevalence, distribution, and interrelations of variables within a population. Political opinion polls are examples of surveys. Survey data are used primarily in correlational studies and are often used to gather information from nonclinical populations (e.g., college students, nurses).

Surveys obtain information about people's actions, knowledge, intentions, and opinions by self-report. Surveys may be either cross-sectional or longitudinal. Any information that can reliably be obtained by direct questioning can be gathered in a survey, although surveys include mostly closed-ended questions and thus yield quantitative data primarily.

Survey data can be collected in various ways, but the most respected method is through personal interviews in which interviewers meet in person with respondents to ask them questions. Personal interviews are expensive because they involve a lot of personnel time, but they yield high-quality data and refusal rates tend to be low. Telephone interviews are less costly, but when the interviewer is unknown, respondents may be uncooperative on the phone. Self-administered questionnaires (especially those delivered over the Internet) are an economical approach to doing a survey but are not appropriate for surveying certain populations (e.g., the elderly, children) and tend to yield especially low response rates.

The greatest advantage of surveys is their flexibility and broadness of scope. Surveys can be used with many populations and can focus on a wide range of topics. The information obtained in surveys, however, tends to be relatively superficial: Surveys rarely probe deeply into complexities of human behavior and feelings.

Example of a survey •
Dall'Ora and colleagues (2020) examined whether nurses working 12-hour shifts or more were less likely than nurses working shifts of 8 hours or less to pursue continuing education and to report that they had time to discuss patient care with other nurses. They gathered their data through a survey of 31,627 nurses in 12 European countries.

A Few Other Types of Research

Most quantitative nursing studies are the types described thus far in this and earlier chapters. However, nurse researchers have pursued a few other specific types of research, as briefly described here. The supplement for this chapter on thePoint° website provides more details about each type.

- **Secondary analysis**. Secondary analyses involve the use of existing data from a previous or ongoing study to test new hypotheses or answer questions that were not initially envisioned. Secondary analyses are often based on quantitative data from a large data set (e.g., from national surveys), but secondary analyses of data from qualitative studies are also undertaken.
- **Delphi surveys**. Delphi surveys were developed as a tool for short-term forecasting. The technique involves a panel of experts who are asked to complete several rounds of questionnaires focusing on their judgments about a topic of interest. Multiple iterations are used to achieve consensus.
- **Methodological studies**. Nurse researchers have undertaken many methodological studies, which focus on the development, validation, and assessment of methodological tools or strategies (e.g., the psychometric testing of a new scale).

Box 12.1 Guidelines for Critically Appraising Studies Described in Chapter 12

1. Was the study exclusively qualitative or exclusively quantitative? If so, could the study have been strengthened by incorporating both approaches?
2. If the study used an MM design, did the inclusion of both approaches contribute to enhanced validity? In what other ways (if any) did the inclusion of both types of data strengthen the study and further the aims of the research?
3. If the study used an MM approach, what was the design—how were the components sequenced, and which had priority? Was this approach appropriate?
4. In a QI project, were adequate methods used to identify the root cause of the problem being addressed? Was PDSA (or another QI model) used to guide the process, and was it used appropriately? Was a good research design used to assess the effects of the QI changes?
5. If the study was a clinical trial or intervention study, was adequate attention paid to developing an appropriate intervention? Was there a well-conceived intervention theory that guided the endeavor? Was the intervention adequately pilot tested?
6. If the study was a clinical trial, evaluation, or intervention study, was there an effort to understand how the intervention was implemented (i.e., a process-type analysis)? Were the financial costs and benefits assessed? If not, should they have been?
7. If the study was outcomes research, which segments of the structure–process–outcomes model were examined? Would it have been desirable (and feasible) to expand the study to include other aspects? Do the findings suggest possible improvements to structures or processes that would be beneficial to patient outcomes?
8. If the study was a survey, was the most appropriate method used to collect the data (i.e., in-person interviews, telephone interviews, mail or Internet questionnaires)?

CRITICAL APPRAISAL OF STUDIES DESCRIBED IN THIS CHAPTER

It is difficult to provide guidance on appraising the types of studies described in this chapter because they are so varied and because many fundamental methodological issues require an appraisal of the overall design. Guidelines for evaluating design-related issues were presented in previous chapters.

You should, however, consider whether researchers took appropriate advantage of the possibilities of an MM design. Collecting both qualitative and quantitative data is not always necessary or practical, but in appraising studies, you can consider whether the study would have been strengthened by integrating different types of data. In studies in which MM were used, you should carefully consider whether the inclusion of both types of data was justified and whether the researcher really made use of both types of data to enhance knowledge on the research topic. Box 12.1 offers a few specific questions for appraising the types of studies included in this chapter.

RESEARCH EXAMPLES WITH CRITICAL THINKING EXERCISES

The nursing literature abounds with studies of the types described in this chapter. Here, we describe an example. Read the summary and then answer the critical thinking questions that follow, referring to the full research report if necessary. Answers to the questions for Exercise 1 are available to instructors on thePoint®. The critical thinking questions for Exercise 2 are based on the study that appears in its entirety in Appendix C of this book. Our comments for this exercise are in the Student Resources section on thePoint®.

EXAMPLE 1: MIXED METHODS STUDY WITH A SURVEY

Study: Secondary traumatic stress in NICU nurses: A mixed-methods study (Beck et al., 2017)

Statement of Purpose: The purposes of this study were to assess the pervasiveness of secondary traumatic stress (STS) in NICU nurses and to explore nurses' traumatic experiences caring for critically ill infants. The researchers asked three research questions: (1) What are the prevalence and severity of STS in nurses who care for critically ill infants in the NICU? (2) What are the traumatic experiences of nurses who care for critically ill infants in the NICU? and (3) How do the quantitative and qualitative sets of results develop a more complete picture of STS in NICU nurses?

Methods: Beck and colleagues used a convergent design (QUAL + QUAN). The 7,500 members of the National Association of Neonatal Nurses were sent an e-mail invitation that included a link to an online survey. A total of 175 nurses completed the survey, which included the 17-item Secondary Traumatic Stress Scale (STSS) to measure the existence and severity of STS. Respondents were also asked to respond to the following probing question: "Please describe in as much detail as you can remember your traumatic experiences caring for critically ill infants in the NICU. Specific examples of points that you are making are extremely valuable" (p. 480). A nested sample of 109 nurses provided in-depth answers to the QUAL question.

Data Analysis and Integration: Statistical methods were used to answer the first research question. For example, descriptive statistics were used to characterize the prevalence and severity of STS, and correlation procedures were used to assess the relationship between the nurses' background characteristics and their STSS scores. Question 2 was addressed using a content analysis of the qualitative data on the nurses' actual experiences. Some qualitative data were also "quantitized." For example, the researchers coded qualitative segments according to their correspondence to the three subscales of the STSS—Arousal, Intrusion, and Avoidance. These codes were then counted for presence/absence in the in-depth responses to the open-ended question. The mixed methods question was addressed by integrating quotes and statistics and by creating joint displays of the MM data.

Key Findings: In this sample, 29% of the NICU nurses reported high to severe STS; 35% screened positive for post-traumatic stress disorder (PTSD) due to attending traumatic births. The total STSS scores were unrelated to any demographic characteristics, such as gender, age, or years practicing in the NICU. The subscale with the highest mean score was Arousal (e.g., "I had trouble sleeping"). The next highest score was for the Intrusion subscale (e.g., "I thought about my work with patients when I didn't want to"). Intrusion-related comments from the nurses' narrative descriptions were especially frequent. Figure 12.1 shows a side-by-side joint display that shows quantitative subscale results on the left and illustrative qualitative results on the right. In the content analysis of the qualitative data, five themes emerged: What intensified NICU nurses' traumatic experiences: multiple scenarios; Parents insisting on aggressive treatment: so distressing; Baby torture: performing painful procedures; Questioning their skills: Did I do enough? and The grief of the family: It is contagious. Thus, the integrated QUAL and QUAN results provided a richer and more complete picture of both the prevalence of STS in NICU nurses and their complex experiences with it.

Critical Thinking Exercises

1. Answer the relevant questions from Box 12.1 regarding this study.
2. What might be an advantage of using a sequential rather than a concurrent design in this study?
3. If the results of this study are valid, what are some of the uses to which the findings might be put in clinical practice?

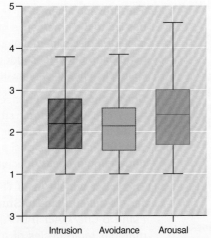

A highly traumatic experience that continues to haunt me in my dreams. These situations pop into my head randomly, even when I'm not at work, and continue to upset me enough to bring tears.

I have anxiety every time I enter that room and try to avoid caring for infants there. I go home wanting to hide and not talk to anyone about the event.

I can't sleep before going to work. I'm impulsive and irritable around others. I feel mentally drained and have difficulty concentrating. It takes me longer to finish a task.

Figure 12.1 Joint display from Beck et al.'s (2017) study of secondary traumatic stress in NICU nurses. The vertical axis shows values of scale item responses, from 1 (*never*) to 5 (*very often*). Each box plot represents the middle 50% of cases, between the 25th and 75th percentiles. The right side includes illustrative quotes from the NICU nurses' qualitative data. Color coding of the boxplot and the quotes helps to match the quantitative and qualitative responses. (Adapted with permission from Beck, C. T., Cusson, R., & Gable, R. [2017]. Secondary traumatic stress in NICU nurses: A mixed-methods study. *Advances in Neonatal Care, 17,* 478–488.)

EXAMPLE 2: MIXED METHODS STUDY IN APPENDIX C

Read the report of the mixed methods study by Bail and colleagues ("Cancer-related symptoms and cognitive intervention adherence among breast cancer survivors") in Appendix C and then address the following suggested activities.

1. Answer questions 1 to 3 in Box 12.1 regarding this study.
2. What was the sampling design in this study? Was this sampling design appropriate and effective?
3. Did the researchers take steps to integrate their qualitative and quantitative data?
4. If the results of this study are valid, what are some of the uses to which the findings might be put in clinical practice?

WANT TO KNOW MORE?

A wide variety of resources to enhance your learning and understanding of this chapter is available on thePoint°.

- Chapter Supplement on Other Specific Types of Research
- Answer to the Critical Thinking Exercises for Example 2
- Internet Resources with useful websites for Chapter 12
- A Wolters Kluwer journal article on a topic related to this chapter

Additional study aids, including eight journal articles and related questions, are also available in *Study Guide for Essentials of Nursing Research, 10e.*

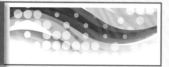

Summary Points

- **Mixed methods research** involves the collection, analysis, and integration of both qualitative and quantitative data within a study or series of studies, often with an overarching goal of achieving both discovery and verification.

- Mixed methods (MM) research has numerous advantages, including the complementarity of qualitative and quantitative data and the practicality of using methods that best address a question. MM research has many applications, including the development and testing of instruments, theories, and interventions.

- The paradigm most often associated with MM research is **pragmatism**, which has as a major tenet "the dictatorship of the research question."

- Key decisions in designing an MM study involve how to sequence the components and which strand (if either) will be given priority. In terms of sequencing, MM designs are either **concurrent** (both strands occurring in one simultaneous phase) or **sequential** (one strand occurring prior to and informing the second strand).

- Notation for MM research often designates priority—all capital letters for the dominant strand and all lowercase letters for the non-dominant strand—and sequence. An arrow is used for sequential designs, and a "+" is used for concurrent designs. QUAL → quan, for example, is a sequential, qualitative-dominant design.

- Core MM designs include the **convergent design** (QUAL + QUAN), **explanatory design** (e.g., QUAN → qual), and **exploratory design** (e.g., QUAL → quan).

- Sampling in MM studies can involve the same or different people in the different strands. *Nesting* is a common sampling approach in which a subsample of the participants in the QUAN strand also participates in the QUAL strand.

- **Quality improvement (QI)** projects are designed to improve practices in a specific organization.

- The growing interest in rigorous QI projects has led to the emergence of **improvement science**, the discipline devoted to the systematic generation of evidence for cultivating positive changes in health care institutions.

- During the planning phase of a QI study, the team can use various strategies to understand the problem, such as a **root cause analysis (RCA)**, which is designed to understand underlying process deficiencies.

- The most widely used QI model in health care is called **Plan-Do-Study-Act (PDSA)** (or *Plan-Do-Check-Act* [PDCA]), which involves multiple *rapid cycles* of improvements and testing. Designs for QI projects are usually quasi-experimental.

- Different disciplines have developed different approaches to (and terms for) efforts to evaluate interventions. **Clinical trials**, which are studies designed to assess clinical interventions, often involve a series of phases. *Phase I* is designed to finalize features of the intervention. In *Phase II*, researchers seek preliminary evidence of efficacy and feasibility. *Phase III* is a full experimental test of treatment *efficacy*. In *Phase IV*, the researcher focuses primarily on generalized *effectiveness*.

- **Evaluation research** focuses on the efficacy of a program, policy, or procedure to assist decision makers in choosing a course of action. Evaluations can answer a variety of questions. **Process analyses** describe the process by which a program gets implemented and how it functions in practice. **Economic (cost) analyses** seek to determine whether the monetary costs of a program are outweighed by benefits. *Realist evaluations* constitute a theory-driven approach to evaluating programs; the focus is on understanding why certain groups benefited from an intervention and others did not.

- **Intervention research** is a term sometimes used to refer to a distinctive *process* of planning, developing, testing, and disseminating interventions—especially *complex interventions*. The construct validity of an emerging intervention is enhanced through efforts to develop an **intervention theory** that conceptualizes what must be done to achieve desired outcomes.

- **Comparative effectiveness research (CER)** involves direct comparisons of health interventions to gain insights into which work best for which patients—as well as which have greater risks of harm. The *Patient-Centered Outcomes Research Institute* (PCORI) is a major funder of CER, which is sometimes referred to as **patient-centered outcomes research**.

- **Outcomes research** (a subset of **health services research**) is undertaken to document the quality and effectiveness of health care and nursing services. A model of health care quality encompasses several broad concepts: *structure* (e.g., nursing skill mix), *process* (nursing interventions and actions), and *outcomes* (the specific end results of patient care in terms of patient functioning). Efforts have been made to identify **nursing sensitive outcomes**.

- **Survey research** examines people's characteristics, behaviors, intentions, and opinions by asking them to answer questions. Surveys can be administered through personal (face-to-face) interviews, telephone interviews, or self-administered questionnaires.

REFERENCES FOR CHAPTER 12

Bauer, K., Agruss, J., & Mayefsky, J. (2020). Partnering with parents to remove barriers and improve influenza immunization rates for young children. *Journal of the American Association of Nurse Practitioners*. Advance online publication. doi:10.1097/JXX.0000000000000381

**Beck, C. T., Cusson, R., & Gable, R. (2017). Secondary traumatic stress in NICU nurses: A mixed-methods study. *Advances in Neonatal Care*, 17, 478–488.

Caldwell, B., Ordway, M., Sadler, L., & Redeker, N. (2020). Parent perspectives on sleep and sleep habits among young children living with economic adversity. *Journal of Pediatric Health Care*, 34, 10–22.

Chambers, C., Petrie, J., Lindsie, S., & Makic, M. B. (2014). How to use quality improvement processes to implement evidence-based practice. In R. Fink, K. Oman, & B. B. Makic (Eds.), *Research & evidence-based practice manual* (3rd ed., pp. 37–48). Aurora, CO: University of Colorado Hospital Authority.

Creswell, J. W., & Plano Clark, V. L. (2018). *Designing and conducting mixed methods research* (3rd ed.). Thousand Oaks, CA: Sage.

*Dall'Ora, C., Griffiths, P., Emmanuel, T., Rafferty, A., & Ewings, S. (2020). 12-hr shifts in nursing: Do they remove unproductive time and information loss or do they reduce education and discussion opportunities for nurses? A cross-sectional study in 12 European countries. *Journal of Clinical Nursing*, 29, 53–59.

Donabedian, A. (1987). Some basic issues in evaluating the quality of health care. In L. T. Rinke (Ed.), *Outcome measures in home care* (Vol. I, pp. 3–28). New York, NY: National League for Nursing.

Dove-Medows, E., Deriemacker, A., Dailey, R., Nolan, T., Walker, D., Misra, D., . . . Giurgescu, C. (2020). Pregnant African American women's perceptions of neighborhood, racial discrimination, and psychological distress as influences on birth outcomes. *MCN: The American Journal of Maternal/Child Nursing*, 45, 49–56.

Griffith, A., Haverstick, S., Blissick, D., Colaianne, T., Shields, H., Johnson, C., . . . Knott, K. (2020). Bridging the communication gap: A quality improvement project of a ventricular assist device program. *Dimensions of Critical Care Nursing*, 39, 4–11.

Haxby, E., & Shuldham, C. (2018). How to undertake a root cause analysis investigation to improve patient safety. *Nursing Standard*, 32, 41–46.

*Institute of Medicine. (2009). *Initial priorities for comparative effectiveness research*. Washington, DC: The National Academies Press.

Johnson, J. (2012). Quality improvement. In G. Sherwood & J. Barnsteiner (Eds.), *Quality and safety in nursing: A competency approach to improving outcomes* (pp. 113–132). New York, NY: John Wiley & Sons.

Kalanlar, B., & Kuru Alici, N. (2020). The effect of care burden on formal caregiver's quality of work life: A mixed-methods study. *Scandinavian Journal of Caring Sciences*. Advance online publication. doi:10.1111/scs.12808

Kinser, P., Moyer, S., Mazzeo, S., York, T., Amstadter, A., Thacker, L., & Starkweather, A. (2020). Protocol for pilot study on self-management of depressive symptoms in pregnancy. *Nursing Research*, 69, 82–88.

Magnowski, S., & Cleveland, S. (2020). The impact of milieu nurse-client shift assignments on monthly restraint rates on an inpatient child/adolescent psychiatric unit. *Journal of the American Psychiatric Nurses Association*, 26, 86–91.

Makic, M., Gilbert, D., Jankowski, C., Reeder, B., Al-Salmi, N., Starr, W., & Cook, P. (2020). Sensor and survey measures associated with daily fatigue in HIV: Findings from a mixed-method study. *Journal of the Association of Nurses in AIDS Care*, 31, 12–24.

Marshall, M., Pronovost, P., & Dixon-Woods, M. (2015). Promotion of improvement as a science. *Lancet (London England)*, 381, 419–421.

*Mitchell, B., Fasugba, O., Cheng, A., Gergory, V., Koerner, J., Collignon, P., . . . Graves, N. (2019). Chlorhexidine versus saline in reducing the risk of catheter associated urinary tract infection: A cost-effectiveness analysis. *International Journal of Nursing Studies*, 97, 1–6.

Mitchell, P., Ferketich, S., & Jennings, B. (1998). Quality health outcomes model. *Image: The Journal of Nursing Scholarship*, 30, 43–46.

Morse, J. M. (1991). Approaches to qualitative-quantitative methodological triangulation. *Nursing Research*, 40, 120–123.

Redeker, N., Ordway, M., Banasiak, N., Caldwell, B., Canapari, C., Crowley, A., . . . Sadler, L. (2018). Community partnership for healthy sleep: Research protocol. *Research in Nursing & Health*, 41, 19–29.

Shirey, M., Hauck, S., Embree, J., Kinner, T., Schaar, G., Phillips, L., . . . McCool, I. (2011). Showcasing differences between quality improvement, evidence-based practice, and research. *Journal of Continuing Education in Nursing*, 42, 57–68.

*A link to this open-access article is provided in the Internet Resources section on thePoint® website.

**This journal article is available on thePoint® for this chapter.

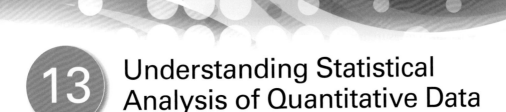

13 Understanding Statistical Analysis of Quantitative Data

Learning Objectives

On completing this chapter, you will be able to:

- Describe the four levels of measurement and identify which level was used for measuring specific variables
- Describe characteristics of frequency distributions and identify and interpret various descriptive statistics
- Describe the logic and purpose of parameter estimation and interpret confidence intervals
- Describe the logic and purpose of hypothesis testing and interpret *p* values
- Specify appropriate applications for *t*-tests, analysis of variance, chi-squared tests, and correlation coefficients and interpret the meaning of the calculated statistics
- Identify several types of multivariate statistics and describe situations in which they could be used
- Identify indexes used in assessments of reliability and validity
- Understand the results of simple statistical procedures described in a research report
- Define new terms in the chapter

Key Terms

- Absolute risk (AR)
- Absolute risk reduction (ARR)
- Alpha (α)
- Analysis of covariance (ANCOVA)
- Analysis of variance (ANOVA)
- Central tendency
- Chi-squared test
- Coefficient alpha
- Cohen's kappa
- Confidence interval (CI)
- Continuous variable
- Correlation
- Correlation coefficient
- Crosstabs table
- *d* statistic
- Descriptive statistics
- Effect size
- *F* ratio
- Frequency distribution
- Hypothesis testing
- Inferential statistics
- Interval measurement
- Intraclass correlation coefficient
- Level of measurement
- Level of significance
- Logistic regression
- Mean
- Median
- Mode
- Multiple correlation coefficient
- Multiple regression

- Multivariate statistics
- N
- Negative relationship
- Nominal measurement
- Nonsignificant result (NS)
- Normal distribution
- Number needed to treat (NNT)
- Odds ratio (OR)
- Ordinal measurement
- p value
- Parameter
- Parameter estimation
- Pearson's r
- Positive relationship
- Predictor variable
- R
- R^2
- Range
- Ratio measurement
- Repeated measures ANOVA
- Skewed distribution
- Standard deviation
- Statistic
- Statistical test
- Statistically significant
- Symmetric distribution
- Test statistic
- t-test
- Type I error
- Type II error
- Variability

Statistical analysis is used in quantitative research for four main purposes—to describe the data (e.g., sample characteristics), to estimate population values, to test hypotheses, and to provide evidence regarding measurement properties of quantified variables. This chapter provides a brief overview of statistical procedures for these purposes. We begin, however, by explaining levels of measurement.

 TIP Although the thought of learning about statistics may be anxiety-provoking, consider Florence Nightingale's view of statistics: "To understand God's thoughts we must study statistics, for these are the measure of His purpose."

LEVELS OF MEASUREMENT

Statistical operations depend on a variable's **level of measurement**. There are four major levels of measurement.

Nominal measurement, the lowest level, involves using numbers simply to categorize attributes. Gender is an example of a nominally measured variable (e.g., females = 1, males = 2, other = 3). The numbers used in nominal measurement do not have quantitative meaning and cannot be treated mathematically. It makes no sense to compute a sample's average gender.

Ordinal measurement ranks people on an attribute. For example, consider this ordinal scheme to measure ability to perform activities of daily living (ADL): 1 = completely dependent; 2 = needs another person's assistance; 3 = needs mechanical assistance; and 4 = completely independent. The numbers signify incremental ability to perform ADL independently, but they do not tell us how much greater one level is than another. As with nominal measures, the mathematic operations with ordinal-level data are restricted.

Interval measurement occurs when researchers can rank people on an attribute *and* specify the distance between them. Most psychological scales and tests yield interval-levels measures. For example, the Stanford-Binet Intelligence (IQ) test is an interval measure. The difference between a score of 140 and 120 is equivalent to the difference between 120 and 100. Some statistical procedures require interval data.

Ratio measurement is the highest level. Ratio scales, unlike interval scales, have a meaningful zero and provide information about the absolute magnitude of the attribute. Many physical measures, such as a person's weight, are ratio measures. It is meaningful to say that someone who weighs 200 pounds is twice as heavy as someone who weighs 100 pounds. Statistical procedures suitable for interval data are also appropriate for ratio-level data. Variables with interval and ratio measurements often are called **continuous variables**.

Example of different measurement levels •
Lee and colleagues (2020) tested the effect of a fatigue management intervention for adults living with HIV. Gender and race were measured as nominal-level variables. Age (45–49, 50–59, 60+ years) was an ordinal measurement. Several variables (sleep quality, anxiety and depression, and physical and cognitive function) were measured on interval-level scales. Other variables were measured at the ratio level (e.g., body mass index, years of HIV duration, CD4 cell count).

Researchers usually strive to use the highest levels of measurement possible because higher levels yield more information and are amenable to more powerful analyses.

HOW-TO-TELL TIP How can you tell a variable's measurement level? A variable is *nominal* if the values could be interchanged (e.g., 1 = male, 2 = female OR 1 = female, 2 = male). A variable is usually *ordinal* if there is a quantitative ordering of values AND if there are a small number of values (e.g., excellent, good, fair, poor). A variable is usually considered *interval* if it is measured with a composite scale or test. A variable is *ratio* level if it makes sense to say that one value is twice as much as another (e.g., 100 mg is twice as much as 50 mg).

DESCRIPTIVE STATISTICS

Statistical analysis enables researchers to make sense of numeric information. **Descriptive statistics** are used to synthesize and describe data. When indexes such as averages and percentages are calculated with population data, they are **parameters**. A descriptive index from a sample is a **statistic**. Most research questions are about parameters; researchers calculate statistics to estimate parameters and use *inferential statistics* to make inferences about the population.

Descriptively, data for a continuous variable can be depicted in terms of three characteristics: the shape of the distribution of values, central tendency, and variability.

Frequency Distributions

Data that are not organized are overwhelming. Consider the 60 numbers in Table 13.1. Assume that these numbers are the scores of 60 preoperative patients on an anxiety scale. Visual inspection of these numbers provides little insight into patients' anxiety.

A **frequency distribution** is an arrangement of values from lowest to highest and a count or percentage of how many times each value occurred. A frequency distribution for the 60 anxiety scores (Table 13.2) makes it easy to see the highest and lowest scores, where scores clustered, and how many patients were in the sample (total sample size is designated as *N* in research reports).

Frequency data can be displayed graphically in a *frequency polygon* (Fig. 13.1). In such graphs, scores typically are on the horizontal line, and counts or percentages are on the

TABLE 13.1 Patients' Anxiety Scores

22	27	25	19	24	25	23	29	24	20	26	16	20	26	17
22	24	18	26	28	15	24	23	22	21	24	20	25	18	27
24	23	16	25	30	29	27	21	23	24	26	18	30	21	17
25	22	24	29	28	20	25	26	24	23	19	27	28	25	26

TABLE 13.2 **Frequency Distribution of Patients' Anxiety Scores**

Score	Frequency	Percentage (%)
15	1	1.7
16	2	3.3
17	2	3.3
18	3	5.0
19	2	3.3
20	4	6.7
21	3	5.0
22	4	6.7
23	5	8.3
24	9	15.0
25	7	11.7
26	6	10.0
27	4	6.7
28	3	5.0
29	3	5.0
30	2	3.3
	$N = 60$	100.0%

vertical axis. Distributions can be described by their shapes. **Symmetric distribution** occurs if, when folded over, the two halves of a frequency polygon would be superimposed (Fig. 13.2). In an *asymmetric* or **skewed distribution**, the peak is off center and one tail is longer than the other. When the longer tail points to the right, the distribution has a *positive skew*, as in Figure 13.3A. Personal income is positively skewed: Most people have moderate incomes, with relatively few people with high incomes at the distribution's right end. If the longer tail points to the left, the distribution has a *negative skew* (Fig. 13.3B). Age at death is

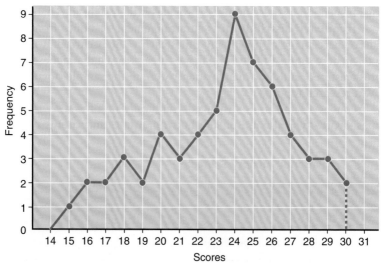

Figure 13.1 Frequency polygon of patients' anxiety scores.

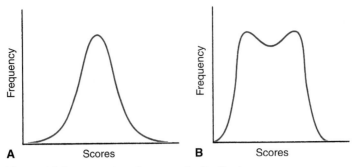

Figure 13.2 Examples of symmetric distributions.

negatively skewed: Most people are at the right end of the distribution, with fewer people dying young.

Another aspect of a distribution's shape concerns how many peaks it has. A *unimodal distribution* has one peak (Fig. 13.2A), whereas a *multimodal distribution* has two or more peaks—two or more values of high frequency. A distribution with two peaks is *bimodal* (Fig. 13.2B). A special distribution called the **normal distribution** (*a bell-shaped curve*) is symmetric, unimodal, and not very peaked (Fig. 13.2A). Many human attributes (e.g., height, intelligence) approximate a normal distribution.

Central Tendency

Frequency distributions clarify patterns, but an overall summary often is desired. Researchers ask questions such as "What is the *average* daily calorie consumption of nursing home residents?" Such a question seeks a single number to summarize a distribution. Indexes of **central tendency** indicate what is "typical." There are three indexes of central tendency: the mode, the median, and the mean.

- **Mode:** The mode is the number that occurs most frequently in a distribution. In the following distribution, the mode is 53:

  50 51 51 52 53 53 53 53 54 55 56

  The value of 53 occurred four times, more than any other number. The mode of the patients' anxiety scores in Table 13.2 was 24. The mode identifies the most "popular" value.

- **Median:** The median is the point in a distribution that divides scores in half. Consider the following set of values:

  2 2 3 3 4 5 6 7 8 9

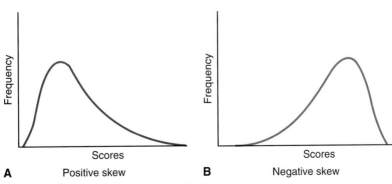

A Positive skew   **B** Negative skew

Figure 13.3 Examples of skewed distributions.

The value that divides the cases in half is midway between 4 and 5; thus 4.5 is the median. The median anxiety score is 24, the same as the mode. The median does not take into account individual values and is insensitive to extremes. In the given set of numbers, if the value of 9 were changed to 99, the median would remain 4.5.

- **Mean:** The mean equals the sum of all values divided by the number of participants—what we usually call the average. The mean of the patients' anxiety scores is 23.4 (1405 / 60). As another example, here are the weights of eight people:

$$85 \quad 109 \quad 120 \quad 135 \quad 158 \quad 177 \quad 181 \quad 195$$

In this example, the mean is 145. Unlike the median, the mean is affected by the value of every score. If we exchanged the 195-pound person for a person weighing 275 pounds, the mean would increase from 145 to 155 pounds. In research articles, the mean is often symbolized as M or $\overline{X}$ (e.g., $\overline{X} = 145$).

For continuous variables, the mean is usually reported. Of the three indexes, the mean is most stable: If repeated samples were drawn from a population, the means would fluctuate less than the modes or medians. Because of its stability, the mean usually is the best estimate of a population's central tendency. When a distribution is skewed, however, the median is preferred. For example, the median is a better index for a sample's average (typical) income than the mean because income is usually positively skewed.

Variability

Two distributions with identical means could differ with respect to how spread out the data are—how people are different from one another on the attribute. This section describes the **variability** of distributions.

Consider the two distributions in Figure 13.4, which represent hypothetical scores for students from two schools on an IQ test. Both distributions have a mean of 100, but school A has a wider range of scores, with some below 70 and some above 130. In school B, there are few low or high scores. School A is more *heterogeneous* (i.e., more varied) than school B, and school B is more *homogeneous* than school A. Researchers compute an index of variability to express the extent to which scores in a distribution differ from one another. Two common indexes are the range and standard deviation.

- **Range:** The range is the highest minus the lowest score in a distribution. In our anxiety score example, the range is 15 (30 − 15). In the distributions in Figure 13.4, the range for school A is about 80 (140 − 60), whereas the range for school B is about 50 (125 − 75). The chief virtue of the range is ease of computation. Because it is based on only two

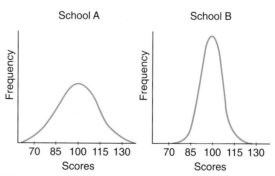

Figure 13.4 Two distributions of different variability.

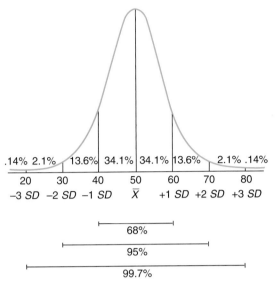

Figure 13.5 Standard deviations in a normal distribution.

scores, however, the range is unstable: From sample to sample drawn from a population, the range can fluctuate greatly.

 Standard deviation: The most widely used variability index is the standard deviation. Like the mean, the standard deviation is calculated based on every value in a distribution. The standard deviation summarizes the *average* amount of deviation of values from the mean.* In the example of patients' anxiety scores (Table 13.2), the standard deviation is 3.725. In research reports, the standard deviation is often abbreviated as *SD*.

TIP *SD*s sometimes are shown in relation to the mean without a label. For example, the anxiety scores might be shown as *M* = 23.4 (3.7) or *M* = 23.4 ± 3.7, where 23.4 is the mean and 3.7 is the standard deviation.

A standard deviation is more difficult to interpret than the range. For the *SD* of anxiety scores, you might ask, 3.725 *what?* What does the number mean? We can answer these questions from several angles. First, the *SD* is an index of how variable the scores in a distribution are and so if (for example) male and female patients had means of 23.0 on the anxiety scale, but their *SD*s were 7.0 and 3.0, respectively, it means that females were more homogeneous (i.e., their scores were more similar to one another) than males.

The *SD* represents the *average* of deviations from the mean. The mean tells us the best value for summarizing an entire distribution, and an *SD* tells us how much, on average, the scores deviate from the mean. A standard deviation can be interpreted as our degree of error when we use a mean to describe an entire sample.

In normal and near-normal distributions, there are roughly three *SD*s above and below the mean. For example, for a normal distribution with a mean of 50 and an *SD* of 10 (Fig. 13.5), a fixed percentage of cases fall within certain distances from the mean.

---

*Formulas for computing the standard deviation and other statistics discussed in this chapter are not shown in this textbook. The emphasis here is on helping you to understand statistical applications. Polit (2010) or Polit and Beck (2021) can be consulted for computation formulas.

Sixty-eight percent of all cases fall within 1 *SD* above and below the mean. Thus, nearly 7 of 10 scores are between 40 and 60. In a normal distribution, 95% of the scores fall within 2 *SD*s of the mean. Only a handful of cases—about 2% at each extreme—lie more than 2 *SD*s from the mean. Using this figure, we can see that a person with a score of 70 achieved a higher score than about 98% of the sample.

 TIP Descriptive statistics (percentages, means, *SD*s) are most often used to describe sample characteristics and key research variables and to document methodological features (e.g., response rates). They are seldom used to answer research questions; inferential statistics usually are used for this purpose.

Example of descriptive statistics •
Wang and colleagues (2020) studied the relationship between the care needs of patients with oral cancer and their postoperative health-related quality of life. Their report presented descriptive statistics about participants' characteristics. For example, the mean age of the 126 study participants was 57.6 years (*SD* = 8.7), the mean number of comorbidities was 1.7 (*SD* = 1.1), 43.7% had Stage IV cancer, and 50.8% had had two or more surgeries.

Bivariate Descriptive Statistics

So far, our discussion has focused on *univariate* (one-variable) *descriptive statistics*. *Bivariate* (two-variable) *descriptive statistics* describe relationships between two variables.

Crosstabulations

A **crosstabs table** is a two-dimensional frequency distribution in which the frequencies of two variables are *crosstabulated*. Suppose we had data on patients' gender and whether they were nonsmokers, light smokers (<1 pack of cigarettes a day), or heavy smokers (≥1 pack a day). The question is whether men smoke more heavily than women, or vice versa (i.e., whether there is a *relationship* between smoking and gender). Fictitious data for this example are shown in Table 13.3. Six *cells* are created by placing one variable (gender) along one dimension and the other variable (smoking status) along the other dimension. After participants' data are allocated to the appropriate cells, percentages are computed. The crosstab shows that women in this sample were more likely than men to be nonsmokers (45.4% vs. 27.3%) and less likely to be heavy smokers (18.2% vs. 36.4%). Crosstabs are used with nominal data or ordinal data with few values. In this example, gender is nominal, and smoking, as operationalized, is ordinal.

TABLE 13.3 Crosstabs Table for Relationship Between Gender and Smoking Status

	Gender					
	Women		Men		Total	
Smoking Status	*n*	*%*	*n*	*%*	*N*	*%*
Nonsmoker	10	45.4	6	27.2	16	36.4
Light smoker	8	36.4	8	36.4	16	36.4
Heavy smoker	4	18.2	8	36.4	12	27.2
TOTAL	22	100.0	22	100.0	44	100.0

Correlation

Relationships between two variables can be described by **correlation** methods. The correlation question is To what extent are two variables related to each other? For example, to what degree are anxiety scores and blood pressure values related? This question can be answered by calculating a **correlation coefficient**, which describes *intensity* and *direction* of a relationship.

Two variables that are related are height and weight: Tall people tend to weigh more than short people. The relationship between height and weight would be a *perfect relationship* if the tallest person in a population was the heaviest, the second tallest person was the second heaviest, and so on. A correlation coefficient indicates how "perfect" a relationship is. Possible values for a correlation coefficient range from -1.00 through .00 to $+1.00$. If height and weight were perfectly correlated, the correlation coefficient would be 1.00 (the actual correlation coefficient is in the vicinity of .50 to .60 for a general population). Height and weight have a **positive relationship** because greater height tends to be associated with greater weight.

When two variables are unrelated, the correlation coefficient is zero. One might anticipate that women's shoe size is unrelated to their intelligence. Women with large feet are as likely to perform well on IQ tests as those with small feet. The correlation coefficient summarizing such a relationship would be in the vicinity of .00.

Correlation coefficients between .00 and -1.00 express a **negative (*inverse*) relationship**. When two variables are inversely related, higher values on one variable are associated with lower values in the second. For example, there is a negative correlation between depression and self-esteem. This means that, on average, people with *high* self-esteem tend to be *low* on depression. If the relationship were perfect (i.e., if the person with the highest self-esteem score had the lowest depression score and so on), then the correlation coefficient would be -1.00. In actuality, the relationship between depression and self-esteem is moderate—usually in the vicinity of $-.30$ or $-.40$. Note that the higher the *absolute value* of the coefficient (i.e., the value disregarding the sign), the stronger the relationship. A correlation of $-.50$, for instance, is stronger than a correlation of $+.30$.

The most widely used correlation statistic is **Pearson's r**, the *product–moment correlation coefficient*, which is computed with continuous measures. (*Spearman's rho* is a correlation index used for ordinal-level data, or when sample sizes are very small.) There are no guidelines on what should be interpreted as strong or weak correlations because it depends on the variables. If we measured patients' body temperature orally and rectally, an r of .70 between the two measurements would be low. For most psychosocial variables (e.g., stress and depression), however, an r of .70 would be high.

TIP Correlation coefficients are sometimes reported in tables displaying a two-dimensional *correlation matrix*, in which every variable is displayed in both a row and a column, and coefficients between pairs of variables are displayed at the intersections. An example is presented later in this chapter.

Example of correlations •
Turan and colleagues (2020) studied the relationships between nursing students' levels of Internet addiction, loneliness, and life satisfaction. In their sample of 160 nursing students, they found that scores on the Internet addiction scale were very modestly and negatively related to loneliness ($r = -.15$) and not related at a meaningful level with life satisfaction scores ($r = -.02$).

TABLE 13.4 Indexes of Risk and Association in a 2 × 2 Table

	Outcome		
Exposure	**Undesirable Outcome**	**Desirable Outcome**	**Total**
Yes, exposed (E) to intervention–experimentals (or, NOT exposed to a risk factor)	a	b	$a + b$
No, not exposed (NE) to intervention–controls (or, exposed to a risk factor)	c	d	$c + d$
TOTAL	$a + c$	$b + d$	$a + b + c + d$

Absolute risk, exposed group (AR_E)	$= a / (a + b)$
Absolute risk, nonexposed group (AR_{NE})	$= c / (c + d)$
Absolute risk reduction (ARR)	$= AR_{NE} - AR_E$
Odds ratio (OR)	$= \dfrac{a/b}{c/d}$
Number needed to treat (NNT)	$= \dfrac{1}{ARR}$

Describing Risk

The evidence-based practice (EBP) movement has made decision making based on research findings an important issue. Several descriptive indexes can be used to facilitate such decision making. Many of these indexes involve calculating risk differences—for example, differences in risk before and after exposure to a beneficial intervention.

We focus on describing dichotomous outcomes (e.g., had a fall/did not have a fall) in relation to exposure or nonexposure to a beneficial treatment or protective factor. This situation results in a 2 × 2 crosstabs table with four cells. The four cells in the crosstabs table in Table 13.4 are labeled so that various indexes can be explained. *Cell a* is the number of cases with an undesirable outcome (e.g., a fall) in an intervention/protected group, *cell b* is the number with a desirable outcome (e.g., no fall) in an intervention/protected group, and *cells c* and *d* are the two outcome possibilities for a nontreated/unprotected group. We can now explain the meaning and calculation of some indexes of interest to clinicians.

Absolute Risk

Absolute risk can be computed for those exposed to an intervention/protective factor and for those not exposed. **Absolute risk (AR)** is simply the proportion of people who experienced an undesirable outcome in each group. Suppose 200 smokers were randomly assigned to a smoking cessation intervention or to a control group (Table 13.5). The outcome is smoking status 3 months later. Here, the absolute risk of continued smoking is .50 in the intervention group and .80 in the control group. Without the intervention, 20% of those in the experimental group would presumably have stopped smoking anyway, but the intervention boosted the rate to 50%.

Absolute Risk Reduction

The **absolute risk reduction (ARR)** index, a comparison of the two risks, is computed by subtracting the absolute risk for the exposed group from the absolute risk for the unexposed group.

TABLE 13.5 **Hypothetical Data for Smoking Cessation Intervention Example, Risk Indexes**

Exposure to Smoking Cessation Intervention	Outcome		Total
	Continued Smoking	**Stopped Smoking**	
Yes, exposed: E (experimental group)	50 (*a*)	50 (*b*)	100
No, not exposed: NE (control group)	80 (*c*)	20 (*d*)	100
TOTAL	130	70	200
Absolute risk, exposed group (AR$_E$)	= 50 / 100 = .50		
Absolute risk, nonexposed group (AR$_{NE}$)	= 80 / 100 = .80		
Absolute risk reduction (ARR)	= .80 − .50 = .30		
Odds ratio (OR)	$= \dfrac{(50 / 50)}{(80 / 20)}$ = .25		
Number needed to treat (NNT)	= 1 / .30 = 3.33		

This index is the estimated proportion of people who would be spared the undesirable outcome through exposure to an intervention/protective factor. In our example, the value of ARR is .30: 30% of the control group subjects would presumably have stopped smoking if they had received the intervention, over and above the 20% who stopped without it.

Odds Ratio

The odds ratio is a widely reported risk index. The *odds*, in this context, is the proportion of people *with* the adverse outcome relative to those *without* it. In our example, the odds of continued smoking for the intervention group is 1.0: 50 (those who continued smoking) divided by 50 (those who stopped). The odds for the control group is 80 divided by 20, or 4.0. The **odds ratio (OR)** is the ratio of these two odds—here, .25. The estimated odds of continuing to smoke are one fourth as high among intervention group members as for control group members. Turned around, the estimated odds of continued smoking is 4 times higher among smokers who do not get the intervention than among those who do.

Example of odds ratios •
Dos Santos and colleagues (2019) studied factors associated with risk-taking behavior among people who had been involved in a motorcycle accident. Many results were reported as odds ratios (ORs). For example, the OR for the relationship between feeling tired at work and failure to use a helmet at the time of the accident was 4.0—that is, those who felt tired were 4 times more likely than those who did not feel tired to not use a helmet.

Number Needed to Treat

The **number needed to treat (NNT)** index estimates how many people would need to receive an intervention to prevent one undesirable outcome. NNT is computed by dividing 1 by the absolute risk reduction. In our example, ARR = .30, and so NNT is 3.33. About three smokers would need to be exposed to the intervention to avoid one person's continued smoking. The NNT is valuable because it can be integrated with monetary information to show if an intervention is likely to be cost-effective.

TIP Another risk index is known as *relative risk* (RR). The RR is the estimated proportion of the original risk of an adverse outcome (in our example, continued smoking) that persists when people are exposed to the intervention. In our example, RR is .625 (.50 / .80): the risk of continued smoking is estimated as 62.5% of what it would have been without the intervention.

INTRODUCTION TO INFERENTIAL STATISTICS

Descriptive statistics are useful for summarizing data, but researchers usually do more than describe. **Inferential statistics**, based on the *laws of probability*, provide a means for drawing inferences about a population, given data from a sample. Inferential statistics are used to test research hypotheses.

Sampling Distributions

Inferential statistics are based on the assumption of random sampling of cases from populations—although this assumption is widely ignored. Even with random sampling, however, sample characteristics are seldom identical to those of the population. Suppose we had a population of 100,000 nursing home residents whose mean score on a physical function (PF) test was 500 with an *SD* of 100. We do not know these parameters—assume we must estimate them based on scores from a random sample of 100 residents. It is unlikely that we would obtain a mean of exactly 500. Our sample mean might be, say, 505. If we drew a new random sample of 100 residents, the mean PF score might be 497. Sample statistics fluctuate and are unequal to the parameter because of *sampling error*. Researchers need a way to assess whether sample statistics are good estimates of population parameters.

To understand the logic of inferential statistics, we must perform a mental exercise. Consider drawing 5,000 consecutive samples of 100 residents from the population of all residents. If we calculated a mean PF score each time, we could plot the distribution of these sample means, as shown in Figure 13.6. This distribution is a *sampling distribution of the mean*. A sampling distribution is theoretical: No one *actually* draws consecutive samples from a population and plots their means. Statisticians have shown that sampling distributions of

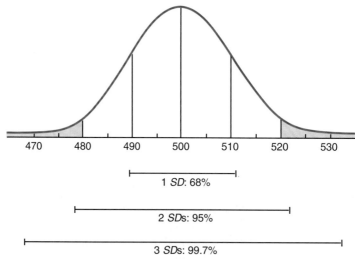

Figure 13.6 Sampling distribution of a mean.

means are normally distributed, and their mean equals the population mean. In our example, the mean of the sampling distribution is 500, the same as the population mean.

For a normally distributed sampling distribution of means, the probability is 95 out of 100 that a sample mean lies between $+2\ SD$ and $-2\ SD$ of the population mean. The SD of the sampling distribution—called the *standard error of the mean* (or SEM)—can be estimated using a formula that uses two pieces of information: the SD for the sample and sample size. In our example, the SEM is 10 (Fig. 13.6), which is the estimate of how much sampling error there would be from one sample mean to another in an infinite number of samples of 100 residents.

We can now estimate the probability of drawing a sample with a certain mean. With a sample size of 100 and a population mean of 500, the chances are 95 out of 100 that a sample mean would fall between 480 and 520—2 SDs above and below the mean. Only 5 times out of 100 would the mean of a random sample of 100 residents be less than 480 or greater than 520.

The SEM is partly a function of sample size, so a larger sample improves the accuracy of the estimate. If we used a sample of 400 residents to estimate the population mean, the SEM would be only 5. The probability would be 95 in 100 that a sample mean would be between 490 and 510. The chance of drawing a sample with a mean very different from that of the population is reduced as sample size increases.

You may wonder why you need to learn about these abstract statistical notions. Consider, though, that we are talking about the accuracy of researchers' results. As an intelligent consumer, you need to evaluate critically how believable research evidence is so that you can decide whether to incorporate it into your nursing practice.

Parameter Estimation

Statistical inference consists of two techniques: parameter estimation and hypothesis testing. **Parameter estimation** is used to estimate a population parameter—for example, a mean, a proportion, or a difference in means between two groups (e.g., smokers vs. nonsmokers). *Point estimation* involves calculating a single statistic to estimate the parameter. In our example, if the mean PF score for a sample of 100 nursing home residents were 510, this would be the point estimate of the population mean.

Point estimates convey no information about the estimate's margin of error. *Interval estimation* of a parameter provides a range of values within which the parameter has a specified probability of lying. With interval estimation, researchers construct a **confidence interval (CI)** around the point estimate. The CI around a sample mean establishes a range of values for the population value and the probability of being right. By convention, researchers use either a 95% or a 99% CI.

As noted previously, 95% of the scores in a normal distribution lie within about 2 SDs (more precisely, 1.96 SDs) from the mean. In our example, if the point estimate for mean scores is 510 with an $SD = 100$, the SEM for a sample of 100 would be 10. We can build a 95% CI using this formula: 95% CI = $(\overline{X} \pm 1.96 \times SEM)$. The confidence is 95% that the population mean lies between the values equal to 1.96 times the SEM, above and below the sample mean. In our example, with an SEM of 10, the 95% CI around the sample mean of 510 is between 490.4 and 529.6.

CIs reflect how much risk of being wrong researchers take. With a 95% CI, researchers risk being wrong 5 times out of 100. A 99% CI sets the risk at only 1% by allowing a wider range of possible values. In our example, the 99% CI around 510 is 484.2 to 535.8. With a lower risk of being wrong, precision is reduced. For a 95% interval, the CI range is about 39 points; for a 99% interval, the range about 52 points. The acceptable risk of error depends on the nature of the problem, but for most studies, a 95% CI is sufficient.

Example of confidence intervals around odds ratio •
Kamp and colleagues (2020) conducted a study to describe symptoms among emerging adults (aged 18 to 29 years) with inflammatory bowel disease. Those with severe abdominal pain were about 50% more likely to report fatigue as a symptom (OR = 1.57, 95% CI [1.16, 2.14]).

Hypothesis Testing

With statistical **hypothesis testing**, researchers use objective criteria to decide whether hypotheses should be accepted or rejected. Suppose we hypothesized that maternity patients who received online interactive breastfeeding support would breastfeed longer than mothers who did not. The mean number of days of breastfeeding is 131.5 for 25 intervention group mothers and 125.1 for 25 control group mothers. Should we conclude that our hypothesis has been supported? Group differences are in the predicted direction, but in another sample, the group means might be more similar. Two explanations for the observed outcome are possible: (1) The intervention was effective in encouraging breastfeeding or (2) the mean difference in this sample was due to chance (sampling error).

The first explanation is the *research hypothesis*, and the second is the *null hypothesis*, which is that there is no relationship between the independent variable (the intervention) and the dependent variable (breastfeeding duration). Statistical hypothesis testing is a process of disproof. It cannot be demonstrated directly that the research hypothesis is correct. But it is possible to show that the null hypothesis has a high probability of being incorrect, and such evidence lends support to the research hypothesis. Hypothesis testing helps researchers to make objective decisions about whether results are likely to reflect chance differences or hypothesized effects. Researchers use **statistical tests** in the hope of rejecting the null hypothesis.

Null hypotheses are accepted or rejected based on sample data, but hypotheses are about population values. The interest in testing hypotheses, as in all statistical inference, is to use a sample to make inferences about a population.

Type I and Type II Errors

Researchers decide whether to accept or reject the null hypothesis by estimating how probable it is that observed group differences are due to chance. Without population data, it cannot be asserted that the null hypothesis is or is not true. Researchers must be content to say that hypotheses are either *probably* true or *probably* false.

Researchers can make two types of error: rejecting a true null hypothesis or accepting a false null hypothesis. Figure 13.7 summarizes possible outcomes of researchers' decisions. Researchers make a **Type I error** by rejecting a null hypothesis that is, in fact, true.

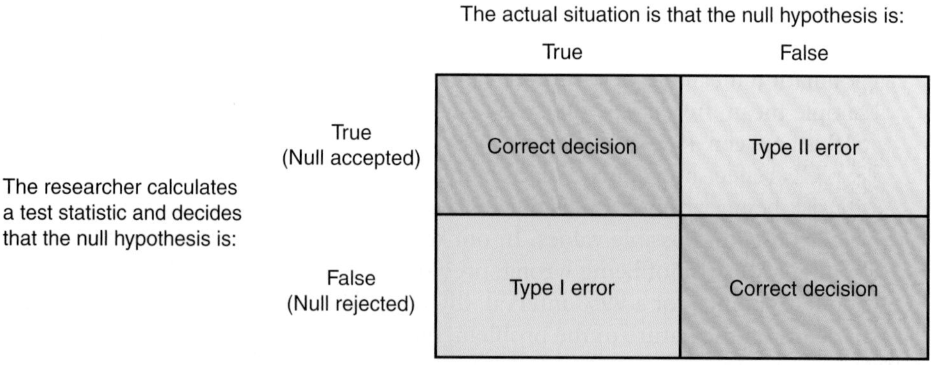

Figure 13.7 Outcomes of statistical decision making.

For instance, if we decided that online support effectively promoted breastfeeding when, in fact, group differences were merely due to sampling error, we would be making a Type I error—a false-positive conclusion. If we decided that differences in breastfeeding were due to sampling fluctuations, when the intervention actually *did* have an effect, we would be making a **Type II error**—a false-negative conclusion.

Level of Significance

Researchers do not know when they have made an error in statistical decision making. However, they control the risk for a Type I error by selecting a **level of significance**, which is the probability of making a Type I error. The two most frequently used levels of significance (referred to as **alpha** or α) are .05 and .01. With a .05 significance level, we accept the risk that out of 100 samples from a population, a true null hypothesis would be wrongly rejected 5 times. In 95 out of 100 cases, however, a true null hypothesis would be correctly accepted. With a .01 significance level, the risk of a Type I error is lower: In only 1 sample out of 100 would we wrongly reject the null. By convention, the minimal acceptable alpha level is .05.

 TIP Levels of significance are analogous to the CI values described earlier—an alpha of .05 is analogous to the 95% CI, and an alpha of .01 is analogous to the 99% CI.

Researchers would like to reduce the risk of committing both types of error, but unfortunately, lowering the risk of a Type I error increases the risk of a Type II error. Researchers can reduce the risk of a Type II error, however, by increasing the sample size. The probability of committing a Type II error can be estimated through *power analysis*, the procedure we mentioned in Chapter 9 for estimating sample size needs. *Power* is the ability of a statistical test to detect true relationships. Researchers ideally use a sample size that gives them a minimum power of .80, and thus, a risk for a Type II error of no more than .20 (i.e., a 20% risk).

 TIP If a report indicates that a research hypothesis was not supported by the data, consider whether a Type II error might have occurred as a result of an inadequate sample size.

Tests of Statistical Significance

In hypothesis testing, researchers use study data to compute a **test statistic**. For every test statistic, there is a theoretical sampling distribution. Hypothesis testing uses theoretical distributions to establish *probable* and *improbable* values for the test statistics, which are used to accept or reject the null hypothesis.

An example can illustrate this process. In our example of a physical functioning test for nursing home residents, suppose that there are population *norms*, which are values derived from large, representative samples. Let us assume that in the sampling distribution for the norming data, the mean is 500 with an SEM of 10, as in Figure 13.6. Now let us say that we recruited 100 nursing home residents to participate in an intervention to improve physical functioning. The null hypothesis is that those receiving the intervention have mean posttest scores that are not different from those in the overall population—i.e., 500—but the research hypothesis is that they will have higher average scores. After the intervention, the mean PF score for the sample is 528. As we can see by examining Figure 13.6, a mean score of 528 is more than 2 standard deviations above the population mean—it is a value that is *improbable* if the null hypothesis is true. Thus, we accept the research hypothesis that the intervention resulted in higher physical functioning scores than those in the population.[†]

[†]The design for our fictitious example is highly flawed, with several serious threats to internal validity. We used this contrived example purely as a simple way to illustrate hypothesis testing.

We would not be justified in saying that we had *proved* the research hypothesis because the possibility of a Type I error remains—but the possibility is less than 5 in 100. Researchers reporting the results of hypothesis tests state whether their findings are **statistically significant**. The word *significant* does not mean important or meaningful. In statistics, the term *significant* means that results are not likely to have been due to chance, at some specified level of probability. A **nonsignificant result** means that any observed difference or relationship could have been the result of chance.

Overview of Hypothesis Testing Procedures

In the next section, a few statistical tests are discussed. We emphasize applications and interpretations of statistical tests, not computations. Each statistical test can be used with specific kinds of data, but the overall hypothesis testing process is similar for all tests:

1. *Select an appropriate statistical test.* Researchers select a test based on such factors as the variables' level of measurement.
2. *Specify the level of significance.* An α level of .05 is usually chosen.
3. *Compute a test statistic.* The value for a test statistic is calculated with study data.
4. *Determine degrees of freedom.* The term *degrees of freedom (df)* refers to the number of observations free to vary about a parameter. The concept can be confusing, but computing degrees of freedom is easy.
5. *Compare the test statistic to a theoretical value.* Theoretical distributions exist for all test statistics. The computed value of the test statistic is compared to a theoretical value to establish significance or nonsignificance.

When a computer is used for the analysis, as is almost always the case, researchers follow only the first step. The computer calculates the test statistic, degrees of freedom, and the actual probability that the relationship being tested is due to chance. For example, the printout may indicate that the probability (p) of an intervention group having a higher mean number of days of breastfeeding than a control group on the basis of chance alone is .025. This means that fewer than 3 times out of 100 (only 25 times out of 1,000) would a group difference of the size observed occur by chance. The computed p **value** is then compared with the desired alpha. In this example, if we had set the significance level to .05, the results would be significant because .025 is more stringent than .05. Any computed probability greater than .05 (e.g., .15) indicates a nonsignificant relationship (*NS*), i.e., one that could have occurred by chance in more than 5 out of 100 samples.

 TIP Most tests discussed in this chapter are *parametric tests*, which are ones that focus on population parameters and involve certain assumptions about variables in the analysis, notably the assumption that they are normally distributed in the population. *Nonparametric tests*, by contrast, do not estimate parameters and involve less restrictive assumptions about the distribution's shape.

BIVARIATE STATISTICAL TESTS

Researchers use a variety of statistical tests to make inferences about their hypotheses. Several frequently used bivariate tests are briefly described and illustrated.

t-Tests

Researchers frequently compare two groups of people on an outcome. A *t*-**test** is a parametric test for testing differences in two group means.

TABLE 13.6 **Fictitious Data for *t*-Test Example: Scores on a Perceived Maternal Competence Scale**

Regular Discharge Mothers		Early Discharge Mothers	
30	32	23	26
27	17	17	16
25	18	22	13
20	28	18	21
24	29	20	14
Mean = 25.0		Mean = 19.0	
t = 2.86, *df* = 18, *p* = .011			

Suppose we wanted to test the effect of early discharge of maternity patients on perceived maternal competence. We administer a scale of perceived maternal competence at discharge to 20 primiparas who had a vaginal delivery: 10 who remained in the hospital 25 to 48 hours (regular discharge group) and 10 who were discharged 24 hours or less after delivery (early discharge group). Data for this example are presented in Table 13.6. Mean scores on the perceived maternal competence measure for these two groups are 25.0 and 19.0, respectively. Are these differences *real* (i.e., Do they exist in the population of early- and regular-discharge mothers?), or do group differences reflect chance fluctuations? The 20 scores vary from one mother to another, ranging from a low of 13 to a high of 30. Some variation reflects individual differences in maternal competence; some might result from participants' moods on a particular day, and so forth. The research question is whether a significant amount of the variation is associated with the independent variable—time of hospital discharge. The *t*-test allows us to make inferences about this question objectively.

The formula for calculating the *t* statistic uses group means, variability, and sample size. The computed value of *t* for the data in Table 13.6 is 2.86. Degrees of freedom here is the total sample size minus 2 (*df* = 20 − 2 = 18). For an α level of .05, the cutoff value for *t* with 18 degrees of freedom is 2.10. *This value is the upper limit to what is probable if the null hypothesis is true.* Thus, the calculated *t* of 2.86, which is larger than the theoretical value of *t*, is improbable (i.e., statistically significant). The primiparas discharged early had significantly lower perceived maternal competence than those who were not discharged early. In fewer than 5 out of 100 samples would a difference in means this large be found by chance. In fact, the actual *p* value is .011: Only in about 1 sample out of 100 would a mean difference of 6.0 on the dependent variable be found by chance.

The situation we just described requires an *independent groups t-test*: Mothers in the two groups were different people, independent of each other. There are situations for which this type of *t*-test is not appropriate. For example, if means for a single group of people measured before and after an intervention were being compared, researchers would compute a *paired t-test* (also called a *dependent groups t-test*), using a different formula.

Example of *t*-tests •
Bekdemír and İlhan (2019) studied factors associated with caregiver burden among those caring for bedridden patients. They used independent groups *t*-tests to compare scores on a caregiver burden scale for various subgroups of caregivers. For example, they found that mean scores on the burden scale were significantly higher for women than for men (*t* = 2.71, *p* < .01) and for caregivers who had their own health problems than for those who did not (*t* = 6.69, *p* < .001).

In lieu of t-tests, CIs can be constructed around the difference between two means. In the example in Table 13.6, we can construct CIs around the mean difference of 6.0 in maternal competence scores ($25.0 - 19.0 = 6.0$). For a 95% CI, the confidence limits are 1.6 and 10.4: We can be 95% confident that the difference between population means for early and regular discharge mothers lies between these values. With CI information, we can also see that the mean difference is significant at $p < .05$ *because the range does not include 0*. There is a 95% probability that the mean difference is not lower than 1.6, so this means that there is less than a 5% probability that there is no difference at all—thus, the null hypothesis can be rejected.

Analysis of Variance

Analysis of variance (ANOVA) is used to test mean group differences of three or more groups. ANOVA sorts out the variability of an outcome variable into two components: variability due to the independent variable (e.g., experimental group status) and variability due to all other sources (e.g., individual differences). Variation *between* groups is contrasted with variation *within* groups to yield an **F ratio** statistic.

Suppose we were comparing the effectiveness of interventions to help people stop smoking. Group A smokers receive nurse counseling; Group B smokers receive a nicotine patch; and a control group (Group C) gets no intervention. The outcome is 1-day cigarette consumption 1 month after the intervention. Thirty smokers are randomly assigned to one of the three groups. The null hypothesis is that the population means for posttreatment cigarette smoking are the same for all three groups, and the research hypothesis is inequality of means. Table 13.7 presents fictitious data for the 30 participants. The mean numbers of posttreatment cigarettes consumed are 16.6, 19.2, and 34.0 for groups A, B, and C, respectively. These means are different, but are they significantly different—or do differences reflect random fluctuations?

An ANOVA applied to these data yields an F ratio of 4.98. For $\alpha = .05$ and $df = 2$ and 27 (2 df between groups and 27 df within groups), the theoretical F value is 3.35. Because our obtained F value of 4.98 exceeds 3.35, we reject the null hypothesis that the population means are equal. The *actual* probability, as calculated by a computer, is .014. In only 14 samples out of 1,000 would group differences this great be obtained by chance alone.

ANOVA results support the hypothesis that different treatments were associated with different cigarette smoking, but we cannot tell from these results whether treatment A was significantly more effective than treatment B. Statistical analyses known as *post hoc tests* (or *multiple comparison procedures*) are used to isolate the differences between group means that result in the rejection of the overall null hypothesis.

TABLE 13.7 Fictitious Data for One-Way ANOVA Example: Number of Cigarettes Smoked in 1 Day Postintervention

Group A Nurse Counseling		Group B Nicotine Patch		Group C Untreated Controls	
28	19	0	27	33	35
0	24	31	0	54	0
17	0	26	3	19	43
20	21	30	24	40	39
35	2	24	27	41	36
Mean$_A$ = 16.6		Mean$_B$ = 19.2		Mean$_C$ = 34.0	
F = 4.98; *df* = 2, 27; *p* = .01					

A type of ANOVA known as **repeated measures ANOVA** (RM-ANOVA) can be used when the means being compared are means at different points in time (e.g., mean blood pressure at 2, 4, and 6 hours after surgery). When two or more groups are measured several times, a repeated measures ANOVA provides information about a main effect for time (Do the measures change significantly over time, irrespective of group?), a main effect for groups (Do the group means differ significantly, irrespective of time?), and an *interaction effect* (Do the groups differ more at certain times?).

Example of an ANOVA ●

Yilmaz and Günes (2019) examined factors related to sacral skin temperature and pressure ulcer development among patients hospitalized in an intensive care unit in Turkey. One-way ANOVA was used, for example, to compare the sacral skin temperature of patients in different age groups (38 to 64 years, 65 to 74 years, and 75 to 90 years). The difference was statistically significant ($F = 13.22$, $p < .001$).

Chi-Squared Test

The **chi-squared (χ^2) test** is used to test hypotheses about differences in proportions, as in a crosstabs. For example, suppose we were studying the effect of nursing instruction on patients' compliance with self-medication. Nurses implement a new instructional strategy with 50 patients, whereas 50 control group patients get usual care. The research hypothesis is that a higher proportion of people in the intervention than in the control condition will be compliant. Some fictitious data for this example are presented in Table 13.8, which shows that 60% of those in the intervention group were compliant, compared to 40% in the control group. But is this 20 percentage point difference statistically significant—i.e., likely to be "real"?

The value of the χ^2 statistic for the data in Table 13.8 is 4.00, which we can compare with the value from a theoretical chi-squared distribution. In this example, the theoretical value that must be exceeded to establish significance at the .05 level is 3.84. The obtained value of 4.00 is larger than would be expected by chance (the actual $p = .046$). We can conclude that a significantly larger proportion of experimental than control patients were compliant.

Example of chi-squared test ●

Tongpeth and colleagues (2020) tested the effectiveness of an Avatar application for teaching heart attack recognition and response. They used chi-squared tests to study group differences on several outcomes. For example, a significantly higher percentage of people in the intervention group (41.9%) than in the usual care group (3.2%) got 100% of the "Action Plan" questions right at the 1-month follow-up ($p < .001$).

TABLE 13.8 Observed Frequencies for Chi-Squared Example: Rates of Compliance With Medications

	Group				
	Experimental		Control		Total
Patient Compliance	*n*	%	*n*	%	*N*
Compliant	30	60.0	20	40.0	50
Noncompliant	20	40.0	30	60.0	50
TOTAL	50	100.0	50	100.0	100

$\chi^2 = 4.0$, $df = 1$, $p = .046$.

As with means, we can construct CIs around the difference between two proportions. In our example, the group difference in proportion compliant was .20 (.60 − .40 = .20). The 95% CI around .20 is .06 to .34. We can be 95% confident that the true population difference in compliance rates between the groups is between 6% and 34%. This interval does not include 0%, so we can be 95% confident that group differences in the population are "real."

Correlation Coefficients

Pearson's r is both descriptive and inferential. As a descriptive statistic, r summarizes the magnitude and direction of a relationship between two variables. As an inferential statistic, r tests hypotheses about population correlations; the null hypothesis is that there is no relationship between two variables, i.e., that the population correlation = .00.

Suppose we were studying the relationship between patients' self-reported level of stress (higher scores indicate more stress) and the pH level of their saliva. With a sample of 50 patients, we find that $r = -.29$. This value indicates a tendency for people with high stress to have lower pH levels than those with low stress. But is the r of −.29 a random fluctuation observed only in this sample, or is the relationship significant? Degrees of freedom for correlation coefficients equal N minus 2—48 in this example. The theoretical value for r with $df = 48$ and $\alpha = .05$ is .28. Because the absolute value of the calculated r is .29, the null hypothesis is rejected: The relationship between patients' stress level and the acidity of their saliva is statistically significant.

> **Example of Pearson's r** •
> Huang and an interprofessional team (2020) studied factors associated with quality of life (QoL) in 150 patients with diabetic hypoglycemia. They found, for example, that QoL scores were positively correlated with participants' social support ($r = .27$, $p < .001$), but not significantly correlated with their age ($r = -.14$, $p = .09$), their weight ($r = -.07$, $p = .37$), or their hemoglobin A_{1c} (HbA_{1c}) levels ($r = -.04$, $p = .65$).

Effect Size Indexes

Effect size indexes are estimates of the magnitude of effects of an "I" component on an "O" component in PICO questions—an important issue in EBP. Effect size information can be crucial because, with large samples, even miniscule effects can be statistically significant. *P* values tell you whether results are likely to be *real*, but effect sizes suggest whether they are important. Effect size plays an important role in systematic reviews.

It is beyond our scope to explain effect sizes in detail, but we offer an illustration. A frequently used effect size index is the **d statistic**, which summarizes the magnitude of differences in two means, such as the difference between intervention and control group means on an outcome. Thus, d can be calculated to estimate effect size when t-tests are used. When d is zero, it means that there is no effect—the means of the two groups being compared are the same. By convention, a d of .20 or less is considered *small*, a d of .50 is considered *moderate*, and a d of .80 or greater is considered *large*.

Different effect size indexes and interpretive conventions are associated with different situations. For example, the r statistic can be interpreted directly as an effect size index, as can the odds ratio (OR). The key point is that they encapsulate information about how powerful the effect of an independent variable is on an outcome.

 TIP   Researchers who conduct a *power analysis* to estimate how big a sample size they need to adequately test their hypotheses (i.e., to avoid a Type II error) must estimate in advance how large the effect size will be—usually based on prior research or a pilot study.

TABLE 13.9 **Guide to Major Bivariate Statistical Tests**

Name	Test Statistic	Purpose	Measurement Level Independent Variable	Measurement Level Dependent Variable
t-Test for independent groups	*t*	To test the difference between the means of two independent groups (e.g., experimental vs. control, men vs. women)	Nominal	Continuous*
t-Test for paired groups	*t*	To test the difference between the means of a paired group (e.g., pretest vs. posttest for the same people)	Nominal	Continuous*
Analysis of variance (ANOVA)	*F*	To test the difference among the means of 3+ independent groups	Nominal	Continuous*
Repeated measures ANOVA	*F*	To test differences among the means for the same group over time or to compare 2+ groups over time	Nominal	Continuous*
Pearson's correlation coefficient	*r*	To test the existence and strength of a relationship between two variables	Continuous*	Continuous*
Chi-squared test	χ^2	To test the difference in proportions in 2+ independent groups	Nominal (or ordinal, few categories)	Nominal (or ordinal, few categories)

*Continuous measures are on an interval- or ratio-level scale.

Example of calculated effect size •
Kim and colleagues (2020) developed an exercise intervention to reduce pain and improve function among people with chronic lower back pain. In a pilot test of the intervention with 12 patients, the effect size for physical activity improvement was large: *d* = .92.

Guide to Bivariate Statistical Tests

The selection of a statistical test depends on several factors, such as number of groups and the levels of measurement of the research variables. To aid you in evaluating the appropriateness of statistical tests used by nurse researchers, Table 13.9 summarizes key features of the bivariate tests mentioned in this chapter.

 TIP Every time a report presents information about statistical tests such as those described in this section, it means that the researcher was testing hypotheses—whether those hypotheses were formally stated in the introduction or not.

MULTIVARIATE STATISTICAL ANALYSIS

We wish we could avoid discussing complex statistical methods in this introductory-level book. The fact is, however, that many quantitative nursing studies today rely on **multivariate statistics** that involve the analysis of three or more variables simultaneously. The increased use of sophisticated analytic methods has resulted in greater rigor in nursing studies, but it can be challenging for those without statistical training to fully understand research reports.

Given the introductory nature of this book and the fact that many of you are not proficient with even basic statistical tests, we present only a brief description of three widely used multivariate statistics. The supplement to this chapter on thePoint® website expands on this presentation.

Multiple Regression

Correlations enable researchers to make predictions. For example, if the correlation between secondary school grades and nursing school grades were .60, nursing school administrators could make predictions—albeit imperfect ones—about applicants' performance in nursing school. Researchers can improve their prediction of an outcome by performing a **multiple regression** in which several independent variables are included in the analysis. As an example, we might predict infant birth weight (the outcome) from such variables as mothers' smoking status, amount of prenatal care, and gestational period. In multiple regression, outcome variables are continuous variables. Independent variables (often called **predictor variables** in regression) are either continuous variables or dichotomous nominal-level variables, such as does/does not smoke.

The statistic used in multiple regression is the **multiple correlation coefficient**, symbolized as R. Unlike Pearson's r, R does not have negative values. R varies from .00 to 1.00, showing the *strength* of the relationship between several predictors and an outcome but not *direction*. Researchers can test whether R is statistically significant—i.e., different from .00. R, when squared, can be interpreted as the proportion of the variability in the outcome that is explained by the predictors. In predicting birth weight, if we achieved an R of .50 ($R^2 = .25$), we could say that the predictors accounted for one fourth of the variation in birth weights. Three fourths of the variation, however, resulted from factors not in the analysis. Researchers usually report multiple correlation results in terms of R^2 rather than R.

Example of multiple regression analysis •
Landi and colleagues (2020) studied factors that predicted child psychological development at 3 months in at-risk families. In their multiple regression analysis, they found that maternal depressive symptoms during pregnancy and a maternal personality trait (social conformity) were significant predictors of poorer scores on a child development measure. The overall R^2 of .24 was significant ($p < .05$).

Analysis of Covariance

Analysis of covariance (ANCOVA), which combines features of ANOVA and multiple regression, is used to control confounding variables statistically—that is, to attempt to "equalize" groups being compared. This approach is valuable in certain situations, like when a nonequivalent control group design has been used. When control through randomization is lacking, ANCOVA offers the possibility of statistical control.

In ANCOVA, the confounding variables being controlled are called *covariates*. ANCOVA tests the significance of differences between group means on an outcome after removing the effect of covariates. ANCOVA yields F statistics for testing the significance of group differences.

Example of ANCOVA •
Liu and colleagues (2020) tested the effect of creativity training for nursing faculty on their teaching skills for creativity using a nonequivalent control group quasi-experimental design. They measured self-efficacy for teaching creativity and creative teaching behaviors before and after the intervention. In their analysis, they used the baseline scores on these measures as the covariates.

Logistic Regression

Logistic regression analyzes relationships between multiple independent variables and a nominal-level outcome (e.g., compliant vs. noncompliant). It is similar to multiple regression, although it employs a different statistical estimation procedure. Logistic regression transforms the probability of an event occurring (e.g., that a woman will practice breast self-examination or not) into its *odds*. After further transformations, the analysis examines the relationship of the predictor variables to the transformed outcome variable. For each predictor, the logistic regression yields an *odds ratio*, which is the factor by which the odds change for a unit change in the predictors after controlling other predictors. Logistic regression yields odds ratios for each predictor, as well as CIs around the ORs.

Example of logistic regression ••
Van der Wal and colleagues (2020) studied thirst in patients with heart failure in Sweden, the Netherlands, and Japan. They used logistic regression to study factors that predicted high thirst and found that a higher dose of loop diuretics (OR = 3.47) and fluid restriction (OR = 2.21) were significant predictors.

MEASUREMENT STATISTICS

In Chapter 9, we described two measurement properties that are key aspects of measurement quality—reliability and validity. When a new measure is developed, researchers undertake a psychometric assessment to estimate its reliability and validity. Such psychometric assessments rely on statistical analyses, using indexes that we briefly describe here. Researchers often report measurement statistics when they describe the measures they opted to use, to provide evidence that their data can be trusted.

Reliability Assessment

Reliability, it may be recalled, is the extent to which scores on a measure are consistent across repeated measurements if the trait itself has not changed. In Chapter 9, we mentioned three major types of reliability, each of which relies on different statistical indexes: test–retest reliability, interrater reliability, and internal consistency reliability.

- *Test–retest reliability*, which concerns the stability of a measure, is assessed by making two separate measurements of the same people, often 1 to 2 weeks apart, and then testing the extent to which the two sets of scores are consistent. Some researchers use Pearson's *r* to correlate the scores at Time 1 with those at Time 2, but the preferred index for test–retest reliability is the **intraclass correlation coefficient (ICC)**, which can range in value from .00 and 1.00.
- *Interrater reliability* is used to assess the extent to which two independent raters or observers assign the same score in measuring an attribute. When the ratings are dichotomous classifications (e.g., presence vs. absence of infusion phlebitis), the preferred index is **Cohen's kappa**, whose values also range from .00 to 1.00. If the ratings are continuous scores, the ICC is usually used.
- *Internal consistency reliability* concerns the extent to which the various components of a multicomponent measure (e.g., items on a psychosocial scale) are consistently measuring the same attribute. Internal consistency is estimated by an index called **coefficient alpha** (or *Cronbach's alpha*). If a psychosocial scale includes several subscales, coefficient alpha is usually computed for each subscale separately.

For all of these reliability indexes, the closer the value is to 1.00, the stronger is the evidence of good reliability. Although opinions about minimally acceptable values vary, values of .80 or higher are usually considered good. Researchers try to select measures with previously demonstrated high levels of reliability, but if they are using a multi-item scale, they usually compute coefficient alpha with their own data as well.

Validity Assessment

Validity is the measurement property that concerns the degree to which an instrument is measuring what it purports to measure. Like reliability, validity has several aspects. Unlike reliability, however, it is challenging to establish a measure's validity. Validation is a process of evidence building, and typically multiple forms of evidence are sought.

Content Validity

Content validity is relevant for composite measures, such as multi-item scales. The issue is whether the content of the items adequately reflects the construct of interest. Content validation usually relies on expert ratings of each item, and the ratings are used to compute an index called the *content validity index (CVI)*. A value of .90 or higher has been suggested as providing evidence of good content validity.

Criterion Validity

Criterion validity concerns the extent to which scores on a measure are consistent with a "gold standard" criterion. The methods used to assess criterion validity depend on the level of measurement of the focal measure and the criterion.

When both the focal measure and the criterion are continuous, researchers administer the two measures to a sample and then compute a Pearson's r between the two scores. Larger coefficients are desirable, but there is no threshold value that is considered a minimum. Usually, statistical significance is the standard for concluding that criterion validity is adequate.

If both the measure and the gold standard are dichotomous variables, researchers often use methods of assessing *diagnostic accuracy*. **Sensitivity** is the ability of a measure to correctly identify a "case," that is, to correctly screen in or diagnose a condition. A measure's sensitivity is its rate of yielding *true positives*. **Specificity** is the measure's ability to correctly identify noncases, that is, to screen *out* those without the condition. Specificity is an instrument's rate of yielding *true negatives*.

To assess an instrument's sensitivity and specificity, researchers need a highly reliable and valid criterion of "caseness" against which scores on the instrument can be assessed. For example, if we wanted to test the validity of adolescents' self-reports about smoking (yes/no in past 24 hours), we could use urinary cotinine level, using a cutoff value for a positive test of ≥200 ng/mL as the gold standard. Sensitivity would be calculated as the proportion of teenagers who said they smoked *and* who had high concentrations of cotinine, divided by all real smokers as indicated by the urine test. Specificity would be the proportion of teenagers who accurately reported they did not smoke, or the true negatives, divided by all *real* negatives. Both sensitivity and specificity can range from .00 to 1.00. It is difficult to set standards of acceptability for sensitivity and specificity, but both should be as high as possible.

When the focal measure is continuous and the gold standard is dichotomous, researchers often use a statistical tool called a *receiver operating characteristic (ROC) curve*. An ROC curve involves plotting each score on the focal measure against its sensitivity and specificity for correct classification based on a dichotomous criterion. A discussion of ROC curves is beyond the scope of this book, but interested readers can consult Polit and Yang (2016).

Construct Validity

Construct validity concerns the extent to which a measure is truly measuring the target construct and is often assessed using hypothesis testing procedures like those described earlier in this chapter. For example, a researcher might hypothesize that scores on a new measure (e.g., a scale of fear of hospitalization) would correlate with scores on another established measure (e.g., an anxiety scale). Pearson's r would be used to test this hypothesis, and a significant correlation would provide some evidence of construct validity. For known-groups validity, which involves testing hypotheses about expected group differences on a new measure, an independent groups t-test could be used. Both bivariate and multivariate statistical tests are appropriate in assessments of a new measure's construct validity.

READING AND UNDERSTANDING STATISTICAL INFORMATION

Unless researchers are reporting a psychometric assessment, measurement statistics are most likely to be presented in the methods section of a report, in their descriptions of the measures they used. Statistical *findings* for a substantive study, however, are communicated in the results section, both in the text and in tables (or, less frequently, in figures). This section offers assistance in reading and interpreting statistical information.

Tips on Reading Text With Statistical Information

Both descriptive and inferential statistics are presented in research reports. Descriptive statistics typically summarize sample characteristics. Information about the participants' background helps readers to draw conclusions about the people to whom the findings can be applied. Researchers may provide statistical information for evaluating biases. For example, when a quasi-experimental or case-control design has been used, researchers may test the equivalence of the groups being compared on baseline or background variables, using tests such as t-tests.

For hypothesis testing, the text of research articles usually provides the following information about statistical tests: (1) the test used, (2) the value of the calculated statistic, and (3) level of statistical significance. Examples of how the results of various statistical tests might be reported in the text are shown below.

1. t-Test: $t = 1.68, p = .09$
2. Chi-squared: $\chi^2 = 16.65, p < .001$
3. Pearson's r: $r = .36, p < .01$
4. ANOVA: $F = 0.18, NS$

The preferred approach is to report significance as the computed probability that the null hypothesis is correct, as in example 1. In this case, the observed group mean differences could be found by chance in 9 out of 100 samples. This result is not statistically significant because the mean difference had an unacceptably high chance of being spurious. The probability level is sometimes reported simply as falling below or above the certain thresholds (examples 2 and 3). Both these results are significant because the probability of obtaining such results by chance is less than 1 in 100. You must be careful to read the symbol following the p value correctly: The symbol $<$ means *less than*. The symbol $>$ means *greater than*—i.e., the results are not significant if the p value is .05 or greater. When results do not achieve statistical significance at the desired level, researchers may simply indicate that the results were not significant (*NS*), as in example 4.

Statistical information often is noted parenthetically in a sentence describing the findings, as in "Patients in the intervention group had a significantly lower rate of infection than those in the control group ($\chi^2 = 5.41, p = .02$)." In reading research reports, the values of the test statistics (e.g., $\chi^2 = 5.41$) are of no inherent interest. What is important is whether the statistical tests indicate that the research hypotheses were accepted as probably true (as demonstrated by significant results) or rejected as probably false (as demonstrated by nonsignificant results).

Tips on Reading Statistical Tables

Tables allows researchers to condense a lot of statistical information. Consider, for example, putting information about dozens of correlation coefficients in the text. Tables are efficient but they may be daunting for novice readers, partly because of the absence of standardization. There is no universally accepted format for presenting t-test results, for example. Thus, each table may present a new deciphering challenge.

We have a few suggestions for helping you to comprehend statistical tables. First, read the text and the tables simultaneously—the text may help your figure out what the table is communicating. Second, before trying to understand the numbers in a table, try to glean information from the accompanying words. Table titles and footnotes often present critical information. Table headings should be carefully scrutinized because they indicate what the variables in the analysis are (often listed as row labels in the first column, as in Table 13.10) and what statistical information is included (often specified as column headings). Third, you may find it helpful to consult the glossary of symbols on the inside back cover of this book to check the meaning of a statistical symbol. Not all symbols in this glossary were described in this chapter, so it may be necessary to refer to a statistics textbook, such as that of Polit (2010), for further information.

 TIP In tables, probability levels associated with significance tests are sometimes presented directly in the table, in a column labeled "p" (e.g., $p = .03$). However, researchers sometimes indicate significance levels in tables with asterisks placed next to the value of the test statistic. One asterisk usually signifies $p < .05$, two asterisks signify $p < .01$, and three asterisks signify $p < .001$. (There should be a key at the bottom of the table indicating what the asterisks mean.) Thus, a table might show: $t = 3.00$ in one column and $p < .01$ in another. Alternatively, the table might show $t = 3.00^{**}$. The absence of an asterisk would signify a nonsignificant result.

CRITICAL APPRAISAL OF QUANTITATIVE ANALYSES

It is often difficult to critically appraise statistical analyses. We hope this chapter has helped to demystify statistics, but we recognize the limited scope of our coverage. It would be unreasonable to expect you to be adept at evaluating statistical analyses, but you can be on the lookout for certain things in reviewing research articles. Some guidance is presented in Box 13.1.

One aspect of the appraisal should focus on which analyses were reported. You should assess whether the statistical information adequately describes the sample and reports the results of statistical tests for all hypotheses. Another presentational issue concerns the researcher's judicious use of tables to summarize statistical information.

Box 13.1 Guidelines for Critically Appraising Statistical Analyses

1. Did the descriptive statistics in the report sufficiently describe the major variables and background characteristics of the sample? Were appropriate descriptive statistics used—for example, was a mean presented when percentages would have been more informative?
2. Were statistical analyses undertaken to assess threats to the study's validity (e.g., to test for selection bias or attrition bias)?
3. Did the researchers report any inferential statistics? If inferential statistics were not used, should they have been?
4. Was information provided about both hypothesis testing and parameter estimation (i.e., confidence intervals)? Were effect sizes reported? Overall, did the reported statistics provide readers with sufficient information about the study results?
5. Were any multivariate procedures used? If not, should they have been used—for example, would the internal validity of the study be strengthened by statistically controlling confounding variables?
6. Were the selected statistical tests appropriate, given the level of measurement of the variables and the nature of the hypotheses?
7. Were the results of any statistical tests significant? What do the tests tell you about the plausibility of the research hypotheses? Were effects sizeable?
8. Were the results of any statistical tests nonsignificant? Is it possible that these reflect Type II errors? What factors might have undermined the study's statistical conclusion validity?
9. Was information about the reliability and validity of measures reported? Did the researchers use measures with good measurement properties?
10. Was there an appropriate amount of statistical information? Were findings clearly and logically organized? Were tables or figures used judiciously to summarize large amounts of statistical information? Are the tables clear, with good titles and row/column labels?

A thorough critical appraisal also addresses whether researchers used the appropriate statistics. Table 13.9 provides guidelines for some frequently used bivariate statistical tests. The major issues to consider are the number of independent and dependent variables, the levels of measurement of the research variables, and the number of groups (if any) being compared.

If researchers did not use multivariate statistics, you should consider whether the bivariate analysis adequately tests the relationship between the independent and dependent variables. For example, if a *t*-test or ANOVA was used, could the internal validity of the study have been enhanced through the statistical control of confounding variables, using ANCOVA? The answer will often be "yes."

Finally, you can be alert to possible exaggerations or subjectivity in the reported results. Researchers should never claim that the data proved, verified, confirmed, or demonstrated that the hypotheses were correct or incorrect. Hypotheses should be described as being *supported* or *not supported*, *accepted* or *rejected*.

The main task for beginning consumers in reading a results section of a research report is to understand the meaning of the statistical tests. What do the quantitative results indicate about the researcher's hypothesis? How believable are the findings? The answer to such questions form the basis for interpreting the research results, a topic discussed in Chapter 14.

RESEARCH EXAMPLES WITH CRITICAL THINKING EXERCISES

In this section, we provide details about the analysis in a nursing study, followed by some questions to guide critical thinking. Read the summary and then answer the critical thinking questions that follow, referring to the full research report if necessary. Answers to the questions for Exercise 1 are available to instructors on thePoint*. The critical thinking questions for Exercises 2 and 3 are based on studies that appear in their entirety in Appendices A and C of this book. Our comments for these exercises are in the Student Resources section on thePoint*. ⤳

EXAMPLE 1: DESCRIPTIVE AND INFERENTIAL STATISTICS

Study: Factors related to self-care behaviours among patients with diabetic foot ulcers (Kim & Han, 2020)

Statement of Purpose: The study aim was to examine the level of self-care behaviors among patients with diabetic foot ulcers (DFU) and to identify factors associated with those self-care behaviors.

Methods: The researchers used a descriptive correlational design. They collected data from a sample of 131 patients diagnosed with DFU at two Korean hospitals. Study participants completed self-report questionnaires that included background questions and psychological scales to measure perceived stress, coping, and family support. Participants also completed a 20-item scale to measure diabetic self-management as well as a 9-item scale to measure diabetic foot care. The report indicated that the internal consistency for these two self-care scales was good (coefficient alpha = .90 and .80, respectively). Excellent internal consistency was also found for the psychological scales (e.g., perceived stress scale: α = .91, perceived family support: α = .92). The researchers also retrieved information from medical records (e.g., erythrocyte sedation rate or ESR, HbA_{1C} values).

Descriptive Statistics: The researchers presented descriptive statistics (means, *SDs*, ranges, and percentages) to describe the characteristics of sample members, in terms of both demographic characteristics and scores on the psychological scales. Table 13.10 presents descriptive information for selected variables. The participants ranged in age from 37 to 79 years, and their mean age was 60.0 years, (±10.0). The typical participant was married (73.3%) and not employed (58.8%). A sizable percentage (38.2%) stated that they had not had diabetes education.

Bivariate Inferential Statistics: The researchers used a variety of bivariate inferential statistics to examine factors that related to participants' self-care behavior. For example, they used independent groups *t*-tests to compare those who did and those who did not have diabetes education. On both diabetes self-management scales, those who had diabetes education had significantly better self-care scores than those who had not: $t = 5.11$, $p < .001$ for the diabetes management scale and $t = 4.67$, $p < .001$ for the foot care scale. The researchers also used Pearson's *r* to examine interrelationships between the psychological scale scores and the self-care scale scores. Table 13.11 presents a correlation matrix that shows the values of *r* for pairs of selected variables. This table lists, on the left, six variables: Variables 1 to 4 are for the scores on the stress, coping, and family support scales, and Variables 5 and 6 are for scores on the two self-care scales, which are the dependent variables in these analyses. The correlation matrix shows, in column 1, the correlation coefficient between perceived stress scores and all other variables. At the intersection of row 1–column 1, we find 1.00, which

TABLE 13.10 Selected Demographic, Clinical, and Psychological Characteristics of Participants in Study on Self-Care Behavior in Patients With Diabetic Foot Ulcers ($N = 131$)

Sample Characteristic	Frequency (n)	Percentage	or Mean (SD)	Range of Values
Gender				
Male	91	69.5%		
Female	40	30.5%		
Marital status				
Married	96	73.3%		
Not married	35	26.7%		
Employment status				
Employed	54	41.2%		
Not employed	77	58.8%		
Diabetic education				
Has had	81	61.8%		
Has not had	50	38.2%		
Age			60.0 (9.9)	37–79
Erythrocyte sedimentation rate (ESR)			49.7 (30.1)	6.0–119.0
HbA$_{1C}$			7.3 (1.4)	4.8–12.0
Perceived stress scores			3.29 (0.93)	1.0–5.0
Problem-focused coping scores			2.41 (0.57)	1.0–4.0
Emotion-focused coping scores			2.51 (0.50)	1.0–4.0
Perceived family support scores			3.70 (0.80)	1.0–5.0
Diabetes self-management scores			3.04 (0.72)	1.0–5.0
Diabetic foot care scores			3.11 (0.72)	1.0–5.0

Adapted from Tables 1 and 2 of Kim, E., & Han, K. (2020). Factors related to self-care behaviours among patients with diabetic foot ulcers. *Journal of Clinical Nursing, 29*(9–10), 1712–1722.

TABLE 13.11 Correlation Matrix for Selected Study Variables in Study on Self-Care Behavior in Patients With Diabetic Foot Ulcers ($N = 131$)

Variable	1	2	3	4	5	6
1 Perceived stress	1.00					
2 Problem-focused coping	.19*	1.00				
3 Emotion-focused coping	.20*	.33***	1.00			
4 Perceived family support	−.30**	.09	.04	1.00		
5 Diabetes self management	−.31***	.24**	−.14	.42***	1.00	
6 Diabetic foot care	−.11	−.20*	−.05	.33***	−.69***	1.00

*$p < .05$. **$p < .01$. *** $p < .001$.
Adapted from Table 5 of Kim, E., & Han, K. (2020). Factors related to self-care behaviours among patients with diabetic foot ulcers. *Journal of Clinical Nursing, 29*(9–10), 1712–1722.

indicates that the scores are perfectly correlated with themselves. The next entry in column 1 is the *r* between perceived stress and problem-solving coping scores. The value of .19 indicates a modest, positive relationship between these two variables—a relationship that was significant at the .05 level. The strongest correlation between a psychological scale and self-care behaviors was for perceived family support, $r = .42$, $p < .001$ for diabetes management.

Multivariate Analyses: The researchers used multiple regression to predict self-care behaviors, using variables that were correlated with scores on the two self-care scales in bivariate analyses. They found, for example, that four factors were significantly correlated with the diabetes foot care scale scores: perceived family support, receipt of diabetic education, HbA_{1C} values, and ESR values. The R^2 for these four predictor variables was .36, $p < .001$. Having had diabetic education made the largest contribution, indicating the importance of such education.

Critical Thinking Exercises

1. Answer the relevant questions from Box 13.1 regarding this study.
2. What is the strongest correlation in Table 13.11? What is the weakest correlation in this table? What do the correlations indicate?
3. What might be some of the uses to which the findings could be put in clinical practice?

EXAMPLE 2: STATISTICAL ANALYSIS IN THE STUDY IN APPENDIX A

1. Read the Results section of Swenson and colleagues' study ("Parents' use of praise and criticism in a sample of young children seeking mental health services") in Appendix A of this book and then answer the relevant questions in Box 13.1.
2. Also consider the following targeted questions:
   a. Looking at Table 1, what percentage of parents had graduated from college? What was the mean score (and the *SD*) of the parents on the CES-D depression scale?
   b. In Table 2, what percentage of parents reported that they "almost never" praised their child? And what percentage reported that they "almost never" criticized their child?
   c. In Table 4, what was the correlation coefficient between parents' self-reported use of criticism and their score on the depressive symptom scale? Was the correlation statistically significant?

EXAMPLE 3: STATISTICAL ANALYSIS IN THE STUDY IN APPENDIX C

Answer the following targeted questions with regard to Bail and colleagues' quantitative analysis for their mixed methods study in Appendix C ("Cancer-related symptoms and cognitive intervention adherence among breast cancer survivors").

   a. Looking at Table 1, what was the mean, *SD*, and range for the following variables: age, years of survivorship, and current weight?
   b. In Table 1, what percentage of women had received chemotherapy? Radiation? Does the table show what percentage of women received neither chemotherapy nor radiation?
   c. Based on the results reported in the text and on the information in Table 2, how many women met the researchers' definition of adherence to the intervention?
   d. The researchers tested the correlation between the women's adherence and depressive symptoms, perceived cognitive impairment, and sleep quality. Which statistical test did they use? Were any of the correlations statistically significant? Is there a possibility that a Type II error occurred?

WANT TO KNOW MORE?

A wide variety of resources to enhance your learning and understanding of this chapter is available on thePoint®.

- Chapter Supplement on Multivariate Statistics
- Answer to the Critical Thinking Exercise for Examples 2 and 3
- Internet Resources with useful websites for Chapter 13
- A Wolters Kluwer journal article on a topic related to this chapter

Additional study aids, including eight journal articles and related questions, are also available in *Study Guide for Essentials of Nursing Research, 10e.*

Summary Points

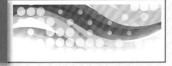

- There are four **levels of measurement**: (1) **nominal measurement**—the classification of attributes into mutually exclusive categories, (2) **ordinal measurement**—the ranking of people based on their relative standing on an attribute, (3) **interval measurement**—indicating not only people's rank order but also the distance between them, and (4) **ratio measurement**—distinguished from interval measurement by having a rational zero point. Interval- and ratio-level measures are often called **continuous**.

- **Descriptive statistics** are used to summarize and describe quantitative data.

- In **frequency distributions**, numeric values are ordered from lowest to highest, together with a count of the number (or percentage) of times each value was obtained.

- Data for a continuous variable can be described in terms of the shape of the distribution, central tendency, and variability.

- A distribution's shape can be **symmetric** or **skewed**, with one tail longer than the other; it can also be unimodal with one peak (i.e., one value of high frequency) or multimodal with more than one peak. A **normal distribution** (bell-shaped curve) is symmetric, unimodal, and not too peaked.

- Indexes of **central tendency** represent average or typical value of a set of scores. The **mode** is the value that occurs most frequently, the **median** is the point above which and below which 50% of the cases fall, and the **mean** is the arithmetic average of all scores. The mean is the most stable index of central tendency.

- Indexes of **variability**—how spread out the data are—include the range and standard deviation. The **range** is the distance between the highest and lowest scores. The **standard deviation** (*SD*) indicates how much, on average, scores deviate from the mean.

- In a normal distribution, 95% of values lie within 2 *SD*s above and below the mean.

- A **crosstabs table** is a two-dimensional frequency distribution in which the frequencies of two nominal- or ordinal-level variables are cross-tabulated.

- **Correlation coefficients** describe the direction and magnitude of a relationship between two variables; they range from −1.00 (perfect **negative correlation**) through .00 to +1.00 (perfect **positive correlation**). The most frequently used correlation coefficient is **Pearson's *r***, used with continuous variables.

- Statistical indexes that describe the effects of exposure to risk factors or interventions provide useful information for clinical decisions. A widely reported risk index is the **odds ratio**

(OR), which is the ratio of the odds for an exposed versus unexposed group, with the *odds* reflecting the proportion of people with an adverse outcome relative to those without it.

- **Inferential statistics**, based on laws of probability, allow researchers to make inferences about population **parameters** based on data from a sample.

- The *sampling distribution of the mean* is a theoretical distribution of the means of an infinite number of same-sized samples drawn from a population. Sampling distributions are the basis for inferential statistics.

- The *standard error of the mean (SEM)*—the standard deviation of this theoretical distribution—indicates the degree of average error of a sample mean; the smaller the SEM, the more accurate are estimates of the population value.

- Statistical inference consists of two approaches: hypothesis testing and **parameter estimation** (estimating a population value).

- *Point estimation* is a single value of a population estimate (e.g., a mean). *Interval estimation* provides a range of values—a **confidence interval (CI)**—within which the population value is expected to fall, at a specified probability. Most often, the 95% CI is reported, which indicates that there is a 95% probability that the true population value lies between the lower and upper confidence limits.

- **Hypothesis testing** through statistical tests enables researchers to make objective decisions about relationships between variables.

- The *null hypothesis* is that no relationship exists between variables; rejection of the null hypothesis lends support to the research hypothesis. In testing hypotheses, researchers compute a **test statistic** and then see if the statistic falls beyond a critical region on the theoretical distribution. The value of the test statistic indicates whether the null hypothesis is "improbable."

- A **Type I error** occurs if a null hypothesis is wrongly rejected (false positives). A **Type II error** occurs when a null hypothesis is wrongly accepted (false negatives).

- Researchers control the risk of making a Type I error by selecting a **level of significance** (or **alpha** level), which is the probability that such an error will occur. The .05 level (the conventional standard) means that in only 5 out of 100 samples would the null hypothesis be rejected when it should have been accepted.

- The probability of committing a Type II error is related to *power*, the ability of a statistical test to detect true relationships. The standard criterion for an acceptable level of power is .80. Power increases as sample size increases.

- Results from hypothesis tests are either significant or nonsignificant; **statistically significant** means that the obtained results are not likely to be due to chance fluctuations at a given probability (*p* **value**).

- Both the *t*-**test** and **analysis of variance (ANOVA)** can be used to test the significance of the difference between group means; ANOVA is used when there are three or more groups. **Repeated measures ANOVA** (RM-ANOVA) is used when data are collected at multiple time points.

- The **chi-squared test** is used to test hypotheses about group differences in proportions.

- Pearson's *r* can be used to test whether a correlation is significantly different from zero.

- **Effect size** indexes (such as the *d* **statistic**) summarize the strength of the effect of an independent variable (e.g., an intervention) on an outcome variable.

- **Multivariate statistics** are used in nursing research to untangle complex relationships among three or more variables.

- **Multiple regression analysis** is a method for understanding the effect of two or more **predictor** (independent) **variables** on a continuous dependent variable. The squared **multiple correlation coefficient** (R^2) is an estimate of the proportion of variability in the outcome variable accounted for by the predictors.

- **Analysis of covariance (ANCOVA)** controls confounding variables (called *covariates*) before testing whether differences in group means are statistically significant.

- **Logistic regression** is used to predict an outcome that is dichotomous on the basis of two or more predictor variables.

- Statistical methods are also used is psychometric assessments to quantify a measure's reliability and validity.

- For test–retest reliability, the preferred index is the **intraclass correlation coefficient (ICC)**. **Cohen's kappa** is used to estimate interrater reliability when the ratings of two independent raters are dichotomous. The index used to estimate internal consistency reliability is **coefficient alpha (α)**. Reliability coefficients of .80 or higher are desirable.

- In terms of content validity, expert ratings of items on a scale are used to compute a *content validity index* (*CVI*).

- Criterion validity is assessed with different statistical methods depending on the measurement level of the focal measure and the criterion. When both are dichotomous, sensitivity and specificity are usually calculated. **Sensitivity** is the instrument's ability to identify a case correctly (i.e., its rate of yielding true positives). **Specificity** is the instrument's ability to identify noncases correctly (i.e., its rate of yielding true negatives).

- Construct validity is evaluated using hypothesis-testing procedures, so statistical test such as those described in this chapter (e.g., Pearson's *r*, *t*-tests) are appropriate.

REFERENCES FOR CHAPTER 13

*Bekdemír, A., & İlhan, N. (2019). Predictors of caregiver burden in caregivers of bedridden patients. *The Journal of Nursing Research*, 27, e24.

*Dos Santos, W., Cêlho, V., Santos, G., & de Ceballos, A. (2019). Work overload and risk behaviors in motorcyclists. *Revista Brasileira de Enfermagem*, 72, 1479–1484.

Huang, M., Hung, C., Chen, C., Hung, W., & Liang, H. (2020). Factors associated with quality of life in patients with diabetic hypoglycaemia. *Journal of Clinical Nursing*, 29(9–10), 1704–1711.

Kamp, K., Dudley-Brown, S., Heitkemper, M., Wyatt, G., & Given, B. (2020). Symptoms among emerging adults with inflammatory bowel disease: A descriptive study. *Research in Nursing & Health*, 43, 48–55.

Kim, E., & Han, K. (2020). Factors related to self-care behaviours among patients with diabetic foot ulcers. *Journal of Clinical Nursing*, 29(9–10), 1712–1722.

Kim, K., Ramesh, D., Perry, M., Bernier, K., Young, E., Walsh, S., & Starkweather, A. (2020). Effects of physical activity on neurophysiological and gene expression profiles in chronic back pain: Study protocol. *Nursing Research*, 69, 74–81.

Landi, I., Giannotti, M., Venuti, P., & de Falco, S. (2020). Maternal and family predictors of infant psychological development in at-risk families: A multilevel longitudinal study. *Research in Nursing & Health*, 43, 17–27.

Lee, K., Jong, S., & Gay, C. (2020). Fatigue management for adults living with HIV: A randomized controlled pilot study. *Research in Nursing & Health*, 43, 56–67.

*Liu, H., Wang, I., Chen, N., & Chao, C. (2020). Effect of creativity training on teaching for creativity for nursing faculty in Taiwan: A quasi-experimental study. *Nurse Education Today*, 85, 104231.

Polit, D. F. (2010). *Statistics and data analysis for nursing research* (2nd ed.). Upper Saddle River, NJ: Pearson.

Polit, D. F., & Beck, C. T. (2021). *Nursing research: Generating and assessing evidence for nursing practice* (11th ed.). Philadelphia, PA: Wolters Kluwer.

Polit, D. F., & Yang, F. (2016). *Measurement and the measurement of change: A primer for health professionals*. Philadelphia, PA: Wolters Kluwer.

Tongpeth, J., Du, H., Barry, T., & Clark, R. (2020). Effectiveness of an Avatar application for teaching heart attack recognition and response: A pragmatic randomized control trial. *Journal of Advanced Nursing*, 76, 297–311.

Turan, N., Durgun, H., Kaya, H., Aşti, T., Yilmaz, Y., Gündüz, G., . . . Ertaş, G. (2020). Relationship between nursing students' levels of internet addiction, loneliness, and life satisfaction. *Perspectives in Psychiatric Care*, 56(3), 598–604.

**Van der Wal, M., Waldréus, N., Jaarsma, T., & Kato, N. (2020). Thirst in patients with heart failure in Sweden, the Netherlands, and Japan. *The Journal of Cardiovascular Nursing*, 35, 19–25.

Wang, T., Li, Y., Chen, L., Chou, C., & Yang, S. (2020). Correlation between postoperative health-related quality of life and care needs of oral cancer patients. *Cancer Nursing*, 43, 12–21.

*Yilmaz, İ., & Günes, Ü. (2019). Sacral skin temperature and pressure ulcer development: A descriptive study. *Wound Management & Prevention*, 65, 30–37.

*A link to this open-access article is provided in the Internet Resources section on thePoint® website.

**This journal article is available on thePoint® for this chapter.

Interpreting Quantitative Findings and Evaluating Clinical Significance

Learning Objectives

On completing this chapter, you will be able to:

- Describe dimensions for interpreting quantitative research results
- Describe the mindset conducive to a critical interpretation of research results
- Identify approaches to an assessment of the credibility of quantitative results and undertake such an assessment
- Distinguish statistical and clinical significance
- Identify some methods of drawing conclusions about clinical significance at the group and individual levels
- Critically appraise researchers' interpretation of their results in discussion sections of research reports
- Define new terms in the chapter

Key Terms

- Benchmark
- Change score
- Clinical significance
- CONSORT guidelines
- Minimal important change (MIC)
- Responder analysis
- Results

In this chapter, we consider approaches to interpreting researchers' statistical results, which require consideration of the various theoretical, methodological, and practical decisions that researchers make in undertaking a study. We also discuss an important but seldom discussed topic: clinical significance.

INTERPRETATION OF QUANTITATIVE RESULTS

Statistical **results** are summarized in the results section of a research article. Researchers present their *interpretations* of the results in the discussion section. It is difficult for the researchers to be totally objective, though, so you should develop your own interpretations.

Aspects of Interpretation

Interpreting study results involves attending to different but overlapping considerations.

- The credibility and accuracy of the results
- The precision of the estimate of effects

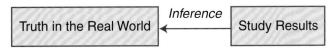

Figure 14.1 Inferences in interpreting research results.

- The magnitude of effects and importance of the results
- The meaning of the results, especially with regard to causality
- The generalizability and applicability of the results
- The implications of the results for nursing practice, theory development, or further research

Before discussing these considerations, we want to remind you about the role of inference in research thinking and interpretation.

Inference and Interpretation

An *inference* involves drawing conclusions based on limited information, using logical reasoning. Interpreting research findings entails making multiple inferences. In research, virtually everything is a "stand-in" for something else. A sample is a stand-in for a population, a scale score is a proxy for the magnitude of an abstract attribute, and so on.

Research findings are meant to reflect "truth in the real world"—the findings are proxies for the true state of affairs (Fig. 14.1). Inferences about the real world are valid to the extent that researchers make good decisions in selecting proxies. This chapter offers several vantage points for assessing whether study findings really reflect "truth in the real world."

The Interpretive Mindset

Evidence-based practice (EBP) involves integrating research evidence into clinical decision making. EBP encourages clinicians to think critically about clinical practice and to challenge the status quo when it conflicts with "best evidence." Thinking critically and demanding evidence are also part of a research interpreter's job. Just as clinicians should ask, "What *evidence* is there that this intervention will be beneficial?" so must interpreters ask, "What *evidence* is there that the results are real and true?"

To be a good interpreter of research results, you can profit by starting with a skeptical ("show me") attitude and a null hypothesis. *The "null hypothesis" in interpretation is that the results are wrong and the evidence is flawed.* The "research hypothesis" is that the evidence reflects the truth. Interpreters decide whether the null hypothesis has merit by critically examining methodological evidence. The greater the evidence that the researcher's design and methods were sound, the less plausible is the null hypothesis that the evidence is inaccurate.

CREDIBILITY OF QUANTITATIVE RESULTS

A critical interpretive task is to assess whether the results are *right*. If the results are not judged to be credible, the remaining interpretive issues (the meaning, magnitude, precision, generalizability, and implications of results) are unlikely to be relevant.

A credibility assessment requires a careful analysis of the study's methodological and conceptual limitations and strengths. To come to a conclusion about whether the results closely approximate "truth in the real world," each aspect of the study—its design, sampling plan, data collection, and analyses—must be subjected to critical scrutiny.

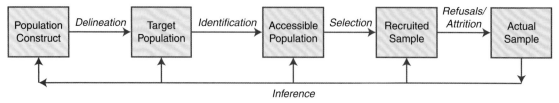

Figure 14.2   Inferences about populations: from final sample to the population.

There are various ways to approach the issue of credibility, including the use of the critical appraisal guidelines we have offered throughout this book and the overall appraisal protocol presented in Table 3.1. We share some additional perspectives in this section.

Proxies and Interpretation

Researchers begin with constructs and then devise ways to operationalize them. The constructs are linked to actual research tactics in a series of approximations; the better the proxies, the more credible the results are likely to be. In this section, we illustrate successive proxies using sampling concepts to highlight the potential for inferential challenges.

When researchers formulate research questions, the population of interest is often abstract. For example, suppose we wanted to test the effectiveness of an intervention to increase physical activity in low-income women. Figure 14.2 shows the series of steps between the abstract population construct (low-income women) and actual study participants. Using data from the actual sample on the far right, the researcher would like to make inferences about the effectiveness of the intervention for a broader group, but each proxy along the way represents a potential problem for achieving the desired inference. In interpreting a study, readers must consider how *plausible* it is that the actual sample reflects the recruited sample, the accessible population, the target population, and the population construct.

Table 14.1 presents a description of a hypothetical scenario in which the researchers moved from the population construct (low-income women) to a sample of 163 participants

TABLE 14.1 Example of Successive Series of Proxies in Sampling

Element	Description	Possible Inferential Challenges
Population construct	Low-income women	
Target population	All women who receive public assistance (cash welfare) in California	• Why only welfare recipients? Why not the working poor? • Why California?
Accessible population	All women who receive public assistance in Los Angeles and who speak English or Spanish	• Why Los Angeles? • What about non-English/non-Spanish speakers?
Recruited sample	A consecutive sample of 282 female public assistance recipients (English or Spanish speaking) who applied for benefits in January 2022 at 2 welfare offices in Los Angeles; 267 were deemed eligible	• Why only new applicants? What about women with long-term receipt? • Why only two offices? Are these representative? • Is January a typical month?
Randomized sample	200 women from the recruited sample who agreed to participate in the study	• How did the 200 participants differ from the 67 who declined to participate?
Final actual sample	163 women who were included in the analysis sample	• How did dropouts differ from those in the final sample?

(recent public assistance recipients from two neighborhoods in Los Angeles) who provided postintervention data. The table identifies questions that could be asked in drawing inferences about the study results. Answers to these questions would affect the interpretation of whether the intervention *really* is effective with low-income women or only with recent recipients of public assistance in Los Angeles who cooperated in the study.

Researchers make methodological decisions that affect inferences, but prospective participants' behavior also needs to be considered. In our example, only 200 of the 267 eligible women agreed to participate in the study, and only 163 provided data for the analysis. The sample of 163 women almost surely would differ in important ways from the 104 who either declined to participate in the study or who dropped out.

Fortunately, researchers are increasingly documenting participant flow in their studies—especially in intervention studies. Guidelines called the Consolidated Standards of Reporting Trials or **CONSORT guidelines** have been adopted by major health care journals to help readers track study participants. CONSORT flow charts, when available in a report, should be scrutinized in interpreting study results. Figure 14.3 provides an example of such a flowchart for the intervention study just described. The chart shows that 282 people were assessed for eligibility, but 82 either did not meet eligibility criteria or refused to be in the study. Of the 200 people who agreed to participate, half were randomized to the intervention group and

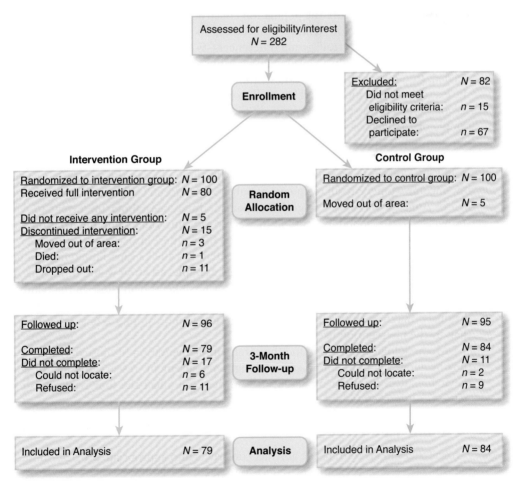

Figure 14.3 Example of CONSORT guidelines flowchart: progression of participants in an intervention study.

the other half to the control group ($N = 100$ per group). However, only 80 in the experimental group received the full intervention. At the 3-month follow-up, researchers attempted to obtain data from 96 people in the intervention group and 95 in the control group (everyone who did not move or die). They obtained follow-up data from 79 in the intervention group and 84 in the control group, and these 163 comprised the analysis sample.

Credibility and Validity

Inference and validity are inextricably linked. To be careful interpreters, readers must search for evidence that the desired inferences are, in fact, valid. Part of this process involves considering alternative competing hypotheses about the credibility and meaning of the results.

In Chapter 8, we discussed four types of validity that relate to the credibility of study results: statistical conclusion validity, internal validity, external validity, and construct validity. We use our sampling example (Fig. 14.2 and Table 14.1) to demonstrate the relevance of methodological decisions to all four types of validity—and hence to inferences about study results.

In our example, the population construct is *low-income women*, which was translated into population eligibility criteria stipulating California public assistance recipients. Yet, there are alternative operationalizations of the population construct (e.g., women living below the official poverty level). Construct validity, it may be recalled, involves inferences from the particulars of the study to higher-order constructs. So it is fair to ask: Do the eligibility criteria adequately capture the population construct, low-income women?

Statistical conclusion validity—the extent to which correct inferences can be made about the existence of "real" group differences—is also affected by sampling decisions. Ideally, researchers would do a power analysis at the outset to estimate how large a sample they needed. In our example, let us assume (based on previous research) that the effect size for the exercise intervention would be small to moderate, with $d = .40$. For a power of .80, with risk of a Type I error set at .05, we would need a sample of about 200 participants. The actual sample of 163 yields a nearly 30% risk of a Type II error, i.e., wrongly concluding that the intervention was not successful.

External validity—the generalizability of the results—is affected by sampling. To whom would it be safe to generalize the results in this example—to the population construct of low-income women? to all recipients of public assistance in California? to all new recipients in Los Angeles who speak English or Spanish? Inferences about the extent to which the study results correspond to "truth in the real world" must take sampling decisions and sampling problems (e.g., recruitment and attrition difficulties) into account.

Finally, the study's internal validity (the extent to which a causal inference can be made) is also affected by sample composition. In this example, attrition would be a concern. Were those in the intervention group more likely (or less likely) than those in the control group to drop out of the study? If so, any observed differences in outcomes could be caused by individual differences in the groups (e.g., differences in motivation to stay in the study), rather than by the intervention itself.

Methodological decisions and the careful implementation of those decisions—whether they be about sampling, intervention design, measurement, research design, or analysis—inevitably affect the rigor of a study. All of them can affect the four types of validity, and hence the interpretation of the results.

Credibility and Bias

A researcher's job is to translate abstract constructs into appropriate proxies. Another major job concerns efforts to eliminate, reduce, or control biases—or, as a last resort, to detect and understand them. As a reader of research reports, your job is to be on the lookout for biases and to factor them into your assessment about the credibility of the results.

TABLE 14.2 Selected List of Major Biases or Errors in Quantitative Studies in Four Research Domains

Research Design	Sampling	Measurement	Analysis
Expectation bias	Sampling error	Social desirability bias	Type I error
Hawthorne effect	Volunteer bias	Acquiescence bias	Type II error
Contamination of treatments	Nonresponse bias	Naysayers bias	
Carryover effects		Extreme response bias	
Noncompliance bias		Recall/memory bias	
Selection bias		Reactivity	
Attrition bias		Observer biases	
History bias			

Biases create distortions and undermine researchers' efforts to reveal "truth in the real world." Biases are pervasive and virtually inevitable. It is important to consider what types of bias might be present and how extensive, sizeable, and systematic they are. We have discussed many types of bias in this book—some reflect design inadequacies (e.g., selection bias), others reflect recruitment problems (nonresponse bias), and others relate to measurement (social desirability bias). Table 14.2 presents biases and errors mentioned in this book. This table is meant to serve as a reminder of some of the problems to consider in interpreting study results.

 TIP The supplement to this chapter on thePoint® website includes a longer list of biases, including some not described in this book; we offer definitions for all biases listed. Different disciplines, and different writers, use different names for the same or similar biases. The actual names are unimportant—but it is important to reflect on how different forces can distort results and affect inferences.

Credibility and Corroboration

Earlier, we noted that research interpreters should seek evidence to disconfirm the "null hypothesis" that research results are wrong. Some evidence to discredit this null hypothesis comes from the quality of the proxies that stand in for abstractions. Ruling out biases also undermines the null hypothesis. Another strategy is to seek corroboration for the results.

Corroboration can come from internal and external sources, and the concept of *replication* is an important one in both cases. Interpretations are aided by considering prior research on the topic, for example. Interpreters can examine whether the study results are congruent with those of other studies. Consistency across studies tends to discredit the "null hypothesis" of erroneous results.

Researchers may have opportunities for replication themselves. For example, in multi-site studies, if the results are similar across sites, this suggests that something "real" is occurring. Triangulation can be another form of replication. We are strong advocates of mixed methods studies (see Chapter 12). When findings from the analysis of qualitative data are consistent with the results of statistical analyses, internal corroboration can be especially powerful and persuasive.

OTHER ASPECTS OF INTERPRETATION

If an assessment leads you to accept that the results of a study are probably "real," you have made important progress in interpreting the study findings. Other interpretive tasks depend on a conclusion that the results are likely credible.

Precision of the Results

Results from statistical hypothesis tests indicate whether a relationship or group difference is probably "real." A p value in hypothesis testing offers information that is important (whether the null hypothesis is probably false) but incomplete. Confidence intervals (CIs), by contrast, communicate information about how precise the study results are. Dr. David Sackett, a founding father of the EBP movement, and his colleagues (2000) said this about CIs: "P values on their own are . . . not informative . . . By contrast, CIs indicate the strength of evidence about quantities of direct interest, such as treatment benefit. They are thus of particular relevance to practitioners of evidence-based medicine" (p. 232). Hopefully, nurse researchers will increasingly report CI information because of its value for interpreting study results.

Magnitude of Effects and Importance

In quantitative studies, results that support the researcher's hypotheses are described as *significant*. A careful analysis of study results involves evaluating whether, in addition to being statistically significant, the effects are large and clinically important.

Attaining statistical significance does not necessarily mean that the results are meaningful to nurses and clients. Statistical significance indicates that the results are unlikely to be due to chance—not that they are important. With large samples, even modest relationships are statistically significant. For instance, with a sample of 500, a correlation coefficient of .10 is significant at the .05 level, but a relationship this weak may have little practical relevance. Estimating the magnitude and importance of effects is relevant to the issue of clinical significance, a topic we discus later in this chapter.

The Meaning of Quantitative Results

In quantitative studies, statistical results are in the form of p values, effect sizes, and CIs, to which researchers and consumers must attach meaning. Questions about the meaning of statistical results often reflect a desire to interpret causal connections. Interpreting what descriptive results mean is not typically a challenge. For example, suppose we found that, among patients undergoing electroconvulsive therapy, the percentage who experience an electroconvulsive therapy–induced headache is 59.4% (95% CI = 56.3, 63.1). This result is directly interpretable. But if we found that headache prevalence is significantly lower in a cryotherapy intervention group than among patients given acetaminophen, we would need to interpret what the results mean. In particular, we need to interpret whether it is plausible that cryotherapy *caused* the reduced prevalence of headaches. In this section, we discuss the interpretation of research outcomes within a hypothesis testing context, with an emphasis on causal interpretations.

Interpreting Hypothesized Results

Interpreting statistical results is easiest when hypotheses are supported—i.e., when there are *positive results*—because existing evidence and theory presumably laid the foundation for the hypotheses. Nevertheless, a few caveats should be kept in mind.

It is important to avoid the temptation of going beyond the data to explain what results mean. For example, suppose we hypothesized that pregnant women's anxiety level about childbearing is correlated with the number of children they have. The data reveal a significant negative relationship between anxiety levels and parity ($r = -.40$). We interpret this to mean that increased experience with childbirth results in decreased anxiety. Is this conclusion supported by the data? The conclusion appears logical, but in fact, there is nothing in the results that leads to this interpretation. An important, indeed critical, research precept is *correlation does not prove causation*. The finding that two variables are related offers no evidence suggesting which of the two variables—if either—caused the other. In our example, perhaps causality runs in the opposite direction, i.e., a woman's anxiety level influences how many children she bears. Or maybe a third variable, such as the woman's relationship with her husband, influences both anxiety and number of children. Inferring causality is especially difficult in studies that have not used an experimental design.

Empirical evidence supporting research hypotheses never constitutes *proof* of their veracity. Hypothesis testing is probabilistic. There is always a possibility that observed relationships resulted from chance—that is, that a Type I error has occurred. Researchers (and consumers) should be tentative about interpreting results—even when the results are in line with expectations.

Example of corroboration of a hypothesis ••••••••••••••••••••••••••••

Wargo-Sugleris and colleagues (2018) tested hypotheses about the relationship between acute care nurses' job satisfaction, successful aging, and delaying retirement. Consistent with hypotheses, successful aging (a construct that incorporated good health, self-assessments of work ability, and use of sick leave) was associated with job satisfaction and intention to delay retirement. The researchers concluded that "environment and successful aging are important areas that have an impact on job satisfaction and delay of retirement in older nurses" (p. 911).

This study is an example of the challenges of interpreting findings in correlational studies. The researchers' interpretation was that successful aging had an *impact* on job satisfaction—a word that implies a causal connection. This is a conclusion supported by earlier research and consistent with theory. Yet, nothing in the data rules out the possibility that nurses' job satisfaction affects nurses' successful aging, or that a third factor might cause both job dissatisfaction and health issues captured in the successful aging measure. The researchers' interpretation is plausible, but their cross-sectional design makes it difficult to rule out other explanations. A major threat to the internal validity of the inference in this study is temporal ambiguity—that is, whether job dissatisfaction preceded indicators of successful aging.

Interpreting Nonsignificant Results

Nonsignificant results pose interpretative challenges. Statistical tests are geared toward disconfirmation of the null hypothesis. Failure to reject a null hypothesis can occur for many reasons, and the real reason may be hard to figure out.

The null hypothesis *could* actually be true, accurately reflecting the absence of a relationship among research variables. On the other hand, the null hypothesis could be false. Retention of a false null hypothesis (a Type II error) can result from such methodological problems as poor internal validity, an anomalous sample, a weak statistical procedure, or unreliable measures. In particular, failure to reject null hypotheses is often a consequence of insufficient power, reflecting too small a sample.

It is important to recognize that a null hypothesis that is not rejected does not confirm the *absence* of relationships among variables. *Nonsignificant results provide no evidence of the truth or the falsity of the hypothesis.*

Because statistical procedures are designed to test support for rejecting null hypotheses, they are not well suited for testing *actual* research hypotheses about the absence of relationships or about equivalence between groups. Yet sometimes, this is exactly what researchers want to do, especially in clinical situations in which the goal is to test whether one's practice is as effective as another—but perhaps less painful or costly. When the actual research hypothesis is null (e.g., a prediction of *no* group difference), stringent additional strategies must be used to provide supporting evidence. It is useful for the researchers to compute effect sizes or CIs to illustrate that the risk of a Type II error was small.

Example of support for a hypothesized nonsignificant result • • • • • • • • • • • • • •
Smith and colleagues (2020) conducted a trial to test the hypothesis that the Orve+wrap thermal blanket is not less safe or effective than forced-air warming in restoring normothermia in the postanesthesia care unit. A total of 129 patients were randomized to receive one or the other treatment. Group differences in temperature and adverse event rates were, as predicted, nonsignificant. The researchers had established a predefined noninferiority margin of 0.3°C, which was not reached. The average temperature was 36.2°C for those receiving the Orve+wrap blanket and 36.3°C for those receiving forced-air warming.

Interpreting Unhypothesized Significant Results

Unhypothesized significant results can occur in two situations. The first involves results from analyses that were not considered when the study was designed. For example, in examining correlations among research variables, a researcher might notice that two variables that were not central to the research questions were nevertheless significantly correlated and interesting.

Example of a serendipitous significant finding •
In a secondary analysis of data from a national survey, Must and colleagues (2017) studied the effect of age on the prevalence of obesity among American youth with and without autism spectrum disorder (ASD). Consistent with expectations, they found that the odds of obesity among children with ASD, but not among those without ASD, increased from ages 10 to 17 years. Unexpectedly, they found that although white children with ASD experienced increases in obesity, minority children with ASD experienced declines.

The second situation is more perplexing: obtaining results *opposite* to those hypothesized. For instance, a researcher might hypothesize that individualized teaching about AIDS risks is more effective than group instruction, but the results might indicate that the group method was better. Although this might seem disconcerting, research should not be undertaken to corroborate predictions but to arrive at truth. When significant findings are opposite to what was hypothesized, the interpretation should involve comparisons with other research, a consideration of alternate theories, and a critical scrutiny of the research methods.

Example of significant results contrary to hypotheses • • • • • • • • • • • • • • • • • • •
Griggs and Crawford (2017) studied the relationship between hope, emotional well-being, and health-risk behaviors in a sample of nearly 500 university freshmen. Contrary to the researchers' hypothesis, higher levels of hope were associated with more—not less—sexual risk-taking behaviors and alcohol use.

In summary, interpreting the meaning of research results is a demanding task, but it offers the possibility of intellectual rewards. Interpreters must play the role of scientific detectives, trying to make pieces of the puzzle fit together so that a coherent picture of the truth emerges.

Generalizability and Applicability of the Results

Researchers typically seek evidence that can be used by others. If a new nursing intervention is found to be successful, others might want to adopt it. Therefore, another interpretive question is whether the intervention will "work" or whether the relationships will "hold" in other settings, with other people. Part of the interpretive process involves asking the question

"To what groups, environments, and conditions can the results reasonably be applied?" In interpreting a study's generalizability, it is useful to consider our earlier discussion about proxies. For which higher order constructs, which populations, which settings, or which versions of an intervention were the study operations good "stand-ins"? This issue is discussed at greater length in Chapter 18.

Implications of the Results

Once you have reached conclusions about the credibility, precision, importance, meaning, and generalizability of the results, you are ready to think about their implications. You might consider the implications of the findings with respect to future research: What should other researchers in this area do—what is the right "next step"? You are most likely to consider the implications for nursing practice: How should the results be used by nurses in their practice?

All of the interpretive dimensions we have discussed are critical in evidence-based nursing practice. With regard to generalizability, it may not be enough to ask a broad question about to whom the results could apply—you need to ask, "Are these results relevant to *my* clinical situation?"

CLINICAL SIGNIFICANCE

It has long been recognized that statistical hypothesis testing provides limited information for interpretation purposes. In particular, attaining statistical significance does not address the question of whether a finding is clinically meaningful or relevant. With a large enough sample, a trivial relationship can be statistically significant. Broadly speaking, we define **clinical significance** as the practical importance of research results in terms of whether they have genuine, palpable effects on the daily lives of patients or on the health care decisions made on their behalf.

In fields other than nursing, notably in medicine and psychotherapy, attention has been paid to defining clinical significance and developing ways to operationalize it. There has been no consensus on either front, but a few conceptual and statistical solutions are being used with some regularity. Here, we provide a brief overview of recent advances in defining and operationalizing clinical significance; further information is available in Polit and Yang (2016).

In statistical hypothesis testing, consensus was reached decades ago—for better or worse—that a p value of .05 would be the standard criterion for statistical significance. It is unlikely that a uniform standard will ever be adopted for clinical significance, however, because of its complexity. For example, in some cases, *no change* over time could be clinically significant if it means that a group with a progressive disease has not deteriorated. In other cases, clinical significance is associated with improvements. Another issue concerns whose *perspective* on clinical significance is relevant. Sometimes, clinicians' perspective is key because of implications for health management. For other outcomes, the patient's view is what matters (e.g., improved quality of life). Two other issues concern whether clinical significance is for group-level findings or about individual patients, and whether clinical significance is attached to point-in-time outcomes or to change scores. Most recent work is about the clinical significance of **change scores** for individual patients (e.g., a change from a baseline measurement to a follow-up measurement). We begin, however, with a brief discussion of group-level clinical significance.

Clinical Significance at the Group Level

Many studies concern group-level comparisons. For example, one-group pretest–posttest designs involve comparing a group at two or more points in time, to examine whether or not a change in outcomes has, on average, occurred. In randomized controlled trials and case-control studies, the central comparison is about average differences for different groups of people. Group-level clinical significance typically involves using statistical information other than *p* values to draw conclusions about the meaningfulness. The most widely used statistics for this purpose are effect size indexes, CIs, and number needed to treat (NNT).

Effect size indexes summarize the magnitude of a change or a relationship and thus provide insights into how a group, *on average*, might benefit from a treatment. In most cases, a clinically significant finding at the group level means that the effect size is sufficiently large to have relevance for patients. CIs are espoused by several writers as useful tools for understanding clinical significance; CIs provide the most plausible range of values, at a given level of confidence, for the unknown population parameter. NNTs are sometimes promoted as good indicators of clinical significance because the information is relatively easy to understand. For example, if the NNT for an important outcome is found to be 2.0, only two patients have to receive a particular treatment in order for one patient to benefit. If the NNT is 10.0, however, 9 patients out of 10 receiving the treatment would get no benefit.

With any of these group-level indexes, researchers should designate in advance what would constitute clinical significance—just as they would establish an alpha value for statistical significance. For example, would an effect size of .20 (for the *d* index described in Chapter 13) be considered clinically significant? A *d* of .20 has been described as a "small" effect, but sometimes, small improvements can have clinical relevance. Claims about attainment of clinical significance for groups should be based on defensible criteria.

Example of clinical significance at the group level •
Johnson and colleagues (2020) studied factors associated with abnormal weight gain in a sample of youth childhood brain tumor survivors. They found relationships with children's fatigue, tumor location, cranial radiation, and chemotherapy. They computed effect size estimates and concluded that the effects were sufficiently large to suggest that the findings were clinically significant.

Clinical Significance at the Individual Level

Clinicians usually are not interested in what happens in a *group* of people—they are concerned with individual patients. A key goal in EBP is to personalize "best evidence" into decisions for a specific patient's needs, within a particular clinical context.

Dozens of approaches to defining and operationalizing clinical significance at the individual level have been developed, but they share one thing in common: They involve establishing a **benchmark** (or *threshold*) that designates the score value on a measure (or the value of a change score) that would be considered clinically important. With an established benchmark for clinical significance, each person in a study can be classified as having or not having a score or change score that is clinically significant.

Example of an individual benchmark for clinical significance • • • • • • • • • • • • • •
Tsai and colleagues (2020) studied the relationships between sleep quality in mothers of children with epilepsy and such factors as child sleep disturbances and maternal depression. The researchers used an established benchmark on the children's sleep disturbance scale and found that 94.7% of the children had a clinically significant sleep disturbance score.

Conceptual Definitions of Clinical Significance

Numerous definitions of clinical significance can be found in the health literature, most of which concern change scores on measures of patient outcomes (e.g., a score at Time 1 subtracted from a score at Time 2). One approach to conceptualizing clinical significance dominates medical research. In a paper cited hundreds of times in the medical literature,

Jaeschke and colleagues (1989) offered the following definition: "The minimal clinically important difference (MCID) can be defined as the smallest difference in score in the domain of interest which patients perceive as beneficial and which would mandate, in the absence of troublesome side effects and excessive cost, a change in the patient's management" (p. 408). Although these researchers referred to the conceptual threshold for clinical significance as a minimal clinically important *difference*, we follow an influential group of measurement experts in using the term **minimal important change (MIC)** because the focus is on individual change scores, not differences between groups.

Operationalizing Clinical Significance: Establishing the Minimal Important Change Benchmark

The Jaeschke and colleagues' (1989) definition of change score benchmarks has inspired researchers to go in different directions to quantify it. The MIC benchmark is usually operationalized as a value for the amount of change in score points on a measure that an individual patient must achieve to be considered as having a clinically important change.

A traditional approach to setting a benchmark for health outcomes is to obtain input from a panel of health care experts—sometimes called a *consensus panel*. For example, a consensus panel that was convened to establish the clinical significance of changes in self-reported pain intensity (e.g., on a visual analog scale) established the benchmark as a 30% reduction in pain.

Another approach is to undertake a study to determine what patients themselves think is a minimally important change on a focal measure. The developers of some new multi-item scales now use this approach to estimate the MIC as part of the psychometric assessment of their instrument. Calculating an MIC using patient ratings of important change requires a careful research design with a large sample of people whose change over time is expected to vary.

A third approach to defining the MIC is based on the distributional characteristics of a measure. Most often, the MIC using this approach is set to a threshold of 0.5 *SDs*—i.e., one half a standard deviation (*SD*) on a distribution of baseline scores. For example, if the baseline *SD* for a scale were 6.0, then the MIC using the 0.5 *SD* criterion would be 3.0. This value, like any MIC, can be used as the benchmark to classify individual patients as having or not having experienced clinically meaningful change.

Many researchers have used the MIC to interpret group-level findings. The MIC is, however, an index of *individual* change, not group differences. Experts have warned that it is inappropriate to interpret mean differences in relation to the MIC. For example, if the MIC on an important outcome has been established as 4.0, this value should not be used to interpret the clinical significance of the mean difference between two groups. If the mean group difference were found to be 3.0, for instance, it would be wrong to conclude that the results were not clinically significant. A mean difference of 3.0 suggests that a sizeable percentage of participants *did* achieve a clinically meaningful benefit—i.e., an improvement of 4 points or more.

MIC thresholds can be used to calculate rates of clinical significance for individual study participants. Once the MIC is known, researchers can classify all people in a study in terms of their having attained or not attained the threshold. Then, researchers can compare the percentage of people who "responded" at clinically important levels in the study groups (e.g., those in the intervention and those in the control group). Such a **responder analysis** is easy to understand and has strong implications for EBP.

Example of a responder analysis •
Evans and colleagues (2018) studied the effects of a yoga intervention for teens with irritable bowel syndrome. Teens in the yoga group were divided into responders and nonresponders using an established threshold for the MIC on a pain scale. The two groups were compared on several quantitative measures (e.g., psychological distress, sleep quality) and on qualitative data obtained in semi-structured interviews.

CRITICAL APPRAISAL OF INTERPRETATIONS

Researchers interpret their findings and discuss what the findings might imply for nursing in the discussion section of research articles. When critically appraising a study, your own interpretation can be contrasted against those of the researchers.

A good discussion section should point out study limitations. Researchers are in the best position to detect and assess sampling deficiencies, data quality problems, and so on, and it is a professional responsibility to alert readers to these difficulties. Of course, researchers are unlikely to note all relevant limitations. Your task as reviewer is to develop your own interpretation and assessment of methodological problems and to challenge conclusions that do not appear to be warranted.

You should also carefully scrutinize causal interpretations, especially in nonexperimental studies. Sometimes, even the titles of reports suggest potential problems. If the title of a nonexperimental study includes terms like "the effect of . . .," or "the impact of . . .," this may signal the need for critical scrutiny of the researcher's inferences.

In addition to comparing your interpretation with that of the researchers, your appraisal should also draw conclusions about the stated implications of the study. Some researchers make grandiose claims or offer unfounded recommendations based on modest results.

The conceptualization and operationalization of clinical significance have not received much attention in nursing, and so studies that do not mention clinical significance should not be faulted for this omission—but researchers who do address clinical significance should be lauded. We hope that nurse researchers will pay more attention to this issue in the years ahead.

Some guidelines for evaluating researchers' interpretation are offered in Box 14.1.

Box 14.1 Guidelines for Critically Appraising Interpretations/Discussions in Quantitative Research Reports

Interpretation of the Findings
1. Were all the important results discussed?
2. Did the researchers discuss any study limitations and their possible effects on the credibility of the findings? In discussing limitations, were key threats to the study's validity and possible biases reviewed? Did the interpretations take limitations into account?
3. What types of evidence were offered in support of the interpretation, and was that evidence persuasive? Were results interpreted in light of findings from other studies?
4. Did the researchers make any unjustifiable causal inferences? Were alternative explanations for the findings considered? Were the rationales for rejecting these alternatives convincing?
5. Did the interpretation take into account the precision of the results and/or the magnitude of effects?
6. Did the researchers draw any unwarranted conclusions about the generalizability of the results?

Implications of the Findings and Recommendations
7. Did the researchers discuss the study's implications for clinical practice or future nursing research? Did they make specific recommendations?
8. If yes, are the stated implications appropriate, given the study's limitations and the magnitude of the effects as well as evidence from other studies? Are there important implications that the report neglected to include?

Clinical Significance
9. Did the researchers mention or assess clinical significance? Did they make a distinction between statistical and clinical significance?
10. If clinical significance was examined, was it assessed in terms of group-level information (e.g., effect sizes) or individual-level results? How was clinical significance operationalized?

RESEARCH EXAMPLES WITH CRITICAL THINKING EXERCISES

In this section, we provide details about the interpretive portion of a quantitative study. Read the summary and then answer the critical thinking questions that follow, referring to the full research report if necessary. Answers to the questions for Exercise 1 are available to instructors on thePoint®. The critical thinking questions for Exercises 2 and 3 are based on the studies that appear in their entirety in Appendices A and D of this book. Our comments for Exercises 2 and 3 are in the Student Resources section on thePoint®.

EXAMPLE 1: INTERPRETATION IN A QUANTITATIVE STUDY

Study: Neurobehavioral effects of aspartame consumption (Lindseth et al., 2014)

Statement of Purpose: The purpose of this study was to examine the effects of consuming diets with higher amounts of aspartame (25 mg/kg body weight/day) versus lower amounts of aspartame (10 mg/kg body weight/day) on neurobehavioral outcomes.

Method: The researchers used a randomized crossover design to assess the effects of aspartame amounts. Study participants were 28 healthy adults, university students, who consumed study-prepared diets. Participants were randomized to orderings of the aspartame protocol (i.e., some received the high-aspartame diet first, others received the low amount first). Participants were blinded to which diet they were receiving. They consumed one of the diets for an 8-day period, followed by a 2-week washout period. Then, they consumed the alternative diet for another 8 days. At the end of each 8-day session, measurements were made for such neurobehavioral outcomes as cognition (working memory, spatial visualization), depression, and irritability.

Analyses: Within-subjects tests (paired t-tests, repeated measures analysis of variance) were used to test the statistical significance of differences in outcomes for the two dietary protocols, with alpha set at .05. In terms of clinical significance, a participant was considered to have a clinically significant neurobehavioral effect if his or her score was $2+$ SDs outside the mean score for normal functioning based on norms for each measure. Thus, change scores for participants were not computed. Rather, each score was assessed for crossing the benchmark value for a normative state—a criterion that is used in many trials of psychotherapeutic interventions.

Results: Statistically significant differences, favoring the low-aspartame diet, were observed for three neurobehavioral outcomes: spatial orientation, depression, and irritability. Despite the fact that the participants were healthy adult students, a few of them experienced clinically significant outcomes in the high-aspartame condition. For example, two participants had clinically significant cognitive impairment (two with working memory deficits and two others with spatial orientation impairment) after 8 days of consuming the high-aspartame diet. Three other participants had clinically relevant levels of depression at the end of the high-aspartame condition. None of the scores was clinically significant after 8 days on the low-aspartame diet.

Discussion: The researchers devoted a large portion of their discussion to the issue of *corroboration*. They pointed out ways in which their findings were consistent with (or diverged from) other studies on the effects of aspartame. In keeping with the researchers' used of a strong experimental design, they concluded that there was a causal relationship between high amounts of aspartame consumption and negative neurobehavioral effects: "A high dose of aspartame caused more irritability and depression than a low-aspartame dose consumed by the same participants, supporting earlier study findings . . ." (p. 191).

The researchers also commented on the clinical significance findings: "Additionally, three participants in our study scored in the clinically depressed category while consuming the high-aspartame diet, despite no previous histories of depression" (p. 191). The researchers concluded their discussion with remarks about the limitations of their study, which included problems of generalizability: "Limitations of our study included the small homogeneous sample, which may make it difficult to apply our conclusions to other study populations. Also, our sample size of 28 participants resulted in statistical power of .72, which is on the lower end of the acceptable range. A washout period before the baseline assessments and using food diaries during the between-treatment washout period to verify that aspartame was not consumed would have strengthened the design" (p. 191).

Critical Thinking Exercises

1. Answer the relevant questions from Box 14.1 regarding this study. (We encourage you to read the report in its entirety, especially the discussion, to answer these questions.)
2. Also consider the following targeted questions:
   a. Comment on the statistical conclusion validity of this study.
   b. Would this study benefit from the inclusion of a CONSORT-type flow chart?
3. What might be some of the uses to which the findings could be put in clinical practice?

EXAMPLE 2: DISCUSSION SECTION IN THE STUDY IN APPENDIX A

1. Read the "Discussion" section of Swenson and colleagues' study ("Parents' use of praise and criticism in a sample of young children seeking mental health services") in Appendix A of this book, and then answer the relevant questions in Box 14.1.
2. Also consider the following targeted questions:
   a. Was a CONSORT-type flow chart used in this study?
   b. Can you think of any limitations that the researchers did not mention?

EXAMPLE 3: QUANTITATIVE STUDY IN APPENDIX D

Read Wilson and colleagues' study ("A randomized controlled trial of an individualized preoperative education intervention for symptom management after total knee arthroplasty") in Appendix D and then address the following suggested activities or questions.

1. Before reading our critical appraisal, which accompanies the full report, write your own critical appraisal or prepare a list of what you think are the study's major strengths and weaknesses. Pay particular attention to validity threats and bias. Then, contrast your appraisal with ours. Remember that you (or your instructor) do not necessarily have to agree with all of the points we made and you may identify strengths and weaknesses that we overlooked. You may find the broad guidelines in Table 3.1 helpful.
2. Write a short summary of how credible, important, and generalizable you find the study results to be. Your summary should conclude with your interpretation of what the results mean and what their implications are for nursing practice. Contrast your summary with the discussion section in the report itself.
3. In selecting studies to include with this textbook, we deliberately chose studies with many strengths. In the following questions, we offer some "pretend" scenarios in which the researchers for the study in Appendix D made different methodological decisions than the ones they in fact did make. Write a paragraph or two critiquing these "pretend" decisions, pointing out how these alternatives would have affected the rigor of the study and the inferences that could be made.
   a. Pretend that the researchers had been unable to randomize subjects to treatments. The design, in other words, would be a nonequivalent control group quasi-experiment.
   b. Pretend that 143 participants were randomized (this is actually what did happen), but that only 80 participants remained in the study at Time 3.

WANT TO KNOW MORE?

A wide variety of resources to enhance your learning and understanding of this chapter is available on the Point.

- Chapter Supplement on Research Biases
- Answers to the Critical Thinking Exercise for Examples 2 and 3
- Internet Resources with useful websites for Chapter 14
- A Wolters Kluwer journal article on a topic related to this chapter

Additional study aids, including eight journal articles and related questions, are also available in *Study Guide for Essentials of Nursing Research, 10e.*

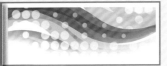

Summary Points

- The interpretation of quantitative **results** (the outcomes of the statistical analyses) typically involves consideration of (1) the credibility of the results, (2) precision of estimates of effects, (3) magnitude of effects, (4) underlying meaning, (5) generalizability, and (6) implications for nursing practice and future research.

- The particulars of the study—especially the methodological decisions made by researchers—affect the inferences that can be made about the correspondence between study results and "truth in the real world."

- A cautious outlook is appropriate in drawing conclusions about the credibility and meaning of study results.

- An assessment of a study's credibility can involve various approaches, one of which involves an evaluation of the degree of congruence between abstract constructs or idealized methods on the one hand and the proxies actually used on the other.

- Credibility assessments also involve an assessment of study rigor through an analysis of validity threats and biases that could undermine the accuracy of the results.

- Corroboration (replication) of results, through either internal or external sources, is another approach in a credibility assessment.

- Researchers can facilitate interpretations by carefully documenting methodological decisions and the outcomes of those decisions (e.g., by using the **CONSORT guidelines** to document participant flow).

- Broadly speaking, **clinical significance** refers to the practical importance of research results—i.e., whether the effects are genuine and palpable in the daily lives of patients or in the management of their health.

- Clinical significance for group-level results is often evaluated based on such statistics as effect size indexes, confidence intervals, and number needed to treat. However, clinical significance is most often discussed in terms of effects for individual patients—especially, whether they have achieved a clinically meaningful change.

- Definitions and operationalizations of clinical significance for individuals typically involve a **benchmark** or threshold to designate a meaningful amount of change. This benchmark is often called a **minimal important change (MIC)**, which is a value for the amount of **change score** points on a measure that an individual patient must achieve to be classified as having clinically meaningful change.

- MIC benchmarks can be used to ascertain whether each person in a sample has or has not achieved a change greater than the MIC, and then a **responder analysis** can be undertaken to compare the percentage of people meeting the threshold in different study groups.

- In their discussions of study results, researchers should themselves point out known study limitations, but readers should draw their own conclusions about the rigor of the study and about the plausibility of alternative explanations for the results.

REFERENCES FOR CHAPTER 14

*Evans, S., Seidman, L., Lung, K., Sternlieb, B., & Zeltzer, L. (2018). Yoga for teens with irritable bowel syndrome: Results from a mixed-methods pilot study. *Holistic Nursing Practice, 32,* 253–260.

Griggs, S., & Crawford, S. (2017). Hope, core self-evaluations, emotional well-being, health-risk behaviors, and academic performance in university freshmen. *Journal of Psychosocial Nursing and Mental Health Services, 55,* 33–42.

Jaeschke, R., Singer, J., & Guyatt, G. H. (1989). Measurement of health status. Ascertaining the minimal clinically important difference. *Controlled Clinical Trials, 10,* 407–415.

Johnson, A., Phillips, S., & Rice, M. (2020). Abnormal weight gain with fatigue and stress in early survivorship after childhood brain tumor diagnosis. *Journal for Specialists in Pediatric Nursing, xx,* yy–zz.

Lindseth, G. N., Coolahan, S., Petros, T., & Lindseth, P. (2014). Neurobehavioral effects of aspartame consumption. *Research in Nursing & Health, 37,* 185–193.

Must, A., Eliasziw, M., Phillips, S., Curtin, C., Kral, T., Segal, M., . . . Bandinit, L. (2017). The effect of age on the prevalence of obesity among US youth with autism spectrum disorder. *Childhood Obesity, 13,* 25–35.

Polit, D. F., & Yang, F. M. (2016). *Measurement and the measurement of change: A primer for health professionals.* Philadelphia, PA: Lippincott Williams & Wilkins.

Sackett, D. L., Straus, S., Richardson, W., Rosenberg, W., & Haynes, R. (2000). *Evidence-based medicine: How to practice and teach EBM* (2nd ed.). Edinburgh, United Kingdom: Churchill Livingstone.

Smith, N., Abernethy, C., Allgar, V., Foster, L., Martinson, V., & Stones, E. (2020). An open-label, randomised controlled trial on the effectiveness of the Orve + wrap® versus forced air warming in restoring normothermia in the postanaesthetic care unit. *Journal of Clinical Nursing, 29,* 1085–1093.

Tsai, S., Lee, W., Lee, C., Jeng, S., & Weng, W. (2020). Sleep in mothers of children with epilepsy and its relation to their children's sleep. *Research in Nursing & Health, 43,* 168–175.

Wargo-Sugleris, M., Robbins, W., Lane, C., & Phillips, L. (2018). Job satisfaction, work environment and successful ageing: Determinants of delaying retirement among acute care nurses. *Journal of Advanced Nursing, 74,* 900–913.

*A link to this open-access article is provided in the Internet Resources section on thePoint® website.

**This journal article is also available on thePoint® for this chapter.

15 Understanding the Analysis of Qualitative Data

Learning Objectives

On completing this chapter, you will be able to:

- Describe activities that qualitative researchers perform to manage and organize their data
- Discuss the procedures used to analyze qualitative data, including both general procedures and those used in ethnographic, phenomenological, and grounded theory, and qualitative descriptive research
- Assess the adequacy of researchers' descriptions of their analytic procedures and evaluate the suitability of those procedures
- Define new terms in the chapter

Key Terms

- Axial coding
- Basic social process (BSP)
- Central category
- Coding scheme
- Constant comparison
- Core category
- Domain
- Emergent fit
- Hermeneutic circle
- Metaphor
- Open coding
- Paradigm case
- Qualitative content analysis
- Selective coding
- Substantive codes
- Taxonomy
- Thematic analysis
- Theme
- Theoretical codes

Qualitative research data are derived from such narrative materials as transcripts of audio-taped interviews or participant observers' field notes. This chapter describes methods for analyzing such qualitative data.

INTRODUCTION TO QUALITATIVE ANALYSIS

Qualitative data analysis is challenging, for several reasons. First, there are no universal rules for analyzing qualitative data. Second, an enormous amount of work is required. Qualitative analysts must organize and make sense of hundreds of pages of narrative materials. Qualitative researchers typically scrutinize their data carefully, often reading the data over and over in a search for understanding. Also, doing qualitative analysis proficiently requires creativity and strong inductive skills (generating universals from particulars). A qualitative analyst must be adept at discerning patterns and weaving them together into an integrated whole.

Another challenge comes in reducing data for reporting purposes. Quantitative results can often be summarized in a few tables. Qualitative researchers, by contrast, must balance the need to be concise with the need to maintain the richness of their data.

TIP   Qualitative analyses are more difficult to *do* than quantitative ones, but qualitative findings are easier to understand than quantitative ones because the stories are told in everyday language. Qualitative analyses are often hard to critically appraise, however, because readers cannot know if researchers adequately captured thematic patterns in the data.

QUALITATIVE DATA MANAGEMENT AND ORGANIZATION

Qualitative analysis is supported by several tasks that help to organize and manage the mass of narrative data.

Developing a Coding Scheme

Qualitative researchers usually begin their analysis by developing a method to classify and index their data. Researchers must be able to access parts of the data, without having repeatedly to reread the data set in its entirety. The usual procedure is to create a **coding scheme**, based on actual data, and then code data according to the categories in the coding scheme. Developing a good coding scheme involves a careful reading of the data, with an eye to identifying underlying concepts.

Saldaña (2016) identified 27 different types of coding approaches that vary along several dimensions, such as amount of detail and level of abstraction. Here are some examples, with coded excerpts from a study of food insecurity in low-income families (Polit et al., 2000):

- **Descriptive coding** uses mainly nouns as codes and is often used by beginning qualitative researchers; it does not, however, provide much insight into meaning.
  - *Excerpt:* "The other day, we ran out of everything and we had to go to a church and get food."
  - *Code:* food pantry use
- **Process coding** often involves using gerunds as codes to connote action and observable activity in the data.
  - *Excerpt:* "The other day, we ran out of everything and we had to go to a church and get food"
  - *Code:* dealing with food shortages
- **Concept coding** involves using a word or phrase to represent symbolically a broad meaning beyond observable facts or behaviors; the codes are usually nouns or gerunds.
  - *Excerpt:* "The other day, we ran out of everything and we had to go to a church and get food."
  - *Code:* coping with the risk of hunger
- **In vivo coding** involves using participant-generated words and phrases; it is used as initial coding in many grounded theory studies.
  - *Excerpt:* "The other day, we <u>ran out of everything</u> and we <u>had to go to a church and get food.</u>"
  - *Codes:* ran out of everything; had to go to a church for food
- **Holistic coding** involves using codes to grasp broad ideas in large "chunks" of data rather than coding smaller segments.
  - *Excerpt:* "I buy on deals. I learned how to, you know, what to buy and what not to buy. Where to shop, where to look for sales. I'll go to all the stores. And I clip coupons from the paper and stuff. But sometimes that's not enough. The other day, we ran out of everything and we had to go to a church and get food."
  - *Code:* food management strategies

As these examples show, the same excerpt can be coded in various ways—there is no single "right" way to code data, and two people are unlikely to develop identical codes for the same data. The nature of the research question and the desired end product influence the type of codes that get created. For example, if the research question were "What is it like for poor families to experience food insecurity?" descriptive coding is unlikely to be productive, but it might be suitable if the research question were "What strategies do poor families use to manage food insecurity?" Descriptive qualitative studies are especially likely to use descriptive or process coding.

Example of a descriptive coding scheme •••••••••••••••••••••••••••••

Dykeman and colleagues (2018) used individual and focus group interviews to explore the views of community service providers regarding the implementation of older adult fall prevention interventions. The data were coded into categories of barriers to such interventions and possible implementation strategies.

Coding Qualitative Data

After a coding scheme has been developed, the data are read in their entirety and coded for correspondence to the categories. This can be a difficult task—it sometimes takes several readings of the material to grasp its nuances. Researchers often discover during coding that the initial coding scheme needs to be modified. Ideas may emerge for new codes, for example. In such a case, it would be necessary to reread all previously coded material to check if the new code should be applied.

Paragraphs from transcribed interviews often contain elements relating to three or four different codes. Figure 15.1 shows an example of a paragraph with multiple codes—this is an excerpt from Beck and Gable's (2012) study about secondary traumatic stress experienced by nurses during traumatic births.

Data Extract	Codes
"One of the most traumatic birth experiences happened a few year ago but I still remember it as though it were yesterday. A grand multipara came to labor and delivery in labor. This was her 9th pregnancy. The doctor, who I don't really get along with, treated her like a piece of dirt. He delivered the baby with no complications. He immediately put the baby in the warmer without letting the mom see or hold her baby. He then proceeded to put his hand inside of her practically halfway up his arm to start pulling her placenta out! She was yelling 'something's not right, it's never hurt like this before!' I walked away from the bed but went back to be with her because she was still screaming. I felt like I was watching a rape! I **felt so helpless**. He's one of those doctors that for whatever reason seems to get away with anything. I talked to my case manager about it and how upset I was. Nothing was ever done. I felt **so powerless**. I really **feel that I failed my patient**. She was counting on me to keep her safe. **I let her down**. To this day I **still think about it and what I could have done differently. I should have protected my patient and advocated for her, but I didn't.**"	**Felt helpless** **Felt powerless** **Feel like I failed my patient** **What could have been done differently?** **I let my patient down**

Figure 15.1 Example of a coded excerpt. From the author's records for the study reported in the following paper: Beck, C., & Gable, R. (2012). A mixed methods study of secondary traumatic stress in labor and delivery nurses. *Journal of Obstetric, Gynecologic, & Neonatal Nursing, 41,* 747–760.

Methods of Organizing Qualitative Data

Before the advent of software for qualitative data management, analysts used *conceptual files* to organize their data. This approach involves creating a physical file for each category and then cutting out and inserting all the materials relating to that code into the file. Researchers then retrieve the content on a particular topic by reviewing the applicable file folder. Creating conceptual files is cumbersome, particularly when segments of the narratives have multiple codes. For example, for the data in Figure 15.1, five copies of the paragraph, corresponding to the five codes, would be needed.

Computer-assisted qualitative data analysis software (CAQDAS) removes the work of cutting and pasting pages of narrative material. These programs permit an entire data set to be entered onto a computer and coded; text corresponding to specified codes can then be retrieved for analysis. Computer programs (e.g., NVivo) offer many advantages for managing qualitative data, but some people prefer manual methods because they allow researchers to get closer to the data. Others object to having a cognitive process turned into a technological activity. Despite concerns, many researchers have switched to computerized data management because it frees up their time and permits them to devote more attention to conceptual issues.

ANALYTIC PROCEDURES

Data *management* in qualitative research is reductionist in nature: It involves converting masses of data into smaller, more manageable segments. By contrast, qualitative data *analysis* is constructionist: It involves putting segments together into meaningful conceptual patterns. Various approaches to qualitative data analysis exist, but some elements are common to several of them.

A General Analytic Overview

The analysis of qualitative materials often begins with the identification of broad *categories*, which are clusters of codes that are connected conceptually. In Figure 15.1, which shows a coded excerpt from Beck and Gable's (2012) study of nurses' secondary traumatic stress, two of the codes ("Feel like I failed my patient" and "I let my patient down") were clustered with other codes to form the category "Failing to Protect the Patient." Ideas for categories usually begin to emerge during coding and would likely be documented in analytic memos.

In many qualitative studies, the next phase involves the identification of themes. In their review of how the term *theme* is used among qualitative researchers, DeSantis and Ugarriza (2000) offered this definition: "A **theme** is an abstract entity that brings meaning and identity to a current experience and its variant manifestations. As such, a theme captures and unifies the nature or basis of the experience into a meaningful whole" (p. 362).

The search for themes involves not only discovering commonalities across participants but also seeking variation. Themes are never universal. Researchers must attend not only to what themes arise but also to how they are patterned. Does the theme apply only to certain types of people or in certain contexts? Thus, qualitative analysts must be sensitive to patterns and relationships within the data.

 TIP Qualitative researchers often use major themes as subheadings in the Results section of their reports. For example, in their analysis of interview data for a study of practitioners' perspectives on interdisciplinary rounding practices, Beaird and colleagues (2020) identified three main themes that were used to organize their qualitative results: "setting the stage," "the work of the team," and benefits to patient care."

Researchers' search for themes and patterns in the data can sometimes be facilitated by devices that enable them to chart the evolution of behaviors and processes. For example, for qualitative studies that focus on dynamic experiences (e.g., decision making), flow charts or timelines can be used to highlight time sequences or major decision points.

Some qualitative researchers use metaphors as an analytic strategy. A **metaphor** is a symbolic comparison, using figurative language to evoke a visual analogy. Metaphors can be expressive tools for qualitative analysts, but they can run the risk of "supplanting creative insight with hackneyed cliché masquerading as profundity" (Thorne & Darbyshire, 2005, p. 1111).

Example of a metaphor •
Peet and colleagues (2019) explored the context and culture of nursing surveillance on an acute care ward using workplace observations and in-depth interviews. They offered the metaphor of nursing surveillance as "the threads that support the very fabric of acute care nursing work" (p. 2924).

In the final analysis stage, researchers strive to weave the thematic pieces into an integrated whole. The various themes are integrated to provide an overall structure (such as a theory or a taxonomy) to the data. Successful integration demands creativity and intellectual rigor.

 TIP Although relatively few qualitative researchers make formal efforts to quantify features of their data, be alert to quantitative implications when you read a qualitative report. Qualitative researchers routinely use words like "some," "most," or "many" in characterizing participants' experiences and actions, which implies some level of quantification.

Qualitative Content Analysis and Thematic Analysis

In the remainder of this section, we discuss analytic procedures used by ethnographers, phenomenologists, and grounded theory researchers. Qualitative researchers who conduct descriptive qualitative studies may, however, simply say that they performed a content analysis or a thematic analysis.

Qualitative content analysis involves analyzing the content of narrative data to identify prominent themes and patterns among the themes. Qualitative content analysis involves breaking down data into smaller *units*, coding and naming the units according to the content they represent, and grouping coded material based on shared concepts. The literature on content analysis often refers to *meaning units*. A meaning unit, essentially, is the smallest segment of a text that contains a recognizable piece of information.

Content analysts often make the distinction between manifest and latent content. *Manifest content* is what the text actually says. In purely descriptive studies, qualitative researchers may focus mainly on summarizing the manifest content communicated in the text. Often, however, content analysts also analyze what the text talks *about*, which involves interpretation of the meaning of its *latent content*. Interpretations vary in depth and level of abstraction and are usually the basis for themes.

Example of a content analysis •
Ak and colleagues (2020) did a content analysis of semi-structured interviews with 18 Muslim women regarding their sexuality after a diagnosis of gynecological cancer. Three overarching categories emerged: situations that make sexual life difficult, impact of cancer on sexual life, and coping.

Many qualitative nurse researchers use the **thematic analysis** methods suggested by Braun and Clarke (2006). In their widely cited article, these psychologists argued that thematic analysis is "an accessible and theoretically flexible approach to analysing qualitative data" (p. 77). They maintained that thematic analysis should be seen as a foundational method for qualitative analysis. Their proposed approach described several important decisions that analysts must make, such as What counts as a theme? Their step-by-step guide covers an analytic process with six phases: familiarizing oneself with the data, generating initial codes, searching for themes, reviewing themes, defining and naming themes, and producing the report.

Example of a thematic analysis ●
Sørensen and colleagues (2020) studied fear of needle injections among children with rheumatic diseases and parental communication approaches during home administration. Using thematic analysis, the researchers identified four overarching themes, each of which had several subthemes. For example, for the theme "Children's efforts to become involved," the subthemes were asking questions, suggesting coping strategies, and showing engagement.

Ethnographic Analysis

In an ethnography, analysis typically begins the moment ethnographers set foot in the field. Ethnographers are continually looking for *patterns* in the behavior and thoughts of participants, comparing one pattern against another. As they analyze patterns of everyday life, ethnographers acquire a deeper understanding of the culture being studied. Maps, flowcharts, and organizational charts are also useful tools that help to crystallize and illustrate the data being collected. Matrices (two-dimensional displays) can also help to highlight a comparison graphically and to discover emerging patterns.

Spradley's (1979) classic approach is sometimes used for ethnographic data analyses. His 12-step sequence included strategies for both data collection and data analysis. In Spradley's method, there are four levels of data analysis: *domain analysis, taxonomic analysis, componential analysis*, and *theme analysis*. **Domains** are broad categories that represent units of cultural knowledge. During this first level of analysis, ethnographers identify relational patterns among terms in the domains that are used by members of the culture. The ethnographer focuses on the cultural meaning of terms and symbols (objects and events) used in a culture and their interrelationships.

In *taxonomic analysis*, the second level in Spradley's data analytic method, ethnographers decide how many domains the analysis will encompass. After making this decision, a **taxonomy**—a system of classifying and organizing terms—is developed to illustrate the internal organization of a domain.

In *componential analysis*, multiple relationships among terms in the domains are examined. The ethnographer analyzes data for similarities and differences among cultural terms in a domain. Finally, in *theme analysis*, cultural themes are uncovered. Domains are connected in cultural themes, which help to provide a holistic view of the culture being studied. The discovery of cultural meaning is the outcome.

Example using Spradley's method ●
You and Yang (2020) explored the survival trajectory and meanings of health of married immigrant women in Korea, within Newman's Theory of Health as Expanding Consciousness. They used Spradley's method of ethnographic analysis and identified and analyzed four domains related to participants' health: spatial-temporality, relationships with family and community, coping strategies, and health resources. In the theme analysis, they analyzed how participants' consciousness changed over time.

Other approaches to ethnography have been developed. For example, in Leininger's ethnonursing method, as described in McFarland and Wehbe-Alamah (2015), ethnographers follow a four-phase data analysis guide. In the first phase, ethnographers collect, describe, and record data. The second phase involves identifying and categorizing descriptors. In phase 3, data are analyzed to discover repetitive patterns in their context. The fourth and final phase involves abstracting major themes and presenting findings.

Example using Leininger's method •
Wahid and colleagues (2019) used Leininger's four-step ethnographic framework in a study that explored the Bugis culture in Indonesia relating to feeding practices for children aged 0 to 23 months. The researchers' analysis revealed three major themes: giving sweet food, choosing a qualified person to give the first bribe, and delayed feeding of animal-sourced food.

Phenomenological Analysis

Schools of phenomenology have developed different approaches to data analysis. Three frequently used methods for descriptive phenomenology are the methods of Colaizzi (1978), Giorgi (1985), and van Kaam (1966), all of whom are from the *Duquesne School* of phenomenology, based on Husserl's philosophy.

The basic outcome of all three methods is the description of the essential nature of an experience, often through the identification of essential themes. Some important differences among these three approaches exist. Colaizzi's (1978) method, for example, is the only one that calls for a validation of results by querying study participants. Giorgi's (1985) view is that it is inappropriate either to return to participants to validate findings or to use external judges to review the analysis. Van Kaam's (1966) method requires that intersubjective agreement be reached with other expert judges. Figure 15.2 provides an illustration of the steps involved in Colaizzi's data analysis approach.

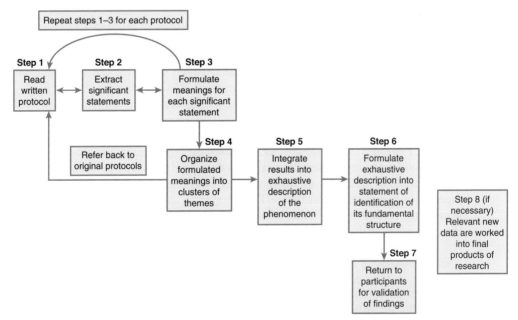

Figure 15.2 Colaizzi's procedural steps in phenomenological data analysis. (Reprinted with permission from Beck, C. T. [2009]. The arm: There is no escaping the reality for mothers of children with obstetric brachial plexus injuries. *Nursing Research, 58,* 237–245.)

Example of a study using Colaizzi's method •
İnan and Üstün (2020) explored the nature of posttraumatic growth in Turkish breast cancer survivors in the first 2 years after treatment. The data from in-depth interviews with 13 breast cancer survivors were analyzed using Colaizzi's (1978) method. Each transcript was read several times and significant statements were extracted and then formulated meanings were identified. Two main themes emerged: making sense of cancer and positive restoring.

Phenomenologists from the *Utrecht School*, such as van Manen (1997), combine characteristics of descriptive and interpretive phenomenology. According to van Manen, thematic aspects of experience can be uncovered from participants' descriptions of the experience by three methods: the holistic, selective, or detailed approach. In the *holistic approach*, researchers view the text as a whole and try to capture its meanings. In the *selective* (or highlighting) *approach*, researchers pull out statements that seem essential to the experience under study. In the *detailed* (or line-by-line) *approach*, researchers analyze every sentence. Once themes have been identified, they become the objects of interpretation through follow-up interviews with participants. Through this process, essential themes are discovered.

Example of a study using van Manen's method •
Olano-Lizarraga and colleagues (2020) provided a thorough description of their use of van Manen's (1997) methods in their study of redefining a "new normality" in patients with chronic heart failure. Examples of holistic, selective, and detailed analyses were provided in the report.

In addition to identifying themes from participants' descriptions, van Manen (1997) also called for gleaning thematic descriptions from artistic sources. Van Manen urged qualitative researchers to keep in mind that literature, painting, and other art forms can provide rich experiential data that can increase insights into the essential meaning of the experience being studied.

A third school of phenomenology is an interpretive approach called Heideggerian hermeneutics. Central to analyzing data in a hermeneutic study is the notion of the **hermeneutic circle**. The circle signifies a methodological process in which, to reach understanding, there is continual movement between the parts and the whole of the text being analyzed.

Benner (1994) offered an analytic approach for hermeneutic analysis that involves three interrelated processes: the search for paradigm cases, thematic analysis, and analysis of exemplars. **Paradigm cases** are "strong instances of concerns or ways of being in the world" (Benner, 1994, p. 113). Paradigm cases are used early in the analytic process as a strategy for gaining understanding. Thematic analysis is done to compare and contrast similarities across cases. Paradigm cases and thematic analysis can be enhanced by *exemplars* that illuminate aspects of a paradigm case or theme. Paradigm cases and exemplars presented in research reports allow readers to play a role in consensual validation of the results by deciding whether the cases support the researchers' conclusions.

Example using Benner's hermeneutical analysis •
Benner and her colleagues (2018) used her own approach in a hermeneutic study that focused on understanding posttraumatic stress disorder in the context of war experience. Nurses who provided care for soldiers injured in the Iraq and Afghanistan wars and 67 wounded servicemen were interviewed. One paradigm case involved a soldier recovering from extreme trauma after being blown up in the air.

Grounded Theory Analysis

Grounded theory methods emerged in the 1960s when two sociologists, Glaser and Strauss, were studying dying in hospitals (Glaser & Strauss, 1967). The two co-originators eventually split and developed divergent approaches. A third analytic approach by Charmaz (2014), constructivist grounded theory, has also emerged.

Glaser's Grounded Theory Method

Grounded theory in all three analytic systems uses **constant comparison,** a method that involves comparing elements present in one data source (e.g., in one interview) with those in another. The process continues until the content of all sources has been compared so that commonalities are identified. The concept of "fit" is an important element in Glaserian grounded theory analysis. *Fit* has to do with how closely the emerging concepts fit with the incidents they are representing—which depends on how thoroughly constant comparison was done.

Coding in the Glaserian approach is used to conceptualize data into patterns. Coding helps the researcher to discover the basic problem with which participants must contend. The substance of the topic under study is conceptualized through **substantive codes,** of which there are two types: open and selective. **Open coding,** used in the first stage of constant comparison, captures what is going on in the data. Open codes may be the actual words participants used. There are three levels of open coding that vary in degree of abstraction. *Level I codes* (or *in vivo codes*) are derived directly from the language of the substantive area. They have vivid imagery and "grab." Table 15.1 presents five level I codes and illustrative interview excerpts from Beck's (2002) grounded theory study on mothering twins.

TABLE 15.1 Collapsing Level I Codes Into the Level II Code of "Reaping the Blessings" (Beck, 2002)

Excerpt	Level I Code
I enjoy just watching the twins interact so much. Especially now that they are mobile. They are not walking yet but they are crawling. I will tell you they are already playing. Like one will go around the corner and kind of peek around and they play hide and seek. They crawl after each other.	Enjoying twins
With twins it's amazing. She was sick and she had a fever. He was the one acting sick. She didn't seem like she was sick at all. He was. We watched him for like 6 to 8 hours. We gave her the medicine and he started calming down. Like WOW! That is so weird. 'Cause you read about it but it's like, Oh come on! It's really neat to see.	Amazing
These days it's really neat 'cause you go to the store or you go out and people are like, "Oh, they are twins, how nice." And I say, "Yeah they are. Look, look at my kids."	Getting attention
I just feel blessed to have two. I just feel like I am twice as lucky as a mom who has one baby. I mean that's the best part. It's just that instead of having one baby to watch grow and change and develop and become a toddler and school-age child, you have two.	Feeling blessed
It's very exciting. It's interesting and it's fun to see them and how the twin bond really is. There really is a twin bond. You read about it and you hear about it, but until you experience it, you just don't understand. One time they were both crying and they were fed. They were changed and burped. There was nothing wrong. I couldn't figure out what was wrong. So I said to myself, "I am just going to put them together and close the door." I put them in my bed together, and they patty-caked their hands and put their noses together and just looked at each other and went right to sleep.	Twin bonding

From the author's records for the study reported in the following paper: Beck, C. T. (2002). Releasing the pause button: Mothering twins during the first year of life. *Qualitative Health Research, 12,* 593–608.

As researchers constantly compare new level I codes with previously identified ones, they condense them into broader *level II codes*. For example, in Table 15.1, Beck's (2002) five level I codes were collapsed into a single level II code, "Reaping the Blessings." *Level III codes* (or theoretical constructs) are the most abstract. Collapsing level II codes aids in identifying constructs.

    TIP   Additional material relating to Beck's (2002) twin study is presented in the supplement to this chapter on thePoint® website.

Open coding ends when the core category is discovered and then selective coding begins. The **core category** (or *core variable*) is a pattern of behavior that is relevant and/or problematic for study participants. In **selective coding**, researchers code only those data that are related to the core category. One kind of core category is a **basic social process (BSP)** that evolves over time in two or more phases. All BSPs are core categories, but some core categories are not BSPs.

Glaser (1978) provided criteria to help researchers decide on a core category. Here are a few examples: It must be central, meaning that it is related to many categories; it must reoccur frequently in the data; it relates meaningfully and easily to other categories; and it has clear and grabbing implications for formal theory.

Theoretical codes provide insights into how substantive codes relate to each other. Theoretical codes help grounded theorists to weave the broken pieces of data back together again. Glaser (1978) proposed 18 families of theoretical codes that researchers can use to conceptualize how substantive codes relate to each other (although he subsequently expanded possibilities in 2005). Four examples of his families of theoretical codes include the following:

- Process: stages, phases, passages, transitions
- Strategy: tactics, techniques, maneuverings
- Cutting point: boundaries, critical junctures, turning points
- The six C's: causes, contexts, contingencies, consequences, covariances, and conditions

Throughout coding and analysis, grounded theory analysts document their ideas about the data and emerging conceptual scheme in *memos*. Memos encourage researchers to reflect on and describe patterns in the data, relationships between categories, and emergent conceptualizations.

The product of a typical Glaserian grounded theory analysis is a theoretical model that endeavors to explain a pattern of behavior that is relevant for study participants. Once the basic problem emerges, the grounded theorist goes on to discover the process these participants experience in coping with or resolving this problem.

Example of a Glaserian grounded theory analysis •
Figure 15.3 presents Beck's (2002) model from a study in which "Releasing the Pause Button" was conceptualized as the core category and process through which mothers of twins progressed as they tried to resume their lives after giving birth. The process involves four phases: Draining Power, Pausing own Life, Striving to Reset, and Resuming Own Life. Beck used 10 coding families in her theoretical coding for the study. The family *cutting point* offers an illustration. Three months seemed to be a turning point for mothers, when life started to be more manageable. Here is an excerpt from an interview that Beck coded as a cutting point: "Three months came around and the twins sort of slept through the night and it made a huge, huge difference."

Glaser cautioned against consulting the literature before a framework is stabilized, but he also saw the benefit of scrutinizing other work. Glaser (1978) discussed the evolution of grounded theories through the process of **emergent fit** to prevent individual substantive theories from being "respected little islands of knowledge" (p. 148). As he noted, generating

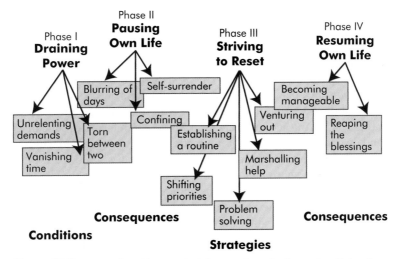

Figure 15.3   Beck's (2002) grounded theory of mothering twins: Releasing the Pause Button. (Reprinted with permission from Beck, C. T. [2002]. Releasing the pause button: Mothering twins during the first year of life. *Qualitative Health Research, 12*, 593–608.)

grounded theory does not necessarily require discovering all new categories or ignoring ones previously identified in the literature. Through constant comparison, researchers can compare concepts emerging from the data with similar concepts from existing theory or research to evaluate which parts have emergent fit with the theory being generated.

Strauss and Corbin's Approach

The Strauss and Corbin approach to grounded theory analysis, most recently described in Corbin and Strauss (2015), differs from the original Glaser and Strauss method with regard to method, processes, and outcomes. Table 15.2 summarizes major analytic differences between the Glaser, Corbin and Strauss, and Charmaz grounded theory analysis methods.

Glaser (1978) stressed that to generate a grounded theory, the basic problem must emerge from the data—it must be discovered. The theory is, from the very start, grounded

TABLE 15.2 Comparison of Alternative Grounded Theory Approaches

	Glaser	Corbin and Strauss	Charmaz
Initial data analysis	Breaking down and conceptualizing data, with comparisons so that patterns emerge	Breaking down and conceptualizing data, which includes taking apart a single sentence, observation, or incident	Creating link between collecting data and developing emergent theory; defining what is occurring in data and beginning to analyze what it means
Types of coding	Open, selective, theoretical	Open, axial	Initial, focused
Connections between categories: strategies	18 coding families plus theoretical codes from different disciplines	Paradigm (conditions, actions–interactions, and consequences or outcomes) and the conditional/consequential matrix	Analytic strategies are emergent rather than procedural application; categories, subcategories, and links
Outcome	Emergent theory (discovery)	Conceptual description (verification)	An interpretive theory constructed through researcher's past and present involvement with persons, perspectives, and research practices.

in the data rather than starting with a preconceived problem. Strauss and Corbin, however, argued that the research itself is only one of four possible sources of a research problem. Research problems can, for example, come from the literature or a researcher's personal and professional experience.

The Corbin and Strauss (2015) method involves two types of coding: open and axial coding. In *open coding*, data are broken down into parts and concepts identified for interpreted meaning of the raw data. In **axial coding**, the analyst codes for context. Here, the analyst is "locating and linking action-interaction within a framework of subconcepts that give it meaning and enable it to explain what interactions are occurring, and why and what consequences real or anticipated are happening" (Corbin & Strauss, 2015, p. 156). The *paradigm* is used as an analytic strategy to help integrate structure and process. The basic components of the paradigm include conditions, actions–interactions, and consequences or outcomes. Corbin and Strauss suggested the conditional/consequential matrix as an analytic strategy for considering the range of possible conditions and consequences that can enter into the context.

The first step in integrating the findings is to decide on the **central category** (sometimes called the *core category*), which is the main construct in the research. The outcome of the Corbin and Strauss approach is a full conceptual description. The original grounded theory method, by contrast, generates a theory that explains how a basic social problem that emerged from the data is processed in a social setting.

Example of Strauss and Corbin grounded theory analysis • • • • • • • • • • • • • • •
Nasu and colleagues (2020) investigated the end-of-life nursing care practice process in long-term care settings for older adults in Japan. Data from interviews with 22 nurses from eight long-term care settings were analyzed using Corbin and Strauss's (2015) approach. The researchers provided an excellent description of their analytic process in a table that identified the analytic stage, the methods used, which researcher was involved in that stage, and examples of the outcomes of that stage. Their core category was "Guiding the rebuilt care community to assist the dying resident."

Constructivist Grounded Theory Approach

The constructivist approach to grounded theory is in some ways similar to Glaserian methods. According to Charmaz (2014), in constructivist grounded theory, the "coding generates the bones of your analysis. Theoretical integration will assemble these bones into a working skeleton" (p. 113). Charmaz offered guidelines for different types of coding: word-by-word coding, line-by-line coding, and incident-to-incident coding. Unlike Glaser's grounded theory approach in which theory is discovered from data separate from the researcher, Charmaz's position is that researchers construct grounded theories by means of their past and current involvements and interactions with individuals and research practices.

Charmaz (2014) distinguished *initial coding* and *focused coding*. In initial coding, the pieces of data (e.g., words, lines, segments, incidents) are studied so the researcher can learn what the participants view as problematic. In focused coding, the analysis is directed toward identifying the most significant initial codes, which are then theoretically coded.

Example of constructivist grounded theory analysis • • • • • • • • • • • • • • • • • • •
Hultstrand and colleagues (2020) used constructivist methods to develop a grounded theory about cancer patients' presentation of bodily sensations in primary care encounters. They discovered a core category that they called *negotiation bodily sensations to legitimize access*, relying primarily on observational data. Their article provided examples of their coding scheme and their approach to analysis.

TIP Grounded theory researchers often present conceptual maps or models to summarize their results, such as the one in Figure 15.3, especially when the central phenomenon is a dynamic or evolving process.

CRITICAL APPRAISAL OF QUALITATIVE ANALYSIS

Evaluating a qualitative analysis is not easy to do. Readers do not have access to the information they would need to assess whether researchers exercised good judgment and critical insight in coding and interpreting the narrative materials, developing a thematic analysis, and integrating materials into a meaningful whole. Researchers are seldom able to include more than a handful of examples of actual data in a journal article. Moreover, the process they used to inductively abstract meaning from the data is difficult to describe and illustrate.

In a critical appraisal of qualitative analyses, one focus should be on whether the researchers adequately documented the analytic process and explained their approach. For example, a report for a grounded theory study should indicate whether the researchers used the Glaser, Corbin and Strauss, or constructivist method.

Another aspect of a qualitative analysis that can be appraised is whether the researchers have documented that they used one approach consistently and were faithful to the integrity of its procedures. Thus, for example, if researchers say they are using the Glaserian approach to grounded theory analysis, they should not also include elements from the Strauss and Corbin method. An even more serious problem occurs when, as sometimes happens, the researchers "muddle" traditions. For example, researchers who describe their study as a grounded theory study should not present *themes* because grounded theory analysis does not yield themes. Researchers who attempt to blend elements from two traditions may not have a clear grasp of the analytic precepts of either one.

Some further guidelines that may be helpful in evaluating qualitative analyses are presented in Box 15.1.

Box 15.1 Guidelines for Critically Appraising Qualitative Analyses

1. Was the data analysis approach appropriate for the research design or tradition?
2. Was the coding scheme described? If so, does the scheme appear logical and complete?
3. Did the report adequately describe the process by which the actual analysis was performed? Did the report indicate whose approach to data analysis was used (e.g., that of Glaser, Corbin and Strauss, or Charmaz in grounded theory studies)?
4. What major themes or processes emerged? Were relevant excerpts from the data provided, and do the themes or categories appear to capture the meaning of the narratives? Is the analysis parsimonious—could two or more themes be collapsed into a broader and perhaps more useful conceptualization?
5. Was a conceptual map, model, or diagram effectively displayed to communicate important processes?
6. Was the context of the phenomenon adequately described? Did the report give you a clear picture of the social or emotional world of study participants?
7. Did the analysis yield a meaningful and insightful picture of the phenomenon under study? Is the resulting theory or description trivial or obvious?

RESEARCH EXAMPLES WITH CRITICAL THINKING EXERCISES

This section describes the analytic procedures used in a qualitative study. Read the summary and then answer the critical thinking questions that follow, referring to the full research report if necessary. Answers to the questions for Exercise 1 are available to instructors on thePoint®. The critical thinking questions for Exercises 2 and 3 are based on studies that appear in their entirety in Appendices B and C of this book. Our comments for these exercises are in the Student Resources section on thePoint®.

EXAMPLE 1: A CONSTRUCTIVIST GROUNDED THEORY ANALYSIS

Study: Protecting: A grounded theory study of younger children's experiences of coping with maternal cancer (Furlong, 2017)

Statement of Purpose: The purpose of this study was to develop a theory of children's day-to-day struggles living with their mothers who had been diagnosed with early-stage breast cancer and were receiving cancer treatment.

Method: This study used classic (Glaserian) grounded theory methods. The researcher collected data through in-depth interviews with 28 7- to 11-year-old children (14 boys and 14 girls) whose mothers had been diagnosed with breast cancer in the previous 4 months. The interviews, which lasted between 25 and 55 minutes, were conducted in the children's homes. The children were asked to describe their experience of having a mother with breast cancer. An interview guide was used but was continually revised as the ongoing analysis identified additional threads of inquiry. Sampling and data collection continued until theoretical saturation was achieved.

Analysis: The data for the study included interview transcripts, field notes, and memos that documented the researcher's analytic insights. Data were analyzed using constant comparison: "data, codes, and categories were compared with each other on an ongoing basis throughout data collection and analysis" (p. 15). NVivo was used for the storage and organization of the data. The analysis began with line-by-line open coding and then the open codes were used to generate categories that were collapsed and refined. Relationships among the categories were also identified. Theoretical coding was performed based on memos that had been written throughout the analysis.

Key Findings: The children's main concern was navigating through the uncertainties in their lives and navigating complex changes. "Protecting" accounted for how these children problematized their experiences living with mothers with early-stage breast cancer. The children used the strategy of protecting (the core category), which mediated three cyclical and iterative processes, which were labeled *shifting normality, shielding,* and *transitioning*. The researcher stated that *protecting* met the criteria for a core category "in that it constantly recurred in the data" and had "the most explanatory power to integrate all other categories" (p. 15). Furlong's conceptual map for the theory of protecting is shown in the supplement to this chapter on thePoint®.

Critical Thinking Exercises

1. Answer the relevant questions from Box 15.1 regarding this study.
2. In her discussion, the author made the following statement: ". . . because few studies have explored the children's experiences during the actual period of when their mothers are receiving treatment, these findings provide new understanding from which to develop hypotheses to test interventions aimed at facilitating healthcare professionals, parents, and children to help them cope and adapt to chronic illness in a parent." Can you develop a hypothesis based on the study results?
3. What might be some of the uses to which the findings could be put in clinical practice?

EXAMPLE 2: A PHENOMENOLOGICAL ANALYSIS IN APPENDIX B

1. Read the method and results sections from Beck and Watson's phenomenological study ("Posttraumatic growth after birth trauma") in Appendix B of this book and then answer the relevant questions from Box 15.1 regarding this study.
2. Also, comment on the amount of data that had to be analyzed in this study. Do you think saturation was achieved?

EXAMPLE 3: A QUALITATIVE ANALYSIS IN APPENDIX C

Read the Method and Results sections for phase II (the qualitative strand) for Bail et al.'s mixed method study ("Cancer-related symptoms and cognitive intervention adherence among breast-cancer survivors") in Appendix C of this book. Then, answer the following questions:

1. Did the researchers explain their coding process?
2. Was computer software used in the analysis?
3. What type of product (e.g., a taxonomy, themes, theory) resulted from the analysis?
4. Did the report incorporate verbatim quotes from study participants to support their analysis and interpretation?

WANT TO KNOW MORE?

A wide variety of resources to enhance your learning and understanding of this chapter is available on thePoint.

- Chapter Supplement on a Glaserian Grounded Theory Study: Illustrative Materials
- Answer to the Critical Thinking Exercise for Examples 2 and 3
- Internet Resources with useful websites for Chapter 15
- A Wolters Kluwer journal article on a topic related to this chapter

Additional study aids, including eight journal articles and related questions, are also available in *Study Guide for Essentials of Nursing Research, 10e.*

Summary Points

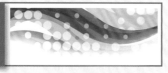

- Qualitative analysis is a challenging, labor-intensive activity, with few fixed rules.

- Qualitative analysis usually begins with efforts to understand and manage the mass of narrative data by developing a **coding scheme**. Analysts use *codes* to identify an interesting, salient, or essential feature of the data in relation to the central phenomenon. Data segments can be coded in different ways, depending on research goals.

- Traditionally, researchers organized their data by developing *conceptual files*, which are physical files into which coded excerpts of data for specific codes are placed. Now, however, computer software (CAQDAS) is widely used to perform basic indexing functions and to facilitate data analysis.

- The analysis of qualitative data often involves a search for broad **categories**, which are clusters of codes that are connected conceptually. In many qualitative studies, the next phase involves the identification of themes. A **theme**, which often cuts across several categories, is a recurring regularity that captures meaningful patterns in the data. Identifying themes involves the discovery not only of commonalities across participants but also of natural variation and patterns in the data.

- Researchers whose goal is qualitative description often say they used **qualitative content analysis**. Content analysis can vary in terms of an emphasis on *manifest content* or *latent content*. **Thematic analysis** is another broad approach to extracting themes from descriptive qualitative data.

- In ethnographies, analysis begins as the researcher enters the field. One analytic approach is Spradley's method, which involves four levels of analysis: *domain analysis* (identifying **domains**, or units of cultural knowledge), *taxonomic analysis* (selecting key domains and constructing **taxonomies**), *componential analysis* (comparing and contrasting terms in a domain), and a *theme analysis* (to uncover cultural themes).

- There are numerous approaches to phenomenological analysis, including the descriptive methods of Colaizzi, Giorgi, and van Kaam, in which the goal is to find common patterns of experiences shared by particular instances.

- In van Manen's approach, which involves efforts to grasp the essential meaning of the experience being studied, researchers search for themes, using either a *holistic approach* (viewing text as a whole), a *selective approach* (pulling out key statements and phrases), or a *detailed approach* (analyzing every sentence).

- Central to analyzing data in a hermeneutic study is the notion of the **hermeneutic circle**, which signifies a process in which there is continual movement between the parts and the whole of the text under analysis.

- Benner's approach consists of three processes: searching for **paradigm cases**, thematic analysis, and the analysis of *exemplars*.

- Grounded theorists use the **constant comparative** method of data analysis, a method that involves comparing elements present in one data source (e.g., in one interview) with those in another. *Fit* has to do with how closely concepts fit with incidents they represent, which is related to how thoroughly constant comparison was done.

- One grounded theory approach is the Glaser and Strauss method, in which there are two broad types of codes: **substantive codes** (in which the empirical substance of the topic is conceptualized) and **theoretical codes** (in which the relationships among the substantive codes are conceptualized).

- Substantive coding involves **open coding** to capture what is going on in the data, and then **selective coding**, in which only variables relating to a core category are coded. The **core category**, a behavior pattern that has relevance for participants, is sometimes a **basic social process (BSP)** that involves a process of coping or adaptation.

In the Glaserian method, open codes begin with *level I (in vivo) codes*, which are collapsed into a higher level of abstraction in *level II codes*. Level II codes are then used to formulate *level III codes*, which are theoretical constructs. Through constant comparison, researchers compare concepts emerging from the data with similar concepts from existing theory or research to see which parts have **emergent fit** with the theory being generated.

Corbin and Strauss's method is an alternative grounded theory method whose outcome is a full conceptual description. This approach to grounded theory analysis involves two types of coding: open coding (in which categories are generated) and **axial coding** (where categories are linked with subcategories and integrated).

In Charmaz's constructivist grounded theory, coding can be word-by-word, line-by-line, or incident-by-incident. Initial coding leads to *focused coding*, which is then followed by theoretical coding.

REFERENCES FOR CHAPTER 15

Ak, P., Günüşen, N., Türkcü, S., & Őzkan, S. (2020). Sexuality in Muslim women with gynecological cancer. *Cancer Nursing, 43*, E47–E53.

Beaird, G., Baernholdt, M., & White, K. (2020). Perceptions of interdisciplinary rounding practices. *Journal of Clinical Nursing, 29*, 1141–1150.

Beck, C. T. (2002). Releasing the pause button: Mothering twins during the first year of life. *Qualitative Health Research, 12*, 593–608.

Beck, C. T. (2009). The arm: There is no escaping the reality for mothers of children with obstetric brachial plexus injuries. *Nursing Research, 58*, 237–245.

Beck, C. T., & Gable, R. (2012). A mixed methods study of secondary traumatic stress in labor and delivery nurses. *Journal of Obstetric, Gynecologic, and Neonatal Nursing, 41*, 747–760.

Benner, P. (1994). The tradition and skill of interpretive phenomenology in studying health, illness, and caring practices. In P. Benner (Ed.), *Interpretive phenomenology: Embodiment, caring, and ethics in health and illness* (pp. 99–127). Thousand Oaks, CA: Sage.

Benner, P., Halpern, J., Gordon, D., Popell, C., & Kelley, P. (2018). Beyond pathologizing harm: Understanding PTSD in the context of war experience. *The Journal of Medical Humanities, 39*, 45–72.

Braun, V., & Clarke, V. (2006). Using thematic analysis in psychology. *Qualitative Research in Psychology, 3*, 77–101.

Charmaz, K. (2014). *Constructing grounded theory* (2nd ed.). Thousand Oaks, CA: Sage.

Colaizzi, P. (1978). Psychological research as the phenomenologist views it. In R. Valle & M. King (Eds.), *Existential-phenomenological alternatives for psychology* (pp. 48–71). New York, NY: Oxford University Press.

Corbin, J., & Strauss, A. (2015). *Basics of qualitative research: Techniques and procedures for developing grounded theory* (4th ed.). Thousand Oaks, CA: Sage.

DeSantis, L., & Ugarriza, D. N. (2000). The concept of theme as used in qualitative nursing research. *Western Journal of Nursing Research, 22*, 351–372.

*Dykeman, C., Markle-Reid, M., Boratto, L., Bowes, C., Gagné, H., McGugan, J., & Orr-Shaw, S. (2018). Community service provider perceptions of implementing older adult fall prevention in Ontario, Canada: A qualitative study. *BMC Geriatrics, 18*, 34.

**Furlong, E. P. (2017). Protecting: A grounded theory study of younger children's experiences of coping with maternal cancer. *Cancer Nursing, 40*, 13–21.

Giorgi, A. (1985). *Phenomenology and psychological research*. Pittsburgh, PA: Duquesne University Press.

Glaser, B. G. (1978). *Theoretical sensitivity: Advances in the methodology of grounded theory*. Mill Valley, CA: Sociology Press.

Glaser, B. G. (2005). *The grounded theory perspective III: Theoretical coding*. Mill Valley, CA: Sociology Press.

Glaser, B. G., & Strauss, A. (1967). *The discovery of grounded theory: Strategies for qualitative research*. New York, NY: Aldine de Gruyter.

*Hultstrand, C., Coe, A., Lilja, M., & Hajdarevic, S. (2020). Negotiating bodily sensations between patients and GPs in the context of standardized cancer patient pathways: An observational study in primary care. *BMC Health Services Research, 20*, 46.

*İnan, F., & Üstün, B. (2020). Post-traumatic growth in the early survival phase: From Turkish breast cancer survivors' perspective. *European Journal of Breast Health, 16*, 66–71.

McFarland, M. R., & Wehbe-Alamah, H. B. (2015). *Leininger's culture care diversity and universality: A worldwide nursing theory* (3rd ed.). Burlington, MA: Jones & Bartlett Learning.

Nasu, K., Sato, K., & Fukahori, H. (2020). Rebuilding and guiding a care community: A grounded theory of end-of-life nursing care practice in long-term care settings. *Journal of Advanced Nursing, 76*, 1009–1018.

Olano-Lizarraga, M., Zaragoza-Salcedo, A., Martín-Martín, J., & Saracíbar-Razquin, M. (2020). Redefining a new normality: A hermeneutic phenomenological study of the experiences of patients with chronic heart failure. *Journal of Advanced Nursing, 76*, 275–286.

Peet, J., Theobald, K., & Douglas, C. (2019). Strengthening nursing surveillance in general wards: A practice development approach. *Journal of Clinical Nursing, 28*, 2924–2933.

Polit, D. F., London, A., & Martinez, J. (2000). *Food insecurity and hunger in poor, mother-headed families in four U.S. cities*. New York, NY: Manpower Demonstration Research.

Saldaña, J. (2016). *The coding manual for qualitative researchers* (3rd ed.). Thousand Oaks, CA: Sage.

*Sørensen, K., Skibekk, H., Kvarstein, G., & Wøien, H. (2020). Children's fear of needle injections: A qualitative study of training sessions for children with rheumatic diseases before home administration. *Pediatric Rheumatology, 18*, 13.

Spradley, J. P. (1979). *The ethnographic interview*. New York, NY: Holt, Rinehart, and Winston.

Thorne, S., & Darbyshire, P. (2005). Land mines in the field: A modest proposal for improving the craft of qualitative health research. *Qualitative Health Research*, *15*, 1105–1113.

Van Kaam, A. (1966). *Existential foundations of psychology*. Pittsburgh, PA: Duquesne University Press.

Van Manen, M. (1997). *Researching lived experience* (2nd ed.). Ontario, Canada: The Althouse Press.

Wahid, N., Wanda, D., & Hayati, H. (2019). An ethnographic study on feeding Bugis children aged 0-23 months in Palopo, South Sulawesi, Indonesia. *Comprehensive Child and Adolescent Nursing*, *42*, 234–244.

You, K., & Yang, J. (2020). Health as expanding consciousness: Survival trajectory of married immigrant women in Korea. *Applied Nursing Research*, *51*, 151–230.

*A link to this open-access article is provided in the Internet Resources section on thePoint® website.

**This journal article is available on thePoint® for this chapter.

16 Appraising Trustworthiness and Integrity in Qualitative Research

Learning Objectives

On completing this chapter, you will be able to:

- Discuss some controversies relating to the issue of quality and integrity in qualitative research
- Identify the criteria proposed in a major framework for evaluating quality in qualitative research
- Discuss strategies for enhancing quality in qualitative research
- Describe different dimensions relating to the interpretation of qualitative results
- Define new terms in the chapter

Key Terms

- Audit trail
- Authenticity
- Confirmability
- Credibility
- Data triangulation
- Dependability
- Disconfirming cases
- Inquiry audit
- Investigator triangulation
- Member check
- Method triangulation
- Negative case analysis
- Peer debriefing
- Persistent observation
- Prolonged engagement
- Reflexivity
- Researcher credibility
- Thick description
- Transferability
- Triangulation
- Trustworthiness

Integrity in qualitative research is a critical issue for both those doing the research and those considering the use of qualitative evidence.

PERSPECTIVES ON QUALITY IN QUALITATIVE RESEARCH

Qualitative researchers agree on the importance of doing high-quality research, yet defining "high quality" has been controversial. We offer a brief overview of the arguments of the debate.

Debates About Rigor and Validity

One controversial issue concerns use of the terms *rigor* and *validity*—terms some people avoid because they are associated with the positivist paradigm. For these critics, the concept of rigor is by its nature a term that does not fit into an interpretive paradigm that values insight and creativity.

Others disagree with those opposing these terms. Morse (2015), for example, has argued that qualitative researchers should return to the terminology of the social sciences—i.e., rigor, reliability, validity, and generalizability.

This debate has given rise to several positions. At one extreme are those who think that validity is an appropriate quality criterion in both qualitative and quantitative studies, although qualitative researchers use different methods to achieve it. At the opposite extreme are those who berate the "absurdity" of validity. A widely adopted stance is what has been called a *parallel perspective*. This position was proposed by Lincoln and Guba (1985), who created standards for the **trustworthiness** of qualitative research that parallel the quality standards in quantitative research.

Generic Versus Specific Standards

Another controversy concerns whether there should be a generic set of quality standards, or whether specific standards are needed for different qualitative traditions. Some writers believe that research conducted within different disciplinary traditions must attend to different concerns and that techniques for enhancing integrity vary. Thus, different writers have offered standards for specific forms of qualitative inquiry, such as grounded theory, phenomenology, ethnography, and critical research. Some writers believe, however, that some quality criteria are fairly universal within the constructivist paradigm. For example, Whittemore and colleagues (2001) prepared a synthesis of criteria that they viewed as essential to all qualitative inquiry.

Terminology Proliferation and Confusion

The result of these controversies is that there is no common vocabulary for quality criteria in qualitative research. Terms such as *truth value*, *goodness*, *integrity*, and *trustworthiness* abound, but each proposed term has been refuted by some critics. With regard to actual *criteria* for evaluating quality in qualitative research, dozens have been suggested. Establishing a consensus on what the quality criteria should be, and what they should be named, remains elusive.

Given the lack of consensus, and the heated arguments supporting and contesting various frameworks, it is challenging to provide guidance about quality standards. We present information about *criteria* from the Lincoln and Guba (1985) framework in the next section. (Criteria from another framework are described in the supplement to this chapter on thePoint® website). We then describe *strategies* that researchers use to strengthen integrity in qualitative research. These strategies should provide guidance for considering whether a qualitative study is sufficiently rigorous/trustworthy/valid.

LINCOLN AND GUBA'S QUALITY CRITERIA

Although not without critics, the criteria often viewed as the "gold standard" for qualitative research are those outlined by Lincoln and Guba (1985). These researchers suggested four criteria for enhancing the trustworthiness of a qualitative inquiry: credibility, dependability, confirmability, and transferability. These criteria represent parallels to the positivists' criteria of internal validity, reliability, objectivity, and external validity, respectively. In later writings, responding to critics and to their own evolving views, a fifth criterion more distinctively aligned with the constructivist paradigm was added: authenticity (Guba & Lincoln, 1994).

Credibility

Credibility refers to confidence in the truth value of the data and interpretations of them. Qualitative researchers must strive to establish confidence in the truth of the findings.

Lincoln and Guba (1985) pointed out that credibility involves two aspects: first, carrying out the study in a way that enhances the believability of the findings, and second, taking steps to *demonstrate* credibility to external readers. Credibility is a crucial criterion in qualitative research that has been proposed in several quality frameworks.

Dependability

Dependability refers to the stability (reliability) of data over time and over conditions. The dependability question is Would the study findings be repeated if the inquiry were replicated with the same (or similar) participants in the same (or similar) context? Credibility cannot be attained in the absence of dependability, just as validity in quantitative research cannot be achieved in the absence of reliability.

Confirmability

Confirmability refers to objectivity—the potential for congruence between two or more independent people about the data's accuracy, relevance, or meaning. This criterion is concerned with establishing that the data represent the information participants provided and that the interpretations of those data are not imagined by the inquirer. For this criterion to be achieved, the findings must reflect the participants' voice and the conditions of the inquiry, and not the researcher's biases.

Transferability

Transferability, analogous to generalizability, is the extent to which qualitative findings have applicability in other settings or groups. Lincoln and Guba (1985) noted that the investigator's responsibility is to provide sufficient descriptive data that readers can evaluate the relevance of the data to other contexts: "Thus the naturalist cannot specify the external validity of an inquiry; he or she can provide only the thick description necessary to enable someone interested in making a transfer to reach a conclusion about whether transfer can be contemplated as a possibility" (p. 316).

Authenticity

Authenticity emerges in a report when it conveys the feeling tone of participants' lives as they are lived. A text has authenticity if it invites readers into a vicarious experience of the lives being described and enables readers to develop a heightened sensitivity to the issues being depicted. When a text achieves authenticity, readers are better able to understand the lives being portrayed "in the round," with some sense of the mood, experience, language, and context of those lives.

STRATEGIES TO ENHANCE QUALITY IN QUALITATIVE INQUIRY

This section describes some strategies that qualitative researchers use to establish trustworthiness in their studies. We hope this description will prompt you to carefully assess the steps researchers did or did not take to enhance quality.

We have not organized strategies according to the five criteria just described (e.g., strategies researchers use to enhance *credibility*) because many strategies simultaneously address multiple criteria. Instead, we have organized strategies by phase of the study—data collection, coding and analysis, and report preparation. Table 16.1 indicates how various quality-enhancement strategies map onto Lincoln and Guba's (1985) criteria.

TABLE 16.1 Quality-Enhancement Strategies in Relation to Lincoln and Guba's Quality Criteria for Qualitative Inquiry

Strategy	Credibility	Dependability	Confirmability	Transferability	Authenticity
Throughout the Inquiry					
Reflexivity/reflexive journaling	X				X
Careful documentation, audit trail		X	X		
Data Collection					
Prolonged engagement	X				X
Persistent observation	X				X
Comprehensive field notes	X			X	
Audio recording and verbatim transcription	X				X
Triangulation (data, method)	X	X			
Saturation of data	X			X	
Member checking	X	X			
Data Coding/Analysis					
Transcription rigor/data cleaning	X				
Intercoder reliability checks	X		X		
Triangulation (investigator)	X	X	X		
Search for disconfirming cases/negative case analysis	X				
Peer review/debriefing	X		X		
Inquiry audit		X	X		
Presentation of Findings					
Documentation of quality-enhancement efforts	X			X	
Thick, vivid description				X	X
Impactful, evocative writing					X
Documentation of researcher credentials, background	X				
Documentation of reflexivity	X				

Quality-Enhancement Strategies During Data Collection

Some of the strategies that qualitative researchers use are difficult to discern in a report. For example, intensive listening during an interview, careful *probing* to obtain rich and comprehensive data, and taking pains to gain participants' trust are all strategies to enhance data quality that cannot easily be communicated in a report. In this section, we focus on some strategies that can be described to readers to increase their confidence in the integrity of the study results.

Prolonged Engagement and Persistent Observation

An important step in establishing integrity in qualitative studies is **prolonged engagement**—the investment of sufficient time collecting data to have an in-depth understanding of the culture, language, or views of the people or group under study; to test for misinformation; and to ensure saturation of important categories. Prolonged engagement is also important for building trust with informants, which in turn makes it more likely that useful and rich information will be obtained.

> **Example of prolonged engagement** •
> Schuessler and colleagues (2020) conducted an in-depth study of the perceptions and experiences of perioperative nurses and nurse anesthetists regarding nursing care in robotic-assisted laparoscopic surgery (RALS). Schuessler and colleagues conducted interviews with 17 nurses and spent "sufficient time with each participant to achieve a deep understanding of the phenomenon" (p. 63). Additionally, they spent time in the field observing 5 RALS procedures to become thoroughly familiar with the setting and nursing roles.

High-quality data collection in qualitative studies also involves **persistent observation**, which concerns the salience of the data being gathered. Persistent observation refers to the researchers' focus on the characteristics or aspects of a situation that are relevant to the phenomena being studied. As Lincoln and Guba (1985) noted, "If prolonged engagement provides scope, persistent observation provides depth" (p. 304).

> **Example of persistent observation** •
> Rissardo and colleagues (2019) conducted an in-depth evaluation of elderly care dynamics in an emergency care unit. In addition to interviews with 33 social actors (health professionals, elderly patients, family members), the researchers conducted participant observation that involved 460 hours of fieldwork, with observations taking place in all three work shifts.

Reflexivity Strategies

Reflexivity involves awareness that the researcher as an individual brings to the inquiry a unique background, set of values, and a professional identity that can affect the research process. Reflexivity requires attending continually to the researcher's effect on the collection, analysis, and interpretation of data.

The most widely used strategy for maintaining reflexivity is to maintain a reflexive journal or diary. Reflexive writing can be used to record, in an ongoing fashion, thoughts about how previous experiences and readings about the phenomenon are affecting the inquiry. Through self-interrogation and reflection, researchers seek to be well positioned to probe deeply and to grasp the experience, process, or culture under study through the lens of participants.

TIP Researchers sometimes begin a study by being interviewed themselves regarding the phenomenon under study.

Data and Method Triangulation

Triangulation refers to the use of multiple referents to draw conclusions about what constitutes truth. The aim of triangulation is to "overcome the intrinsic bias that comes from single-method, single-observer, and single-theory studies" (Denzin, 1989, p. 313). Triangulation can also help to capture a more complete, contextualized picture of the phenomenon under study. Denzin (1989) identified four types of triangulation (data triangulation, investigator triangulation, method triangulation, and theory triangulation), and other types have been proposed. Two types are relevant to data collection.

Data triangulation involves the use of multiple data sources for the purpose of validating conclusions. There are three types of data triangulation: time, space, and person. *Time triangulation* involves collecting data on the same phenomenon or about the same people at different points in time (e.g., at different times of the year). This concept is similar to test–retest reliability assessment—the point is not to study a phenomenon longitudinally to assess change but to establish the congruence of the phenomenon across time. *Space triangulation* involves collecting data on the same phenomenon in multiple sites, to test for cross-site consistency. Finally, *person triangulation* involves collecting data from different types or levels of people (e.g., patients, health care staff), with the aim of validating data through multiple perspectives on the phenomenon.

Method triangulation involves using multiple methods of data collection. In qualitative studies, researchers often use a rich blend of unstructured data collection methods (e.g., interviews, observations, documents) to develop a comprehensive understanding of a phenomenon. Diverse data collection methods provide an opportunity to evaluate the extent to which a consistent and coherent picture of the phenomenon emerges.

Example of person, space, and method triangulation ••••••••••••••••••••
De Kok and an interdisciplinary team (2020) conducted an ethnographic study of respectful maternity care in Malawi. Data were collected through interviews and focus group interviews with midwives, recently delivered mothers, and "guardians" (the women's relatives or neighbors). Observations were conducted in five facilities in Malawi.

Comprehensive and Vivid Recording of Information

In addition to taking steps to record interview data accurately (e.g., via careful transcriptions of recorded interviews), researchers ideally prepare field notes that are rich with descriptions of what transpired in the field—even if interviews are the only source of data.

Some researchers specifically develop an **audit trail**—a systematic collection of materials that would allow an independent auditor to draw conclusions about the data. An audit trail might include the raw data (e.g., interview transcripts), methodological and reflexive notes, topic guides, and data reconstruction products (e.g., drafts of the final report). Similarly, the maintenance of a *decision trail* that articulates the researcher's decision rules for categorizing data and making analytic inferences is a useful way to enhance the dependability of the study. When researchers share decision trail information in their reports, readers can better evaluate the soundness of the decisions.

Example of an audit trail •
Chua and colleagues (2020) explored the experiences of junior doctors and nurses in medical emergency teams in escalating care for clinically deteriorating patients in general wards. The researchers maintained an audit trail of the entire research process.

Member Checking

In a **member check**, researchers provide participants with feedback about emerging interpretations and elicit participants' reactions. The argument is that participants should have an opportunity to assess and validate whether the researchers' interpretations are good representations of their realities. Member checking can be carried out as data are being collected (e.g., through probing to ensure that interviewers have properly interpreted participants' meanings) and more formally after data have been analyzed in follow-up interviews.

Despite the potential that member checking has for enhancing credibility, it has potential drawbacks. For example, member checks can lead to erroneous conclusions if participants share a common façade or a desire to "cover up." Also, some participants might agree with researchers' interpretations out of politeness or in the belief that researchers are "smarter" than they are. Thorne and Darbyshire (2005) cautioned against what they called *adulatory validity*, "a mutual stroking ritual that satisfies the agendas of both researcher and researched" (p. 1110). They noted that member checking tends to privilege interpretations that place participants in a charitable light.

Few strategies for enhancing data quality are as controversial as member checking. Nevertheless, it is a strategy that has the potential to enhance credibility if it is done in a manner that encourages candor and reflection by participants.

Example of member checking •
Haex and an interprofessional team (2020) studied how older clients and their caregivers experienced quality in home care. A sample of 6 home care clients and 10 formal and informal caregivers participated in in-depth interviews. The analysis revealed several key attributes contributing to experienced quality of home care (e.g., a small number of caregivers, a caring atmosphere). Preliminary results were shared during two group meetings with 9 participants to verify the researchers' interpretations.

Strategies Relating to Coding and Analysis

Excellent qualitative inquiry is likely to involve the simultaneous collection and analysis of data, and so several of the strategies described earlier also contribute to analytic integrity. Member checking, for example, can occur in an ongoing fashion during data collection, but typically also involves participants' review of preliminary analytic constructions. In this section, we introduce a few additional quality-enhancement strategies associated with the coding, analysis, and interpretation of qualitative data.

Investigator Triangulation

Investigator triangulation refers to the use of two or more researchers to make data collection, coding, and analysis decisions. The premise is that through collaboration, investigators can reduce the possibility of biased decisions and idiosyncratic interpretations.

Conceptually, investigator triangulation is analogous to interrater reliability in quantitative studies; it is a strategy often used in coding qualitative data. Some researchers take formal steps to compare two or more independent category schemes or independent coding decisions.

Example of independent coding •••••••••••••••••••••••••••••••••••••
Kim and colleagues (2020) studied the dyadic experience of managing heart failure. In-depth interviews were conducted with 17 patients and their family caregivers. The research team developed a coding scheme, and two authors coded the interview transcripts independently. The codes were checked for interrater agreement, and discrepancies were discussed and resolved.

Collaboration can also be used at the analysis stage. If investigators bring to the analysis task a complementary blend of skills and expertise, the analysis and interpretation can potentially benefit from divergent perspectives.

Searching for Disconfirming Evidence and Competing Explanations

A powerful verification procedure involves a systematic search for data that will challenge a categorization or explanation that emerged early in the analysis. The search for **disconfirming cases** occurs through purposive or theoretical sampling methods. This strategy depends on concurrent data collection and data analysis: Researchers cannot look for disconfirming data unless they have a sense of what they need to know.

Lincoln and Guba (1985) discussed the related activity of **negative case analysis**. This strategy (sometimes called *deviant case analysis*) is a process by which researchers search for cases that appear to disconfirm earlier hypotheses and then revise their interpretations as necessary. The goal of this procedure is to continuously refine a conceptualization or theory until it accounts for *all* cases.

Example of a negative case analysis ••••••••••••••••••••••••••••••••••
Ong and colleagues (2018) studied the trajectory of critical care nurses' experience in providing end-of-life care. Ten nurses in a medical intensive care unit were interviewed. Two researchers analyzed the data independently and then came to a consensus. Negative case analysis was "carried out by inspecting the themes in detail for issues that were internally conflicting with the themes, and themes were reframed to suit the data better" (p. 259).

Peer Review and Debriefing

Peer debriefing involves external validation, often in face-to-face sessions with the researchers' peers to review aspects of the inquiry. Peer debriefing exposes researchers to the searching questions of others who are experienced in either the methods of constructivist inquiry, the phenomenon being studied, or both.

In a peer review or debriefing session, researchers might present written or oral summaries of their data, categories and themes that are emerging, and interpretations of the data. In some cases, recorded interviews might be played. Among the questions that peer reviewers might address are the following:

- Do the gathered data adequately portray the phenomenon?
- If there are important omissions, what strategies might remedy this problem?
- Are there any apparent errors of fact or errors of interpretation?
- Is there evidence of researcher bias?
- Are the themes and interpretations knit together into a cogent, useful, and creative conceptualization of the phenomenon?

Example of peer review •
Brown and colleagues (2020) studied the experiences of the parents of young adults
with intellectual disabilities in transitioning from child to adult health services. The researchers established an Advisory Group of peers, who reviewed the study findings.

Inquiry Audits

A similar, but more formal, approach is to undertake an **inquiry audit**, a procedure that
involves a scrutiny of the actual data and relevant supporting documents by an external
reviewer. Such an audit requires careful documentation of all aspects of the inquiry. Once
the *audit trail* materials are assembled, the inquiry auditor proceeds to audit, in a fashion
analogous to a financial audit, the trustworthiness of the data and the meanings attached to
them. Such audits are a good tool for persuading others that qualitative data are worthy of
confidence. Relatively few comprehensive inquiry audits have been reported in the literature, but some studies report partial audits.

Strategies Relating to Presentation

This section describes some aspects of the qualitative report itself that can help to persuade
readers of the high quality of the inquiry.

Thick and Contextualized Description

Thick description refers to a rich, thorough, and vivid description of the research context,
study participants, and events and experiences observed during the inquiry. Transferability cannot occur unless investigators provide information for judging contextual similarity.
Lucid and textured descriptions, with judicious inclusion of verbatim quotes from study
participants, contribute to the authenticity of a qualitative study.

 TIP Sandelowski (2004) cautioned that "the phrase *thick description* likely ought not
to appear in write-ups of qualitative research at all, as it among those qualitative research words that should be seen but not written" (p. 215).

In high-quality qualitative studies, descriptions typically go beyond a faithful render-
ing of information. Powerful description is evocative and has the capacity for emotional
impact. Qualitative researchers must be careful, however, not to misrepresent their findings
by sharing only the most poignant stories. Thorne and Darbyshire (2005) warned against
"lachrymal validity," a criterion for evaluating research by the extent to which the report can
wring tears from its readers. At the same time, they noted the opposite problem with reports
that are "bloodless." Bloodless findings are characterized by a tendency of some researchers
to "play it safe in writing up the research, reporting the obvious . . . (and) failing to apply any
inductive analytic spin to the sequence, structure, or form of the findings" (p. 1109).

Researcher Credibility

Another aspect of credibility is **researcher credibility**. In qualitative studies, researchers
are the data-collecting instruments—as well as creators of the analytic process—and so their
qualifications, experience, and reflexivity are relevant in establishing confidence in the data.
Patton (2015) argued that trustworthiness is enhanced if the report contains information
about the researchers, including information about credentials and any personal connections the researchers had to the people, topic, or community under study. For example, it is
relevant for a reader of a report on the coping mechanisms of patients with AIDS to know

that the researcher is HIV positive. Researcher credibility is also enhanced when reports describe the researchers' efforts to be reflexive.

Example of researcher credibility •
Currie and Szabo (2020) studied the experiences of parents caring for the complex needs of children who have rare neurodevelopmental disorders (NDD). The report noted that both researchers worked with parents and children with NDDs as pediatric nurses, and that one researcher was herself the mother of a child with a rare NDD.

INTERPRETATION OF QUALITATIVE FINDINGS

It is difficult to describe the interpretive process in qualitative studies, but there is considerable agreement that the ability to "make meaning" from qualitative texts depends on researchers' immersion in and closeness to the data. *Incubation* is the process of *living* the data, a process in which researchers must try to understand their meaning, find essential patterns, and draw insightful conclusions. Another ingredient in interpretation and meaning-making is researchers' self-awareness and the ability to reflect on their own worldview—that is, reflexivity. Creativity also plays an important role in uncovering meaning in the data. Researchers need to devote sufficient time to achieve the *aha* that comes with making meaning beyond the facts.

For *readers* of qualitative reports, interpretation is hampered by having limited access to the data and no opportunity to "live" the data. Researchers are selective in the amount and types of information to include in their reports. Nevertheless, you should strive to consider some of the same interpretive dimensions for qualitative studies as for quantitative ones (see Chapter 14).

The Credibility of Qualitative Results

As with quantitative reports, you should consider whether the results of a qualitative inquiry are believable. It is reasonable to expect authors of qualitative reports to provide *evidence* of the credibility of the findings. Because consumers view only a portion of the data, they must rely on researchers' efforts to corroborate findings through such strategies as peer debriefings, member checks, audits, triangulation, and negative case analysis. They must also rely on researchers' frankness in acknowledging known limitations.

In considering the believability of qualitative results, it makes sense to adopt the posture of a person who needs to be persuaded about the researcher's conceptualization and to expect the researcher to present evidence with which to persuade you. It is also appropriate to consider whether the researcher's conceptualization is consistent with your own clinical insights.

The Meaning of Qualitative Results

The researcher's interpretation and analysis of qualitative data occur virtually simultaneously in an iterative process. Unlike quantitative analyses, the meaning of the data flows directly from qualitative analysis. Efforts to validate the analysis are necessarily efforts to validate interpretations as well. Nevertheless, prudent qualitative researchers hold their interpretations up for closer scrutiny—self-scrutiny as well as review by external reviewers.

The Importance of Qualitative Results

Qualitative research is especially productive when it is used to describe and explain poorly understood phenomena. However, the phenomenon must be one that merits scrutiny.

You should also consider whether the findings themselves are trivial. Perhaps the topic is worthwhile, but you may feel after reading a report that nothing has been learned beyond what is everyday knowledge—this can happen when the data are "thin" or when the conceptualization is shallow. Readers, like researchers, want to have an *aha* experience when they read about participants' lives. Qualitative researchers often attach catchy labels to their themes, but you should ask yourself whether the labels have really portrayed an insightful construct.

The Transferability of Qualitative Results

Qualitative researchers do not strive for generalizability, but the possible application of the results to other settings is important to evidence-based practice. Thus, in interpreting qualitative results, you should consider how transferable the findings are. In what types of settings and contexts would you expect the phenomena under study to be manifested in a similar fashion? Of course, to make such an assessment, the researchers must have described the participants and context in sufficient detail. Because qualitative studies are context bound, it is only through a careful analysis of the key features of the study context that transferability can be assessed.

The Implications of Qualitative Results

If the findings are judged to be believable and important and if you are satisfied with the interpretation of the results, you can begin to consider what the implications of the findings might be. First, you can consider implications for further research: Should a similar study be undertaken in a different setting? Has an important construct been identified that merits the development of a formal measuring instrument? Do the results suggest hypotheses that could be tested through controlled quantitative research? Second, do the findings have implications for nursing practice? For example, could the health care needs of a subculture (e.g., the homeless) be addressed more effectively as a result of the study? Finally, do the findings shed light on fundamental processes that could play a role in nursing theories?

CRITICAL APPRAISAL OF QUALITY AND INTEGRITY IN QUALITATIVE STUDIES

For qualitative research to be judged trustworthy, investigators must earn the trust of their readers. In a world that is conscious about the quality of research evidence, qualitative researchers need to be proactive in doing high-quality research and persuading others that they were successful.

Demonstrating integrity to others involves providing a good description of the quality-enhancement activities that were undertaken—and yet, many qualitative reports fail to do so. Just as clinicians seek *evidence* for clinical decisions, research consumers need evidence that findings are trustworthy. Researchers should include enough information about their quality-enhancement strategies for readers to draw conclusions about study quality.

Part of the difficulty that qualitative researchers face in demonstrating trustworthiness is that page constraints in journals impose conflicting demands. It takes a precious amount of space to present quality-enhancement strategies adequately and convincingly. Using space for such documentation means that there is less space for the thick description of context and rich verbatim accounts that support authenticity and vividness. It is well to keep the need for compromise in mind in appraising qualitative research reports.

An important point in thinking about quality in qualitative inquiry is that attention needs to be paid to both "art" and "science" and to interpretation and description. Creativity and

> ### Box 16.1 Guidelines for Critically Appraising Quality and Integrity in Qualitative Studies
>
> 1. Did the report discuss efforts to enhance or evaluate the quality of the data and the overall inquiry? If so, was the description sufficiently detailed and clear? If not, was there other information that allowed you to draw inferences about the quality of the data, the analysis, and the interpretations?
> 2. Which specific techniques (if any) did the researcher use to enhance the trustworthiness and integrity of the inquiry? What quality-enhancement strategies were *not* used? Would additional strategies have strengthened your confidence in the study and its evidence?
> 3. Did the researcher adequately represent the multiple realities of those being studied? Do the findings seem *authentic*?
> 4. Given the efforts to enhance data quality, what can you conclude about the study's validity/integrity/rigor/trustworthiness?
> 5. Did the report discuss any study limitations and their possible effects on the credibility of the results or on interpretations of the data?
> 6. Did the researchers discuss the study's implications for clinical practice or future research? Were the implications well grounded in the study evidence and in evidence from earlier research?

insightfulness need to be attained but not at the expense of soundness. And the quest for soundness cannot sacrifice inspiration, or else the results are likely to be "perfectly healthy but dead" (Morse, 2006, p. 6). Good qualitative work is both descriptively accurate and explicit and interpretively rich and innovative. Some guidelines that may be helpful in evaluating qualitative methods and analyses are presented in Box 16.1.

RESEARCH EXAMPLES WITH CRITICAL THINKING EXERCISES

This section describes quality-enhancement efforts in a grounded theory study. Read the summary and then answer the critical thinking questions that follow, referring to the full research report if necessary. Answers to the questions for Exercise 1 are available to instructors on thePoint®. The critical thinking questions for Exercise 2 are based on the study that appears in its entirety in Appendix B of this book. Our comments for these exercises are in the Student Resources section on thePoint®.

EXAMPLE 1: TRUSTWORTHINESS IN A GROUNDED THEORY STUDY

Study: The psychological process of breast cancer patients receiving initial chemotherapy: Rising from the ashes (Chen et al., 2016)

Statement of Purpose: The purpose of this study was to explore patients' suffering and adverse effects during the process of receiving the first course of chemotherapy for breast cancer.

Method: The researchers used Glaser's grounded theory methods. Twenty Taiwanese women, ranging in age from 39 to 62 years, were interviewed in a private room in a hospital within 6 months of completing the first course of chemotherapy. Purposive sampling was used initially, and then, theoretical sampling was used to select additional participants until categories were saturated. The interviews included such broad questions as the following: During chemotherapy, what was on your mind? How did the chemotherapy affect your life? The audiorecorded interviews were transcribed for analysis.

Quality-Enhancement Strategies: The researchers' report provided good detail about efforts to enhance the trustworthiness of their study, as described in a subsection of their Method section labeled "Rigor." The researchers noted that the lead investigator participated in the care of the women during their hospitalization and during follow-up visits, thereby contributing to prolonged engagement—and to the development of a good therapeutic relationship. The researchers continued to observe the verbal and nonverbal expressions of these patients during follow-up visits; this strategy was described as persistent observation but could also be considered data triangulation if the analysis was informed by both the interview data and the informal observations. Three experts were invited to review and discuss the emerging conceptualization (peer debriefing). Two study participants reviewed the findings in a member check effort. The lead researcher also maintained a reflexive journal that guided her during data collection. During the interviews, the questioning was informed by ongoing data analysis, so that questions were linked to emergent categories to achieve saturation. The report also included explicit statements about the researchers' credentials and experience, thus supporting researcher credibility. In terms of thick description, the researchers provided many vivid excerpts from the interviews. Moreover, they provided a table that described each individual participant in terms of age, marital status, religion, occupation, breast cancer stage, and type of chemotherapy.

Key Findings: The researchers concluded that the core category was "Rising from the ashes." Four categories represented four stages of the psychological process experienced by these patients: the fear stage, the hardship stage, the adjustment stage, and the relaxation stage. The authors noted that each stage is likely to occur repeatedly.

Critical Thinking Exercises

1. Answer the relevant questions from Box 16.1 regarding this study.
2. Also consider the following targeted questions:
   a. Which quality-enhancement strategy used by Chen et al. gave you the *most* confidence in the integrity and trustworthiness of their study? Why?
   b. Think of an additional type of triangulation that the researchers could have used in their study and describe how this could have been implemented.
3. What might be some of the uses to which the findings could be put in clinical practice?

EXAMPLE 2: TRUSTWORTHINESS IN THE PHENOMENOLOGICAL STUDY IN APPENDIX B

1. Read the method and results sections from Beck and Watson's phenomenological study ("Posttraumatic growth after birth trauma") in Appendix B of this book and then answer the relevant questions from Box 16.1 regarding this study.
2. Also consider the following targeted questions:
   a. Suggest one or two ways in which triangulation could have been used in this study.
   b. Which quality-enhancement strategy used by Beck and Watson gave you the *most* confidence in the integrity and trustworthiness of their study? Why?

WANT TO KNOW MORE?

A wide variety of resources to enhance your learning and understanding of this chapter is available on thePoint®.

- Chapter Supplement on Whittemore and Colleagues' Framework of Quality Criteria in Qualitative Research
- Answer to the Critical Thinking Exercise for Example 2
- Internet Resources with useful websites for Chapter 16
- A Wolters Kluwer journal article on a topic related to this chapter

Additional study aids, including eight journal articles and related questions, are also available in *Study Guide for Essentials of Nursing Research, 10e*.

Summary Points

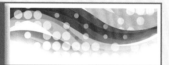

- One controversy regarding *quality* in qualitative studies involves terminology. Some argue that *rigor* and *validity* are quantitative terms that are not suitable as goals in qualitative inquiry, but others believe these terms are appropriate. Other controversies involve what criteria to use as indicators of integrity and whether there should be generic or tradition-specific criteria.

- Lincoln and Guba (1985) proposed a framework for evaluating **trustworthiness** in qualitative inquiries, using five criteria: credibility, dependability, confirmability, transferability, and authenticity.

- **Credibility**, which refers to confidence in the truth value of the findings, has been viewed as the qualitative equivalent of internal validity. **Dependability**, the stability of data over time and over conditions, is somewhat analogous to reliability in quantitative studies. **Confirmability** refers to the objectivity of the data. **Transferability**, the analog of external validity, is the degree to which findings can be transferred to other settings or groups. **Authenticity** is the extent to which researchers faithfully show a range of different realities and convey the feeling tone of lives as they are lived.

- Strategies for enhancing quality during qualitative data collection include **prolonged engagement**, which strives for adequate scope of data coverage; **persistent observation**, which is aimed at achieving adequate depth; comprehensive recording of information (including maintenance of an **audit trail**); triangulation; and **member checks** (asking study participants to review and react to emerging conceptualizations).

- **Triangulation** is the process of using multiple referents to draw conclusions about what constitutes the truth. This includes **data triangulation** (using multiple data sources to validate conclusions) and **method triangulation** (using multiple methods to collect data about the same phenomenon).

- Strategies for enhancing quality during the coding and analysis of qualitative data include **investigator triangulation** (independent coding and analysis of data by two or more researchers), searching for **disconfirming evidence**, undertaking a **negative case analysis** (revising interpretations to account for cases that appear to disconfirm early conclusions), external validation through **peer debriefings** (exposing the inquiry to the searching questions of peers), and launching an **inquiry audit** (a formal scrutiny of audit trail documents by an independent auditor).

- Strategies that can be used to convince readers of the high quality of qualitative inquiries include using **thick description** to vividly portray contextualized information about study participants and the focal phenomenon and making efforts to be transparent

about researchers' credentials and reflexivity so that **researcher credibility** can be established.

- Interpretation in qualitative research involves "making meaning"—a process that is difficult to describe or appraise. Yet interpretations in qualitative inquiry need to be reviewed in terms of credibility, importance, transferability, and implications.

REFERENCES FOR CHAPTER 16

Brown, M., Higgins, A., & MacArthur, J. (2020). Transition from child to adult health services: A qualitative study of the views and experiences of families of young adults with intellectual disabilities. *Journal of Clinical Nursing, 29,* 195–207.

**Chen, Y. C., Huang, H., Kao, C., Sun, C., Chiang, C., & Sun, F. (2016). The psychological process of breast cancer patients receiving initial chemotherapy: Rising from the ashes. *Cancer Nursing, 39,* E36–E44.

Chua, W., Legido-Quigley, H., Jones, D., Hassan, N., Tee, A., & Liaw, S. (2020). A call for better doctor-nurse collaboration: A qualitative study of the experiences of junior doctors and nurses in escalating care for deteriorating ward patients. *Australian Critical Care, 33,* 54–61.

*Currie, G., & Szabo, J. (2020). Social isolation and exclusion: The parents' experience of caring for children with rare neurodevelopmental disorders. *International Journal of Qualitative Studies on Health and Well-Being, 15,* 1725362.

de Kok, B., Uny, I., Immamura, M., Bell, J., Geddes, J., & Phoya, A. (2020). From global rights to local relationships: Exploring disconnects in respectful maternity care in Malawi. *Qualitative Health Research, 30,* 341–355.

Denzin, N. K. (1989). *The research act* (3rd ed.). New York, NY: McGraw-Hill.

Guba, E., & Lincoln, Y. (1994). Competing paradigms in qualitative research. In N. Denzin & Y. Lincoln (Eds.), *Handbook of Qualitative Research* (pp. 105–117). Thousand Oaks, CA: Sage.

Haex, R., Thoma-Lürken, T., Beurskens, A., & Zwakhalen, S. (2020). How do clients and (in)formal caregivers experience quality of home care? A qualitative approach. *Journal of Advanced Nursing, 76,* 264–274.

Kim, J. S. R., Risbud, R., Gray, C., Banerjee, D., & Trivedi, R. (2020). The dyadic experience of managing heart failure: A qualitative investigation. *The Journal of Cardiovascular Nursing, 35,* 12–18.

Lincoln, Y. S., & Guba, E. G. (1985). *Naturalistic inquiry.* Newbury Park, CA: Sage.

Morse, J. M. (2006). Insight, inference, evidence, and verification: Creating a legitimate discipline. *International Journal of Qualitative Methods, 5*(1).

Morse, J. M. (2015). Critical analysis of strategies for determining rigor in qualitative inquiry. *Qualitative Health Research, 25,* 1212–1222.

Ong, K., Ting, K., & Chow, Y. (2018). The trajectory of experience of critical care nurses in providing end-of-life care: A qualitative descriptive study. *Journal of Clinical Nursing, 27,* 257–268.

Patton, M. Q. (2015). *Qualitative research & evaluation methods* (4th ed.). Thousand Oaks, CA: Sage.

*Rissardo, L., Kantorski, L., & Carreira, L. (2019). Evaluation of elderly care dynamics in an emergency care unit. *Revista Brasileira de Enfermagem, 72,* 161–168.

Sandelowski, M. (2004). Counting cats in Zanzibar. *Research in Nursing & Health, 27,* 215–216.

Schuessler, Z., Stiles, A., & Mancuso, P. (2020). Perceptions and experiences of perioperative nurses and nurse anaesthetists in robotic-assisted surgery. *Journal of Clinical Nursing, 29,* 60–74.

Thorne, S., & Darbyshire, P. (2005). Land mines in the field: A modest proposal for improving the craft of qualitative health research. *Qualitative Health Research, 15,* 1105–1113.

Whittemore, R., Chase, S. K., & Mandle, C. L. (2001). Validity in qualitative research. *Qualitative Health Research, 11,* 522–537.

*A link to this open-access article is provided in the Internet Resources section on thePoint® website.

**This journal article is available on thePoint® for this chapter.

17

Learning From Systematic Reviews

Learning Objectives

On completing this chapter, you will be able to:

- Discuss alternative approaches to integrating research evidence and advantages to using systematic methods
- Describe key decisions and steps in doing a systematic review of quantitative and qualitative study findings
- Critically appraise key aspects of a written systematic review
- Define new terms in the chapter

Key Terms

- Effect size (ES)
- Forest plot
- Frequency effect size
- GRADE
- Intensity effect size
- Manifest effect size
- Meta-aggregation
- Meta-analysis
- Meta-ethnography
- Meta-summary
- Metasynthesis
- Primary study
- Publication bias
- Qualitative evidence synthesis (QES)
- Statistical heterogeneity
- Subgroup analysis
- Systematic review

Systematic reviews, a cornerstone of evidence-based practice (EBP), are inquiries that follow many of the same rules as those for **primary studies**, i.e., original research investigations. This chapter provides guidance in helping you to understand and evaluate the systematic integration of research evidence.

RESEARCH INTEGRATION AND SYNTHESIS

In a **systematic review**, researchers carefully and transparently integrate research evidence about a specific research question using methodical procedures that are spelled out in advance. The review process is disciplined and transparent, so that readers of a systematic review can assess the integrity of the conclusions.

Originally, systematic reviews in health care fields were mainly syntheses of evidence from randomized controlled trials (RCTs) that addressed Therapy/intervention questions. Systematic reviews of findings from RCTs—which are at the pinnacle of most evidence hierarchies for Therapy questions (see Fig. 1.2)—often involve the statistical integration of evidence in a **meta-analysis**. The Cochrane Collaboration is a premiere organization for creating and disseminating reviews of research evidence; most reviews in the Cochrane Collaboration database involve meta-analyses. Systematic reviews of all types of quantitative evidence—including findings from studies addressing Etiology, Prognosis, or Diagnosis questions—have also burgeoned.

Qualitative researchers have also created techniques to integrate evidence from multiple studies. Their products are often called *metasyntheses*. Metasyntheses typically involve integrations of studies focused on abstract phenomena and experiences (e.g., grief following a miscarriage). However, there is an emerging interest among health care researchers on synthesizing information on the qualitative aspects of interventions, such as patient acceptance, implementation processes and contexts, and barriers to implementation (e.g., Shaw et al., 2014). Such reviews are often called *qualitative evidence syntheses*.

 TIP In the evolving field of evidence synthesis, special types of review are emerging. For example, in a *rapid review* the reviewers follow streamlined procedures designed to produce an evidence synthesis in a timely (but less rigorous) manner than a standard systematic review. *Umbrella reviews* integrate findings from multiple systematic reviews on a topic. Also, the emergence of mixed methods research (see Chapter 12) has given rise to *systematic mixed studies reviews* (also called *mixed research syntheses*), which use disciplined procedures to integrate and synthesize findings from qualitative, quantitative, and mixed methods studies.

SYSTEMATIC REVIEWS OF QUANTITATIVE EVIDENCE

In systematic reviews, the "data" are the findings from studies that addressed a specific question (e.g., mean pain levels following receipt of a pain-reducing intervention). Data from the included studies can be integrated in a narrative fashion or statistically in a meta-analysis.

Basics of Meta-Analysis

The essence of a meta-analysis is that findings from each study are used to compute a common index, an *effect size*. Effect sizes are *averaged* across studies, yielding aggregated information about not only the existence of a relationship between variables but also an estimate of its magnitude.

Advantages of Meta-Analysis

Meta-analysis offers a simple advantage as an integration method: *objectivity*. It is difficult to draw objective conclusions about a body of evidence using narrative methods when results are inconsistent, as they often are. Narrative reviewers make subjective decisions about how much weight to give findings from different studies, and so different reviewers may reach different conclusions in reviewing the same set of studies. Meta-analysts make decisions that are explicit and open to scrutiny. The integration itself is objective because it uses statistical formulas. Readers of a meta-analysis can be confident that another analyst using the same data set and analytic decisions would reach the same conclusions.

Another advantage of meta-analysis concerns *power*, i.e., the probability of detecting a true relationship between variables (see Chapter 13). By combining effects across multiple studies, power is increased. In a meta-analysis, it is possible to conclude that a relationship is real (e.g., that an intervention is effective), even when several small studies yielded nonsignificant findings. In a narrative review, 10 nonsignificant findings would almost surely be interpreted as lack of evidence of effectiveness, which could be the wrong conclusion.

Criteria for Undertaking a Meta-Analysis

Despite its advantages, meta-analysis is not always appropriate, so reviewers need to decide whether statistical integration is suitable. A basic criterion is that the research question should be nearly identical across studies. This means that the independent and dependent variables, and the study populations, are sufficiently similar to merit integration.

Another criterion concerns whether there is a sufficient knowledge base for statistical integration. If there are only a few studies, or if all studies are weakly designed, it usually would not make sense to compute an "average" effect.

One other issue concerns the consistency of the evidence. When the same hypothesis has been tested in multiple studies and the results are highly conflicting, meta-analysis is likely not appropriate. As an extreme example, if half the studies testing an intervention found benefits for those in the intervention group, but the other half found benefits for the controls, it would be misleading to compute an average effect. In this situation, it would be better to do an in-depth narrative analysis of *why* the results are conflicting.

Example of decision not to conduct a meta-analysis • • • • • • • • • • • • • • • • • • •
Chao and colleagues (2020) undertook a systematic review of taste differences among people with eating disorders. They identified 49 studies that met the inclusion criteria. They found that, due to the diverse range of methods and designs used in these studies and the heterogeneity of results among the studies, they were unable to complete a meta-analysis.

Steps in a Quantitative Systematic Review

Unlike literature reviews, systematic reviews require a team. The team usually includes content experts, statisticians (if there is a meta-analysis), and a librarian or information specialist. Putting together a good team is essential. This section describes major steps in a quantitative systematic review so that you can understand the decisions a review team makes—decisions that affect the quality of the review.

Formulation of the Review Question

A focused systematic review begins with a carefully framed question. Review questions sometimes follow the PICO format described in Chapter 1, with specification of the Population, the Intervention or Influence, the Comparison against which the intervention/influence is contrasted, and Outcomes. The careful definition of key constructs is critical for deciding whether a primary study qualifies for the synthesis.

Example of a question from a meta-analysis •
Sherifali and an interprofessional team (2018) conducted a systematic review and meta-analysis that addressed the question (using the PICO framework described in Chapter 1) of whether Internet-based interventions (I), compared to the absence of an Internet-based intervention (C), have positive effects on the mental health (O) of caregivers caring for adults with a chronic health problem (P).

A strategy that is gaining momentum is to undertake a *scoping review* to refine the specific question for a systematic review. A scoping review is a preliminary investigation that clarifies the range and nature of the evidence base, using flexible procedures. Such scoping reviews can identify strategies for a full systematic review and can also indicate whether a meta-analysis is feasible.

The Design of a Quantitative Systematic Review

Sampling is an important design issue. In a systematic review, the sample consists of the primary studies that have addressed the research question, and eligibility criteria must be stated. Substantively, the criteria specify the population (P) and the variables (I, C, and O). For example, if the reviewer is integrating findings about the effectiveness of an intervention, which outcomes *must* the researchers have studied? With regard to the population, will (for example) certain age groups be excluded? The criteria might also specify that only studies that used a randomized design will be included. On practical grounds, reports not written in English might be excluded. Another decision is whether to include both published and unpublished reports.

Example of sampling criteria for a quantitative review • • • • • • • • • • • • • • • • • •
Huang and colleagues (2020) did a systematic review of RCTs to assess the effect of removing an indwelling urinary catheter at different times on urinary retention and urinary tract infection (UTI) in surgical patients. To be eligible, a study had to be an RCT involving participants undergoing gynecological surgery with varying times of catheter removal (e.g., immediate, ≤6 hours) and had to include the outcomes of urinary retention and UTI after extubation.

Researchers sometimes use study quality as a sampling criterion. Screening out studies of lower quality can occur indirectly if the review team excludes studies that did not use a randomized design. More directly, each potential primary study can be rated for quality and excluded if the quality score falls below a threshold. Alternative ways of dealing with study quality are discussed in a later section. Suffice it to say, however, that evaluations of study quality are part of the integration process, and so reviewers must decide how to assess quality and what to do with assessments.

In reviews involving a meta-analysis, another design issue concerns the **statistical heterogeneity** of results in the primary studies. For each study, meta-analysts compute an index to summarize the strength of relationship between an independent variable and a dependent variable. Just as there is inevitably variation *within* studies (not all people in a study have identical scores on outcomes), so there is inevitably variation in effects *across* studies. If the results are highly variable (e.g., results across studies are conflicting), a meta-analysis may be inappropriate. If the results are moderately variable, different analytic techniques might be required.

 TIP Review teams are increasingly expected to prepare a *protocol* of a proposed systematic review. Protocols are often registered in an international database called PROSPERO—so if you are searching for evidence for an EBP project, it is a good idea to check in PROSPERO to see if a review is forthcoming.

The Search for Evidence in the Literature

Systematic reviewers typically aim for an exhaustive search of primary studies that meet the eligibility criteria, but they must decide whether their review will include unpublished findings. Although there is not total agreement about the scope of the search, reviewers are increasingly likely to cast as wide a net as possible and include *grey literature*—that is, studies with a more limited distribution, such as dissertations or unpublished reports. Some people restrict their sample to reports in peer-reviewed journals, arguing that the peer review system is a tried-and-true screen for findings worthy of consideration as evidence.

Excluding nonpublished findings, however, runs the risk of biased results. **Publication bias** is the tendency for published studies to systematically overrepresent statistically significant findings. This bias is widespread: Authors may refrain from submitting manuscripts for studies with nonsignificant results, reviewers and editors tend to reject such reports when they are submitted, and users of evidence may ignore the findings if they are published. The exclusion of grey literature in a meta-analysis can lead to the overestimation of effects.

Meta-analysts can use various search strategies to locate grey literature, in addition to the usual methods for a literature review. These include contacting key researchers in the field to see if they have done studies (or know of studies) that have not been published and reviewing abstracts from conference proceedings.

> **Example of a search strategy from a systematic review** ● ● ● ● ● ● ● ● ● ● ● ● ● ● ● ●
> Leach and colleagues (2020) did a systematic review of the association between community mental health nursing and hospital admissions for people with serious mental illness. Their search strategy included a search of 10 bibliographic databases and 2 clinical trial registries of studies in progress. The reference lists of included publications were also searched to identify potentially eligible studies.

Evaluations of Study Quality

In systematic reviews, the evidence from primary studies needs to be evaluated to assess how much confidence to place in the findings. Evaluations of study quality sometimes involve overall ratings of study features on a multi-item scale. Dozens of quality assessment rating scales exist, but their use is not universally endorsed. Quality criteria vary from scale to scale, and so study quality can be rated differently with different assessment scales—or by different raters using the same scale.

The Cochrane Collaboration takes an approach that emphasizes risk of bias, using a "domain" approach (Higgins et al., 2019). *Risk of bias* in intervention studies refers to a potential bias in conclusions about a causal effect. In Cochrane reviews, reviewers rate each study for such internal validity threats as selection bias and attrition bias; each is rated low risk, high risk, or unclear risk of bias. Although this Cochrane's risk-of-bias tool is primarily relevant for studies addressing Therapy questions, a comparable domain-based tool for nonrandomized studies has been developed.

Quality assessments of primary studies, regardless of approach, should be done by two or more qualified individuals. If there are disagreements between the raters, there should be a discussion until a consensus has been reached or until another rater helps to resolve the difference.

> **Example of quality assessments in a systematic review** ● ● ● ● ● ● ● ● ● ● ● ● ● ● ● ●
> Zhang and colleagues (2020) did a systematic review to assess the effectiveness of culturally tailored interventions to promote mammography screening among Chinese American women. The methodological quality of studies was evaluated using an instrument developed by the Joanna Briggs Institute that uses 10 quality criteria (e.g., randomization, blinding). Two reviewers independently rated quality, and differences were resolved by consensus.

Extraction and Encoding of Data for Analysis

The next step is to extract and record relevant information about the findings, methods, and study characteristics. If a meta-analysis is being undertaken, the goal is to create a data set amenable to statistical analysis. Basic source information must be recorded (e.g., journal, year of publication). Important methodological features include sample size, whether participants were randomized to treatments, whether blinding was used, rates of attrition, and length of follow-up. Characteristics of participants must be encoded as well (e.g., their mean age). Finally, information about findings must be extracted. For a meta-analysis, reviewers must either calculate effect sizes (discussed in the next section) or must record sufficient statistical information that computer software can compute them.

As with other decisions, extraction and coding of information should be completed by two or more people, at least for a portion of the studies in the sample. This allows for an assessment of interrater agreement, which should be sufficiently high to persuade readers of the review that the data are accurate.

Example of data extraction and intercoder agreement • • • • • • • • • • • • • • • • •
Fang and colleagues (2020) conducted a systematic review of studies that examined the association between heart rate variability and the risk of cardiovascular events and all-cause death. Two researchers independently extracted data from 28 studies. Discrepancies were resolved through discussion with a third investigator.

Calculation of Effects in Meta-Analyses

Meta-analyses depend on the calculation of an **effect size (ES)** index that encapsulates in a single number the relationship between the independent and outcome variable in each study. Effects are captured differently depending on the measurement level of variables. The three most common scenarios for meta-analysis involve comparisons of two groups such as an intervention versus a control group on a continuous outcome (e.g., body mass index), comparisons of two groups on a dichotomous outcome (e.g., stopped smoking vs. continued smoking), or correlations between two continuous variables (e.g., between blood pressure levels and anxiety scores).

The first scenario, comparison of two group means, is especially common. When the outcomes across studies are on identical scales (e.g., all outcomes are measures of weight in pounds), the effect is captured by simply subtracting the mean for one group from the mean for the other. For example, if the mean postintervention weight in an intervention group were 182.0 pounds and that for a control group were 194.0 pounds, the ES would be −12.0. Typically, however, outcomes are measured on different scales (e.g., a scale of 0 to 10 vs. 0 to 100 to measure pain). Mean differences across studies cannot in such situations be combined and averaged; researchers need an index that is neutral to the original metric. Cohen's *d*, the effect size index most often used, transforms all effects into standard deviation units. If *d* were computed to be .50, it means that the group mean for one group was one half a standard deviation higher than the mean for the other group—regardless of the original measurement scale.

 TIP The term *effect size* (ES) is widely used for *d* in the nursing literature, but the term usually used for Cochrane reviews is *standardized mean difference* or SMD.

When the outcomes in the primary studies are dichotomies, meta-analysts usually use the odds ratio (OR) or the relative risk (RR) index as the ES statistic. In nonexperimental studies, a common effect size statistic is Pearson's *r*, which indicates the magnitude and direction of effect.

Analysis of Data in a Meta-Analysis

After an effect size is computed for each study, as just described, a pooled effect estimate is computed as a *weighted average* of the individual effects. The bigger the weight given to any study, the more that study will contribute to the weighted average. A widely used approach is to give more weight to studies with larger samples.

An important decision concerns how to deal with the heterogeneity of findings— i.e., differences from one study to another in the magnitude and direction of effects. Statistical heterogeneity should be formally tested, and meta-analysts should report their results.

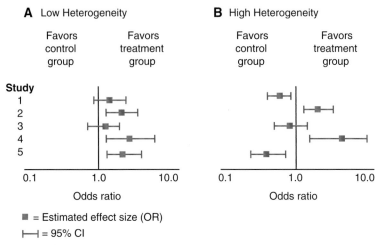

A Low Heterogeneity   **B** High Heterogeneity

Figure 17.1   Two forest plots.

Visual inspection of heterogeneity usually relies on the construction of **forest plots**, which are often included in meta-analytic reports. A forest plot graphs the effect size for each study, together with the 95% confidence interval (CI) around each estimate. Figure 17.1 illustrates forest plots for situations in which there is low heterogeneity (A) and high heterogeneity (B) for five studies. In panel A, all five effect size estimates (here, odds ratios) favor the intervention group. The CI information indicates the intervention effect is statistically significant (does not encompass 1.0) for studies 2, 4, and 5. In panel B, by contrast, the results are "all over the map." Two studies favor the control group at significant levels (studies 1 and 5) and two favor the treatment group (studies 2 and 4). Meta-analysis is not appropriate for the situation in panel B.

 TIP   Heterogeneity affects not only whether a meta-analysis is appropriate but also which statistical model should be used in the analysis. When findings are similar, the researchers may use a *fixed effects model.* When results are more varied, it is better to use a *random effects model.*

Some meta-analysts seek to understand *why* effect size estimates vary across studies. Differences could be the result of clinical characteristics. For example, in intervention studies, variation in effects across studies could be related to whether the intervention agents were nurses or other health care professionals. Or, variation in results could be explained by differences in participant characteristics (e.g., patients in different age groups). One strategy for exploring systematic differences in effect size is to do **subgroup analyses**. Such analyses (sometimes called *moderator* analyses) involve splitting the sample into distinct categorical groups—for example, based on gender. Effects for studies with all-male (or predominantly male) samples could be compared to those for studies with all or predominantly female samples.

Example of an investigation of heterogeneity •
Amirshahi and an interdisciplinary team (2020) conducted a systematic review to estimate the global prevalence of postoperative nausea and vomiting. In addition to estimating overall prevalence, the reviewers undertook a subgroup analysis to examine whether prevalence differed by age, type of surgery, and gender. None of these factors was related to prevalence rates, which were estimated at 31.4% for nausea and 16.8% for vomiting.

Another analytic issue concerns study quality. There are several strategies for dealing with study quality in a meta-analysis. One is to establish a quality threshold for sampling studies (e.g., omitting studies with a poor quality score). A second strategy is to undertake analyses to evaluate whether excluding lower quality studies changes the results (this is called a *sensitivity analysis*). Another approach is to use quality as the basis for a subgroup analysis. For example, do randomized designs yield different average effect size estimates than quasi-experimental designs? A mix of strategies is probably a prudent approach to dealing with differences in study quality.

Assessment of Degree of Confidence: GRADE

Until a few year ago, reviewers typically moved from analyzing their data to writing a report. Now, many reviewers undertake a systematic procedure to draw conclusions about how much *confidence* can be placed in the results of the review. Internationally, numerous organizations, including the Cochrane Collaboration, have adopted the Grades of Recommendation, Assessment, Development, and Evaluation (**GRADE**) approach to grading the quality of evidence (Guyatt et al., 2008).

GRADE involves a two-part process that was designed to guide the development of clinical guidelines for interventions. In the first step, the quality of evidence about an intervention's effect on specific outcomes is graded. In the second part, a recommendation is made about using or not using the intervention. For those conducting systematic reviews, only the first part is completed—that is, reviewers do not make clinical recommendations.

GRADE ratings are done on an outcome-by-outcome basis and usually are applied to only a subset of outcomes included in a review—the outcomes judged to be critical to those making decisions about adopting an intervention. The GRADE system involves using ratings to make a categorical determination of the *confidence* one can place in the systematic review results—that is, whether confidence in the evidence for a specified outcome (regardless of effect size) is high, moderate, low, or very low. A rating of high, for example, corresponds to high confidence that the *true* effect is close to the effect estimated in the review. The supplement to this chapter on thePoint® provides more information about the GRADE system.

   TIP   There are explicit reporting guidelines for systematic reviews. One is called *PRISMA*, which is used primarily for reporting systematic reviews of randomized controlled trials (RCTs). The PRISMA guidelines call for the inclusion of a flow chart that documents the identification, screening, and inclusion of studies in a systematic review.

SYSTEMATIC REVIEWS OF QUALITATIVE EVIDENCE

Integration of qualitative findings is a burgeoning and evolving field for which there are no standard procedures—dozens of approaches have been proposed. This section provides a brief overview of some major issues.

Aggregative and Interpretive Qualitative Reviews

Several scholars have characterized systematic reviews as being either *aggregative* or *interpretive/configurative* (e.g., Booth et al., 2018; Gough et al., 2012). Most qualitative reviews have elements of both aggregation and interpretation. The decision on which broad (and specific) qualitative synthesis approach to use depends on several factors, including the nature of the question and the reviewers' philosophical leanings.

Aggregative Qualitative Reviews

Qualitative reviews that are predominantly aggregative are similar in many respects to quantitative systematic reviews. Aggregative reviews involve the *pooling* of findings (i.e., themes, categories, or processes) across the qualitative studies in the review. Aggregative qualitative reviews tend to be fairly structured, the questions addressed are fairly focused, and exhaustive searching for primary studies is expected. The goal of most aggregative reviews is to provide direct, usable guidance for action.

Research questions that are especially well suited to an aggregative approach often concern how best to address a specific health care problem or how to design or improve an intervention. Examples of such questions include the following: What strategies do people use in efforts to quit smoking? What are patients' barriers to participating in a smoking cessation intervention? What features of a smoking intervention lead to nonparticipation?

Both the Joanna Briggs Institute (JBI) and the Cochrane Collaboration, who typically use the umbrella term **qualitative evidence synthesis (QES)**, provide guidance for reviews that would best be characterized as aggregative. At JBI, qualitative reviews use an approach to evidence synthesis called *meta-aggregation* (Aromataris & Munn, 2017; Hannes & Lockwood, 2011).

Interpretive Qualitative Reviews

Qualitative reviews that are predominantly interpretive emphasize the creation of theories and integrated conceptualizations by interpreting and reconfiguring findings from qualitative primary studies. Interpretive syntheses tend to be loosely structured and may not involve comprehensive searching or quality assessments.

Interpretive syntheses most often focus on questions about meanings, feelings, experiences, and processes—questions typically addressed through phenomenological, ethnographic, or grounded theory research. Examples of such questions include the following: What is it like for smokers to lose a loved one to lung cancer? What is the process by which previous smokers succeeded in quitting? In nursing, the term **metasynthesis** has predominated as the term for qualitative evidence synthesis, usually referring to syntheses that are interpretive.

Metasynthesis

Over a decade ago, five leading thinkers on qualitative integration used the term *metasynthesis* as an umbrella term that broadly represented "a family of methodologic approaches to developing new knowledge based on rigorous analysis of existing qualitative research findings" (Thorne et al., 2004, p. 1343). Just as there are many different approaches to doing qualitative research, there are diverse approaches to doing a metasynthesis and to defining what it is.

There is more agreement on what a metasynthesis is *not* than on what it *is*. Metasynthesis is not a literature review—a summary of research findings—or is it a concept analysis. Schreiber and colleagues (1997) offered a definition of what metasynthesis *is*, ". . . the bringing together and breaking down of findings, examining them, discovering the essential features and, in some way, combining phenomena into a transformed whole" (p. 314). Most metasynthesis methods involve a transformational process.

Preliminary Steps in a Metasynthesis

Formulation of the Problem

In a metasynthesis, researchers begin with a broad research question or an investigative focus. Booth and colleagues (2018) have described the research question in an aggregative review as an "anchor," but it is more like a "compass" in interpretive reviews. The research question may evolve during the course of the review—it may not be evident at first whether the initial question can be answered, or whether the scope of the review should be expanded or contracted. It is sometimes useful to involve relevant stakeholders in the problem-framing stage of a review. In their reports, metasynthesists sometimes state an overall study purpose rather than a research question.

> **Example of a statement of purpose in a metasynthesis** • • • • • • • • • • • • • • • • •
> Holmen and an interprofessional team (2020) stated the purpose of their metasynthesis as follows: "The present systematic review of qualitative empirical studies aims to provide an in-depth insight regarding how HCPs [health care professionals] experience working with patients with chronic diseases" (p. 3).

> **TIP** Having a team of at least two researchers to design and implement a metasynthesis is often advantageous because of the subjective nature of interpretive efforts. Investigator triangulation is one strategy for enhancing the integrity of metasyntheses.

Development of Sampling and Search Strategies

Metasynthesists must make sampling decisions. One issue is whether the sample of studies will be exhaustive (i.e., including all relevant studies) or purposive. Some approaches to metasynthesis, notably meta-ethnography, may involve purposive strategies in which studies are selected for conceptual purposes. Another issue is whether to include findings from only peer-reviewed journals. An advantage of including alternative sources is that journal articles have page constraints. Finfgeld (2003) noted that in her metasynthesis on *courage*, she used dissertations even when a peer-reviewed journal article was available from the same study because the dissertation had richer information. Metasynthesists must also decide whether to search for studies about a phenomenon in a single versus multiple qualitative traditions.

It is generally more difficult to find qualitative than quantitative studies using mainstream approaches such as searching electronic databases. For example, "qualitative" became a medical subject heading (MeSH) term in MEDLINE in 2003, but it is risky for reviewers to assume that all qualitative studies (e.g., ethnographies) are coded as qualitative.

> **TIP** Sample sizes in nursing metasyntheses are highly variable, ranging from 5 or fewer studies to over 100. Sample size varies as a function of the scope of the inquiry, the extent of prior research, and the type of metasynthesis undertaken. One guideline for sampling adequacy is whether categories in the metasynthesis are saturated.

Evaluations of Study Quality

In general, there is less emphasis on assessing the quality of primary studies in interpretive syntheses than in aggregative ones. Nevertheless, critical appraisal is often used in metasyntheses, sometimes simply to describe the sample of studies in the review but in other cases to make sampling decisions.

Not everyone agrees that study quality should be a criterion for study inclusion. Some have argued that a flawed study does not necessarily invalidate the rich data from those studies. Noblit and Hare (1988), whose meta-ethnographic approach is widely used by nurse researchers, advocated including all relevant studies but suggested giving more weight to higher quality studies. Many nurse researchers use the 10-question assessment tool from the Critical Appraisal Skills Programme (CASP) of the Centre for Evidence-Based Medicine in the United Kingdom.

Example of evaluations and sampling decisions in a metasynthesis • • • • • • •
Wigert and colleagues (2020) conducted a metasynthesis of studies that focused on women's experiences of fear in childbirth. They searched for relevant studies from all qualitative traditions. After excluding 64 studies that had low quality ratings, the 14 primary studies in their review included grounded theory, phenomenology, and descriptive qualitative research.

Extraction of Data

Information about various features of the study need to be abstracted and coded, such as data source information (e.g., year of publication), sample characteristics, and methodological features (e.g., research tradition). Most important, the study findings must be extracted and recorded—typically the key themes, metaphors, or categories from each study.

However, *finding* the findings is not always easy. Qualitative researchers intermingle data with interpretation and findings from other studies with their own. Noblit and Hare (1988) advised that, just as primary study researchers must read and reread their data before they can proceed with their analysis, metasynthesists must read the primary studies multiple times to fully grasp the categories or metaphors being described.

Data Analysis and Interpretation in Metasynthesis

Strategies for metasynthesis diverge most markedly at the analysis stage. We briefly describe two approaches. Regardless of approach, metasynthesis is a complex interpretive task that involves "carefully peeling away the surface layers of studies to find their hearts and souls in a way that does the least damage to them" (Sandelowski et al., 1997, p. 370).

The Noblit and Hare Approach

Noblit and Hare (1988), whose approach is called **meta-ethnography**, argued that integration should be interpretive and not aggregative—i.e., that the synthesis should focus on constructing interpretations rather than descriptions. Their approach includes seven phases that overlap and repeat as the metasynthesis progresses. The first three phases occur before the analysis: (1) deciding on the phenomenon, (2) deciding which studies are relevant for the synthesis, and (3) reading and rereading each study. Phases 4 through 6 concern the analysis:

- *Phase 4*: deciding how the studies are related. In this phase, the researcher lists the key metaphors (or themes/concepts) in each study and their relation to each other. Studies can be related in three ways: *reciprocal* (directly comparable), *refutational* (in opposition to each other), or in a *line of argument* rather than reciprocal or refutational.
- *Phase 5*: translating the qualitative studies into one another. Noblit and Hare (1988) noted that "translations are especially unique syntheses because they protect the particular, respect holism, and enable comparison. An adequate translation maintains the central metaphors and/or concepts of each account in their relation to other key metaphors or concepts in that account" (p. 28).
- *Phase 6*: synthesizing translations. Here, the challenge for the researcher is to make a whole into more than the individual parts imply.

The final phase in the Noblit and Hare (1988) approach involves writing up the synthesis.

Example of Noblit and Hare's approach •
Fernández-Basanta and colleagues (2020) used Noblit and Hare's (1988) approach in their meta-ethnography of 14 studies focused on the coping experiences of parents following perinatal loss. Five themes described the parents' coping strategies, and the themes were synthesized into the metaphor *Staying afloat in the storm*.

The Sandelowski and Barroso Approach

Sandelowski and Barroso (2007) dichotomized integration efforts based on the degree of synthesis and interpretation in the primary studies. Primary studies are called *summaries* if they yield descriptive synopses of the qualitative data, usually with lists and frequencies of themes. *Syntheses*, by contrast, are more interpretive and involve conceptual or metaphorical reframing. Sandelowski and Barroso have argued that only syntheses should be used in a metasynthesis.

Both summaries and syntheses can, however, be used in a **meta-summary**, which can lay a foundation for a metasynthesis. Sandelowski and Barroso (2007) provided an example of a meta-summary, using studies of mothering within the context of HIV infection. The first step, extracting findings, resulted in almost 800 sentences from 45 reports and represented a comprehensive inventory of findings. The 800 sentences were then reduced to 93 thematic statements, or abstracted findings.

The next step involved calculating **manifest effect sizes**, i.e., effect sizes calculated from the manifest content pertaining to mothering in the context of HIV, as represented in the 93 abstracted findings. (Qualitative effect sizes should not be confused with effects in a meta-analysis.) Two types of effect size can be created. A **frequency effect size**, indicating the *magnitude* of the findings, is the number of reports that contain a given finding, divided by all reports (excluding those with duplicated findings from the same data). For example, Sandelowski and Barroso (2007) calculated an overall frequency effect size of 60% for the finding of mothers' struggle about disclosing their HIV status to their children. In other words, 60% of the 45 primary studies had a finding of this nature.

An **intensity effect size** indicates the concentration of findings *within* each study. It is calculated by computing the number of different findings in a given report, divided by the total number of findings in all reports. As an example, one primary study in Sandelowski and Barroso's (2007) meta-summary had 29 out of the 93 total findings, for an intensity effect size of 31%.

Metasyntheses can build upon meta-summaries but require findings that are more interpretive, i.e., from studies characterized as syntheses. The purpose of a metasynthesis is not to summarize but to offer novel interpretations of qualitative findings. Such interpretive integrations require metasynthesists to piece the individual syntheses together to craft a new coherent explanation of a target event or experience.

Example of Sandelowski and Barroso's approach •

Dam and Hall (2016) conducted a meta-summary to understand children's experiences living with a parent with severe mental illness. The findings of 22 qualitative studies were synthesized into the overarching theme of navigating in an unpredictable everyday life, which was composed of three subthemes of "being a responsible and worrying carer," "concealing," and "coping." Each subtheme was further classified into three to four categories. Intrastudy intensity effect sizes for the categories ranged from 66% to 100%. Interstudy frequency effect sizes ranged from 45% to 81%.

Meta-Aggregation

The Joanna Briggs Institute uses an aggregative approach to the synthesis of qualitative evidence that is highly structured. JBI maintains that regardless of whether the evidence is quantitative or qualitative, the same review process should be used, with certain steps tailored to accommodate the special nature of the findings. The JBI **meta-aggregation** method is aimed at delivering synthesized findings to inform clinical decision making or policy development.

The JBI reviewer's manual (Aromataris & Munn, 2017) offers guidance on preparing a *qualitative evidence synthesis* using meta-aggregation. Researchers at JBI also prepared a series of articles describing their approach that appeared in *The American Journal of Nursing* in 2014 (e.g., Munn et al., 2014; Stern et al., 2014). In this section, we briefly mention a few issues relating to the JBI approach.

Preliminary Steps in a Joanna Briggs Institute Qualitative Evidence Synthesis

In a meta-aggregation, an explicit review question is formulated upfront. JBI recommends using the PICo format (**P**opulation, phenomenon of **I**nterest, **Co**ntext) for articulating the question (Stern et al., 2014). Reviewers are expected to do comprehensive searching for relevant evidence, including a search of the grey literature. Data are extracted by two independent reviewers using a JBI extraction form, in which findings and a supporting quote from the study's raw data are recorded.

Quality appraisals of the studies are undertaken using the 10-item JBI Critical Appraisal Checklist for Qualitative Research. In addition to appraising each study for its overall methodological quality, the JBI approach calls for ratings of the *credibility* of each finding in a study. Reviewers assign a rating of *unequivocal* (a finding is beyond a reasonable doubt), *credible* (finding is open to challenge), and *unsupported* (findings not supported by the data).

Analysis Through Meta-Aggregation

Data synthesis using meta-aggregation is a three-step process that begins with the extraction of findings and illustrations from all included studies. In the second step, findings that are sufficiently similar or related conceptually are collapsed into categories. Each category must have two or more findings. In the final step, the reviewers develop one or more synthesized finding that encompass at least two categories. Reviewers are expected to explain what data they considered as a "finding," the process by which findings were identified, and how findings were grouped to create categories.

Munn et al. (2014) illustrated a meta-aggregation of qualitative evidence on how patients experience high-technology medical imaging like magnetic resonance imaging (MRI) scans. Three *findings* were "an alien experience," "being in another world," and "swallowed and sinking," and these were grouped into the *category* "out of this world, alien experience." A *synthesized finding* derived from this and three other categories was "Scanning is a unique, out-of-this world experience that must be experienced by the person to be truly understood" (p. 53).

Assessment of Confidence

Inspired by the GRADE rating system for quantitative reviews, a working group at JBI developed a system to rate confidence in the synthesized findings of a QES. The *ConQual* approach, as it is called, requires a score—on a scale from 4 (high) to 1 (very low)—summarizing the reviewers' confidence in each finding. A synthesized qualitative finding is given an initial score of "high" that can be downgraded because of low credibility (e.g., a mix of unequivocal and credible findings results in the loss of a point) or low dependability. The dependability score is based on answers to five specific questions from the JBI critical appraisal tool.

 TIP   A separate effort was undertaken by a group working with GRADE to develop a means of rating confidence in the findings from a qualitative evidence synthesis—*GRADE-CERQual* (Lewin et al., 2018). Although ConQual and CERQual develop similar rankings, the criteria for scoring in the two systems differ.

CRITICAL APPRAISAL OF SYSTEMATIC REVIEWS

Like all studies, systematic reviews should be thoroughly appraised before the findings are deemed trustworthy and useful in clinical practice. Box 17.1 offers some guidelines for evaluating systematic reviews. We have distinguished questions about analysis separately for quantitative and qualitative reviews. The list of questions is not necessarily comprehensive—supplementary questions might be needed for particular types of review.

Box 17.1 Guidelines for Critically Appraising Systematic Reviews

The Problem
- Did the report state the research problem and/or research questions? Is the scope of the project appropriate? Was the approach to integration described, and was the approach appropriate?

Search Strategy
- Did the report describe criteria for selecting primary studies, and are the criteria reasonable?
- Were the bibliographic databases used by the reviewers identified, and are they appropriate and comprehensive? Were search terms identified?
- Did the reviewers use adequate supplementary efforts to identify relevant studies?

The Sample
- Were inclusion and exclusion criteria clearly articulated?
- Did the search strategy yield a good sample of studies?

Quality Appraisal
- Did the reviewers appraise the quality of the primary studies? Did they use a well-defined set of criteria or a validated quality appraisal scale?
- Did two or more people do the appraisals, and was interrater agreement reported?
- Was quality information used effectively in selecting studies or analyzing results?

Data Extraction
- Was adequate information extracted about the study design, sample characteristics, and study findings?
- Were two or more people used to extract and record information for analysis?

Data Analysis—General
- Did the reviewers explain their method of pooling and integrating the data?
- Were tables, figures, and text used effectively to summarize findings?

Data Analysis—Quantitative
- If a meta-analysis was not performed, was there adequate justification for using narrative integration? If a meta-analysis *was* performed, was this justifiable?
- For meta-analyses, did the report describe how effect sizes were computed?
- Was heterogeneity of effects assessed? Was the decision to use a random effects model versus a fixed effects model sound? Were subgroup analyses undertaken—or was the absence of subgroup analyses justified?

Data Analysis—Qualitative
- Was the analytic approach mainly aggregative or interpretive?
- In a metasynthesis, did the reviewers describe the techniques they used to compare the findings of each study, and did they explain their method of interpreting their data?
- In a metasynthesis, did the synthesis achieve a fuller understanding of the phenomenon to advance knowledge? Do the interpretations seem well-grounded?
- In a meta-aggregation, does the integration of findings into categories and categories into synthesized findings appear insightful and justifiable?

Box 17.1 Guidelines for Critically Appraising Systematic Reviews *(Continued)*

Conclusions
- Did the reviewers draw reasonable conclusions about their results and about the quality of evidence relating to the research question?
- Did the reviewers use GRADE or another system to rate confidence in the review findings?
- Were limitations of the review/synthesis noted?
- Were implications for nursing and health care practice and further research clearly stated?

All systematic reviews   Systematic reviews of quantitative studies   Metasyntheses

In drawing conclusions about a research synthesis, a major issue concerns the nature of the decisions the reviewers made. Sampling decisions, approaches to handling quality of the primary studies, and analytic approaches should be carefully evaluated. In quantitative reviews, the review team should provide a good rationale if a meta-analysis was not undertaken. Reviewers of qualitative studies should explain why they chose to use a primarily interpretive or aggregative approach.

A thorough discussion section is important in systematic reviews. The discussion should include the reviewers' assessment about the strengths and limitations of the body of evidence, suggestions on further research needed to improve the evidence base, and the implications of the review. Critical appraisals should result in envisioning whether and how clinicians could use the evidence in their practice.

RESEARCH EXAMPLES WITH CRITICAL THINKING EXERCISES

We conclude this chapter with a description of two systematic reviews, one with a meta-analysis and one with a metasynthesis. Read the summaries and then answer the critical thinking questions that follow, referring to the full research report if necessary. Answers to the questions for Exercises 1 and 2 are available to instructors on thePoint®. Additionally, a meta-analysis and a metasynthesis appear in their entirety in the *Study Guide* that accompanies this book.

EXAMPLE 1: A META-ANALYSIS

Study: Outcomes of nurse practitioner-led care in patients with cardiovascular disease: A systematic review and meta-analysis (Smigorowsky et al., 2020)

Purpose: The purpose of the systematic review was to assess the impact of nurse practitioner–led cardiovascular (CV) care on patient outcomes, as evaluated in trials that compared the nurse practitioner (NP) model of care to other care models (typically physician-led care).

Eligibility Criteria: A primary study was considered eligible for the systematic review if it met the following criteria (with PICO elements identified): (1) The study used an RCT design to assess the impact of NP-led CV care (I) versus CV care by another health care provider (C); (2) the participants in the trial had to be older than 18 years of age and diagnosed with a CV disease (P); (3) the outcomes of care (O) had be associated with NP-led care specific to the setting and research focus—outcomes such as symptoms (e.g., angina), monitored risk factor reduction variables (e.g., blood pressure), health care system quality (e.g., length of stay), and patient-reported outcomes (e.g., quality of life); and (4) the studies were published in English between 2007 and 2017.

Search Strategy: A search for primary studies was undertaken in seven bibliographic databases (e.g., CINAHL, MEDLINE, EMBASE). Numerous search terms were used, including the MeSH terms *cardiovascular disease*, *atrial fibrillation*, *nurse practitioner*, *coronary artery disease*, and *hypertension*. Additional search methods were used, including ancestry searching, with the assistance of a reference librarian. The reviewers included an appendix that detailed their full search strategy.

Sample: The analysis was based on a sample of 5 studies that met all eligibility criteria: 2 from Canada, 2 from the United States, and 1 from the Netherlands. Initially, 1,563 studies were identified in the electronic search, 958 of which were duplicates and removed. After reviewing titles, another 539 studies were excluded, and a further 56 studies were removed after abstract reviews. The sample sizes for the 5 included studies ranged from 48 to 330 patients, for a total of 887 patients.

Quality Appraisal: The reviewers used the Cochrane risk of bias approach for six domains: random sequence generation, allocation concealment, blinding of outcome assessment; attrition; selective reporting; and other bias. Studies were then categorized on whether they had low risk of bias (at risk in zero to one domain), moderate risk (at risk in two to three domains), or high risk (at risk in four to six domains). Overall, two studies were categorized as low risk, two were moderate risk, and one was high risk of bias.

Data Extraction: Two reviewers independently extracted data; disagreements were resolved by consensus. The extracted data included publication information, sample size, number of patients per group, CV care area; NP role; and associated outcomes of care. Identified outcomes for a meta-analysis included 30-day readmission rate for heart failure, length of stay after cardiac surgery, and patients' scores on a quality of life scale called SF-36, which yields separate physical and mental health scores. One outcome (vascular risk reduction) was available in only one study and was not analyzed in a meta-analysis.

Effect Size Calculation: Odds ratios were used as the effect size index for some outcomes (e.g., 30-day readmission for heart failure), and Cohen's *d*—the standardized mean difference—was used for other outcomes (e.g., length of stay postsurgery, scores on the SF-36).

Statistical Analyses: The researchers found evidence of significant statistical heterogeneity for one outcome (mental health subscale scores). They used a random effects model for their main analysis, in which the effect sizes were weighted by the study sample size. Because there were only five studies in the review, no subgroup analyses were undertaken.

Key Findings: There were no statistically significant differences in effect sizes for NP-led care versus other CV care for 30-day readmissions, length of stay, and scores on the two quality of life subscales. For example, the mean difference for length of stay was −.89, 95% CI = −2.44, 0.66. In the narrative review of vascular risk reduction, the one available study found a 12% reduction in the Framingham risk score for NP-led care. The reviewers also used GRADE to assess confidence in the evidence. In their appraisal, the quality of evidence was low for the absence of an effect for 30-day readmissions, and moderate for other outcomes included in the meta-analysis.

Discussion: The reviewers concluded that, despite the rigorous search and analysis methods used in this systematic review, the findings should be considered inconclusive because of the limited number of relevant primary studies and the moderate-to-high risk of bias in all but two studies. They stated that "[i]t is extremely important for further high-quality research to be conducted to identify clinical outcomes of care associated with NP-led CV care as a model of care" (p. 92).

Critical Thinking Exercises

1. Answer the relevant questions from Box 17.1 regarding this study.
2. How might the nonsignificant effects be interpreted?

EXAMPLE 2: A META-ETHNOGRAPHY

Study: Experiences of people taking opioid medication for chronic non-malignant pain: A qualitative evidence synthesis using meta-ethnography (Nichols et al., 2020)

Purpose: The purpose of this qualitative evidence synthesis was to integrate evidence on the experience of taking opioid medication for chronic nonmalignant pain (CNMP) or coming off the opioids. The protocol for the review was published in PROSPERO.

Eligibility Criteria: A study was included if it (1) used qualitative methods, (2) was published in English in a peer-reviewed journal, (3) included adults (age 18+ years) who were taking or had taken opioid medication in the previous 5 years, and (4) reported patient perspectives on using opioid medication for nonmalignant pain. The researchers placed no limits based on publication date, country of origin, or research tradition.

Search Strategy: A search of seven electronic databases was undertaken by one reviewer, with the assistance of an academic librarian (e.g., CINAHL, MEDLINE, Scopus, PsycINFO). Search terms included MeSH terms for all opioid drugs as well as their generic names. Their search included *qualitative* as well as words used to describe all types of qualitative research. The reviewers included a supplementary appendix detailing their search terms and combinations. Forward citation searches were also conducted. Citations were screened independently by two researchers against the eligibility criteria. Any disagreements were resolved by a third researcher.

Sample: The report presented a flow chart showing the researchers' sampling progression. Of the 5,064 citations initially identified through database searching, a total of 2,129 were screened, and then 153 full-text articles were assessed for eligibility. After removing 122 studies that were not eligible, a total of 31 studies were included in the meta-ethnography. The included studies were from the United States, Canada, the United Kingdom, and Australia.

Quality Appraisal: The researchers used the CASP tool for appraisal of the included studies. One reviewer critically appraised all studies, and another reviewer independently appraised 10% for a consistency check. CASP scores for each included study were shown in a table in the review. The team also used the GRADE-CERQual approach to appraise the reviewers' confidence in the research findings.

Data Analysis: The analysis was based on Noblit and Hare's (1988) meta-ethnographic approach. The lead reviewer read all studies, and two others shared reading all studies. All reviewers extracted concepts independently. The three reviewers met to discuss their extractions and reached agreement. The concepts were sorted into categories, and the categorizations were discussed by all three. Patterns and associations between categories were examined, and a line of argument approach was deemed to be the most useful method of interpreting the data.

Key Findings: The reviewers identified five themes: (1) Reluctant users with little choice, (2) Understanding opioids: the good and the bad, (3) A therapeutic alliance: not always on the same page, (4) Stigma: feeling scared and secretive but needing support, and (5) The challenge of tapering or withdrawal. An overarching theme of "constantly balancing" emerged in their analysis. Using the

GRADE-CERQual system, the reviewers found no major concerns in terms of confidence in the review findings. Minor concerns were noted for the fifth theme regarding the challenge of withdrawal.

Discussion: The reviewers noted that the themes had positive and negative aspects that illustrate "how complex it is for patients to balance decisions at every stage of their journey" (p. 13). The reviewers stated that the findings "demonstrate that the stigma surrounding how patients feel about being on opioids can be compounded by the judgements of others" (p. 13).

Critical Thinking Exercises

1. Answer the relevant questions from Box 17.1 regarding this study.
2. Do you think the researchers should have included non–peer-reviewed studies in their review? Why or why not?
3. What might be some of the uses to which the findings could be put in clinical practice?

WANT TO KNOW MORE?

A wide variety of resources to enhance your learning and understanding of this chapter is available on thePoint.

- Chapter Supplement on Using GRADE in Systematic Reviews
- Internet Resources with useful websites for Chapter 17
- A Wolters Kluwer journal article on a topic related to this chapter

Additional study aids, including eight journal articles and related questions, are also available in *Study Guide for Essentials of Nursing Research, 10e.*

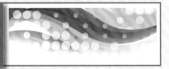

Summary Points

- Evidence-based practice relies on rigorous integration of research evidence through systematic reviews. A **systematic review** involves the methodical and transparent integration of findings from multiple **primary studies** about a specific research question using careful sampling and data collection procedures that are spelled out in advance in a *protocol.*

- Systematic reviews are undertaken to synthesize quantitative, qualitative, or mixed method evidence. Reviews of quantitative studies often involve statistical integration of findings through **meta-analysis**, a procedure whose advantages include objectivity and enhanced power; meta-analysis is not appropriate, however, for broad questions or when there is substantial inconsistency of findings.

- Major steps in a systematic review typically involve formulating a question, defining eligibility criteria, searching for and selecting primary studies, evaluating study quality, extracting data, analyzing the data, interpreting and evaluating confidence in the findings, and reporting the findings.

- Reviewers are increasingly likely to search for *grey literature*—i.e., unpublished reports. The concern is the risk of **publication bias** that stems from the underrepresentation of nonsignificant findings in published literature.

- In meta-analyses, findings from primary studies are represented by an **effect size (ES)** index that quantifies the relationship between the independent and dependent variables. The most common effect size indexes in nursing are *d* (the *standardized mean difference*), the odds ratio, and correlation coefficients.

- Effects from individual studies are pooled in a meta-analysis to yield an estimate of the population effect size by calculating a weighted average of effects, usually giving greater weight to studies with larger samples.

- **Statistical heterogeneity** (diversity in effects across studies) is a major issue in meta-analysis; it affects decisions about which statistical model to use and whether a meta-analysis is justified. Heterogeneity can be examined visually using a **forest plot**.

- Heterogeneity can be explored through **subgroup analyses**, the purpose of which is to see whether effects systematically vary based on clinical, demographic, or methodological attributes.

- Quality assessments (which may involve formal ratings or risk-of-bias assessments) are sometimes used to exclude weak studies from reviews, but they can also be used to differentially weight studies or to evaluate whether including or excluding weaker studies changes conclusions in a *sensitivity analysis*.

- Systematic reviewers are increasingly likely to use the **GRADE** (Grades of Recommendation, Assessment, Development, and Evaluation) approach to assess the degree of *confidence* that the reviewers have in the estimated effect, for specific outcomes in a review.

- Qualitative systematic reviews have been described as either **aggregative** (in which findings from multiple studies are pooled) or **interpretive** (in which the goal is to discover new or enriched ways of understanding phenomena). Aggregative reviews are often called **qualitative evidence syntheses (QES)**. The umbrella term most often used for interpretive reviews is **metasynthesis**. Many qualitative reviews in nursing have elements of both aggregation and interpretation.

- Metasyntheses are more than just summaries of prior qualitative findings; they involve a discovery of essential features of a body of findings and a transformation that yields new interpretations.

- One approach to metasynthesis is called **meta-ethnography**, which was proposed by Noblit and Hare (1988); this approach involves listing key themes or metaphors across studies and then translating them into each other.

- In the approach of Sandelowski and Barroso (2007), a **meta-summary** involves listing abstracted findings from the primary studies and calculating **manifest effect sizes**. A **frequency effect size** is the percentage of reports that contain a given findings. An **intensity effect size** indicates the percentage of all findings that are contained in any given report. A meta-summary can lay the foundation for a metasynthesis.

- The approach to qualitative evidence synthesis used at the Joanna Briggs Institute (JBI) is **meta-aggregation**, which is more structured than a metasynthesis and relies on comprehensive searching and systematic quality appraisals. In a meta-aggregation, similar findings across studies are grouped into *categories*, which in turn are grouped into *synthesized findings*. In JBI qualitative reviews, confidence in the findings is assessed using a rating system called *ConQual*.

REFERENCES FOR CHAPTER 17

*Amirshahi, M., Behnamfar, N., Badakhsh, M., Rafiemanesh, H., Keikhaie, K., Sheyback, M., & Sari, M. (2020). Prevalence of postoperative nausea and vomiting: A systematic review and meta-analysis. *Saudi Journal of Anesthesia*, *14*, 48–56.

*Aromataris, E., & Munn, Z. (Eds.). (2017). *Joanna Briggs Institute reviewer's manual*. Adelaide, Australia: The Joanna Briggs Institute.

Booth, A., Noyes, J., Flemming, K., Gerhardus, A., Wahlster, P., van der Wilt, G., . . . Rehfuess, E. (2018). Structured methodology review identified seven (RETREAT) criteria for selecting qualitative evidence synthesis approaches. *Journal of Clinical Epidemiology*, *99*, 41–52.

*Chao, A., Roy, A., Franks, A., & Joseph, P. (2020). A systematic review of taste differences among people with eating disorders. *Biological Research for Nursing*, *22*, 82–91.

Dam, K., & Hall, E. (2016). Navigating in an unpredictable daily life: A metasynthesis on children's experiences living with a parent with severe mental illness. *Scandinavian Journal of Caring Sciences*, *30*, 442–457.

Fang, S., Wu, Y., & Tsai, P. (2020). Heart rate variability and risk of all-cause death and cardiovascular events in patients with cardiovascular disease: A meta-analysis of cohort studies. *Biological Research for Nursing*, *22*, 45–56.

Fernández-Basanta, S., Coronado, C., & Movilla-Fernández, M. (2020). Multicultural coping experiences of parents following perinatal loss: A meta-ethnographic synthesis. *Journal of Advanced Nursing*, *76*, 9–21.

Finfgeld, D. (2003). Metasynthesis: The state of the art—so far. *Qualitative Health Research*, *13*, 893–904.

*Gough, D., Thomas, J., & Oliver, S. (2012). Clarifying differences between review designs and methods. *Systematic Reviews*, *1*, 28.

*Guyatt, G., Oxman, A. D., Vist, G., Kunz, R., Falck-Ytter, Y., Alonso-Coello, P., & Schünemann, H. (2008). GRADE: An emerging consensus on rating quality of evidence and strength of recommendations. *BMJ*, *336*, 924–926.

Hannes, K., & Lockwood, C. (2011). Pragmatism as the philosophical foundation for the Joanna Briggs meta-aggregative approach to qualitative evidence synthesis. *Journal of Advanced Nursing*, *67*, 1632–1642.

Higgins, J., Chandler, J., Cumpston, M., Li, T., Page, M., & Welch, V. (Eds.). (2019). *Cochrane handbook for systematic reviews of interventions, Version 6.0*. Chichester, United Kingdom: Wiley & Sons.

*Holmen, H., Larsen, M., Sallinen, M., Thoresen, L., Ahlsen, B., Andersen, M., . . . Mengshoel, A. (2020). Working with patients suffering from chronic diseases can be a balancing act for health care professionals—A meta-synthesis of qualitative studies. *BMC Health Services Research*, *20*, 98.

**Huang, H., Dong, L., & Gu, L. (2020). The timing of urinary catheter removal after gynecologic surgery: A meta-analysis of randomized controlled trials. *Medicine*, *99*(2), e18710.

*Leach, M., Jones, M., Bressington, D., Jones, A., Nolan, F., Muyambi, K., . . . Gray, R. (2020). The association between community mental health nursing and hospital admissions for people with serious mental illness: A systematic review. *Systematic Reviews*, *9*, 35.

*Lewin, S., Booth, A., Glenton, C., Munthe-Kaas, H., Rashidian, A., Wainwright, M., . . . Noyes, J. (2018). Applying GRADE-CERQual to qualitative evidence synthesis findings: Introduction to the series. *Implementation Science*, *13*, 2.

Munn, Z., Tufanaru, C., & Aromataris, E. (2014). JBI's systematic reviews: Data extraction and synthesis. *The American Journal of Nursing*, *114*(7), 49–54.

*Nichols, V., Toye, F., Eldabe, S., Sandhu, H., Underwood, M., & Seers, K. (2020). Experiences of people taking opioid medication for chronic non-malignant pain: A qualitative evidence synthesis using meta-ethnography. *BMJ Open*, *10*, e032988.

Noblit, G., & Hare, R. D. (1988). *Meta-ethnography: Synthesizing qualitative studies*. Newbury Park, CA: Sage.

Sandelowski, M., & Barroso, J. (2007). *Handbook for synthesizing qualitative research*. New York, NY: Springer.

Sandelowski, M., Docherty, S., & Emden, C. (1997). Qualitative metasynthesis: Issues and techniques. *Research in Nursing & Health*, *20*, 365–371.

Schreiber, R., Crooks, D., & Stern, P. N. (1997). Qualitative meta-analysis. In J. M. Morse (Ed.), *Completing a qualitative project* (pp. 311–326). Thousand Oaks, CA: Sage.

*Shaw, R., Larkin, M., & Flowers, P. (2014). Expanding the evidence within evidence-based healthcare: Thinking about the context, acceptability and feasibility of interventions. *Evidence-Based Medicine*, *19*, 201–203.

*Sherifali, D., Ali, M., Markle-Reid, M., Ploeg, J., Valaitis, R., Bartholomew, A., . . . McAiney, C. (2018). Impact of internet-based interventions on caregiver mental health: Systematic review and meta-analysis. *Journal of Medical Internet Research*, *20*, e10668.

*Smigorowsky, M., Sebastianski, M., McMurtry, M., Tsuyuki, R., & Norris, C. (2020). Outcomes of nurse practitioner-led care in patients with cardiovascular disease: A systematic review and meta-analysis. *Journal of Advanced Nursing*, *76*, 81–95.

Stern, C., Jordan, Z., & McArthur, A. (2014). JBI's systematic reviews: Developing the review question and inclusion criteria. *The American Journal of Nursing*, *114*(4), 53–56.

Thorne, S., Jensen, L., Kearney, M., Noblit, G., & Sandelowski, M. (2004). Qualitative metasynthesis: Reflections on methodological orientation and ideological agenda. *Qualitative Health Research*, *14*, 1342–1365.

*Wigert, H., Nilsson, C., Dencker, A., Begley, C., Jangsten, E., Sparud-Lundin, C., . . . Patel, H. (2020). Women's experiences of fear of childbirth: A meta-synthesis of qualitative studies. *International Journal of Qualitative Studies in Health and Well-Being*, *15*, 1704484.

Zhang, X., Li, P., Guo, P., Wang, J., Liu, N., Yang, S., . . . Zhang, W. (2020). Culturally tailored intervention to promote mammography screening practice among Chinese American women: A systematic review. *Journal of Cancer Education*. Advance online publication. doi:10.1007/s13187-020-01730-4.

*A link to this open-access article is provided in the Internet Resources section on thePoint® website.

**This journal article is available on thePoint® for this chapter.

18

Putting Research Evidence Into Practice: Evidence-Based Practice and Practice-Based Evidence

Learning Objectives

On completing this chapter, you will be able to:

- Distinguish research utilization and evidence-based practice (EBP)
- Identify several resources available to facilitate EBP in nursing practice
- Identify several models for implementing EBP
- Discuss the five major steps in undertaking an EBP effort
- Describe some limitations of the current EBP model and discuss the concept of practice-based evidence
- Distinguish generalizability and applicability
- Identify some strategies for enhancing applicability
- Define new terms in the chapter

Key Terms

- AGREE II
- Applicability
- Clinical practice guidelines
- Cochrane Collaboration
- Iowa Model
- Knowledge translation
- Practice-based evidence
- Pragmatic clinical trial
- Precision health care
- Research utilization
- Subgroup analysis
- The 5As

Evidence-based practice (EBP) has been a major force in the health professions for the past few decades. In Chapter 1, we offered some preliminary information about EBP—for example, we described EBP-related research purposes, evidence hierarchies, and the PICO framework for asking well-worded clinical questions. This chapter expands the coverage of EBP and introduces some emerging ideas about how to enhance the production and use of **practice-based evidence**. We begin with some background on EBP.

EVIDENCE-BASED PRACTICE AND RELATED CONCEPTS

As we described in Chapter 1, EBP is usually defined as a decision-making process that incorporates three elements: *best evidence*, *clinical expertise*, and *patient preferences and values*. This definition is fairly well established—and yet, several decades ago, there was little discussion of EBP—and perspectives on EBP are still evolving.

During the 1980s, concern about research utilization began to emerge. **Research utilization (RU)** is the use of findings from a study in a practical application. In RU, the emphasis is on translating new knowledge into real-world applications. EBP is a broader concept than RU because it integrates research findings with other factors, as just noted. Also, whereas RU begins with the research itself (How can I put this new knowledge to use in my clinical setting?), the starting point in EBP typically is a clinical question (What does the evidence suggest is the best approach to solving this clinical problem?).

During the 1980s and 1990s, RU projects were undertaken by numerous hospitals and nursing organizations. These projects were institutional attempts to implement changes in nursing practice based on research findings. During the 1990s, however, the call for RU was superseded by the push for EBP.

The EBP movement originated in the fields of medicine and epidemiology during the 1990s. British epidemiologist Archie Cochrane criticized health care practitioners for failing to incorporate research evidence into their decision making. His work led to the establishment of the **Cochrane Collaboration**, an international partnership with centers established in 43 countries. The Collaboration prepares and disseminates reviews of research evidence and has a goal of making Cochrane "the home of evidence" relating to health care decision making.

Also during the 1990s, a group from McMaster University Medical School in Canada (led by Dr. David Sackett) developed a clinical learning strategy they called *evidence-based medicine*. The evidence-based medicine movement has shifted to a broader conception of using best evidence by all health care practitioners (not just physicians) in multidisciplinary teams. EBP is considered a major shift for health care education and practice. In the EBP environment, a skillful clinician can no longer rely on a repository of memorized information but rather must be a lifelong learner who is adept in accessing, evaluating, and using new evidence.

RU and EBP involve activities that can be undertaken at the level of individual nurses or at a higher organizational level. A related movement mainly concerns system-level efforts to bridge the gap between knowledge generation and use. **Knowledge translation** (KT) is a term that is often associated with efforts to enhance systematic change in clinical practice. The World Health Organization (WHO) (2005) has defined KT as "the synthesis, exchange, and application of knowledge by relevant stakeholders to accelerate the benefits of global and local innovation in strengthening health systems and improving people's health."

 TIP   *Translational science* has emerged as a discipline devoted to developing methods to promote knowledge translation. Translational science involves the study of interventions, implementation processes, and contextual factors that affect the uptake of new evidence in health care practice. In nursing, the need for translational research was an impetus for the development of the Doctor of Nursing Practice degree.

RESOURCES FOR EVIDENCE-BASED PRACTICE IN NURSING

Resources to support EBP are increasingly available. We offer some guidance in this section and urge you to explore other ideas with your mentors and health information experts.

Preprocessed and Pre-Appraised Evidence

Searching for best evidence requires skill, especially because of the accelerating pace of evidence production. Thousands of primary studies of relevance to nurses are published each month in professional journals, but they are not pre-appraised for quality or clinical utility.

Fortunately, finding evidence useful for practice is often facilitated by the availability of evidence sources that are preprocessed (synthesized) and sometimes pre-appraised.

DiCenso and colleagues (2009) have created a "6S" hierarchy of evidence *sources*, which is intended as a guide to evidence retrieval. On the first rung above primary studies are synopses of single studies, followed by systematic reviews, and then synopses of systematic reviews. Clinical practice guidelines are near the top of the hierarchy. At each successive step in the hierarchy, there is greater ease in applying the evidence to clinical practice. We described various types of systematic reviews in the previous chapter, so here we focus on clinical practice guidelines.

Evidence-based **clinical practice guidelines** distill a body of evidence into a usable form. Unlike systematic reviews, clinical practice guidelines (which often are *based* on systematic reviews) give specific recommendations for evidence-based decision making. Guideline development typically involves the consensus of a group of researchers, experts, and clinicians. The use or adaptation of a clinical practice guideline is often a good focus for an EBP project.

Finding clinical practice guidelines can be challenging, however, because there is no single guideline repository. A standard search in bibliographic databases such as MEDLINE will yield many references—including a mixture of citations not only to the actual guidelines but also to commentaries and implementation studies.

A recommended approach is to search in guideline databases or through specialty organizations that have sponsored guideline development. For example, in the United States, nursing and health care guidelines are maintained by the National Guideline Clearinghouse (www.guideline.gov). An important nursing guideline resource comes from the Registered Nurses' Association of Ontario (RNAO) (www.rnao.org/bestpractices).

There are many topics for which practice guidelines have not yet been developed, but the opposite problem is also true: Sometimes, there are multiple guidelines on the same topic. Worse yet, because of differences in the rigor of guideline development and interpretation of evidence, different guidelines may offer different or even conflicting recommendations. Thus, those who wish to adopt clinical practice guidelines should appraise them to identify ones that are based on the strongest evidence, have been meticulously developed, are user-friendly, and are appropriate for local use or adaptation.

Several appraisal instruments are available to evaluate clinical practice guidelines. One with broad support is the Appraisal of Guidelines Research and Evaluation (AGREE) instrument, now in its second version (Brouwers et al., 2010). The **AGREE II** instrument has ratings for 23 dimensions within six domains (e.g., scope and purpose, rigor of development, presentation). As examples, a dimension in the scope and purpose domain is "The population (patients, public, etc.) to whom the guideline is meant to apply is specifically described"; and one in the rigor of development domain is "The guideline has been externally reviewed by experts prior to its publication." The AGREE tool should be applied to a guideline by a team of two to four appraisers. For those interested in learning more about the AGREE II instrument, we offer more information in the chapter supplement on thePoint®.

Example of using AGREE II •••••••••••••••••••••••••••••••••••••••
Zhao and colleagues (2020) conducted a systematic review of clinical practice guidelines on uncomplicated birth. Two reviewers independently assessed 11 clinical practice guidelines using the AGREE II instrument. Two guidelines, including one by the WHO, were deemed to have the highest quality.

 TIP The GRADE system for appraising the confidence in systematic review findings, as described in Chapter 17, is increasingly used in the development of clinical practice guidelines.

Models of the Evidence-Based Practice Process

EBP models offer frameworks for designing and implementing EBP projects in practice settings. Some models focus on the use of research by individual clinicians (e.g., the *Stetler Model*, one of the oldest models that originated as an RU model), but most focus on institutional EBP efforts (e.g., the Iowa Model). The many worthy EBP models are too numerous to list comprehensively but include the following:

- Advancing Research and Clinical Practice Through Close Collaboration (ARCC) Model (Melnyk & Fineout-Overholt, 2019)
- Diffusion of Innovations Model (Rogers, 1995)
- Iowa Model of Evidence-Based Practice to Promote Quality Care (Buckwalter et al., 2017; Titler et al., 2001)
- Johns Hopkins Nursing Evidence-Based Practice Model (Dearholt & Dang, 2012)
- Promoting Action on Research Implementation in Health Services (PARIHS) Model (Harvey & Kitson, 2016; Rycroft-Malone et al., 2013)
- Stetler Model of Research Utilization (Stetler, 2010)

For those considering undertaking an EBP effort who wish to follow a formal EBP model, the cited references should be consulted. Several models are also nicely synthesized by Melnyk and Fineout-Overholt (2019), and Schaffer and colleagues (2013) identify features to consider in selecting a model to plan an EBP project. Each model offers different perspectives on how to translate research findings into practice, but several steps and procedures are similar across the models. Figure 18.1 shows a diagram of one prominent EBP model, the revised **Iowa Model** of Evidence-Based Practice (Buckwalter et al., 2017).

> **Example of using an evidence-based practice model** • • • • • • • • • • • • • • • • • • •
> Saqe-Rockoff and colleagues (2018) used the Iowa Model in their EBP project designed to improve thermoregulation for trauma patients in the emergency department. Their article appears in its entirely in this book's *Study Guide* (available for separate purchase).

> **TIP** Several models of EBP distinguish two broad types of stimulus ("triggers") for undertaking an EBP endeavor: (1) *problem-focused triggers*, which are clinical practice problems identified as needing a solution and (2) *knowledge-focused triggers*, which come from readings in the research literature and thus is more akin to research utilization.

INDIVIDUAL AND ORGANIZATIONAL EVIDENCE-BASED PRACTICE

Individual nurses make many decisions and convey important health care information and advice to patients, so they have ample opportunity to put research into practice. Here are three clinical scenarios that provide examples of such opportunities:

- Clinical scenario 1. You work in an allergy clinic and notice how difficult it is for many children to undergo allergy scratch tests. You wonder if an interactive distraction intervention would help reduce children's anxiety when they are being tested.
- Clinical scenario 2. You work in a rehabilitation hospital and one of your elderly patients, who had total hip replacement, tells you she is planning a long airplane trip to visit her daughter after rehabilitation treatments are completed. You know that a long plane ride

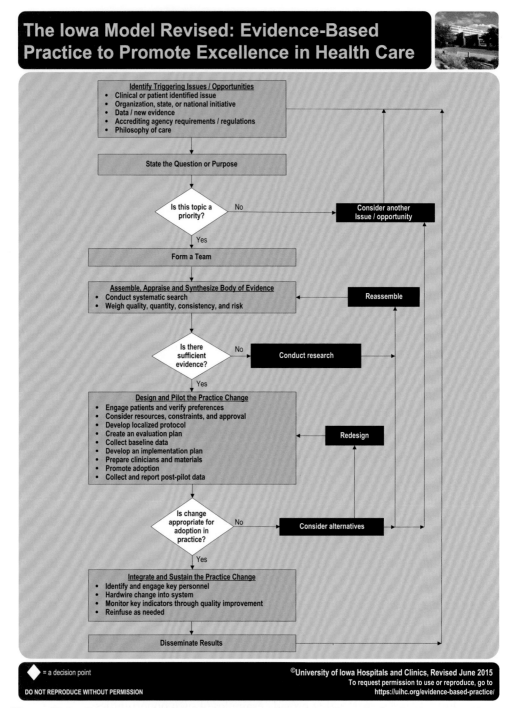

Figure 18.1   Revised Iowa Model of Evidence-Based Practice to Promote Quality Care. Iowa Model Collaborative. (2017). Iowa model of evidence-based practice: Revisions and validation. *Worldviews on Evidence-Based Nursing, 14*(3), 175–182. doi:10.1111/wvn.12223. Used/reprinted with permission from the University of Iowa Hospitals and Clinics, copyright 2015. For permission to use or reproduce, please contact the University of Iowa Hospitals and Clinics at 319-384-9098.

will increase her risk of deep vein thrombosis and wonder if compression stockings are an effective in-flight treatment for her. You decide to look for the best evidence to answer this question.

- Clinical scenario 3. You are caring for a hospitalized cardiac patient who tells you that he has sleep apnea. He confides in you that he is reluctant to undergo continuous positive airway pressure (CPAP) treatment because he worries it will hinder intimacy with his wife. To enable yourself to better address your patient's concerns, you wonder if there is any evidence you could review about what it is like to experience CPAP treatment.

In these and thousands of other clinical situations, research evidence can be put to good use to improve the quality of nursing care. Thus, individual nurses need to have the skills to personally search for, appraise, and apply evidence in their practice.

For some clinical scenarios that trigger an EBP effort, individual nurses have sufficient autonomy to implement research-informed actions on their own (e.g., answering patients' questions about experiences with CPAP). In other situations, however, decisions are best made by a team of nurses (or an interprofessional team) working together to solve a common clinical problem. Institutional EBP efforts typically result in a formal policy or protocol affecting the practice of many nurses and other staff.

Many of the steps in institutional EBP projects are the same as those we describe in the next section, but additional issues are of relevance at the organizational level. For example, some additional activities include assessing whether the question is an organizational priority, forming a team, and conducting a formal evaluation.

 TIP Organizational EBP projects share features with quality improvement efforts, as described in Chapter 12.

MAJOR STEPS IN EVIDENCE-BASED PRACTICE

In this section, we provide an overview of how research evidence can be put to use in clinical settings. In describing the basic steps in the EBP process, we use a mnemonic device (**the 5As**) that we have adapted from several sources (e.g., Guyatt et al., 2015).

- Step 1: **Ask**: Ask a well-worded clinical question that can be answered with research evidence.
- Step 2: **Acquire**: Search for and retrieve the best evidence to answer the clinical question.
- Step 3: **Appraise**: Critically appraise the evidence for validity and applicability to the problem and situation.
- Step 4: **Apply**: After integrating the evidence with clinical expertise, patient preferences, and local context, apply it to clinical practice.
- Step 5: **Assess**: Evaluate the outcome of the practice change.

The EBP process cannot be undertaken in a vacuum, however. A precondition for the entire undertaking is to have an openness to change and a desire to provide the best possible care, based on evidence showing benefits to patient outcomes. Melnyk and Fineout-Overholt (2019) call this Step 0: cultivating a spirit of inquiry. Johnson and Fineout-Overholt (2005) noted that "getting from zero to one" involves having nurses be reflective about their clinical practice. An additional step after Step 5 might be to disseminate information about the EBP project.

Step 1, asking a well-worded question, was described in Chapter 1. We noted that the PICO framework is a widely used system for the wording of clinical questions: (P) Population, (I) Intervention or influence, (C) Comparator to the intervention or influence, and (O) Outcome. We describe features of the other four steps in this section.

Step 2: Acquire Research Evidence

By asking clinical questions in a well-worded form, you should be able to more effectively search the research literature for the information you need. Using the templates we provided in Table 1.3, the information inserted into the blanks constitutes *keywords* for undertaking an electronic search of important bibliographic databases.

We noted earlier in this chapter that pre-appraised sources can be used to facilitate an efficient search for evidence. Starting with pre-appraised evidence might lead you to a quick answer—and potentially to a better answer than would be possible if you had to start with individual studies. Researchers who prepare systematic reviews and synopses usually have excellent research skills and use established standards to evaluate the evidence. Thus, when preprocessed evidence is available to answer a clinical question, you may not need to look any further, unless the review is not recent or is of poor quality. When high-quality preprocessed evidence cannot be located or is old, you will need to look for best evidence in primary studies, using strategies we described in Chapter 6.

 TIP The free Internet resource PubMed offers a special tool for those seeking evidence for clinical decisions. Guidance on conducting a clinical query search is provided in the supplement to Chapter 6 on thePoint®. Another important database, CINAHL, allows users to restrict a search with an "evidence-based practice" limiter.

Step 3: Appraise the Evidence

The evidence acquired in Step 2 of the EBP process should be appraised before taking clinical action. Critical appraisal for EBP may involve several types of assessments. Various criteria have been proposed for EBP appraisals, including the following:

1. *Quality*: To what extent is the evidence valid—how serious is the risk of biases?
2. *Magnitude*: How large is the effect of the intervention or influence (I) on the outcome (O) in the population of interest (P)? Are the effects clinically significant?
3. *Quantity*: How much evidence is there? How many studies have been conducted, and did those studies involve a large number of participants?
4. *Consistency*: How consistent are the findings across various studies?
5. *Applicability*: To what extent is the evidence relevant to my clinical situation and patients?

Evidence Quality

The first appraisal issue is the extent to which the findings in a research report are valid. That is, were the study methods sufficiently rigorous that the evidence has a low risk of bias? Melnyk and Fineout-Overholt (2019) propose the following formula: level of evidence (LOE) from an evidence hierarchy (e.g., Fig. 1.2) + quality of evidence = strength of evidence. Thus, in coming to a conclusion about the quality of the evidence, it is insufficient to simply "level" the evidence using an LOE scale—it must also be appraised. Systematic reviews with a GRADE score of "high confidence" yield evidence of especially high quality. If there are several primary studies and no existing systematic review, you yourself would need to draw conclusions about the body of evidence taken as a whole.

Magnitude of Effects

The appraisal criterion relating to magnitude considers how powerful the effects of an intervention or influence are. Estimating the magnitude of the effect for quantitative findings is especially important when an intervention is costly or when there are potentially negative side effects. If, for example, there is good evidence that an intervention is only modestly effective in improving a health problem, it is important to consider other factors (e.g., evidence regarding its effects on quality of life). There are various ways to quantify the magnitude of effects, such as an *effect size index*, discussed in Chapter 13. The magnitude of effects also has a bearing on *clinical significance*, as we discussed in Chapter 14.

Quantity and Consistency of Evidence

A rigorously conducted primary study of a randomized controlled trial (RCT) offers especially strong evidence about the effect of an intervention on an outcome of interest. But *multiple* RCTs are better than a single study. Large-scale studies (such as multisite studies) with a large number of study participants are especially desirable.

   If there are multiple studies that address your clinical query, however, the strength of the evidence is likely to be diminished if there are inconsistent results across studies. In the GRADE system, inconsistency of results leads to a lower quality-of-evidence grade. When the results of different studies do not corroborate each other, it is likely that further research will have an impact on confidence about an intervention's effect.

Applicability

It is also important to appraise the evidence in terms of its relevance for the clinical situation at hand—that is, for *your* patient in a specific clinical setting. Best practice evidence can most readily be applied to an individual patient in your care if he or she is similar to people in the study or studies under review. Would your patient have qualified for participation in the study—or is there some factor such as age, illness severity, or comorbidity that would have excluded him or her? Practitioners must reach conclusions about the applicability of research evidence, but researchers also bear some responsibility for enhancing the applicability of their work. We discuss applicability at greater length later in this chapter.

 TIP   An appraisal of evidence for use in your practice may involve additional factors. In particular, costs are likely to be an important consideration. Some interventions are expensive, and so the amount of resources needed to put best evidence into practice would need to be factored into any decision. Of course, the cost of *not* taking action is also important.

Actions Based on Evidence Appraisals

Appraisals of the evidence may lead you to different courses of action. You may reach this point and conclude that the evidence is not sufficiently sound, or that the likely effect is too small, or that the cost of applying the evidence is too high. The evidence may suggest that "usual care" is the best strategy. If, however, the initial appraisal of evidence suggests a promising clinical action, then you can proceed to the next step.

Step 4: Apply the Evidence

As the definition for EBP implies, research evidence needs to be integrated with your own clinical expertise and knowledge of your clinical setting. You may be aware of factors that would make implementation of the evidence, no matter how sound or promising, inadvisable. Patient preferences and values are also important. A discussion with the patient may reveal negative attitudes toward a potentially beneficial course of action, contraindications (e.g., comorbidities), or possible impediments (e.g., lack of health insurance).

Armed with rigorous evidence, your own clinical know-how, and knowledge about your patient's circumstances, you can use the resulting information to make an evidence-based decision or provide research-informed advice. Although the steps in the process, as just described, may seem complicated, in reality, the process can be efficient—*if* there is an adequate evidence base, and especially if it has been skillfully preprocessed. EBP is most challenging when findings from research are contradictory, inconclusive, or "thin"—that is to say, when better quality evidence is needed.

One final issue is the importance of integrating evidence from qualitative research, which can provide rich insights about how patients experience a problem, or about barriers to complying with a treatment. A new intervention with strong potential benefits may fail to achieve desired outcomes if it is not implemented with sensitivity and understanding of the patients' perspectives. As Morse (2005) so aptly noted, evidence from an RCT may tell you whether a pill is effective, but qualitative research can help you understand why patients may not swallow the pill.

Step 5: Assess the Outcomes of the Practice Change

One last step in many EBP efforts concerns evaluating the outcomes of the practice change. Did you achieve the desired outcomes? Were patients satisfied with the results?

Straus and colleagues (2011) remind us that part of the ongoing evaluation involves how well you are performing EBP. They offer self-evaluation questions that relate to the EBP steps, such as asking answerable questions (Am I asking any clinical questions at all? Am I asking well-formulated questions?) and acquiring external evidence (Do I know the best sources of current evidence? Am I becoming more efficient in my searching?).

EVIDENCE-BASED PRACTICE AND PRACTICE-BASED EVIDENCE

The EBP movement has made enduring contributions to the well-being of human beings. Clinicians no longer rely exclusively on a repository of knowledge acquired during their training—they are expected to be relentless learners who seek and use evidence from rigorous studies about how best to address pressing health problems.

Yet, EBP has limitations that are not always acknowledged. In particular, concerns have been expressed that EBP fails to provide "evidence to guide decisions in clinical care for individual patients" (Horwitz & Singer, 2017). Several commentators have noted that high-quality patient care requires practice-based evidence—evidence that is developed in real-world settings and is responsive to the needs and circumstances of specific patients and contexts (Horwitz et al., 2017; Sacristán & Dilla, 2018). In this section, we briefly point out some limitations of the current model of EBP with respect to the applicability of research findings for clinical decision making.

Evidence-Based Practice and Population Models of Evidence

EBP is based on evidence about *populations* of people. Systematic reviews of RCTs, at the pinnacle of evidence hierarchies, are the cornerstone of EBP. Yet, systematic reviews of RCTs cannot affirm that *all* patients receiving an effective intervention will benefit from it—only that the "average" patient in a specified population probably would. Clinicians, however, do not treat "average" patients—they care for people with varying and distinctive traits, preferences, and health risks.

Subramanian and colleagues (2018) were especially eloquent about this issue, noting that inferences about *average treatment effects* can be misleading or even harmful when responses to an intervention diverge—a situation called *heterogeneity of treatment effects* (HTE). They noted that the "average patient" is a construct, not a reality, and provided some evidence for their claim that "most people taking RCT-validated, effective treatments derive no benefit from them" (p. 78). Universal treatment effects should seldom be assumed. It is not that trial information about average effects is unimportant, but it is often insufficient. For an individual patient, the average effect is of little interest—an intervention either is or is not beneficial for that patient.

Average treatment effects, such as the ones estimated in systematic reviews, are problematic from another perspective: Averages strip away *context*. Context shapes how interventions get implemented and influences their effectiveness. However, population models of EBP provide context-free conclusions about the delivery of effective care.

Evidence-Based Practice and External Validity

In Chapter 8, we noted the tensions between efforts to enhance a study's internal validity (inferences that an intervention *caused* an effect) and external validity (inferences that causal claims generalize across persons, settings, and time). Strategies to reduce threats to internal validity tend to negatively impact external validity, and vice versa.

Researchers who seek to generate evidence for practice have traditionally resolved the tension between internal and external validity in favor of internal validity. Evidence hierarchies, for example, rank study designs based on their ability to eliminate threats to internal validity; external validity is ignored. In systematic reviews, evaluations of study quality and confidence in the findings (GRADE) focus on internal rather than external validity.

Traditional RCTs undermine the generalizability of the results in diverse ways. RCTs have typically been conducted under ideal conditions rather than in normal, real-world situations. All aspects of the study are tightly controlled, including what the exact intervention is, who the interventionists are, where the study takes place, and who participates in the study.

Sampling in RCTs is particularly troublesome for generalizing the results. To reduce confounding, trialists tend to impose exclusion criteria that eliminate key groups of people—often, older people and those with comorbidities, who might especially benefit from, or be harmed by, the intervention under study. This problem is compounded by low rates of participation in RCTs, with refusal rates sometimes approaching 90%. The bottom line is that patients in general usually are very different from ones included in RCTs.

The combined effect of relying on a population model of average effects and using data from highly select study participants is that EBP is often based on evidence of whether an intervention works for a hypothetical "average" patient under ideal, context-neutral conditions. Although the RCT results may be unbiased from an internal validity standpoint, they may be less useful than one would hope in making decisions about individual patients who are neither "ideal" nor "average."

Generalizability, Applicability, and Relevance

The terms *generalizability* and *applicability* have often been used interchangeably, but there is a growing view that they are distinct (Sacristán & Dilla, 2018). *Generalizability* is a term associated with populations—researchers identify characteristics of a population to which their findings might reasonably be generalized.

We define **applicability** as the degree to which research evidence can be applied to individuals, small groups of individuals, or local contexts. Applicability is relevant to clinical decision making because of human heterogeneity—averages are not of much value as decision guides if there is wide diversity in whether an intervention works or how it is viewed, experienced, adhered to, or incorporated into normal life. Sacristán & Dilla (2018) noted, "As health care decisions are becoming more patient centric, the term 'applicability' should evoke 'individual patient' rather than 'average patient'" (p. 165).

New ideas are emerging about how to enhance applicability, generalizability, and relevance. In the context of practice-based evidence, we define *relevance* as evidence that is important to key stakeholders and has the potential to be actionable. **Patient-centered research**, which focuses on developing evidence that is meaningful and valuable to patients, involves efforts to attain relevance.

New Directions in Health Care Research

Concern about the limitations of current models of EBP for guiding decisions about individuals in real-world contexts has led to the emergence of new ideas and innovative methods for *optimizing* evidence. Efforts at optimization have taken shape under various formulations, such as *precision health care, personalized health care*, and *patient-centered health care*. Research in these domains has gone in broadly similar directions but with different emphases. Such research typically strives for evidence that is practice-based.

In this section, we describe a few strategies that researchers are using to enhance the applicability of their research findings. We encourage you to think about the benefits of such strategies when you are critically appraising research evidence.

Comparative Effectiveness Research

Comparative effectiveness research (CER), described briefly in Chapter 12, is an important manifestation of emerging directions in health care research. CER emphasizes patient-centeredness and involves direct comparisons of clinical interventions to facilitate decision making. As noted by Greenfield and Kaplan (2012), "CER calls for substantial changes in the way clinical research is conducted, interpreted, and practically applied . . . the evolving CER paradigm requires . . . innovations that address three basic questions: what works? for whom? and in whose hands?" (p. 263).

The Institute of Medicine's (2009) report on priorities for CER offered six defining characteristics of CER:

1. *CER's objective is to directly inform clinical decisions.* CER places a high value on the ability to generalize results to real-world decision making. A broad range of relevant stakeholders and decision makers (including patients) should be included in setting priorities, designing studies, and implementing results.
2. *CER involves comparisons of two or more alternative treatments, each of which has potential to be "best practice."* CER avoids the use of placebos, attention controls, or no intervention as comparators in testing an intervention.
3. *CER seeks evidence at both the population and the subgroup level.* A goal of CER is to help providers and patients in individualizing decisions—going beyond "average effects" to effects for people with similar characteristics.
4. *CER uses outcomes that are important to patients.* CER strives to include and give weight to patient-reported outcomes and to attend to benefits, harms, and unintended consequences of health care interventions.
5. *CER uses diverse research designs and methods.* Some comparative effectiveness studies involve experimental designs, but CER also uses other designs, including nonexperimental (observational) approaches.
6. *CER is conducted in real-world settings.* CER studies the effectiveness of interventions in settings similar to those where an intervention would actually be used.

These characteristics of CER diverge in important respects from the research model that has come to be established under EBP, which focuses on internal validity and adheres firmly to evidence from RCTs. Note that these characteristics of CER embody concerns about generalizability (no. 1), applicability (no. 3), and relevance (no. 4).

Pragmatic Clinical Trials

As we noted, features of traditional RCT designs are so tightly controlled that the relevance of the findings to real-life situations can be questioned. Concern about this problem has led to interest in **pragmatic clinical trials (PCTs)**, which have features designed to maximize external validity with minimal negative effect on internal validity (Ford & Norrie, 2016). Tunis and colleagues (2003), in a seminal paper, defined pragmatic (practical) clinical trials as "trials for which the hypotheses and study design are formulated based on information needed to make a decision" (p. 1626). Thus, pragmatic trials are consistent with the goals of CER.

 TIP *Pragmatism* as a construct can be applied in most studies. As noted by Sacristán & Dilla (2018), pragmatism is not so much a design type but a "mindset"—pragmatic attitudes can be used in all types of research.

Compared to more traditional *explanatory trials* conducted under optimal conditions with carefully selected participants, PCTs address practical questions about the benefits and risks of an intervention—as well as its costs—as they would unfold in routine clinical practice. Tunis and coauthors (2003) made these recommendations for PCTs: enrollment of diverse populations with fewer exclusions of high-risk patients, recruitment of participants from a variety of practice settings, follow-up over a longer period, inclusion of economic outcomes, and comparisons of clinically viable alternatives.

Trials cannot readily be categorized as *pragmatic* or *explanatory* because they do not represent a dichotomy—pragmatism can be conceptualized as being on a continuum. A tool called *PRECIS-2* (**PR**eferred **E**xplanatory **C**ontinuum **I**ndicator **S**ummary) has been developed to help researchers evaluate how pragmatic their trial is and to help ensure that their designs are congruent with their intended aims (Loudon et al., 2015). The tool covers nine domains (e.g., patient eligibility, patient recruitment), each of which is rated from 1 (very explanatory) to 5 (very pragmatic). For example, the question for the eligibility domain is, "To what extent are the participants in the trial similar to those who would receive this intervention if it was part of usual care?"

Example of the use of PRECIS-2 ●
Nguyen and colleagues (2018) described the application of the PRECIS-2 tool for the design and implementation of a pragmatic clinical trial of physical activity coaching for patients with chronic obstructive pulmonary disease (COPD) in a real-world setting. They described the tool as "a useful guide for organizing decisions about study designs and implementation approaches to help diverse stakeholders recognize the compromises between internal and external validity with those decisions" (p. 455).

The most promising (and widely used) designs for PCTs include *cluster randomization* (randomization of groups rather than individuals) and delayed treatment designs (everyone gets the intervention eventually). When a delay-of-treatment strategy is combined with cluster randomization, the result is a *stepped wedge design*, which involves having clusters randomized to receive the intervention at different points (Battaglia & Glasgow, 2018).

PCTs protect internal validity by using familiar bias-reducing strategies such as randomization, allocation concealment, and blinding. Moreover, cluster randomized pragmatic trials can promote internal validity by guarding against contamination of treatments. However, pragmatic trials can suffer from certain problems that are not present in traditional explanatory trials. One issue, for example, is that the interventions are usually less standardized in different real-world settings, perhaps resulting in differential "dosing" of the intervention and different degrees of intervention fidelity.

TIP Nurse researchers have demonstrated growing interest in pragmatic clinical trials. A methods conference at the 2017 meeting of the Council for the Advancement of Nursing Science was devoted to pragmatic trials; a special issue of *Nursing Outlook* included several papers based on conference presentations. In that issue, Battaglia and Glasgow (2018) asserted that pragmatic research "is an area of tremendous opportunity for the nursing science community" (p. 430).

Subgroup Analyses

Some researchers try to develop evidence that is applicable to well-defined groups of people (rather than to entire populations) by conducting subgroup analyses. A **subgroup analysis** involves efforts to disentangle HTEs for subpopulations of people. For example, a subgroup analysis might suggest that an intervention is effective for men but not for women, or more effective for people with comorbidities than for those without them.

Subgroup analyses, which are intuitively appealing to those interested in individualizing care, are often undertaken in the context of RCTs. Evidence suggests that the rate of subgroup analysis is increasing perhaps because of its prominence in CER.

Subgroup analyses are, however, controversial, in part because they are frequently not undertaken properly (e.g., Sun et al., 2014). The struggle between wanting to go beyond population averages on the one hand and the statistical challenges of subgroup analysis on the other was described by renowned clinical epidemiologist Alvan Feinstein as a "clinico-statistical tragedy" (Feinstein, 1998, p. 297).

The statistical challenge in subgroup analyses involves addressing the strong risk of both Type I and Type II errors. False positives (Type I errors) are common because researchers often test multiple subgroups without making adjustments to probabilities. The probability of a false positive might be 5% for one test, but for three independent tests, the risk is 14%. This problem has resulted in many reported subgroup effects that could not be replicated. Potential subgroup effects are also at high risk of being missed because of a Type II error. If a study is adequately powered for the entire sample, it will often be underpowered when the sample is divided into subgroups.

Because of increased interest in personalized health care, the number of scholarly papers devoted to subgroup analyses and HTE has burgeoned in recent years. Advice for those who conduct subgroup analyses includes adopting strategies such as the following:

- *Specifying hypotheses in advance.* Subgroup analysis should be a hypothesis-testing effort, not a fishing expedition. Hypotheses about differential effects should be based on sound theoretical reasoning, biological plausibility, or previous empirical evidence.
- *Restricting the number of subgroup analyses.* Burke and colleagues (2015) argued that only rarely should more than one or two primary subgroup analyses be performed—the risk of a false positive increases as the number of tests goes up.
- *Avoiding severely underpowered subgroup analyses.* When subgroup analyses are planned, greater power for the overall analyses should likely be used to estimate sample size needs (e.g., 90% rather than the standard 80%).
- *Basing the analyses on variables defined at baseline.* Subgroup analyses should be based on baseline characteristics, not on ones that emerge during the study (e.g., length of intensive care unit [ICU] stay). Frequently used variables for subgroup analyses in medical RCTs include risk factors for the outcome (e.g., smoking status, disease severity, comorbidity), sex, and age (Gabler et al., 2016).
- *Analyzing for subgroup differences using tests for interactions.* Most analyses for subgroup effects are done incorrectly (e.g., Gabler et al., 2016). The typical approach is to test for intervention effects *within* each subgroup—for example, testing intervention-control group differences separately for men and women—and then comparing the results.

However, such analyses could lead to erroneous conclusions—for example, the differences might simply be the result of differential subgroup sample sizes. The question that should be addressed is *Are subgroup treatment effects significantly different from each other?* The appropriate analysis (too complex to explain here) is to test for an *interaction* between the treatment variable and the subgroup variable.

Because the risk of statistical errors is high, it is wise to be cautious in interpreting subgroup results. The most convincing evidence for a subgroup effect comes from replicated results—especially if the effect is supported by a persuasive biological or theoretic rationale. Corroboration can occur in the context of a systematic review.

Example of a subgroup analysis •
Bowen and an interdisciplinary team (2016) conducted a comparative effectiveness study that involved randomizing 150 adults with type 2 diabetes to either an attention control group or to one of two alternative diabetes self-management nutrition education approaches. The researchers prespecified a subgroup analysis: They hypothesized that patients with a baseline hemoglobin A_{1C} (HbA_{1C}) between 7% and 10% would be most likely to benefit from educational interventions. Using appropriate tests of interaction, the researchers found that, 6 months after baseline, patients with moderately uncontrolled diabetes had improved HbA_{1C} in both intervention groups, which "may allow improved targeting" (p. 1374) of the interventions.

Precision/Personalized Health Care

A fundamental tenet of **precision health care** (a term sometimes used interchangeably with *personalized health care* or *stratified health care*) is that interventions can be individually tailored to people based on their unique genetic, physiological, behavioral, lifestyle, and environmental profile. The goal is not necessarily to develop a unique treatment for every individual but rather to tailor interventions for those with tightly grouped biological and other features—moving beyond what is possible with subgroup analyses. Personalized health care is being driven by advances in molecular genomics and is heavily dependent on data linkages and integration, data analytics, and machine learning for the identification of patterns in large datasets (big data).

The term *precision health care* has been strongly connected with advances in genomics, but a wide range of biomarkers, data from electronic health records, and data from wearable sensors are examples of data with relevance to precision health care. This suggests the inevitability of complex statistical models that will be needed for mapping dynamic factors that affect individual health.

At present, precision health care is only an emerging aspiration rather than a broad reality (Fröhlich et al., 2018), and many challenges remain. However, precision science is advancing rapidly, which bodes well for improving targeted and efficient health care with high levels of applicability. Hickey and colleagues (2019) provide a description of the Nursing Science Precision Health Model.

Concluding Thoughts on Practice-Based Evidence

The push for EBP has led to impressive improvements in health care in all health disciplines, and ongoing commitment to EBP is warranted. However, for maximum benefit, efforts to generate evidence based on population models will have to be integrated with evidence for individualized care.

Several forces in health research are converging to encourage greater demand for and interest in evidence that is patient-centered, practice-based, and personalized. These include frustration about the limitations of the traditional EBP model on the part of many clinicians, the growth of interest in and funding for CER, and the emerging excitement over opportunities that will become available through precision health care research.

New challenges and new rewards are in store for those who wish to facilitate patient-centered care based on patient-centered evidence. Thus, the overall message in this concluding chapter is to think about the applicability and relevance of research findings when coming to conclusions about "best evidence" in your context.

TIP Every nurse can play a role in using research evidence. Here are some strategies:

- *Read widely and critically.* Professionally accountable nurses keep abreast of research developments relating to their specialty by reading professional journals.
- *Attend professional conferences.* Conference attendees have opportunities to meet researchers and to explore practice implications of new research.
- *Insist on evidence that a procedure is effective.* Every time nurses or nursing students are told about a standard nursing procedure, they have a right to ask: Why? Nurses should expect that the clinical decisions they make are based on sound, evidence-based rationales.
- *Become involved in a journal club.* Many organizations that employ nurses sponsor journal clubs that review studies with potential relevance to practice.
- *Pursue and participate in EBP projects.* Several studies have found that nurses who are involved in research activities (e.g., an EBP project or data collection activities) develop more positive attitudes toward research and better research skills.

CRITICAL APPRAISAL OF APPLICABILITY, RELEVANCE, AND GENERALIZABILITY

Box 18.1 provides a few suggestions for those who wish to consider whether researchers have provided sufficient information for coming to conclusions about a study's relevance, applicability, and generalizability.

Box 18.1 Guidelines for Critically Appraising a Study's Generalizability, Applicability, and Relevance*

1. Were patients or other stakeholders involved in codesigning the study? In what way were they involved (e.g., identifying the research question, designing the study, disseminating or using the results)?
2. Did the researchers mention that the study was comparative effectiveness research? If the study was a clinical trial, what was the comparator?
3. If the study was a clinical trial, where on the pragmatic-to-explanatory continuum did the trial lie? To what extent was the study conducted in "real-world" circumstances with a broad range of study participants? Did the researchers claim that the trial was pragmatic?
4. What are some of the constraints on the generalizability of the results? For example, could the study context limit generalizability? Do the eligibility criteria for the sample constrain generalizability? Did a high percentage of people invited to participate in the study decline?
5. Were subgroup effects examined? If yes, were the subgroup analyses done properly (e.g., a priori hypotheses of a small number of subgroup effects; appropriate test for interaction)?
6. Did the discussion section of the report adequately address the issues of generalizability, applicability, and relevance?

*These questions are primarily relevant for quantitative or mixed methods studies, especially for trials of an intervention.

In many cases, the researchers' lack of attention to the issues discussed in the section on practice-based evidence might be disappointing. The absence of information on applicability may reflect page constraints in the journal. It may also reflect the fact that most researchers use conventional standards in preparing their articles—standards that have not taken applicability into account. Moreover, the peer review of most articles is undertaken by researchers who may not yet be attuned to changes taking place in health care research. We hope that in the future, researchers will do more to help clinicians answer questions about relevance, applicability, and generalizability.

RESEARCH EXAMPLES WITH CRITICAL THINKING EXERCISES

This section presents brief summaries of two studies completed by nurse researchers relevant to the content of this chapter. Example 1 describes an evidence-based practice project and Example 2 describes a pragmatic clinical trial. Read the research summaries for these two examples and then answer the critical thinking questions that follow, referring to the full research reports if necessary. Answers to Exercises 1 and 2 are available to instructors on thePoint® website.

EXAMPLE 1: AN EVIDENCE-BASED PRACTICE PROJECT

Study: Implementation of the MEDFRAT to promote quality care and decrease falls in community hospital emergency rooms (McCarty et al., 2018)

Purpose: An interprofessional team undertook an evidence-based practice (EBP) implementation project at a health care delivery system with 12 emergency departments (EDs). The focus of the project was to decrease falls in community hospital EDs.

Framework: The project used the Iowa Model as its guiding framework. The EBP team identified a clinical problem on which to focus—the inconsistent use of fall risk assessments and variation in falls in the EDs.

Approach: The project team assembled relevant literature to identify an appropriate assessment tool for use in EDs. The team selected the Memorial Emergency Department Fall-Risk Assessment Tool (MEDFRAT) because it was simple to use (only six questions) and had been validated for use in EDs. The tool creates two risk stratification levels, and each has suggested fall risk prevention interventions. For example, possible interventions included hourly rounding, bed in low position, bedside alarms, and locating patients into view of the nurses' station. Information systems staff built the MEDFRAT into the electronic medical record. The team then created and implemented a 1-hour education session about falls for nurses in the EDs, and 60 nurses attended the sessions. The participating nurses offered feedback and further suggestions. Several nurses mentioned the lack of bedside alarms, so portable alarms were ordered. Another suggestion concerned the use of different colored grip socks to identify patients at high risk of a fall. Overall, the nurses' reactions to MEDFRAT were unanimously positive.

Evaluation: The MEDFRAT has been implemented in all 12 EDs in the system. McCarty's (2020) team collected fall-related data for a 1-year period before and a 1-year period after implementing MEDFRAT. They reported preliminary outcomes on the screening and fall rate in the 12 months following the implementation. They found that MEDFRAT use varied by hospital, ranging from less than 1% to 95% of patients, but in general documentation of fall risk assessments increased from the pre-MEDFRAT period. Unfortunately, however, increased assessments did not result in decreased falls.

Conclusions: The authors of the report concluded that the Iowa Model was a useful framework for their EBP project. They suggested that qualitative data would help them to better understand the circumstances surrounding falls and to pursue other fall-prevention strategies.

Critical Thinking Exercises

Consider the following targeted questions, which may assist you in assessing aspects of the study's merit:

1. What would you say was the clinical question on which the EBP team focused? (Use the PICO framework).
2. What type of trigger was the impetus for the project?
3. What are the merits and limitations of the design used to evaluate MEDFRAT?

EXAMPLE 2: PRAGMATIC CLINICAL TRIAL

Study: The ACHRU-CPP versus usual care for older adults with type-2 diabetes and multiple chronic conditions and their family caregivers: Study protocol for a randomized controlled trial (Markle-Reid et al., 2017)

Background: An interdisciplinary team in Canada has developed a program of research called the Aging, Community and Health Research Unit (ACHRU). The research program, which is devoted to research on the promotion of optimal aging at home for older adults with multimorbidities, is described as patient oriented and devoted to interagency and intersectoral partnerships with community-based agencies, policy makers, and health and social service agencies (Markle-Reid et al., 2018).

Program Objectives: The research program has numerous objectives, some of which include (1) the codesign of integrated and person-centered interventions with older adults, family/friend caregivers, and providers; (2) the assessment of newly designed interventions; (3) the examination of intervention context and implementation barriers and facilitators; and (4) the development of patient-oriented research strategies. Three pragmatic clinical trials are being undertaken, one of which is described here. (The protocol for another trial has also been published: Markle-Reid et al., 2019).

Trial Description: The research team is undertaking the implementation and testing of an intervention for older adults with type 2 diabetes and multiple comorbidities and their family caregivers. The intervention, a 6-month interprofessional, nurse-led program to promote self-management for older patients and to provide support to their caregivers, is being implemented through a community partnership program (CPP). The multicomponent intervention, involving in-home visits and group meetings, will be delivered by nurses and dietitians in coordination with partnering community organizations. Each client is considered "a key member of the care team and is fully engaged in the development of a care plan that is tailored to their individual needs and preferences" (p. 6). The intervention was pilot tested and then modified based on feedback from clients and interventionists.

Methods: The ACHRU-CPP intervention will be tested in two Canadian provinces. The plan is to enroll 160 participants, who will be randomly assigned to either the program or to usual care. The trial design is mixed methods and pragmatic: The program will be implemented under real-world conditions in community settings, including participants' homes. The intervention is being implemented in "two different jurisdictions and multiple sites" (p. 12). The inclusion criteria "were designed to be minimally stringent in order to facilitate the broad applicability of the results . . . " (p. 5). The sample size was calculated to detect a minimally important difference in the primary outcome. The primary outcome is the change in clients' physical functioning; secondary outcomes included self-efficacy and changes in mental functioning. Caregiver outcomes include quality of life and depressive symptoms. A wide range of implementation outcomes will be monitored. Qualitative data will be collected to examine program implementation and team collaboration. The researchers will also undertake subgroup analyses to identify which clients benefit most from the treatment. Subgroup hypotheses were not stated, but several possible subgroup variables were identified (e.g., based on age, gender, number of comorbidities). The subgroup analyses will be conducted for the primary outcome using interaction terms.

Critical Thinking Exercises

Answer the relevant questions in Box 18.1 regarding this study.

WANT TO KNOW MORE?

A wide variety of resources to enhance your learning and understanding of this chapter is available on thePoint.

- Chapter Supplement on Evaluating Clinical Practice Guidelines—AGREE II
- Internet Resources with useful websites for Chapter 18
- A Wolters Kluwer journal article on a topic related to this chapter

Additional study aids, including eight journal articles and related questions, are also available in *Study Guide for Essentials of Nursing Research, 10e.*

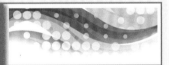
Summary Points

- Two underpinnings of the evidence-based practice (EBP) movement are the **Cochrane Collaboration** (which is based on the work of British epidemiologist Archie Cochrane) and the clinical learning strategy called *evidence-based medicine* developed at the McMaster University Medical School.

- **Research utilization (RU)** and EBP are overlapping concepts that concern efforts to use research as a basis for clinical decisions, but RU *starts* with a research-based innovation that gets evaluated for possible use in practice.

- **Knowledge translation (KT)** is a term used primarily about system-wide efforts to enhance systematic change in clinical practice or policies. *Translational science* is a discipline devoted to developing methods to promote KT and the use of evidence.

- Resources to support EBP are growing at a phenomenal pace. Preprocessed (synthesized) and pre-appraised evidence is especially useful for addressing clinical queries. Evidence-based **clinical practice guidelines** are a major example of pre-appraised evidence. Clinical practice guidelines should be carefully and systematically appraised; for example, using the Appraisal of Guidelines Research and Evaluation (**AGREE II**) instrument.

- Many models of EBP have been developed, including models that provide a framework for individual clinicians (e.g., the *Stetler model*) and others for organizations or teams of clinicians (e.g., the **Iowa Model** of Evidence-Based Practice to Promote Quality Care).

- Although organizational projects include additional steps, the most basic steps in EBP for both individuals and teams are as follows (**the 5As**): *Ask* a well-worded clinical question; *Acquire* the best evidence to answer the question; *Appraise* and synthesize the evidence; *Apply* the evidence, after integrating it with patient preferences and clinical expertise; and *Assess* the effects of the practice change.

- The EBP movement has made significant contributions to health care worldwide. However, a variety of forces is combining to demand greater attention to **practice-based evidence**—*patient-centered evidence* from real-world settings that is responsive to the needs of specific patients and local contexts.

- The standard EBP model is based on evidence about populations of people; it relies heavily on results from randomized controlled trials (RCTs)—which, when integrated in systematic reviews, yield *average treatment effects* within the population of interest.

- *Generalizability* concerns the ability to extrapolate evidence from samples to a specified population. **Applicability** is the degree to which research evidence can be applied to individuals, small groups of individuals, or local contexts.

- *Relevance*, in the context of this discussion, is the degree to which research evidence is important to key stakeholders and has the potential to be actionable. A key strategy for developing practice-based evidence is to involve stakeholders as cocreators of the research process.

- RCTs are seldom designed with the goals of generalizability or applicability in mind. In traditional *explanatory trials*, researchers value internal validity at the expense of external validity and typically focus on average effects at the expense of understanding *heterogeneity of treatment effects* (HTE)—individual variation in response to interventions.

- Researchers have begun to address these issues with innovative methodological strategies. In particular, there is growing interest in *comparative effectiveness research*, whose defining characteristics are in line with person-centered research and practice-based evidence.

- Concerns about features of explanatory RCTs (e.g., restrictive eligibility criteria, tight controls) have led to interest in **pragmatic clinical trials** that enroll diverse people from real-world settings and are designed to enhance external validity. The degree to which a trial is "pragmatic" can be evaluated using a tool called *PRECIS-2*.

- **Subgroup analyses** are efforts to disentangle HTEs for subpopulations. Subgroup analyses have been controversial because of risks of both Type I and Type II errors, but guidance for rigorously conducting them has emerged (e.g., prespecification of hypotheses, limiting analyses to a small number of subgroups, testing for interactions).

- Advances in technology and research methods, coupled with increased interest in personalized and precision health care, will likely advance the promise of practice-based and patient-centered evidence and contribute to its applicability.

REFERENCES FOR CHAPTER 18

Battaglia, C., & Glasgow, R. (2018). Pragmatic dissemination and implementation research models, methods and measures and their relevance for nursing research. *Nursing Outlook, 66*, 430–445.

*Bowen, M., Cavanaugh, K., Wolff, K., Davis, D., Gregory, R., Shintani, A., ... Rothman, R. (2016). The diabetes nutrition education study randomized controlled trial: A comparative effectiveness study of approaches to nutrition in diabetes self-management education. *Patient Education and Counseling, 99*, 1368–1376.

*Brouwers, M., Kho, M., Browman, G., Burgers, J., Cluzeau, F., Feder, G., ... Zitzelsberger, L. (2010). AGREE II: Advancing guideline development, reporting and evaluation in health care. *CMAJ, 182*, E839–E842.

Buckwalter, K., Cullen, L., Hanrahan, K., Kleiber, C., McCarthy, A., Rakel, B., ... Tucker, S. (2017). Iowa model of evidence-based practice: Revisions and validation. *Worldviews on Evidence-Based Nursing, 14*, 175–182.

*Burke, J., Sussman, J., Kent, D., & Hayward, R. (2015). Three simple rules to ensure reasonably credible subgroup analyses. *BMJ, 351*, h5651.

Dearholt, D., & Dang, D. (Eds.). (2012). *Johns Hopkins nursing evidence-based practice: Model and guidelines* (2nd ed.). Indianapolis, IN: Sigma Theta Tau International.

Dicenso, A., Bayley, L., & Haynes, B. (2009). Accessing pre-appraised evidence: Fine-tuning the 5S model into a 6S model. *Evidence-Based Nursing, 12*, 99–101.

Feinstein, A. R. (1998). The problem of cogent subgroups: A clinicostatistical tragedy. *Journal of Clinical Epidemiology, 51*, 297–299.

*Ford, I., & Norrie, J. (2016). The changing face of clinical trials: Pragmatic trials. *New England Journal of Medicine, 375*, 454–463.

*Fröhlich, H., Balling, R., Beerenwinkel, N., Kohlbacher, O., Kumar, S., Lengauer, T., . . . Zupan, B. (2018). From hype to reality: Data science enabling personalized medicine. *BMC Medicine, 16*, 150.

*Gabler, N., Duan, N., Raneses, E., Suttner, L., Ciarametaro, M., Cooney, E., . . . Kravitz, R. (2016). No improvement in the reporting of clinical trial subgroup effects in high-impact general medical journals. *Trials, 17*, 320.

*Greenfield, S., & Kaplan, S. (2012). Building useful evidence: Changing the clinical research paradigm to account for comparative effectiveness research. *Journal of Comparative Effectiveness Research, 1*, 263–270.

Guyatt, G., Rennie, D., Meade, M., & Cook, D. (2015). Users' guides to the medical literature: A manual for evidence-based clinical practice (3rd ed.). New York, NY: McGraw-Hill Education.

*Harvey, G., & Kitson, A. (2016). PARIHS revisited: From heuristic to integrated framework for the successful implementation of knowledge into practice. *Implementation Science, 11*, 33.

Hickey, K., Bakken, S., Byrne, M., Bailey, D., Demiris, G., Docherty, S., . . . Grady, P. (2019). Precision health: Advancing symptom and self-management science. *Nursing Outlook, 67*, 462–475.

Horwitz, R., Hayes-Conroy, A., Caricchio, R., & Singer, B. (2017). From evidence based medicine to medicine based evidence. *The American Journal of Medicine, 130*, 1246–1250.

Horwitz, R., & Singer, B. (2017). Why evidence-based medicine failed in patient care and medicine-based evidence will succeed. *Journal of Clinical Epidemiology, 84*, 14–17.

*Institute of Medicine. (2009). *Initial national priorities for comparative effectiveness research*. Washington, DC: National Academies Press.

Johnston, L., & Fineout-Overholt, E. (2005). Teaching EBP: "Getting from zero to one." Moving from recognizing and admitting uncertainties to asking searchable, answerable questions. *Worldviews on Evidence-Based Nursing, 2*, 98–102.

*Loudon, K., Treweek, S., Sullivan, F., Donnan, P., Thorpe, K., & Zwarenstein, M. (2015). The PRECIS-2 tool: Designing trials that are fit for purpose. *BMJ, 350*, h2147.

*Markle-Reid, M., Ploeg, J., Fraser, K., Fisher, K., Akhtar-Danesh, N., Bartholomew, A., . . . Upshur, R. (2017). The ACHRU-CPP versus usual care for older adults with type-2 diabetes and multiple chronic conditions and their family caregivers: Study protocol for a randomized controlled trial. *Trials, 18*, 55.

*Markle-Reid, M., Ploeg, J., Valaitis, R., Duggleby, W., Fisher, K., Fraser, K., . . . Williams, A. (2018). Protocol for a program of research from the Aging, Community and Health Research Unit: Promoting optimal aging at home for older adults with comorbidities. *Journal of Comorbidity, 8*, 1–16.

*Markle-Reid, M., Valaitis, R., Bartholomew, A., Fisher, K., Fleck, R., Ploeg, J., . . . Thabane, L. (2019). Feasibility and preliminary effects of an integrated hospital-to-home transitional care intervention for older adults with stroke and multimorbidity: A study protocol. *Journal of Comorbidity, 9*, 1–22.

McCarty, C., Harry, M., Woehrle, T., & Kitch, L. (2020). Screening and falls in community hospital emergency rooms in the 12 months following implementation of MEDFRAT. *The American Journal of Emergency Medicine, 38*(8), 1686–1687.

*McCarty, C., Woehrle, T., Waring, S., Taran, A., & Kitch, L. (2018). Implementation of the MEDFRAT to promote quality care and decrease falls in community hospital emergency rooms. *Journal of Emergency Nursing, 44*, 280–284.

Melnyk, B. M., & Fineout-Overholt, E. (2019). *Evidence-based practice in nursing and healthcare* (4th ed.). Philadelphia, PA: Lippincott Williams & Wilkins.

Morse, J. M. (2005). Beyond the clinical trial: Expanding criteria for evidence. *Qualitative Health Research, 15*, 3–4.

Nguyen, H., Moy, M., Fan, V., Gould, M., Xiang, A., Bailey, A., . . . Coleman, K. (2018). Applying the pragmatic-explanatory continuum indicator summary to the implementation of a physical activity coaching trial in chronic obstructive pulmonary disease. *Nursing Outlook, 66*, 455–463.

Rogers, E. M. (1995). *Diffusion of innovations* (4th ed.). New York, NY: Free Press.

*Rycroft-Malone, J., Seers, K., Chandler, J., Hawkes, C., Crichton, N., Allen, C., . . . Strunin, L. (2013). The role of evidence, context, and facilitation in an implementation trial: Implications for the development of the PARIHS framework. *Implementation Science, 8*, 28.

*Sacristán, J., & Dilla, T. (2018). Pragmatic trials revisited: Applicability is about individualization. *Journal of Clinical Epidemiology, 99*, 164–166.

Saqe-Rockoff, A., Schubert, F., Ciardiello, A., & Douglas, E. (2018). Improving thermoregulation for trauma patients in the emergency department: An evidence-based practice project. *Journal of Trauma Nursing, 25*, 14–20.

Schaffer, M. A., Sandau, K., & Diedrick, L. (2013). Evidence-based practice models for organizational change: Overview and practical applications. *Journal of Advanced Nursing, 69*, 1197–1209.

Stetler, C. B. (2010). Stetler model. In J. Rycroft-Malone & T. Bucknall (Eds.), *Models and frameworks for implementing evidence-based practice: Linking evidence to action* (pp. 51–77). Malden, MA: Wiley-Blackwell.

Straus, S. E., Glasziou, P., Richardson, W., & Haynes, R. (2011). *Evidence-based medicine: How to practice and teach it* (4th ed.). Toronto, Canada: Churchill Livingstone.

Subramanian, S., Kim, N., & Christakis, N. (2018). The "average" treatment effect: A construct ripe for retirement. A commentary on Deaton and Cartwright. *Social Science & Medicine, 210*, 77–82.

Sun, X., Ioannidis, J., Agoritsas, T., Alba, A., & Guyatt, G. (2014). How to use a subgroup analysis: Users' guide to the medical literature. *JAMA, 311*, 405–411.

Titler, M. G., Kleiber, C., Steelman, V., Rakel, B., Budreau, G., Everett, L., . . . Goode, C. (2001). The Iowa model of evidence-based practice to promote quality care. *Critical Care Nursing Clinics of North America, 13*, 497–509.

Tunis, S. R., Stryer, D., & Clancy, C. (2003). Practical clinical trials: Increasing the value of clinical research for decision making in clinical and health policy. *JAMA, 290*, 1624–1632.

*World Health Organization. (2005). *Bridging the "know-do" gap: Meeting on knowledge translation in global health*. Retrieved from https://www.measureevaluation.org/resources/training/capacity-building-resources/high-impact-research-training-curricula/bridging-the-know-do-gap.pdf

Zhao, Y., Lu, H., Zang, Y., & Li, X. (2020). A systematic review of clinical practice guidelines on uncomplicated birth. *BJOG, 127*(7), 789–797.

---

*A link to this open-access article is provided in the Internet Resources section on thePoint® website.

**This journal article is available on thePoint® for this chapter.

Parents' Use of Praise and Criticism in a Sample of Young Children Seeking Mental Health Services

Stephanie Swenson, BSN, RN, Grace W. K. Ho, PhD, RN, Chakra Budhathoki, PhD, Harolyn M. E. Belcher, MD, MHS, Sharon Tucker, PhD, RN, FAAN, Kellie Miller, & Deborah Gross, DNSc, RN, FAAN

Stephanie Swenson, Registered Nurse, Children's National Medical Center, Washington, DC.

Grace W. K. Ho, Morton and Jane Blaustein Postdoctoral Fellow in Mental Health & Psychiatric Nursing, School of Nursing, Johns Hopkins University, Baltimore, MD.

Chakra Budhathoki, Assistant Professor, School of Nursing, Johns Hopkins University, Baltimore, MD.

Harolyn M.E. Belcher, Director of Research, Center for Child and Family Traumatic Stress at Kennedy Krieger Institute, and Associate Professor of Pediatrics, Johns Hopkins School of Medicine, Baltimore, MD.

Sharon Tucker, Director of Nursing Research, Evidence-Based Practice & Quality, University of Iowa Hospitals & Clinics, Iowa City, IA.

Kellie Miller, Research Coordinator, School of Nursing, Johns Hopkins University, Baltimore, MD.

Deborah Gross, Leonard and Helen Stulman Professor in Mental Health & Psychiatric Nursing, School of Nursing, Johns Hopkins University, Baltimore, MD.

This study was conducted as part of the first author's research honors project while she was a student at Johns Hopkins University School of Nursing. Data are from a larger study supported by a grant from the National Institute for Nursing Research (R01 NR012444) to Drs. Gross and Belcher.

Conflicts of interest: None to report.

Correspondence: Stephanie Swenson, BSN, RN, c/o Deborah Gross, DNSc, RN, FAAN, School of Nursing, Johns Hopkins University, Ste 531, 525 N Wolfe St, Baltimore, MD 21205; e-mail: stephswenson@gmail.com.

0891-5245/$36.00

Copyright © 2016 by the National Association of Pediatric Nurse Practitioners. Published by Elsevier Inc. All rights reserved.

Published online October 30, 2015.

http://dx.doi.org/10.1016/j.pedhc.2015.09.010

ABSTRACT

Parents' use of praise and criticism are common indicators of parent-child interaction quality and are intervention targets for mental health treatment. Clinicians and researchers often rely on parents' self-reports of parenting behavior, although studies about the correlation of parents' self-reports and actual behavior are rare. We examined the concordance between parents' self-reports of praise and criticism of their children and observed use of these behaviors during a brief parent-child play session. Parent self-report and observational data were collected from 128 parent-child dyads referred for child mental health treatment. Most parents reported praising their children often and criticizing their children rarely. However, parents were observed to criticize their children nearly three times more often than they praised them. Self-reported and observed praise were positively correlated ($r_s = 0.32$, $p < .01$), whereas self-reported and observed criticisms were negatively correlated ($r_s = -0.21$, $p < .05$). Parents' tendencies to overestimate their use of praise and underestimate their use of criticism are discussed. J Pediatr Health Care. (2016) 30, 49-56.

KEY WORDS

Parenting, young children, praise, critical statements, parent self-report

Parents are a powerful source of feedback in shaping their young children's behavior and sense of self. It is within these earliest relationships that children first begin to acquire a sense of themselves as capable, competent, and loved (Bohlin, Hagekull, & Rydell, 2000; Bowlby, 1988; Cassidy, 1988). Two common sources of parental feedback used to shape young

Reprinted with permission from Swenson, S., et al. (2016). Parents' use of praise and criticism in a sample of young children seeking mental health services. *Journal of Pediatric Health Care, 30*, 49–56.

331

children's behavior and self-esteem are *praise* (i.e., positive statements designed to reinforce desirable behaviors in children or communicate pleasure with the child) and *criticism* (i.e., negative statements designed to stop or change children's undesirable behavior or communicate displeasure with the child).

> Parents are a powerful source of feedback in shaping their young children's behavior and sense of self.

Praise from parents has been used as a marker of positive parenting behaviors in numerous studies (Breitenstein et al., 2012; Chorpita, Caleiden, & Weisz, 2005; Wahler & Meginnis, 1997). Praise is often accompanied by other parenting behaviors indicative of parental warmth, responsiveness, and nurturance (Furlong et al., 2013). Although the question of whether excessive use of praise can negatively influence children's intrinsic motivation has been debated (Owens, Slep, & Heyman, 2012), substantial research now shows that praise, used strategically, can boost children's feelings of competence and confidence. Therefore, praise remains an important indicator of positive parenting behavior (Brummelman, Thomaes, Orobio de Castro, Overbeek, & Bushman, 2014; Cimpian, 2010; Henderlong & Lepper, 2002; Mueller & Dweck, 1998; Zentall & Morris, 2010).

Parents may use critical statements to express disapproval with their children's behavior or attitude. However, using criticism can undermine their self-esteem, lead to greater child defiance and aggression, and increase the likelihood of their developing behavioral problems (Barnett & Scaramella, 2013; Lorber & Egeland, 2011; Tung, Li, & Lee, 2012; Webster-Stratton & Hammond, 1998). Thus, contrary to parents' expectations, using critical statements to shape child behavior actually may be counterproductive. In clinical studies of young children in mental health treatment, parents who directed more critical statements at their children were also more likely to drop out of treatment (Fernandez & Eyberg, 2009).

Given their salience in child development research, parent training interventions have been designed to increase parents' use of praise and reduce their use of criticisms with their children (Breitenstein et al., 2012; Brotman et al., 2009; Eyberg et al., 2001; Gross et al., 2009). In clinical practice and research, parents' use of praise and criticism is often assessed using parent self-report. However, some investigators have questioned the accuracy of using self-reports to measure actual parenting behaviors, particularly when those behaviors are susceptible to recall or social desirability biases (Morsbach & Prinz, 2006). These biases may be particularly heightened in a child mental health population,

where parents might be highly sensitive to feeling "blamed" for their child's illness or to the stigma of engaging the mental health system (Meltzer, Ford, Goodman, & Vostanis, 2011; Angold, et al., 1998).

This study examines the extent to which parents' self-reports of praise and criticism are reflected in their observed behavior in a sample of parents of preschool children referred for mental health treatment. We also explore whether two indicators of parents' tendency to hold negative attributions about themselves and their children, depressive symptoms and perceptions of their children as being more behaviorally difficult, moderate the relationship between self-report and observed use of praise and critical statements. Consistent with cognitive attribution theory, depressed parents may develop biases that their children's misbehavior is intentional and within their control, leading them to be less positive and more critical in their interactions (Dix, Ruble, Grusec, & Nixon, 1986; Leung & Slep, 2006; Scott & Dadds, 2009).

Using a descriptive, cross-sectional design, we posed the following research questions:

- What is the relationship between parents' self-reported and observed use of praise based on (a) frequency and (b) the proportion of statements to their child that are praise during a 15-minute free play session?
- What is the relationship between parents' self-reported and observed use of criticism based on (a) number and (b) the proportion of statements to their child that are criticisms during a 15-minute free play session?
- Do parents' depressive symptoms moderate the association between their self-reported and observed use of praise and critical statements?
- Do parents' perception of the severity of their children's behavior problems affect the association between their self-reported and observed used of praise and critical statements?

The goals of this study are to (a) understand the extent to which parents' self-reported use of praise and criticism accurately reflect the appraisals of their observed behavior and (b) offer guidance to practitioners on how to address these two important parenting practices in pediatric primary care with parents of young children at risk for mental health problems.

METHODS

This study is a secondary analysis of baseline parent-report and observation data collected as part of a larger clinical trial comparing two evidence-based parent training programs. The larger clinical trial was conducted in an urban mental health clinic serving low-income families with preschool children (Gross et al., 2014) and was approved by the Johns Hopkins University Medical Institutions Institutional Review Board.

Reprinted with permission from Swenson, S., et al. (2016). Parents' use of praise and criticism in a sample of young children seeking mental health services. *Journal of Pediatric Health Care, 30*, 49–56.

Sampling Design

Data were drawn from a convenience sample of 128 parents seeking treatment at an urban child mental health clinic serving families of young children, birth to 5 years old, who were recruited into the larger clinical trial. Approximately 80% of the clinic population is African American or multiracial, and more than 95% of families receive Medicaid. Criteria for inclusion were that the parent is (a) the biological or adoptive parent or legal guardian for a 2- to 5-year-old child and (b) seeking mental health treatment for their child's behavior problems. Parents were excluded if they had a severe mental illness, substance use disorder, or cognitive impairment that would interfere with their child's treatment. Children were excluded if they were actively suicidal or psychotic, had a diagnosis of autism or pervasive developmental disorder, or had a congenital or genetic anomaly that would interfere with treatment. Parents who met the inclusion criteria and consented to participate in the clinical trial completed a set of baseline measures and were video recorded with their child during a 15-minute free-play session (see the Procedures section).

Variables and Measures

Self-reported praise and criticism

Parents' self-reported use of praise and criticism was measured using two survey items from the Parenting Questionnaire (Gross, Fogg, Garvey, & Julion, 2004; McCabe, Clark, & Barnett, 1999), a 40-item Likert-type measure of parent discipline strategies. One item asks parents to circle the frequency with which they praise their child along a 5-point scale of 1 (*almost never*) to 5 (*very often*). Another item asks parents to circle the frequency with which they criticize their child, using the same 5-point scale of 1 (*almost never*) to 5 (*very often*).

Parent depressive symptoms

The 20-item Center for Epidemiologic Studies Depression Scale–Revised (CESD-R) was used to measure parent depressive symptoms. This version of the CESD was created to better reflect the range of symptoms indicative of major depression (Eaton, Muntaner, Smith, Tien, & Ybarra, 2004). Validity of the CESD-R has been supported by confirmatory factor analysis and positive correlations with other measures of depression and anxiety (Van Dam & Earleywine, 2011). Higher scores are indicative of more depressive symptoms; a score of 16 or higher indicates depressive symptomatology within the clinical range. The Cronbach α for the CESD-R in this sample was 0.92.

Child behavior problems

Parents' reports of their child's behavior problems were measured using the Child Behavior Checklist for ages 1½ to 5 years (CBCL; Achenbach & Rescorla, 2000).

The CBCL measures two dimensions of child behavior problems: externalizing behavior (e.g., aggression, noncompliance, and inattention) and internalizing behavior (e.g., anxiety, depression, and withdrawal). Parents rate their child's behavior problems on a scale of 0 (behavior is not true) to 2 (behavior is very true or often true); higher scores are indicative of more behavior problems. In the current study, only externalizing behavior problems were examined because these behaviors tend to be more aversive to parents. The CBCL externalizing scale contains 24 items, and scores range from 0 to 48. Standardized T scores are used to identify children with externalizing behavior problems in the borderline clinical (93rd percentile) and clinical (98th percentile) range. In low-income racial and ethnic minority populations, α reliabilities for the externalizing scale range from 0.88 to 0.91 (Gross et al., 2006), and validity has been supported (Gross et al., 2007; Sivan, Ridge, Gross, Richardson, & Cowell, 2008).

Observed use of praise and criticism

Frequencies of observed praise and criticism were measured from 15-minute video recorded parent-child free play interactions using a modified version of the Dyadic Parent-Child Interaction Coding System (DPICS; Eyberg & Robinson, 1992). The DPICS measures frequencies of select observed parent and child verbalizations and behavior. Observed parent verbalizations collected in this study include numbers of critical statements, encouraging statements, praise statements, and commands. Parents' use of praise and criticism were estimated in two ways; (a) the *frequency* of observed praise statements or critical statements and (b) the *proportion* of praise statements or critical statements to all observed parent verbalizations during the 15-minute free play session.

Praise statements include both labeled and unlabeled praise. Labeled praise is operationalized as any specific statement by a parent expressing their favorable judgment of an activity, product, or attribute of the child, such as "That's a terrific house you made." Unlabeled praise is operationalized as a nonspecific verbal comment by the parent expressing a favorable judgment of an activity or attribute of the child, such as "Great" or "Good job." In this analysis, these two types of praise were summed to form a single estimate of parents' total use of praise.

Critical statements are operationally defined as parent verbalizations that find fault with the activities, products, or attributes of the child. Blame statements and guilt-inducing statements are also considered to be critical statements. Examples include, "You're being naughty" and "I don't like your attitude."

Procedures

After completing the self-report measures, parents were asked to play with their child for 15 minutes

Reprinted with permission from Swenson, S., et al. (2016). Parents' use of praise and criticism in a sample of young children seeking mental health services. *Journal of Pediatric Health Care, 30,* 49–56.

while the research assistant video recorded the inter-action. Parents were instructed to play with their child as they normally would, and the research assistant would let them know when the 15 minutes was over. Video recordings were then sent electronically to trained DPICS coders who were blinded to study hypotheses. Inter-rater reliability, assessed through intraclass correlation for 10% of DPICS assessments, was 0.98 for praise statements and 0.92 for critical statements.

Data were analyzed using SPSS version 22 (IBM Corp., Armonk, NY). Descriptive statistics were used to summarize parents' self-reports of praise and criti-cism use and observed use of praise and criticism (as frequencies and as proportions of total verbalizations) in a 15-minute play session. Bivariate correlations between parents' self-reported and observed uses of praise or criticism, as well as correlations between self-reported and observed uses of praise and criticism with parent depression and perceived child behavior problems, were calculated using Spearman's rho. Multiple regression analyses were conducted to test the effects of parent depressive symptoms or perceived child behavior problems on parents' self-reports of praise and criticism as predictors of their observed use. To address data skewness, outliers were removed using Mahalanobis distance, Cook's distance, and centered leverage values.

RESULTS

Sample characteristics are summarized in Table 1. A majority of the parents were mothers (75.8%), African American (67.2%), unemployed (64.1%), and economically disadvantaged (95.3% reported a household income less than $20,000 or received Medicaid). The mean parent age was 34 years (SD = 10.3). The mean CESD-R score was 17.8 (SD = 15.6); more than 46% of the parents had depressive symptom scores in the clinical range. The average age of the children was 3.64 years (SD = 1.04). More than half of the children were boys (54.7%). Although all of the children were referred for behavior problems, only 41.7% of the parents reported child externalizing behavior prob-lems in the clinical or borderline clinical range.

Parents' Use of Praise and Criticism

A majority of the parents (86.7%) reported using praise "often" or "very often," and using criticism "rarely" or "almost never" (77.3%). During their observed parent-child play interactions, parents verbalized a median of three praise statements (range = 0-48) and eight critical statements (range = 0-38) in 15 minutes. A higher proportion of parents' total verbalizations consisted of critical state-ments compared with praise statements (13.6% vs. 7.4%). These results are presented in Table 2.

TABLE 1. Sample characteristics

Characteristic	Mean (SD)	n (%)
Parent characteristics (n = 128)		
Age, year	34 (10.3)	
Relationship to child		
Mother		97 (75.8)
Other		31 (24.2)
Race/ethnicity		
African American		86 (67.2)
White		30 (23.4)
Hispanic/Latino		6 (4.7)
Education level		
High school graduate or less		79 (61.7)
Some college		28 (21.9)
College graduate or higher		11 (8.6)
Household income < $20,000 or receive Medicaid		121 (95.3)
Unemployed		82 (64.1)
CESD-R score	17.8 (15.6)	
Score ≥ 16		59 (46.1)
Child characteristics (n = 128)		
Age, year	3.6 (1.0)	
Male		70 (54.7)
Externalizing behavior ≥ borderline clinical range		53 (41.7)

Note. CESD-R, Center for Epidemiologic Studies Depression Scale–Revised; SD, standard deviation.

Relationships Between Parents' Self-Reported and Observed Use of Praise and Criticism

Tables 3 and 4 summarize bivariate correlations between pertinent variables for parent praise and criticism, respectively. We found a positive correlation between parents' self-reported and observed use of praise based on absolute frequency of praise (r_s = 0.32, $p < .01$) and proportion of praise to total parent verbalizations (r_s = 0.23, $p < .01$). In contrast, a negative association was found between parents' self-reported use of criticism and the observed frequency of critical statements (r_s = −0.21, $p < .05$). No relationship was found between parents' self-reports of their use of criticism with their child and the proportion of observed critical statements to total parent verbaliza-tions (r_s = −0.05, not significant).

Moderating Effect of Parent Depressive Symptoms on the Relationship Between Parents' Self-Reported and Observed Behaviors

As shown in Table 3, parent depression scores were not significantly associated with parents' use of praise based on self-report (r = −0.08, not significant) or observation (r = −0.05, not significant). Also based on regression analysis, parents' depressive symptoms did not moderate the relationship between self-reported and observed use of praise (i.e., no significant interac-tion between depressive symptoms and self-reported use of praise was found; β = −0.10, p = not significant).

Reprinted with permission from Swenson, S., et al. (2016). Parents' use of praise and criticism in a sample of young children seeking mental health services. *Journal of Pediatric Health Care, 30,* 49–56.

TABLE 2. Parents' self-reported and observed use of praise and criticism

Variables	f (%)	Median	Mean (SD)	Range	Proportion, %*
Parent self-reports					
"I praise my child…"					
Almost never	1 (0.8)				
Rarely	0 (0)				
Sometimes	16 (12.5)				
Often	46 (35.9)				
Very often	65 (50.8)				
"I criticize my child…"					
Almost never	69 (53.9)				
Rarely	30 (23.4)				
Sometimes	22 (17.2)				
Often	7 (5.5)				
Very often	0 (0)				
Observed parent behaviors					
Total praise statements		3	5.8 (7.7)	0-48	7.4
Labeled praise		0	0.3 (0.7)	0-4	0.3
Unlabeled praise		3	5.5 (7.3)	0-45	7.1
Critical statements		8	8.5 (6.6)	0-38	13.6
Other parent verbalizations		48.5	55.8 (35.7)	1-155	79.0
Total verbal behaviors		61	70.1 (43.4)	2-201	100

*Proportion of praise or critical statements to all parent verbalizations.

As shown in Table 4, parents' depression scores were also unrelated to frequency ($r = -0.05$, not significant) and proportion ($r = 0.07$, not significant) of observed critical statements. However, parents with higher depression scores self-reported using more criticism with their children ($r_s = 0.20$, $p < .05$). Parents' depressive symptoms did not moderate the relationship between parents' self-reported and observed use of critical statements (i.e., depressive symptoms and self-reported use of criticism did not interact significantly; $\beta = -0.12$, p = not significant).

Moderating Effect of Parents' Perceptions of the Severity of Their Child's Behavior Problems on the Relationship Between Their Self-Reported and Observed Behaviors

As shown in Table 3, parents' self-reports of their use of praise was inversely correlated with their perceptions of their child's externalizing behavior problems ($r_s = -0.18$, $p < .05$)—that is, parents who rated their children as having more behavior problems were less likely to report praising their child. However, moderation analysis did not reveal a significant interaction between the child's externalizing behavior and parents' self-reported use of praise in predicting their observed use ($\beta = -0.03$, p = not significant). Children's externalizing behavior problems were also unrelated to parents' use of critical statements based on self-report and observation (see Table 4). Finally, there was no evidence that parents' perceptions of the severity of their children's externalizing behavior problems moderated the relationships between parents' self-reported and observed use of critical statements (i.e., no significant interaction was found between perceived child externalizing behavior problems and self-reported criticism use; $\beta = -0.06$, p = not significant).

TABLE 3. Bivariate Spearman's rank correlation coefficients for main variables related to parent praise

Variables	1	2	3	4	5
1 Self-reported praise		0.32†	0.23†	−0.08	−0.18*
2 Observed praise			0.89†	−0.05	−0.003
3 Praise as proportion				−0.001	−0.02
4 Parent's depressive symptoms					0.31†
5 Child's externalizing behaviors					

*Correlation coefficient significant at p < .05.
†Correlation significant at p < .01.

TABLE 4. Bivariate Spearman's rank correlation coefficients for main variables related to parent criticism

Variables	1	2	3	4	5
1 Self-reported criticism		−0.21*	−0.05	0.20*	0.15
2 Observed criticism			0.65†	−0.05	0.13
3 Criticism as proportion				0.07	0.12
4 Parent depressive symptoms					0.31†
5 Child externalizing behaviors					

*Correlation coefficient significant at p < .05.
†Correlation significant at p < .01.

Reprinted with permission from Swenson, S., et al. (2016). Parents' use of praise and criticism in a sample of young children seeking mental health services. *Journal of Pediatric Health Care, 30*, 49–56.

DISCUSSION

Parents' praise and criticism are powerful sources of feedback in shaping their young children's behavior and development. These parenting behaviors have been a key focus in child development research and serve as important indicators of positive or negative parenting in families of children with mental, emotional, and behavior disorders. Although many studies use parents' self-reports of praise and criticism, the extent to which we can rely on parent report as reliable indicators of their actual use remains unclear. Data obtained from this clinic sample suggest that parents tend to overestimate their use of praise and underestimate their use of criticism with their preschool children.

> Data obtained from this clinic sample suggest that parents tend to overestimate their use of praise and underestimate their use of criticism with their preschool children.

Although parents who reported praising their child more often were observed to use more praise, the magnitude of the effect was small (r_s = 0.32). This modest correlation is consistent with prior literature showing generally small correlations across methods, suggesting that self-report and observation capture different aspects of the same variable (i.e., perceived versus actual parenting behavior; Gardner, 2000).

Despite the positive correlation between self-reported and observed use of praise, praise was not frequently expressed. Parents verbalized a median of only three praise statements in the 15-minute observed play sessions. On average, only 7% of the parents' statements counted from the parent-child interactions qualified as praise, though these sessions were intended to be a positive one. Yet, nearly 87% of parents reported praising their children "often" or "very often."

Parents' self-reports of their use of criticism was modestly though negatively correlated with their actual use. Specifically, parents who reported using criticisms infrequently were actually *more likely* to criticize their children during the 15-minute play session. There are multiple plausible explanations for this finding. First, parents are aware that being critical is a socially undesirable behavior and therefore may have reported a more socially acceptable answer. However, it is also possible that parents are truly unaware of how frequently they criticize their children. Indeed, the parents in this sample criticized their children nearly three times more frequently than they praised them (i.e., eight criticisms versus three praise statements) despite their reports to the contrary (77% reported criticizing their children

"rarely" or "almost never"). Another explanation relates to the artificial conditions under which the observed behavior sample was obtained. Parents with a stronger tendency to criticize their children may have consciously suppressed those comments during the 15-minute play session. Nonetheless, it should be noted that despite the possibility that parents may have modified their behavior while being observed, the proportion of parents' critical statements were still nearly twice those of their praise statements (i.e., 13.6% vs. 7.6%). We also examined whether two indicators of parents' tendency to hold negative attributions about themselves and their children (i.e., parents' depressive symptoms and parents' ratings of their children's externalizing behaviors) affected concordance between self-report and observed behavior. Higher depressive symptom scores were associated with more self-reported use of critical statements. However, parents' depression scores did not moderate the relationships between self-reported and observed used of criticism or praise. In addition, parents who rated their children as having more externalizing behavior problems also reported praising their children less often, but the severity of their child's behavior problems did not moderate the association between self-reported and observed use of criticism or praise. These data suggest that parents' negative attributions affect how they perceive their children and themselves, but these attributions do not appear to account for the lack of concordance between self-reported and observed behavior.

Several study limitations should be noted. First, parents' self-reported use of praise and criticism were each measured from a single item extracted from a parent survey. A single item measure may not be an accurate indicator of parents' perceptions of their use of praise or criticism. Second, the behavior sample used to measure observed parent behavior was derived from a video-recorded 15-minute play session. Parents' behavior in this context may not have been representative of their typical behavior. However, being recorded while playing with one's child would likely elicit more positive behavior than might be typical. Thus, the number of parent praises observed might have actually been higher and the number of critical statements observed lower than was typical for these participants. Finally, this secondary analysis relied on an existing convenience sample of parents seeking mental health services for their children. As a result, the size of the sample, the study measures used, and the representativeness of the sample were all limited. Additional studies evaluating concordance between parents' self-reports and observed behavior with their children using larger and more diverse samples in both mental health and community populations are warranted to better

Reprinted with permission from Swenson, S., et al. (2016). Parents' use of praise and criticism in a sample of young children seeking mental health services. *Journal of Pediatric Health Care, 30*, 49–56.

understand these discrepancies in measurement and best practices for guiding parents in using more positive parenting strategies with their preschool children.

IMPLICATIONS FOR PRACTICE

Chronic mental health problems in children have now surpassed physical illnesses as one of the five most prevalent disabilities affecting children in the United States (Halfon, Houtrow, Larson, & Newacheck, 2012; Slomski, 2012). Their prevalence points to the importance of screening for behavioral and emotional problems in pediatric primary care and identifying appropriate resources for parents (Weitzman & Wegner, 2015).

Thoughtful discussions with parents in primary care settings about positive strategies for supporting their children's behavioral health, supplemented with written materials on how and when to use these strategies, would be an initial step. For example, Bright Futures includes brief handouts on communicating with children in ways that support their self-esteem (www.brightfutures.org). These handouts, in conjunction with discussions on the importance of parents' positive statements supporting their children's efforts and behavior, would be an important addition to well-child visits. Referral to parent training programs that are available in many cities across the country would connect parents to interventions that strengthen parents' use of positive skills, such as praise, and teach alternate strategies for discouraging misbehavior other than criticism. Parent training programs that use brief video-recorded examples of parents using evidence-based parenting strategies to promote positive child behavior may be useful if parents have not previously been exposed to these strategies (e.g., the Chicago Parent Program, the Incredible Years). The National Registry of Evidence-Base Programs and Practices, sponsored by the Substance Abuse and Mental Health Services Administration, lists more than 70 different parent-training programs. The Web site also provides critical evaluations of each program's evidence and readiness for dissemination along with program contact information for providers and consumers seeking additional information (www.nrepp.samhsa.gov).

It is important to note that although the parents in this sample were seeking help for their children's behavior, these parents also represent a highly vulnerable population. Most were unemployed and economically disadvantaged, and more than 46% evidenced high levels of depressive symptoms. It is possible that these parents have experienced little praise and a great deal of criticism in their lives. As a result, their perspective on what constitutes "a lot" of praise and "rare" criticism may be skewed. Moreover, parents raising young children in under-resourced communities may feel the need to "toughen" their children to the realities of life. Thus, critical statements may seem to some parents to be a more responsible and realistic way to prepare their children for adulthood than using praise. The challenge for clinicians is to support parents in preparing their children for life's difficulties by building the self-esteem and resilience that their children will need to grow and thrive despite the difficulties.

> The challenge for clinicians is to support parents in preparing their children for life's difficulties by building the self-esteem and resilience that their children will need to grow and thrive despite the difficulties.

We gratefully acknowledge the support of Mirian Ofonedu, Ivonne Begue De Benzo, and Maria Cecelia Lairet-Michelena.

REFERENCES

Achenbach, T. M., & Rescorla, L. A. (2000). *Manual for the ASEBA preschool forms and profiles.* Burlington, VT: University of Vermont, Department of Psychiatry.

Angold, A., Messer, S. C., Stangl, D., Farmer, E. M. Z., Costello, E. J., & Burns, B. J. (1998). Perceived parental burden and service use for child and adolescent psychiatric disorders. *American Journal of Public Health, 88*(1), 75-80.

Barnett, M. A., & Scaramella, L. V. (2013). Mothers' parenting and child sex differences in behavior problems among African American preschoolers. *Journal of Family Psychology, 27*(5), 773-783.

Bohlin, G., Hagekull, B., & Rydell, A. (2000). Attachment and social functioning: A longitudinal study from infancy to middle childhood. *Social Development, 9*, 24-39.

Bowlby, J. (1988). *A secure base: Parent-child attachment and healthy human development.* New York, NY: Basic Books.

Breitenstein, S. M., Gross, D., Fogg, L., Ridge, A., Garvey, C., Julion, W., & Tucker, S. (2012). The Chicago Parent Program: Comparing 1-year outcomes for African American and Latino parents of young children. *Research in Nursing and Health, 35*(5), 475-489.

Brotman, L. M., O'Neal, C. R., Huang, K. Y., Gouley, K. K., Rosenfelt, A., & Shrout, P. E. (2009). An experimental test of parenting practices as a mediator of early childhood physical aggression. *Journal of Child Psychology and Psychiatry, 50*(3), 235-245.

Brummelman, E., Thomaes, S., Orobio de Castro, B., Overbeek, G., & Bushman, B. J. (2014). "That's not beautiful—that's incredibly beautiful!": The adverse impact of inflated praise on children with low self-esteem. *Psychological Science, 25*(3), 728-735.

Cassidy, J. (1988). Child-mother attachment and the self in six-year-olds. *Child Development, 59*, 121-134.

Chorpita, B. F., Caleiden, E. L., & Weisz, J. R. (2005). Identifying and selecting the common elements of evidence-based interventions: A distillation and matching model. *Mental Health Services Research, 7*(1), 5-20.

Reprinted with permission from Swenson, S., et al. (2016). Parents' use of praise and criticism in a sample of young children seeking mental health services. *Journal of Pediatric Health Care, 30*, 49–56.

Cimpian, A. (2010). The impact of generic language about ability on children's achievement motivation. *Developmental Psychology, 46*(5), 1333-1340.

Dix, T., Ruble, D. N., Grusec, J. E., & Nixon, S. (1986). Social cognition in parents: Inferential and affective reactions to children of three age levels. *Child Development, 57*(4), 879-894.

Eaton, W., Muntaner, C., Smith, C., Tien, A., & Ybarra, M. (2004). Center for Epidemiologic Studies Depression Scale: Review and revisions (CESD and CESD-R). In M. E. Maruish (Ed.), *The use of psychological testing for treatment planning and outcomes assessment* (3rd ed., pp. 363-377). Mahwah, NJ: Lawrence Erlbaum.

Eyberg, S. M., & Robinson, E. (1992). *Manual for the Dyadic Parent-Child Interaction Coding System*. Seattle, WA: University of Washington Department of Nursing.

Eyberg, S. M., Funderburk, B. W., Hembree-Kigin, T. L., McNeil, C. B., Querido, J. G., & Hood, K. K. (2001). Parent-child interaction therapy with behavior problem children: One and two year maintenance of treatment effects in the family. *Child & Family Behavior Therapy, 23*(4), 1-20.

Fernandez, M. A., & Eyberg, S. M. (2009). Predicting treatment and follow-up attrition in parent-child interaction therapy. *Journal of Abnormal Child Psychology, 37*(3), 431-441.

Furlong, M., McGilloway, S., Bywater, T., Hutchings, J., Smith, S. M., & Donnelly, M. (2013). Cochrane review: Behavioural and cognitive-behavioural group-based parenting programmes for early-onset conduct problems in children aged 3 to 12 years. *Evidence-based Child Health, 8*(2), 318-692.

Gardner, F. (2000). Methodological issues in the direct observation of parent-child interaction: Do observational findings reflect the natural behavior of participants? *Clinical Child and Family Psychology Review, 3*(3), 185-198.

Gross, D. A., Belcher, H. M. E., Ofonedu, M. E., Breitenstein, S., Frick, K. D., & Budhathoki, C. (2014). Study protocol for a comparative effectiveness trial of two parent training programs in a fee-for-service mental health clinic: Can we improve mental health services to low-income families? *Trials, 15*, 70.

Gross, D., Fogg, L., Garvey, C., & Julion, W. (2004). Behavior problems in young children: An analysis of cross-informant agreements and disagreements. *Research in nursing & health, 27*(6), 413-425.

Gross, D., Fogg, L., Young, M., Ridge, A., Cowell, J. M., Richardson, R., & Sivan, A. (2006). The equivalence of the Child Behavior Checklist/1-1/2-5 across parent race/ethnicity, income level, and language. *Psychological Assessment, 18*(3), 313-323.

Gross, D., Fogg, L., Young, M., Ridge, A., Cowell, J. M., Sivan, A., & Richardson, R. (2007). Reliability and validity of the Eyberg Child Behavior Inventory with African American and Latino parents of young children. *Research in Nursing & Health, 30*, 213-223.

Gross, D., Garvey, C., Julion, W., Fogg, L., Tucker, S., & Mokros, H. (2009). Efficacy of the Chicago Parent Program with low-income African American and Latino parents of young children. *Prevention Science, 10*, 54-65.

Halfon, N., Houtrow, A., Larson, K., & Newacheck, P. W. (2012). The changing landscape of disability in childhood. *The Future of Children, 22*(1), 13-42.

Henderlong, J., & Lepper, M. R. (2002). The effects of praise on children's intrinsic motivation: A review and synthesis. *Psychological Bulletin, 128*(5), 774-795.

Leung, D. W., & Slep, A. M. (2006). Predicting inept discipline: The role of parental depressive symptoms, anger, and attributions. *Journal of Consulting and Clinical Psychology, 74*(3), 524-534.

Lorber, M. F., & Egeland, B. (2011). Parenting and infant difficult: testing a mutual exacerbation hypothesis to predict early onset conduct problems. *Child Development, 82*(6), 2006-2020.

McCabe, K. M., Clark, R., & Barnett, D. (1999). Family protective factors among urban African American youth. *Journal of Child Clinical Psychology, 28*, 137-150.

Meltzer, H., Ford, T., Goodman, R., & Vostanis, P. (2011). The burden of caring for children with emotional or conduct disorders. *International Journal of Family Medicine, 2011*, 801203.

Mueller, C. M., & Dweck, C. S. (1998). Praise for intelligence can undermine children's motivation and performance. *Journal of Personality and Social Psychology, 75*(1), 33-52.

Morsbach, S. K., & Prinz, R. J. (2006). Understanding and improving the validity of self-report of parenting. *Clinical Child and Family Psychology Review, 9*(1), 1-21.

Owens, D. J., Slep, A. M., & Heyman, R. E. (2012). The effect of praise, positive nonverbal response, reprimand, and negative nonverbal response on child compliance: A systematic review. *Clinical Child and Family Psychological Review, 15*(4), 364-385.

Scott, S., & Dadds, M. R. (2009). Practitioner review: When parent training doesn't work: Theory-driven clinical strategies. *Journal of Child Psychology and Psychiatry and Applied Disciplines, 50*(12), 1441-1450.

Sivan, A. B., Ridge, A., Gross, D., Richardson, R., & Cowell, J. M. (2008). Analysis of two measures of child behavior problems by African American, Latino, and Non-Hispanic Caucasian parents of young children: A focus group study. *Journal of Pediatric Nursing, 23*(1), 20-27.

Slomski, A. (2012). Chronic mental health issues in children now loom larger than physical problems. *Journal of the American Medical Association, 308*(3), 223-225.

Tung, I., Li, J. J., & Lee, S. S. (2012). Child sex moderates the association between negative parenting and childhood conduct problems. *Aggressive Behavior, 28*(3), 239-251.

Van Dam, N. T., & Earleywine, M. (2011). Validation of the Center for Epidemiologic Studies Depression Scale–Revised (CESD-R): Pragmatic depression assessment in the general population. *Psychiatry Research, 186*(1), 128-132.

Wahler, R. G., & Meginnis, K. L. (1997). Strengthening child compliance through positive parenting practices: What works? *Journal of Clinical Child Psychology, 26*(4), 433-440.

Webster-Stratton, C., & Hammond, M. (1998). Conduct problems and level of social competence in Head Start children: Prevalence, pervasiveness, and associated risk factors. *Clinical Child and Family Psychology Review, 1*(2), 101-124.

Weitzman, C., & Wegner, L. (2015). Promoting optimal development: Screening for behavioral and emotional problems. *Pediatrics, 135*(2), 384-395.

Zentall, S. R., & Morris, B. J. (2010). "Good job, you're so smart": The effects of inconsistency of praise type on young children's motivation. *Journal of Experimental Child Psychology, 107*(2), 155-163.

Reprinted with permission from Swenson, S., et al. (2016). Parents' use of praise and criticism in a sample of young children seeking mental health services. *Journal of Pediatric Health Care, 30*, 49–56.

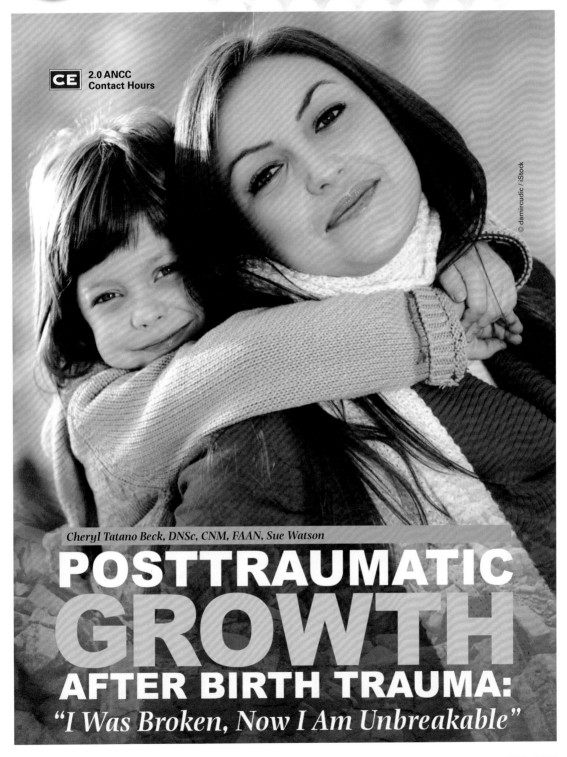

B

CE 2.0 ANCC
Contact Hours

© damircudic / iStock

Cheryl Tatano Beck, DNSc, CNM, FAAN, Sue Watson

POSTTRAUMATIC GROWTH
AFTER BIRTH TRAUMA:
"I Was Broken, Now I Am Unbreakable"

Reprinted with permission from Beck, C. T., & Watson, S. (2016). Posttraumatic growth after birth trauma. *MCN: American Journal of Maternal Child Nursing, 41,* 264-271.

Abstract

Purpose: The aim of this study was to investigate women's experiences of posttraumatic growth following traumatic childbirth.

Study Design and Methods: A descriptive phenomenological study was conducted using Colaizzi's data analysis method. The Internet sample of 15 mothers was recruited from the Trauma and Birth Stress Web site. Women were asked to describe in as much detail as they could remember, their experiences of any positive changes in their beliefs or life as a result of their traumatic childbirth.

Results: Using Calhoun and Tedeschi's metaphor of an earthquake to help explain posttraumatic growth, the seismic waves of birth trauma had enough power to lead to four themes of posttraumatic growth revealed in this phenomenological study: (1) Opening oneself up to a new present, (2) Achieving a new level of relationship nakedness, (3) Fortifying spiritual-mindedness, and (4) Forging new paths.

Clinical Implications: Mothers' experiences of their personal growth after birth trauma can help inform future research that can promote posttraumatic growth in mothers. Clinicians can share results of this study with their patients to provide some hope to mothers struggling with the aftermath of a traumatic birth that some women have reported positive growth. Healthcare providers need to respect trauma survivors' struggles while at the same time permitting mothers to explore possibilities for growth. Clinicians must not, however, create the false expectation that posttraumatic growth will happen in most trauma survivors.

Key words: Parturition; Posttraumatic stress disorder; Qualitative research.

Posttraumatic growth has been reported among persons who have experienced a wide range of traumas. Examples of these trauma survivors include veterans (Tsai, El-Gabalawy, Sledge, Southwick, & Pietrzak, 2015), childhood cancer survivors (Duran, 2013), survivors of intimate partner violence (Valdez & Lilly, 2015), and women with infertility (Yu et al., 2014).

Up to 34% of new mothers have reported experiencing a traumatic birth (Soet, Brack, & DiIorio, 2003). Traumatic childbirth is an event(s) that occurs during labor and birth and involves a woman's perception of (1) an actual or threatened serious injury or death to herself or her infant and/or (2) being treated in a dehumanizing way that strips the woman of her dignity. In a meta-analysis, Grekin and O'Hara (2014) reported prevalence of posttraumatic stress disorder (PTSD) due to birth trauma in community samples was 3.1%. In at-risk samples it was 15.7%.

Traumatic childbirth has both short term and chronic adverse consequences for mothers such as its impact on breastfeeding and subsequent childbirth (Beck, 2015). Only a handful of studies have been conducted on perinatal posttraumatic growth. Examining their personal growth, which involves positive changes in women's lives following birth trauma, can provide a more complete picture of these psychological reactions which in turn can help inform future research that can promote posttraumatic growth in mothers. Clinicians can share results of this study with their patients to provide some hope to women struggling with the aftermath of a traumatic birth that aspects of positive growth in their lives may be possible.

> *Up to 34% of new mothers have reported experiencing a traumatic birth.*

Posttraumatic Growth

Posttraumatic growth is defined as the "positive psychological change experienced as a result of the struggle with highly challenging life circumstances" (Tedeschi & Calhoun, 2004, p. 1). In posttraumatic growth a person's development in some areas surpasses what was present prior to occurrence of the struggle with the crisis. This does not happen as a direct result of the trauma but instead as the result of the person's struggle in the aftermath of the trauma as they attempt to cope or survive. Posttraumatic growth can coexist with the distress of the trauma (Calhoun & Tedeschi, 2013).

Calhoun and Tedeschi (1998) used the metaphor of an earthquake to illustrate posttraumatic growth. Key to this development may be the traumatic event's ability to successfully "shake the foundations" of the person's assumptive world (Calhoun & Tedeschi, 1998, p. 216). The trauma experience needs to be seismic, like in an earthquake, to achieve this severe shaking of a person's understanding of the world. These assumptions about the world that can be shaken include beliefs such as the meaning of life; things that happen to people are fair; why persons think and act the way they do; relationships with others; one's abilities, strengths, weaknesses, and expectations for the future; spiritual or religious beliefs; and a person's worth or value as an individual (Cann et al., 2010). Cognitive rebuilding is necessary after a psychological crisis just as physical structures must be rebuilt after an earthquake.

Tedeschi and Calhoun (1996) identified five dimensions of growth: Appreciation of Life, Relating to Others, Personal Strength, New Possibilities, and Spiritual Change. They developed the Posttraumatic Growth

Reprinted with permission from Beck, C. T., & Watson, S. (2016). Posttraumatic growth after birth trauma. *MCN: American Journal of Maternal Child Nursing, 41,* 264-271.

Inventory (PTGI), which is a 21-item Likert scale that measures these five dimensions. Ratings are made on a 6-point scale from 0 to 5 and can yield a range of possible total scores from 0 to 105 with a higher score indicating greater growth. A person can experience growth in some dimensions but not necessarily in all five domains. It is important to note that not all individuals who experience trauma develop posttraumatic growth.

Perinatal Posttraumatic Growth

Only three studies were found that examined perinatal posttraumatic growth after birth trauma. All these studies used Tedeschi and Calhoun's (1996) PTGI in some manner to measure the five dimensions of growth. In their qualitative study Black and Sandelowski (2010) interviewed women who had been told prenatally of the presence of a severe fetal anomaly. They found that, 1 year later, 12 of the 15 women had experienced positive changes in their lives. The five dimensions of the PTGI were used as the categories to code the interview data. The dimension that showed the earliest and most prolonged change was in Relating to Others.

In the next two studies, conducted in the United Kingdom, community samples were used. To be included in the studies women did not have to perceive their births to be traumatic. A convenience sample of 219 women who had given birth within the previous 36 months, with a mean of 10.95 months (SD = 7.20), participated in an Internet study (Sawyer & Ayers, 2009). In this study, 37.2% of the mothers fulfilled the Diagnostic and Statistical Manual of Mental Disorders' (DSM-IV) (American Psychological Association, 2000) criterion for PTSD of experiencing a traumatic event (in this case, childbirth). At least moderate levels of posttraumatic growth were experienced by 50% of mothers. The researchers defined "at least moderate levels" as a total score on the PTGI of more than 62. The mean total PTGI score for the sample was 58.81. There were no significant differences in posttraumatic growth levels between women who fulfilled the PTSD stressor criterion and those who did not. Appreciation of Life was the most endorsed dimension of posttraumatic growth (80%), followed next by Personal Strength (63%), Relating to Others (52%), New Possibilities (48%), and Spiritual Change (16%).

Sawyer, Ayers, Young, Bradley, and Smith (2012) conducted a longitudinal study with 125 women who completed the PTGI during their third trimester of pregnancy and again at 8 weeks postpartum. Twenty-three percent of the mothers' perception of their birth as traumatic fulfilled the DSM-IV's PTSD stressor criterion. In this study, 48% of the women experienced at least a small degree of positive change after birth that was operationalized as a total score in the PTGI of more than 41. The mean total PTGI score was 39.81. Results mirrored Sawyer and Ayers's (2009) earlier study with Appreciation of Life being the most endorsed dimension (68%). Personal Strength was second (52%), followed by Relating to Others (51%), New Possibilities (45%), and lastly Spiritual Change (22%).

Further research is warranted on perinatal posttraumatic growth. In the only two quantitative studies of posttraumatic growth in mothers, community samples were used. These studies did not specifically assess growth in mothers who perceived their childbirth to be traumatic. There had yet to be a phenomenological study conducted that would explore mothers' experiences of posttraumatic growth without using the PTGI dimensions to guide the analysis. Therefore, the purpose of this descriptive phenomenological study was to investigate women's experiences of posttraumatic growth following traumatic childbirth.

Methods

Research Design

Descriptive phenomenology is an inductive method that attempts to uncover and describe the essential structures of the lived experience of a phenomenon. The essence of a phenomenon is grasped through the study of the particulars of experiences. Husserl's (1970) philosophy of phenomenology underpins the descriptive phenomenological method. The two steps of epoché and reduction are essential to Husserl's philosophy. Epoché means abstention and reduction means to lead back. For Husserl the epoché helps suspend our natural attitude of taken-for-granted beliefs of the phenomenon. He used the term "bracketing" for this first step where one puts asides presuppositions that can stand in our way from being open to the phenomenon. Once bracketing is completed and we open ourselves to the world without our presuppositions, it leads to reduction where one can see what is unique in a phenomenon (Husserl). Colaizzi's (1978) phenomenological method was used in this study.

Sample

Inclusion criteria were that the mother a) perceived her childbirth had been traumatic, (b) experienced some aspect of personal growth after her birth trauma, and (c) was at least 18 years of age. The international Internet sample consisted of 15 mothers who were all married. Six women (40%) were from the United Kingdom, 4 (27%) from New Zealand, 3 (20%) from the United States, and 2 (13%) from Australia. Their ages ranged from 32 to 57. Fourteen women were White and one was Samoan. Eleven mothers (73%) were multiparas, whereas 4 (27%) were primiparas. Ten women had vaginal births and 5 had cesareans. Twelve women reported their education; 1 had a high school diploma, 9 bachelor's degrees, and 2 master's degrees. Examples of types of birth trauma these women experienced included infant death, emergency cesarean, stillborn infant, 4th degree laceration, postpartum hemorrhage, vacuum extraction, and stripped of their dignity. Five women (33%) reported being formally diagnosed with PTSD due to their traumatic births. Length of time since the women's traumatic births ranged from 5 months to 19 years.

Reprinted with permission from Beck, C. T., & Watson, S. (2016). Posttraumatic growth after birth trauma. *MCN: American Journal of Maternal Child Nursing, 41*, 264-271.

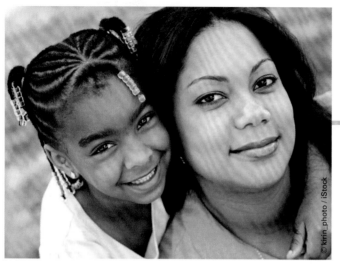

Posttraumatic growth involves positive psychological changes experienced by an individual as a result of struggling with a highly challenging life event.

the participants' descriptions that pertain directly to the phenomenon were extracted and their meanings formulated. Next the formulated meanings were categorized into themes. The themes were then integrated into an exhaustive description of the phenomenon under study. This exhaustive description was then returned to some of the participants for validation. There were no changes suggested by the participants.

Procedure

Recruitment began once receiving the University's Institutional Review Board approval. Women were primarily recruited through Trauma and Birth Stress (TABS), a charitable trust in New Zealand whose mission is to provide support for women who have experienced traumatic childbirth. A recruitment notice was posted on TABS' Web site (www.tabs.org.nz). The second author of this study is the Chairperson of TABS who was actively involved in recruiting participants through her connection with this Web site. Two mothers from other Web sites, such as www.birthtraumaaustralia.com, participated in the study.

Women who wanted information about the study emailed the first author at her university address. Two documents were then sent on attachment via email to the potential participants: an information sheet and directions for the study. Participants were asked to respond to the following statement: Please describe for us in as much detail as you can remember your experiences of any positive changes in your beliefs or life as a result of your traumatic childbirth. Mothers sending their narratives to the first author implied informed consent. After receiving the information sheet and directions, the length of time it took for mothers to send their descriptions of their posttraumatic growth to the researchers ranged from 2 days to 4 months. Data collection continued for 18 months until achieving data saturation. Length of mothers' descriptions of their posttraumatic growth ranged from 1 to 7 single-spaced typed written pages. After reading a mother's description of her experiences of posttraumatic growth, the first author emailed the participant if clarification of some part of her narrative was needed.

Colaizzi's (1978) method was used to analyze mothers' written descriptions of their posttraumatic growth. In this method all the significant statements included in

Trustworthiness

Credibility was enhanced by the first author keeping a reflexive journal throughout data collection and data analysis. Thick description provided by rich quotes was included in the description of each theme to bring it to life and increased authenticity of the findings. Confirmability focused on the congruence between two or more persons regarding the data's meaning. One mother who experienced posttraumatic growth reviewed the findings and shared that "this is excellent. There is nothing I can add. Very, very powerful." The second author confirmed the audit trail of the results starting with reading all the data and following Colaizzi's (1978) data analysis steps. A PhD student who has been a labor and delivery nurse with 20 years' experience followed the audit trail and confirmed findings.

Results

Analysis of the 15 descriptions of posttraumatic growth following birth trauma yielded four themes. Figure 1 uses the metaphor of an earthquake to illustrate the seismic power of a traumatic childbirth that can lead to posttraumatic growth. Though women in this study experienced different types of birth trauma, themes of their personal growth in their lives were all similar. The country where the posttraumatic growth took place did not seem to be a factor in the patterns of positive changes.

Theme 1. Opening Oneself Up to a New Present

Achieving posttraumatic growth was a process. The following quote provides one mother's insight into this process: "At first, the very fabric of your being is shattered, destroyed. Nothing makes sense. The pieces do not go back together again. Rather, it is a gradual, new, very different kind of becoming." A mother's opening herself up to this new present can be "much like the agony a butterfly suffers as it fights through its chrysalis." The

Reprinted with permission from Beck, C. T., & Watson, S. (2016). Posttraumatic growth after birth trauma. *MCN: American Journal of Maternal Child Nursing, 41,* 264–271.

Figure 1. Earthquake Model of Mothers' Posttraumatic Growth after Birth Trauma

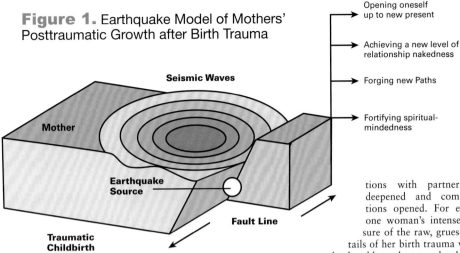

Opening oneself up to new present

Achieving a new level of relationship nakedness

Forging new Paths

Fortifying spiritual-mindedness

personal rewards can be immense for some women as illustrated by this woman's quote: "I was broken. Now I am unbreakable."

Mothers experiencing positive changes in their lives felt that their surviving birth trauma made them a stronger person. There is an inner knowing now that they can survive anything. One mother shared that "no one would wish trauma or subsequent PTSD upon anyone, yet when having had this, one knows you have become CHANGED FOR-EVER yet a better person for it all. Better and stronger and very self-aware undergirds your new daily life."

Heightened empathy was another important area of personal growth for women following birth trauma. Women also learned to become more assertive as part of their personal growth in the aftermath of their traumatic childbirth. Learned was a willingness to use their voice and personal power to fight back both emotionally and physically for themselves and others.

Theme 2. Achieving a New Level of Relationship Nakedness

Posttraumatic growth infused the relationships a woman had on multiple levels: with her husband, her friends, her children, and even sometimes with her patients if she happened to have a career in healthcare. Connec-

Though the women in this study experienced different types of birth trauma, themes of their personal growth in their lives were similar.

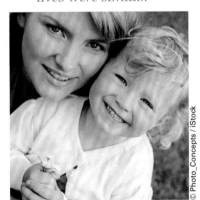

© Photo_Concepts / iStock

tions with partners were deepened and communications opened. For example, one woman's intense disclosure of the raw, gruesome details of her birth trauma with her husband brought a new level of what she described as "relationship nakedness." By relationship nakedness is meant that women no longer covered up what they were thinking or feeling but now felt secure enough in their relationships with their partners to be totally open and "naked" in front of them not hiding behind anything. A deeper level of understanding and a new tenderness between women and their partners developed through their growth after birth trauma.

Posttraumatic growth also involved deeper and closer relationships with longtime girlfriends and also with new friends. Being able to talk intimately with friends about their traumatic births was hugely important to mothers in their growth. New, invaluable friendships began as mothers reached out to other women on traumatic childbirth Web sites.

Relationships with their infants and older children took on an even deeper meaning. Some mothers experienced a heightened need for their children "to know love, to know they are delighted in, to feel safe, to feel empowered and supported, and to feel nurtured." Mothers' relationships with their children involved a new focused meaning on being role models, especially for their daughters.

Theme 3. Fortifying Spiritual-Mindedness

For some mothers their faith became stronger and they developed a better understanding of spiritual and

Reprinted with permission from Beck, C. T., & Watson, S. (2016). Posttraumatic growth after birth trauma. *MCN: American Journal of Maternal Child Nursing, 41,* 264-271.

religious matters in their everyday lives. One mother disclosed "I used to feel that my traumatic birth was something I wanted to take back (to somehow reverse time and change it so I could be 'ME' again) but over time I have learnt to embrace it as it keeps me connected to God and has also been one of the biggest catalysts for positive change in my life."

Another mother shared that "I can honestly say that overall, the most significant thing in my growth has been prayer and my personal relationship with the creator of this universe. I now believe that I was made for a purpose. Not only has He opened the right doors for me to gain healing and growth I specifically needed, but He has also given me huge insight into birth trauma which I hope to use for His glory in helping others with similar experiences." The lyrics from an old hymn were shared by one participant as she introduced them by saying: "These words often bring me to tears when I sing them because I know just how much God had done in my life and just how grateful I am." Here is the verse: "Something beautiful, something good, All my confusion, He understood, All I had to offer Him was brokenness and strife, but He made something beautiful out of my life."

Theme 4. Forging New Paths

New professional and personal goals were established as part of posttraumatic growth following birth trauma. There were two main paths that women followed. One path led to enrolling in and completing university degrees and the second path led to volunteer work. Women reported studying at universities in the fields of nursing, midwifery, and child and family health. As one mother explained, "I then went to the university to complete a nursing degree. I faced a number of fears in my nursing placements. As I did this I became stronger and stronger and after a lot of hard work I achieved my Bachelor of Health Science in Nursing."

Volunteering was another important aspect of positive life changes for some mothers. These women had never volunteered before but now felt the need to not only help other women who have experienced traumatic childbirth but also to try and prevent this from happening to other women. In one mother's narrative she explained, "I need to stress my overwhelming desire to talk about my experience and prevent it from happening again led me to volunteering for the Birth Trauma Association. This in itself was a big area of growth for me." In another woman's narrative she shared that her PTSD due to her traumatic pregnancy and birth "catapulted me into action and that this should not be happening to others." As one of her positive life changes, one woman formed a local International Cesarean Awareness Network chapter and actively

volunteered there. Lastly one participant who is a midwife now volunteers at a crisis pregnancy center to help support women and families in crisis.

Discussion

Traumatic childbirth can certainly be viewed as a psychologically seismic event of a magnitude that can severely shake the foundations of a woman's assumptive world (Beck, 2015). The seismic waves had enough

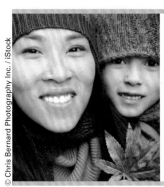

Clinicians need to respect mothers' struggles with traumatic childbirth and help them explore possibilities for growth.

© Chris Bernard Photography Inc. / iStock

power to lead to the four themes of posttraumatic growth revealed in this phenomenological study. The themes that emerged from mothers' descriptions of their experiences of positive life changes in the aftermath of a traumatic childbirth confirmed earlier findings from the qualitative study of growth after severe fetal anomaly diagnosis (Black & Sandelowski, 2010) where increased emotional closeness with partners (Theme 2), recognizing new possibilities such as attending nursing school (Theme 4), and increased spirituality (Theme 3) were reported.

In two quantitative studies measuring perinatal posttraumatic growth using the PTGI the most endorsed domain was Appreciation of Life (Sawyer & Ayers, 2009; Sawyer et al., 2012). The voices of the mothers in this current phenomenological study did express appreciation of life but it was not the strongest essential component of their posttraumatic growth. Personal Strength (Theme 1) and Relating to Others (Theme 2) emerged as the loudest themes that women voiced in their descriptions of positive life changes following birth trauma. In both of Sawyer et al.'s studies Personal Strength and Relating to Others were the second and third most endorsed dimensions. One possible explanation for the differences in the magnitude of the various dimensions experienced by mothers of posttraumatic growth in the Sawyer et al. studies and this current phenomenological study is the differing samples. In both of Sawyer et al.'s quantitative studies community samples were recruited. In this current qualitative study, however, only women who perceived

Reprinted with permission from Beck, C. T., & Watson, S. (2016). Posttraumatic growth after birth trauma. *MCN: American Journal of Maternal Child Nursing, 41,* 264-271.

they had experienced birth trauma followed by positive changes in their lives were included.

Limitations

Only women who had access to the Internet participated in this study. These women used the resources of TABS and other Web sites for traumatic childbirth. It is not known whether mothers who have neither Internet access nor support from online support groups would describe their experiences of posttraumatic growth differently than what emerged for the current study. Because the length of time since participants self-identified their birth trauma ranged for 5 months to 19 years, the potential of recall bias needs to be noted. None of the participants, however, shared any difficulty in remembering the positive changes in their lives following their traumatic births. Literature supports the accuracy of long-term recollections about the birthing experience (Takehara, Noguchi, Shimane, & Misago, 2014).

Implications for Practice

Clinicians can share with mothers struggling with posttraumatic stress some of the results of this qualitative study to alert their patients that some women have reported positive growth. Healthcare providers are in an important position to promote and encourage a focus on potentially positive aspects in mothers' lives in the aftermath of traumatic childbirth.

Calhoun and Tedeschi (2013) proposed that in working with survivors of trauma, clinicians take on the role of an "expert companion." They chose this term to convey a sense of humility that healthcare providers need to have to provide an environment where personal exploration can help occur to promote the survivor's experience of posttraumatic growth. Healthcare providers need to respect the trauma survivor's struggles and difficulties while at the same time permitting the person to explore the possibilities for growth. Calhoun and Tedeschi stressed, however, not to create the false expectation that posttraumatic growth will happen in most trauma survivors. In conclusion, sage advice from an amazingly strong mother who participated in this study is included

Clinical Nursing Implications

- Clinicians can share with women struggling with posttraumatic stress that some mothers have reported positive changes in their lives.

- While respecting women's struggles with traumatic childbirth, healthcare providers can encourage mothers to explore possibilities for growth.

- In working with trauma survivors, clinicians can take on the role of an "expert companion."

- Healthcare providers must not, however, create false hopes in mothers that posttraumatic growth occurs in most trauma survivors.

Achieving posttraumatic growth in mothers' personal lives was a process.

so that it can be used by clinicians who are helping women currently struggling with the devastating aftermath of their traumatic childbirth: "LOVE+STRENGTH+HOPE = Our yellow brick road. This was written in the hope that all survivors will find the path to their own road, with love xxx." ❖

Acknowledgment
Words do not seem enough to thank the mothers from around the world who so willingly shared their stories of birth trauma and their resulting posttraumatic growth in the hopes of helping other women who have experienced birth trauma. Thank you also to Carrie Eaton, MSN, RNC-OB, for reviewing the data analysis process.

Cheryl Tatano Beck is a Distinguished Professor, University of Connecticut, School of Nursing, Storrs, CT. She can be reached via e-mail at Cheryl.beck@uconn.edu

Sue Watson is the Chairperson, Trauma and Birth Stress.

The authors declare no conflict of interest.

DOI:10.1097/NMC.0000000000000259

References
American Psychological Association. (2000). *Diagnostic and statistical manual of mental disorders-Text revision* (4th ed.). Washington, DC: Author.

Beck, C.T. (2015). Middle range theory of traumatic childbirth: The ever-widening ripple effect. *Global Qualitative Nursing Research*, 2, 1-13. doi:10.1177/2333393615575313

Black, B., & Sandelowski, M. (2010). Personal growth after severe fetal diagnosis. *Western Journal of Nursing Research*, 32(8), 1011-1030. doi:10.1177/0193945910371215

Calhoun, L. G., & Tedeschi, R. G. (1998). Posttraumatic growth: Future directions. In R. G. Tedeschi, C. L. Park, & L. G. Calhoun (Eds.), *Posttraumatic growth: Positive change in the aftermath of crisis* (pp. 215-238). Mahwah, NJ: Lawrence Erlbaum Associates.

Calhoun, L. G., & Tedeschi, R. G. (2013). *Posttraumatic growth in clinical practice*. New York: Routledge.

Cann, A., Calhoun, L. G., Tedeschi, R. G., Kilmer, R. P., Gil-Rivas, V., Vishnevsky, T., & Danhauer, S. C. (2010). The Core Beliefs Inventory: A brief measure of disruption in the assumptive world. *Anxiety, Stress, and Coping*, 23(1), 19-34. doi:10.1080/10615800802573013

Colaizzi, P. (1978). Psychological research as the phenomenologist views it. In R. Valle & M. King (Eds.). *Existential phenomenological alternatives for psychology* (pp. 48-71). New York: Oxford University Press.

Duran, B. (2013). Posttraumatic growth as experienced by childhood cancer survivors and their families: A narrative synthesis of qualitative and quantitative research. *Journal of Pediatric Oncology Nursing*, 30(4), 179-197. doi:10.1177/1043454213487433

Grekin, R., & O'Hara, M. W. (2014). Prevalence and risk factors of postpartum posttraumatic stress disorder: A meta-analysis. *Clinical Psychology Review*, 34(5), 389-401. doi:10.1016/j.cpr.2014.05.003

Reprinted with permission from Beck, C. T., & Watson, S. (2016). Posttraumatic growth after birth trauma. *MCN: American Journal of Maternal Child Nursing, 41,* 264-271.

Husserl, E. (1970). *The crisis of European sciences and transcendental phenomenology: An introduction to phenomenology.* Evanston, IL: Northwestern University Press.

Sawyer, A., & Ayers, S. (2009). Post-traumatic growth in women after childbirth. *Psychology and Health, 24*(4), 457-471. doi:10.1080/08870440701864520

Sawyer, A., Ayers, S., Young, D., Bradley, R., & Smith, H. (2012). Post-traumatic growth after childbirth: A prospective study. *Psychology and Health, 27*(3), 362-377. doi:10.1080/08870446.2011.578745

Soet, J. E., Brack, G. A., & Dilorio, C. (2003). Prevalence and predictors of women's experience of psychological trauma during childbirth. *Birth, 30*(1), 36-46.

Takehara, K., Noguchi, M., Shimane, T., & Misago, C. (2014). A longitudinal study of women's memories of their childbirth experiences at five years postpartum. *BMC Pregnancy and Childbirth, 14*, 221-227. doi:10.1186/1471-2393-14-221

Tedeschi, R. G., & Calhoun, L. G. (1996). The Posttraumatic Growth Inventory: Measuring the positive legacy of trauma. *Journal of Traumatic Stress, 9*(3), 455-472.

Tedeschi, R. G., & Calhoun, L. G. (2004). Posttraumatic growth: Conceptual foundations and empirical evidence. *Psychological Inquiry, 15*(1), 1-18.

Tsai, J., El-Gabalawy, R., Sledge, W. H., Southwick, S. M., & Pietrzak, R. H. (2015). Post-traumatic growth among veterans in the USA: Results from the National Health and Resilience in Veterans Study. *Psychological Medicine, 45*(1), 165-179. doi:10.1017/S0033291714001202

Valdez, C. E., & Lilly, M. M. (2015). Posttraumatic growth in survivors of intimate partner violence: An assumptive world process. *Journal of Interpersonal Violence, 30*(2), 215-231. doi:10.1177/0886260514533154

Yu, Y., Peng, L., Chen, L., Long, L., He, W., Li, M., & Wang, T. (2014). Resilience and social support promote posttraumatic growth of women with infertility: The mediating role of positive coping. *Psychiatry Research, 215*(2), 401-405. doi:10.1016/j.psychres.2013.10.032

ONLINE

Trauma and Birth Stress
www.tabs.org.nz

Postpartum Support International
www.postpartum.net

Birth Trauma Association of United Kingdom
www.birthtraumaassociation.org.uk

The Australian Birth Trauma and PTSD Treatment Centre
www.birthtraumaaustralia.com

Birth Trauma of Canada
www.birthtraumacanada.org

Solace for Mothers Healing after Traumatic Childbirth
www.solaceformothers.org

Reprinted with permission from Beck, C. T., & Watson, S. (2016). Posttraumatic growth after birth trauma. *MCN: American Journal of Maternal Child Nursing, 41,* 264-271.

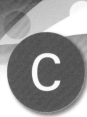

Jennifer R. Bail, PhD, RN

Nataliya Ivankova, PhD, MPH

Karen Heaton, PhD, COHN-S, FNP-BC, FAAN, FAAOHN

David E. Vance, PhD, MGS

Kristen Triebel, PsyD

Karen Meneses, PhD, RN, FAAN

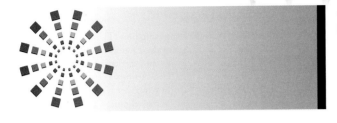

Cancer-Related Symptoms and Cognitive Intervention Adherence Among Breast Cancer Survivors: A Mixed-Methods Study

KEYWORDS

Adherence

Breast cancer survivors

Cancer-related symptoms

Cognitive impairment

Cognitive training

Mixed-methods research

Background: Breast cancer survivors (BCSs) experience long-term symptoms of cancer and treatment, which may exacerbate cognitive function and ability to adhere to interventions aimed at improving cognition. **Objective:** The intent of this study was to explore the relationship between selected cancer-related symptoms and adherence to the **S**peed of Processing in Middle Aged and **O**lder Bre**A**st Cancer Su**R**vivors (SOAR) cognitive training (CT) intervention among BCSs residing in Alabama. **Methods:** A sequential quantitative to qualitative (Quan→Qual) mixed-methods design was used. First, the relationship between selected cancer-related symptoms and adherence to SOAR among BCSs (n = 30) was examined using self-reported questionnaire data. Follow-up semistructured interviews with 15 purposefully selected participants (adherent and nonadherent) were conducted to explore how symptoms contributed to/explained differences in adherence to SOAR. Data were analyzed using RStudio and NVivo software. **Results:** Spearman's ρ correlation suggested relationships between adherence and perceived cognitive impairment, depressive symptoms, and sleep quality. Inductive thematic analysis yielded 4 themes: (1) experiences of cancer-related symptoms, (2) influences of CT, (3) adherence to CT, and (4) environment for CT. Integration of quantitative and qualitative results revealed that experiences of and responses to CT and cancer-related symptoms differently shape adherence to CT among BCSs. **Conclusions:** To aid in cognitive intervention adherence among BCSs, future studies may consider applying a comprehensive approach aimed at addressing

Authors Affiliations: Department of Nutrition Sciences (Dr Bail), School of Health Professions (Dr Ivankova), School of Nursing (Drs Ivankova, Heaton, Vance, and Meneses), and Department of Neurology (Dr Triebel), University of Alabama at Birmingham.

This study was supported by the American Cancer Society Doctoral Degree Scholarship in Cancer Nursing (DSCN-16-066-01; principal investigator: J.R.B.), Susan G. Komen Graduate Traineeship in Disparities Research Award (GTDR 15329376; principal investigator: K.M./Demark-Wahnefried), and Center for Translational Research on Aging and Mobility, Edward R. Roybal Center Project

(P30 AG022838; principal investigator: J.R.B.; pilot principal investigator: K.M.). D.E.V. has served as a paid consultant for Posit Science, Inc (the software used for the cognitive training in this study).

The authors have no conflicts of interest to disclose.

Correspondence: Jennifer R. Bail, PhD, RN, Department of Nutrition Sciences, University of Alabama at Birmingham, WTI 102C, 1824 6th Ave S, Birmingham, AL 35294 (jbail@uab.edu).

Accepted for publication December 27, 2018.

DOI: 10.1097/NCC.0000000000000700

concurrent cancer-related symptoms. **Implications for Practice:** Clinicians can routinely assess cognition and provide education and resources for management of cancer-related symptoms.

With more than 3.5 million breast cancer survivors (BCSs) in the United States,[1] the management of cancer-related symptoms after cancer and its treatment is concerning. One such cancer-related symptom is cognitive impairment. Cognitive impairment is a decline in function in one or multiple cognitive domains (ie, attention, memory, executive function, and information processing speed).[2] Studies among BCSs indicate that cognitive impairment negatively impacts self-esteem, confidence, social relationships, work ability, and overall quality of life.[3–5] Interventions aimed at remediating cognitive impairment among BCSs vary, with the most promising being cognitive training (CT).[6,7] Cognitive training comprises a range of activities focused on memory, speed of processing, attention, and executive function. Cognitive training improves cognition by stimulating the creation of new neurons and strengthening the connections among existing neurons.[6] Cognitive training may even decrease the likelihood of developing dementia. Data from the ACTIVE study, conducted among healthy older adults (N = 2802), revealed a 29% reduced risk of dementia (hazard ratio, 0.71; 95% confidence interval, 0.50-0.998; $P = .049$) among those who had been randomized to the CT (ie, speed of processing training) group as compared with control subjects at 10-year follow-up. Moreover, each additional hour of CT was associated with a 10% lower hazard for dementia (unadjusted hazard ratio, 0.90; 95% confidence interval, 0.85-0.95; $P < .001$),[8] illuminating the importance of CT dosage. These findings are especially relevant for BCSs, who may be more likely than healthy older adults to develop dementia.[9] Other cancer-related symptoms that tend to co-occur among BCSs include depressive symptoms and poor sleep quality. Concurrent cancer-related symptoms may potentially exacerbate cognitive impairment and adherence to interventions aimed at improving cognitive function.[6,10–12] Yet, to date, no research has been reported to examine the relationship between cancer-related symptoms and adherence to a CT intervention among BCSs.

Recently, the parent study (**S**peed of Processing in Middle Aged and **O**lder Bre**A**st Cancer Su**R**vivors [SOAR]) examined the feasibility of a CT intervention among BCSs.[13] Study observations, including nonadherence to CT dosage and comments about cancer-related symptoms, suggested that cancer-related symptoms may be related to BCSs' adherence to SOAR. These observations informed the present study, which aimed to (1) understand the relationship between selected cancer-related symptoms and adherence to the SOAR CT intervention among BCSs and (2) explore potential facilitators and/or barriers to SOAR and how identified symptoms contribute to/explain differences in adherence.

■ Methods

The study protocol received approval from the University of Alabama at Birmingham Institutional Review Board. Participants gave written informed consent prior to data collection.

Theoretical Framework

The Theory of Unpleasant Symptoms (TUS) was used to guide this study.[14] The TUS provides a framework for understanding the complexity of the symptom experience and relationships to potential outcomes. The TUS theorists assert that the nature of multiple symptoms occurring together results in an experience that is not independent, but synergistic. Consequences of the symptom experience include performance, which is the outcome or effect of the symptom experience. For the purposes of this study, symptoms were operationalized as perceived cognitive impairment, depressive symptoms, and poor sleep quality. Performance was operationalized as adherence.

Parent Study

The SOAR participants (N = 60) were recruited across North Central Alabama and randomized to either a home-based CT intervention (n = 30) or a no-contact control group (n = 30). Cognitive training consisted of the "Double Decision" program (www.BrainHQ.com). Participants were instructed to complete 10 hours (2 hours per week) of CT over a period of 6 to 8 weeks, received weekly reminder calls from study staff, and were compensated $20 for each hour of CT completed (up to $200). A detailed description of the SOAR study was previously published.[13]

Study Design

This study used a sequential quantitative-to-qualitative mixed-methods design, consisting of 2 phases.[15,16] Figure 1 provides a diagram of the study design and procedures for the study phases. The rationale for using this design was that the quantitative data and results provide a general picture of the research problem (ie, which selected cancer-related symptoms contributed to and/or impeded BCSs' adherence to a web-based CT intervention), whereas the qualitative data and its analysis refined and explained the statistical results by exploring participants' views in more depth.[15,16] As illustrated in Figure 1, the sequence of procedures in this design was as follows: (1) quantitative data collection and analysis, (2) interview protocol development and participant selection, (3) qualitative data collection and analysis, and (4) interpretation and explanation of the quantitative and qualitative results. The following sections are organized by study phase.

■ Phase I: Quantitative

Participants and Data Collection

Convenience sampling was used to select intervention participants (n = 30) from SOAR (N = 60). Control group participants were excluded from the sample. Data included participant characteristics,

Reprinted with permission from Bail, J., et al. (2020). Cancer-related symptoms and cognitive intervention adherence among breast cancer survivors: A mixed methods study. *Cancer Nursing*, 43(5), 354–365.

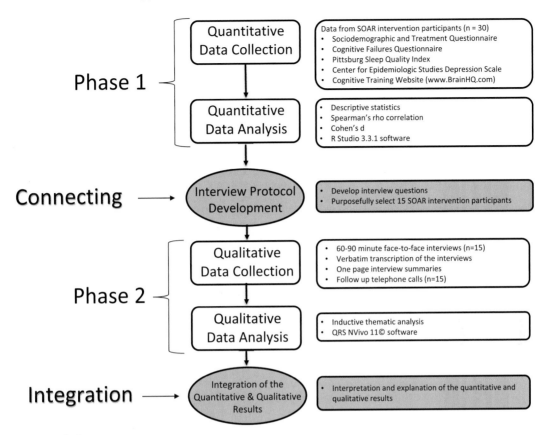

Figure 1. Study design.

perceived cognitive impairment, sleep quality, depressive symptoms (previously collected in SOAR at baseline), and intervention adherence using the following instruments.

PARTICIPANT CHARACTERISTICS

The researchers used a 20-item questionnaire to collect participant characteristics.[13] Items included age, race, education, marital status, employment status, household size and income, date of cancer diagnosis, type of surgery, cancer treatment, weight gain, and use of support services.

PERCEIVED COGNITIVE IMPAIRMENT

Perceived cognitive impairment was measured via the validated Cognitive Failures Questionnaire, a 25-item self-report instrument that measures cognitive failures (ie, memory, attention, and motor function) on a 5-point Likert scale over a 6-month period.[17,18] Scores range from 0 to 100, with higher scores indicating greater perceived cognitive impairment.

SLEEP QUALITY

Sleep quality was measured using the validated Pittsburgh Sleep Quality Index (PSQI), an 11-item self-report instrument assessing sleep quality among adults over a 4-week period.[19,20] Scores range from 0 to 21, with a score of 5 or greater indicative of poor sleep quality.

DEPRESSIVE SYMPTOMS

Depressive symptoms were measured using the validated Center for Epidemiologic Studies–Depression Scale (CES-D), a 20-item self-report instrument that measures the occurrence of depressive symptoms on a 4-point Likert scale over a 1-week period.[21,22] Scores range from 0 to 60, with a score of 5 or greater indicative of depressive symptoms.[23]

INTERVENTION ADHERENCE

The online CT program BrainHQ (www.BrainHQ.com) tracked the duration of each training session. While the SOAR intervention protocol requested participants to complete 10 hours of CT (2 hours a week over 6-8 weeks), consistent with seminal CT studies, participants who completed 8 hours or more of CT were considered adherent to the intervention.[8]

Data Analysis

Data were analyzed using RStudio software version 3.3.1.[24] Descriptive statistics were conducted for the participant characteristics.

Reprinted with permission from Bail, J., et al. (2020). Cancer-related symptoms and cognitive intervention adherence among breast cancer survivors: A mixed methods study. *Cancer Nursing, 43*(5), 354–365.

Frequencies and percentages were used to describe all categorical variables. Means and SDs were generated for scores on all continuous variables. Adherence was dichotomized as adherent (≥8 hours of CT) and nonadherent (<8 hours of CT). Correlations among continuous (perceived cognitive impairment, depressive symptoms, and sleep quality) and categorical (adherence) study variables were analyzed using the nonparametric test Spearman's ρ. Correlation strength was determined using Cohen's standard (small ~0.1, medium ~0.3, large ~0.5 or greater).[25] Formal statistical inference was not conducted because of the exploratory rather than confirmatory nature of the investigation.

Results

Participants had a mean age of 54 years and mean survivorship time of 6 years, and the majority were African American (AA) (Table 1). While the majority of these women were college graduates, fewer than half were employed, with many being retired or disabled. Almost all participants had health insurance, and many had a household income of more than $50 000 per year. Most households included children and/or a spouse. Weight gain since treatment was common among participants, and the majority were on endocrine therapy. Mean instrument scores indicated poor sleep quality, depressive symptoms, and perceived cognitive impairment among participants (Table 2). Four participants had PSQI scores of less than 5, indicating good sleep quality, and 24 participants had PSQI scores of 5 or greater, indicating poor sleep quality. One participant had a CES-D score of less than 5, indicating that they were not likely to be experiencing depressive symptoms; 11 participants had CES-D scores of 5 or greater, indicating depressive symptoms; and 18 participants had CES-D scores of 16 or greater, indicating high depressive symptoms. Cognitive Failures Questionnaire scores ranged from 29 to 80, indicating worse perceived cognitive function. The mean duration of CT was 7.17 hours. Seventeen participants completed 8 hours or more of CT, meeting the defined criterion for adherence. Spearman's ρ correlation suggested relationships between adherence and perceived cognitive impairment, depressive symptoms, and sleep quality. A small to medium inverse correlation occurred with sleep quality and adherence (r_s = −0.24, P = .19). Nonrelevant correlations were seen with depressive symptoms and adherence (r_s = −0.03, P = .87) and perceived cognitive impairment and adherence (r_s = 0.17, P = .85). In addition, sleep quality had a statistically nonsignificant marginal correlation with perceived cognitive impairment (r_s = 0.29, P = .12) and depressive symptoms (r_s = 0.29, P = .11).

▪ Phase II: Qualitative

Interview Protocol Development

Interview questions (Table 3) sought to elicit potential facilitators and/or barriers to CT and how cancer-related symptoms shaped BCSs' intervention adherence. The development of the interview

☀ Table 1 • Sociodemographic and Treatment Data (N = 30)

Variables	Mean (SD) Range	n (%)
Age, y	53.69 (10) 35–71	
Survivorship, y	6.1 (5.69) 1–25	
Race		
African American		16 (53%)
Caucasian		14 (47%)
Education, y	15.10 (2.9) 12-20	
High school or less		6 (20%)
Some college		9 (30%)
College graduate		15 (50%)
Marital status		
Married		18 (60%)
Divorced		6 (20%)
Never married		6 (20%)
Living with others		25 (83%)
Spouse		15 (50%)
Children	1–5	17 (57%)
Parents		2 (12%)
Other relatives		3 (18%)
Employment status		
Employed		14 (46.6%)
Unemployed		4 (13.4%)
Retired/disabled		12 (40%)
Household income		
<$10 000		1 (3%)
$10 000-$50 000		11 (37%)
>$50 000		12 (40%)
Chemotherapy		
Yes		26 (87%)
No		4 (13%)
Radiation		
Yes		24 (80%)
No		6 (20%)
Endocrine therapy		
Yes		20 (67%)
No		10 (33%)
Weight gain[a]		15 (50%)
Weight gained, lb	23 (14) 0–50	
Current weight, lb	192 (40.5) 123–274	
Support services		
Support group		19 (63.4%)
Counseling		3 (10%)
Electronic/blog		1 (3.3%)
None		9 (30%)

[a]Does not equal 100%.

protocol was based on quantitative results and probed for additional factors.[15,16] The interview protocol consisted of 9 open-ended questions to allow participants to fully express their viewpoints and experiences.[26] Follow-up prompts were used for further understanding.[27] The protocol included questions that

Reprinted with permission from Bail, J., et al. (2020). Cancer-related symptoms and cognitive intervention adherence among breast cancer survivors: A mixed methods study. *Cancer Nursing*, *43*(5), 354–365.

Table 2 • Cognitive Training and Self-reported Cancer-Related Symptoms (N = 30)

Variables	Total (N = 30) Mean (SD) Range	r_s
Cognitive training hours[a]	7.17 (4.07) 0–14	—
Perceived cognitive failures[b]	55.60 (12.64) 29–80	0.17
Depressive symptoms[c]	17.87 (9.89) 2–43	−0.03
Sleep disturbances[d]	8.87 (4.38) 1–19	−0.24

[a]Collected from BrainHQ (adherent ≥8 hours of cognitive training < nonadherent).
[b]Measured by the Cognitive Failures Questionnaire, with higher scores indicative of worse perceived cognitive function.
[c]Measured by the Center for Epidemiologic Studies–Depression Scale, with a score of 5 or greater indicative of depressive symptoms and 16 or greater indicative of high depressive symptoms.
[d]Measured by the Pittsburgh Sleep Quality Index, with a score of 5 or greater indicative of poor sleep quality.
r_s is Spearman's ρ correlation with adherence (absolute value): small ~0.1, medium ~0.3, large ~0.5 or greater.

focused on study expectations and impressions, experiences and influences of cancer-related symptoms, experiences and influences of CT, facilitators/barriers to CT, and the environment for CT. The protocol was pilot tested with 2 SOAR participants who were not part of the phase II sample.

Participant Selection

Participants for phase II (Table 4) were selected from phase I participants. To aid in understanding variations in experiences, maximum variation purposeful sampling (based on adherence) was used to select 13 interview participants,[15,16] resulting in a balanced representation of adherent (n = 6) and nonadherent (n = 7) participants. To further explore preliminary phase II (qualitative) findings (eg, experiencing anxiety, frustration, and self-defeating thoughts during CT), 2 additional participants, who had completed 1 hour or less of CT, were selected for interviews. Data saturation occurred at 15 participants.

Data Collection

Participants completed a 1-time face-to-face interview. Interviews were guided by the interview protocol, audio recorded, and lasted

Table 3 • Interview Questions

Question	Follow-up Prompts
1. What expectations did you have when you enrolled in the SOAR study?	• How did the study meet your expectations? • How easy was the study? • How difficult was the study?
2. What is your overall impression of cognitive training?	• Do you think the number of training hours were sufficient? Why or why not? • What did you like about the training? • What did you dislike about the training? • How helpful do you think the training was for you?
3. What changes have you noticed after completing the cognitive training?	• How do you think that your mental abilities have improved? Why? Can you give an example? • How do you think that your mood has improved? Why? Can you give an example? • How do you think that your sleep has improved? Why? Can you give an example?
4. Tell me what helped you complete the cognitive training.	• How did you schedule your training? What day/time worked best? Why? • Where did you do your training? Was it free from distractions? • How comfortable were you using the computer? Did you have assistance from others?
5. Tell me about any challenges you faced with cognitive training.	• Were you able to overcome these challenges? How or why not? • What difficulties did you experience in accessing/navigating the training? • How did daily activities/responsibilities interfere with the training? • What would have made the training easier for you?
6. What support did you receive from others?	• Please describe what your household looks like. • Did anyone in your household support you? How so? • Did anyone at work support you? How so? • Did anyone in your community/church/support group support you? How so?
7. What other factors helped or challenged you with the cognitive training?	• How do you feel that your ability to focus influenced completing the training? • How do you feel that your sleep quality influenced completing the training? • How do you feel that being in a particular mood influenced completing the training?
8. What advice would you give to other breast cancer survivors about this program?	
9. Is there anything else that would you like to share?	

Reprinted with permission from Bail, J., et al. (2020). Cancer-related symptoms and cognitive intervention adherence among breast cancer survivors: A mixed methods study. *Cancer Nursing*, 43(5), 354–365.

✳ **Table 4** • Qualitative Participant Characteristics (n = 15)

Participant ID	CT Hours	Age	Race	Work Status	Household Size	Household Support	CFQ Score	CES-D Score	PSQI Score
Adherent (n = 6)									
2	10	42	CAU	Homemaker	4	Yes	57	13	3
5	10	40	CAU	Employed	4	Yes	56	27	13
6	10	45	AA	Unemployed	3	Yes	47	10	4
7	10	51	AA	Unemployed	8	Yes	60	16	8
8	10	39	CAU	Employed	1	No	53	11	7
10	10	64	CAU	Retired	2	Yes	78	12	9
Nonadherent (n = 9)									
1	3	41	AA	Employed	6	No	44	21	7
3	3	50	CAU	Disabled	3	No	57	13	3
4	7	61	AA	Retired	1	No	56	27	13
9	3	71	AA	Retired	1	No	47	10	4
11	0	65	AA	Employed	5	No	60	16	8
12	7	68	CAU	Retired	7	Yes	53	11	7
13	0.5	55	AA	Employed	1	No	78	12	9
14	0.72	55	AA	Employed	1	No	43	9	10
15	0.33	62	CAU	Employed	2	No	67	39	10

Abbreviations: AA, African American; CAU, Caucasian; CES-D, Center for Epidemiologic Studies–Depression Scale; CFQ, Cognitive Failures Questionnaire; CT, cognitive training; PSQI, Pittsburgh Sleep Quality Index.

an average of 54 minutes. At the end of the interview, participants received a $25 gift card. Audio recordings were transcribed verbatim. A 1-page summative report was generated and sent to each participant to review for accuracy (member checking). Follow-up calls were conducted within 3 days of the interview, lasted an average of 5 minutes, and allowed for (1) verification of summative report accuracy, (2) researcher clarification, and (3) participants to further elaborate or to add anything they did not previously mention. After completion of the call, participants were mailed another $25 gift card.

Data Analysis

Data analysis occurred simultaneously with data collection and followed Creswell and Creswell's[16] step-by-step approach: (1) organizing and preparing data for analysis, (2) reading and getting familiar with the data, (3) coding the data, (4) synthesizing the codes to develop themes, and (5) interpreting the meaning of the themes. These steps were iterative and were repeated until data interpretation was sufficient to answer the research question.[16] Strategies to establish trustworthiness of the data included spending prolonged time with participants, member checking, audit trail, and study team data review meetings.[28] QSR NVivo software version 11 was used to assist with data analysis.[29]

Results

The following 4 themes emerged: (1) experiences of cancer-related symptoms, (2) influences of CT, (3) adherence to CT, and (4) environment for CT. These themes describe how cancer-related symptoms were related to adherence to SOAR among BCSs and variations in participant experiences. The following sections provide descriptions of these themes, supported by participant quotes. To provide confidentiality, BCSs are referred to by their participant number (eg, PT 01). In addition, to aid in identifying differences and/or similarities among

participant responses and in the integration of the findings, identifiers of adherent/nonadherent, AA/Caucasian, older/younger, and employed/unemployed are used.

THEME 1: EXPERIENCES OF CANCER-RELATED SYMPTOMS

This theme included participants' experiences of perceived cognitive impairment, depressive symptoms, and poor sleep quality. Notably, cancer-related symptoms did not occur in isolation; they were often concurrent and exacerbated difficulty in cognition. Other people (ie, family, friends, and coworkers) did not always understand BCSs' experiences of cancer-related symptoms and were not always supportive.

All participants reported experiencing perceived cognitive impairment since cancer and tended to refer to it as chemobrain. Both AA and Caucasian participants described not being able to remember things that they normally would have before cancer, forgetting names, difficulty finding words, and feeling "foggy" (PT 05 and 08) or "cotton headed" (PT 02). The majority of BCSs were not informed by their healthcare provider about cognitive impairment, which led to some BCSs fearing that they were "going crazy" (PT 07). One participant expressed, "I felt like I was just crazy. I couldn't remember anything" (PT 07). Perceived cognitive impairment was described as an "uncontrollable brain" (PT 01 and 02) that made participants feel out of control. Breast cancer survivors saw their mental ability as an essential part of themselves. One older AA participant spoke of losing one of her greatest assets: "My mind is one of my best assets and that if that starts to dysfunction, that's me" (PT 11). A loss of sense of self was a fear voiced by many BCSs. For a younger Caucasian participant, it was terrifying: "I've always had a quick memory, and so it was terrifying to feel like that part of what's been my identity was slipping away" (PT 08). Overall, BCSs felt that "nobody knows how it feels" (PT 07 and PT 12) to experience cognitive impairment.

African American and Caucasian participants reported experiencing depressive symptoms and described feelings of unhappiness. Sources of unhappiness varied. For some, not being able to enjoy

Reprinted with permission from Bail, J., et al. (2020). Cancer-related symptoms and cognitive intervention adherence among breast cancer survivors: A mixed methods study. *Cancer Nursing, 43*(5), 354–365.

leisure activities made them feel sad. Reading was one leisure activity that BCSs reported not getting pleasure from anymore. Difficulties with focus and memory were key factors in their displeasure with reading: "I didn't have the brain to read long passages anymore, especially if it was a book where I was supposed to carry a lot of names in my mind. That made me sad" (PT 15). For others, social activities were no longer joyful. Social activities were now seen as stressful and dreaded and were avoided. One adherent AA participant characterized the distress of socializing this way: "I didn't enjoy it when I went out, I just didn't. I didn't have any joy" (PT 07). A source of unhappiness was not always identifiable for BCSs. For some BCSs, unhappiness was just a way of being: "I find myself sad, and I don't know why I'm sad" (PT 14). One nonadherent AA participant captured the experience of being unhappy: "When I'm not happy, I may not talk a lot. I may isolate myself. I do a lot of self-examination and blaming because I think I'm responsible for the whole condition of the world" (PT 11).

All BCSs reported experiencing poor sleep quality since their cancer diagnosis. African American and Caucasian participants expressed difficulty falling asleep due to constant random thoughts. One unemployed Caucasian participant noted, "Part of the chemobrain is not being able to sleep" (PT 03). Participants described the experience of constant random thoughts as "my mind won't shut down" (PT 01 and 05) or "my brain won't shut up" (PT 15). Trying to force themselves to sleep and tossing and turning until 3:00 in the morning was an ongoing problem for some BCSs. Difficulty falling asleep affected daily activities and work performance for many BCSs. One employed Caucasian participant who works as a teacher explained, "A lot of times, I don't get to sleep until 3 or 4 o'clock in the morning, so I'm tired, lagging, and lacking energy a lot during the day" (PT 15). Participants described having 3 to 6 hours of disrupted sleep per night. For most BCSs, waking up numerous times per night was due to restlessness, hot flashes, and worrying thoughts. Some BCSs described being able to fall asleep and sleeping for several hours, but then waking up and not be able to go back to sleep. For one nonadherent AA participant, this was a daily occurrence: "I literally wake up at 2:00 AM and can't go back to sleep" (PT 13). Several consecutive days of poor sleep quality lead to exhaustion and eventually "crashing" (PT 01, 03, and 15) for some BCSs. One nonadherent Caucasian participant captured this experience as follows: "I will be so tired because I don't sleep all night. I have hot flashes. I get up all through the night, and I stay awake for so long. Then about 3 or 4 nights in, I just crash and I sleep all night, but I only do that like twice a week, because I just can't sleep" (PT 03).

The frequency of reporting experiencing cancer-related symptoms was similar between adherent and nonadherent participants. However, nonadherent participants' descriptions of experiencing cancer-related symptoms tended to be more emotionally charged with angst and despair than those of adherent participants. The description of these experiences elucidated the state of participants, relating to their mental and physical ability to attend to CT.

THEME 2: INFLUENCES OF COGNITIVE TRAINING

Differences in influences of CT, as well as responses to these influences, were seen between adherent and nonadherent participants.

While nonadherent participants tended to describe negative experiences (eg, anxiety, frustration, and/or self-defeating thoughts), adherent participants tended to describe positive experiences of CT (eg, improvement in cognition, mood, and/or sleep). One AA adherent participant described: "I could see a difference as I went along with the study. The more I put in the time [CT] I could see the improvement in my thinking. My memory was better, my forgetfulness was better" (PT 10). For one Caucasian adherent participant, improvements in her thinking led to improved mood: "I feel less frustrated, because I feel like it makes you feel out of control or something when your mind is not working right. I feel less frustrated with that than I did before. That's a positive in the mood realm" (PT 02). Several adherent participants experienced improved sleep, which was attributed to fewer "random thoughts" (PT 01), less "restlessness" (PT 5 and 10), and a "calmer mind" (PT 07). In contrast, nonadherent participants reported experiencing mental agitation. One nonadherent AA participant referred to CT as "frightening" (PT 14). Several AA participants conveyed thoughts of being "not smart enough" (PT 09, 11, and 14) and "failing" (PT 09, 11, and 14). Consequently, self-defeating thoughts thwarted BCSs from doing CT. One nonadherent AA participant explained, "I just didn't like it, because I wasn't going to be able to remember. I had already set myself up to fail, thinking there were too many things for my memory to prioritize. I became unsure of my own ability" (PT 14). All BCSs who communicated self-defeating thoughts were employed, highly educated women. The experience of self-defeating thinking was summarized by a nonadherent AA participant: "This is going to be so hard that I'm not going to be able to do it, and I'm going to feel worse about myself when I finish" (PT 11). Although some Caucasian participants described experiencing anxiety, frustration, and self-defeating thoughts, these experiences were largely described by AA participants.

THEME 3: ADHERENCE TO COGNITIVE TRAINING

The influence of cancer-related symptoms on adherence varied among the BCSs in this study. While the experience of perceived cognitive impairment hindered adherence for nonadherent participants, for adherent participants it was a source of determination to complete the training. Nonadherent participants tended to view CT as frustrating. These feelings of frustration impaired participants' ability to focus, made CT mentally exhausting, and led to avoidance. These participants described not being in the mood to be "fooling" (PT 03) or "fiddling" (PT 15) with CT, and they "just didn't do it" (PT 13 and 12). A nonadherent AA participant explained, "It was frustrating, I couldn't do it [CT]. I couldn't concentrate. I was like, 'I'm not fooling with you today!'" (PT 03). In contrast, adherent participants viewed CT as a tool to improve their cognition. In order to improve their cognition, they persevered through cognitive difficulties, frustration, and sleeplessness to complete the CT. One adherent AA participant wanting to improve her cognition explained, "I knew there was something that the chemo did, and I needed something to improve it" (PT 06). Improving cognition served as a driving force for CT among these BCSs. One adherent participant, who experienced cognitive improvement, described her resolve: "I was just determined to

Reprinted with permission from Bail, J., et al. (2020). Cancer-related symptoms and cognitive intervention adherence among breast cancer survivors: A mixed methods study. *Cancer Nursing*, 43(5), 354–365.

complete it [CT] because I see I was improving" (PT 10). Determination kindled adherence to CT. One adherent AA participant captured the essence of determination: "You just have to have a willingness to stick with it [CT] or it won't work. You can sit back and get frustrated and say I don't want to do it [CT] and give up, or you can just go on and just persevere and just say, 'I'm not going to let this beat me.' That's what I did with the cancer. That's what I did with the CT. Just determined that I will beat this" (PT 07). Differences in frequency of describing influences of depressive symptoms and poor sleep quality on CT adherence were seen between Caucasian and AA participants. That is, Caucasians tended to more frequently describe the influence of depressive symptoms, and AA participants tended to more frequently describe the influence of poor sleep quality. Depressive symptoms and poor sleep quality were noted to negatively influence CT motivation and performance among nonadherent and some adherent participants. Not being in the mood or being too tired made focusing more difficult and CT frustrating. Feelings of frustration and exhaustion resulted in nonadherent participants, and occasionally some adherent participants, not wanting to be bothered with CT and just skipping it.

THEME 4: ENVIRONMENT FOR COGNITIVE TRAINING

Environmental influences included computer access, household dynamics, and support system. Employed Caucasian and AA participants were very "comfortable using the computer" (PT 13 and 14), since they "do it all the time" (PT 05 and 08), and were able to access the CT without any difficulties. One employed AA participant described accessing the CT as "It was easy. The software was easy, self-explanatory, not a problem" (PT 01). Unemployed AA BCSs needed assistance to access the CT. For these participants, using the computer was not a regular activity. However, once receiving assistance, participants were self-sufficient and able to manage on their own. Assistance was provided by children living in the household. One unemployed AA participant described: "I'm not that computer literate, but my daughter helped me. Then after that, it was a go! Once you got started, there was no problem" (PT 09).

Due to "life events" (PT 01, 03, and 12), some nonadherent participants had unexpected changes in the household. Unexpected changes of having extended family members moving in changed the normal household environment and added additional responsibilities, causing some participants to become distressed and sidetracked, which hindered CT. Household support was advantageous to CT. Explaining personal significance of the study (ie, importance of study participation) facilitated receiving support from others. One adherent Caucasian participant who shared her personal significance of the study with her family members and received their support described: "I explained to them about what it was for and what I felt about it contributing and being a part of offering something to help people. They were totally on board and supportive of me doing that because they knew it was important to me" (PT 02). The act of "keeping it to self" hindered AA participants from receiving CT support. Several AA nonadherent participants revealed not sharing with others about participating in the study. Instead, they "kept it to

myself" (PT 01, 04, 09, 13, and 14). They felt CT was something personal and were not comfortable telling others. One nonadherent AA participant remarked, "I'm kind of private on stuff like that. They didn't know" (PT 04). One AA nonadherent participant explained how "you do not tell these things; it is better to keep it to yourself" (PT 01). One nonadherent AA participant described the stigma of "chemobrain" as "shaming" (PT 14). This act of "kept it to myself" impeded AA participants from receiving support from others. One nonadherent AA participant, who did not share the importance of the study and did not receive any household support, described how having support at home matters and how it may have made a difference in her completing the CT: "If I had support, a lot of things might have changed. Just to realize how important that was for me. Yeah, maybe I could have completed those 10 hours [CT]. Yeah, support at home matters" (PT 01).

INTERRELATION OF THEMES

We further explored the interrelationships of the 4 emergent themes: (1) *experiences* of cancer-related symptoms, (2) *influences* of CT, (3) *adherence* to CT, and (4) *environment* for CT. The model presented in Figure 2 illustrates how the themes interact with each other. All BCSs in this study experienced cancer-related symptoms; therefore, cancer-related symptoms appear at the core of the figure. The way BCSs *experience* cancer-related symptoms (ie, feelings of depression, poor sleep quality, and cognitive impairment) *influences* how CT effects cancer-related symptoms. The *influence* of CT on cancer-related symptoms impacts *adherence* to CT. *Adherence* to CT drives how cancer-related symptoms are *experienced*. All of which is transpiring in the *environment* (computer access, household dynamics, support system)

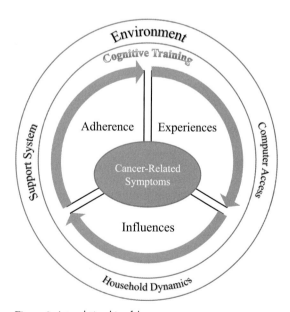

Figure 2. Interrelationship of themes.

Reprinted with permission from Bail, J., et al. (2020). Cancer-related symptoms and cognitive intervention adherence among breast cancer survivors: A mixed methods study. *Cancer Nursing, 43*(5), 354–365.

in which CT occurs. The arrows in the figure capture the dynamic character of how the themes interact with each other.

■ Integration/Discussion of Quantitative and Qualitative Findings

Results of the quantitative and qualitative phases were integrated to provide a more in-depth understanding of the relationship between selected cancer-related symptoms and adherence and how they contribute to differences in adherence to the SOAR CT intervention among BCSs. We discuss the integrated findings as they are related to the 3 cancer-related symptoms (ie, perceived cognitive impairment, depressive symptoms, and poor sleep quality) that collectively influence BCSs' adherence to CT. We developed a statistics-by-themes joint display to help guide the comparison and integrated interpretation of the quantitative and qualitative findings (Table 5). In the following paragraphs, we discuss integrated conclusions using a weaving strategy.[30]

Perceived Cognitive Impairment

Quantitative results revealed the presence of perceived cognitive impairment among participants, which had a nonrelevant correlation with adherence. The qualitative data elucidated that CT challenged participants and raised their awareness of perceived cognitive impairment and confirmed that BCSs' response to this raised awareness differed. Personal determination was pivotal in how BCSs responded to the difficulty of CT and the raised awareness of perceived cognitive impairment and, consequently, in their willingness to persevere to complete the CT. Those who persevered reported experiencing improved cognition. These findings are supported by cognitive studies among other populations. In a study of 32 older adults with mild cognitive impairment (mean age, 67 years; 53% female), Werheid and colleagues[31] reported that participants with more awareness of their cognitive impairment were less likely to participate in a cognitive intervention. However, among traumatic brain injury patients, awareness of cognitive impairment is positively associated with motivation for cognitive interventions.[32] According to Hill and colleagues,[33] this difference in response may be related to personality type. That is, participants who ordinarily would be high-achieving goal setters but are aware of their cognitive impairment might be less willing to risk participation in cognitive interventions where they might not meet their own high expectations. In addition, findings from the present study are consistent with CT studies among BCSs. Becker and colleagues[34] reported a 0% adherence rate to their web-based CT intervention among 20 female BCSs (mean age, 53 years; 85% Caucasian). This lack of adherence was attributed to BCSs' verbal reports of being unmotivated due to awareness of poor CT performance. Von Ah and colleagues[35] reported that 17% of BCSs (mean age, 57 years; 89% Caucasian) indicated that CT was difficult. Yet, evidence exists that continued CT improves perceived cognitive function among BCSs.[34–37] Findings from this study illuminated that BCSs' response to their awareness of perceived cognitive impairment is critical to CT adherence and ultimately improving cognition.

Depressive Symptoms

Breast cancer survivors' descriptions of the experiences of depressive symptoms and CT aid in understanding the relationship between depressive symptoms and adherence to CT. Quantitative results revealed the presence of clinically relevant depressive symptoms (CES-D ≥16) among participants. A correlational analysis identified a nonrelevant inverse correlation between depressive symptoms and adherence. The qualitative data elucidated that CT exacerbated depressive symptoms among some BCSs, resulting in not being in the mood to be "fooling" with CT and just not doing it. Yet, those who persevered experienced improved mood. An inverse relationship between depressive symptoms and adherence is supported by intervention studies aimed at improving quality of life among BCSs. Lack of adherence in these interventions often was attributed to depressive symptoms.[10,11,38,39] Breast cancer survivors who had higher levels of depressive symptoms at baseline were less likely to comply with the intervention protocol than those who did not. For example, Wang and colleagues[11] found that baseline depressive symptoms were associated with lower intervention adherence to the WHEL study, a dietary intervention among 2800 female BCSs (mean age, 53 years; 86% Caucasian). In the Rural Breast Cancer Survivors Study, a population-based psychoeducational support intervention among 432 rural female BCSs (mean age, 63 years; 94% Caucasian), Meneses and colleagues[10] found that depressive symptoms were a significant predictor of attrition. The experience of improvements in mood is supported by findings from other CT interventions among BCSs and healthy older adults. Breast cancer survivors report an improvement in depressive symptoms after CT.[34–37] Among healthy older adults, CT has been demonstrated to reduce the risk of depression and improve internal locus of control.[40,41] Previous cognitive studies among BCSs have reported adherence rates as low as 0% (range, 0%-97%), with attrition rates as high as 22% (range, 3%-22%).[34–37] Von Ah and colleagues[35] reported that some BCSs indicated, via a Likert-based Client Satisfaction Questionnaire, not enjoying CT (23%) and preferring a different cognitive intervention (20%). Yet, participant reactions to CT and influences on depressive symptoms among these studies are unreported and unknown. Findings from this study illuminate that CT exacerbates depressive symptoms among some BCSs, hindering adherence.

Poor Sleep Quality

Breast cancer survivors' description of the experiences of poor sleep quality and CT aided in understanding the relationship between sleep quality and adherence to CT. Quantitative results revealed the presence of poor sleep quality (PSQI ≥5) among participants. A correlational analysis identified a moderate, nonsignificant inverse correlation between sleep quality and adherence. In addition, sleep quality had a moderate, nonsignificant correlation with perceived cognitive impairment and depressive symptoms. The qualitative data elucidated that poor sleep quality aggravated cognition and mood and negatively influenced CT motivation and performance, creating a snowball effect for nonadherent participants. Those who continued CT experienced improved sleep, mood, and ambition. Previous quantitative studies

Reprinted with permission from Bail, J., et al. (2020). Cancer-related symptoms and cognitive intervention adherence among breast cancer survivors: A mixed methods study. *Cancer Nursing*, 43(5), 354–365.

✳ **Table 5 • Integrated Findings by Cancer-Related Symptom**

Quantitative			Qualitative			
Adherence	Hours	Score	Experiences of Cancer-Related Symptoms	Influences of Cognitive Training	Adherence to Cognitive Training	Environment for Cognitive Training
Perceived cognitive impairment[a]						
Adherent	10	78	"Before I was sharp as a tack. I've left the stove on I can't tell you how many times and I used to never do that."	"I was just determined to complete it because I could see the improvement in my thinking."	"It [ability to focus] did influence me doing my brain training. I knew there was something that the chemo did and I needed something to improve it."	"My daughter and my husband really encouraged me to do it."
Nonadherent	3	57	"I used to be pretty sharp. I know that these things that I'm forgetting, I shouldn't be forgetting, I just can't remember anything."	"It was pretty difficult. I felt like I was stressing, because I was trying so hard to get them right. Then it would be over. Thank goodness!"	"You have to be able to focus. If you can't focus, then there's no way you could do it. You can't do it with people walking in, talking to you, and asking you questions. At least once or twice, I had to stop because I just could not focus"	"I had a grandchild that I was taking care of at the time. My husband was out of town working, which didn't help a whole lot."
Depressive symptoms[b]						
Adherent	10	16	"When you can't remember things, it's frustrating and you get angry and you feel bad. I would just cry because some things were just important."	"It really has helped me. Before I couldn't remember things, I just felt inadequate. Now my confidence has come back, and I just feel good. I'm happier now. I smile more."	"Some days, yeah, it frustrated me. I got a little frustrated. I wanted to beat it. I didn't want it to beat me, so I kept on and kept on. I was determined that it wasn't going to beat me."	"My son let me use his computer. My daughter cooked and made sure things were clean so I could do the training. I really had a lot of help."
Nonadherent	0.33	39	"If my husband is telling me directions to a place, and he gives me more than 3 or 4 directions at a time, I can't process it; it makes me nervous."	"The program itself made me nervous and anxious. My breath stops; my heart races."	"I couldn't do it; I couldn't commit to it. It made me anxious."	"I didn't receive any support. I told my husband it made me anxious and crazy. I think his response was, 'Ooh, that sounds awful.'"
Sleep quality[c]						
Adherent	10	4	"I do get up in the night. Sometimes I can't go back to sleep. Sometimes I'm feeling tired during the day."	"When I was doing it, I was staying focused. It was awesome. I just see that it could help. It helped. It was just good."	"I still do it. It was still motivated to do it. If I was tired or sleepy, I was like 'let me get on here.'"	"My daughters were, like, 'Mama, you doing your brain training? How long you going to stay on today?' They wanted me to do it."
Nonadherent	0.5	9	"I still wake up sometimes two, 3 o'clock in the morning and can't go back to sleep. Usually by the end of the day I have to go home and take a nap."	"When I was doing it, it's like my brain hurt. I didn't get a headache per se, but it made me mentally exhausted."	"By the time I did have time to actually do it, I was tired already, physically tired, and then the exercises seemed to make me more mentally tired. And so it was like a bad combination."	"I live alone. Nobody knew I was doing it. I didn't see the need to share."

Hours = cognitive training hours completed and ranged from 0 to 10, with 8 or more considered as adherent.
[a]Measured by the Cognitive Failures Questionnaire, with higher scores indicative of worse perceived cognitive function.
[b]Measured by the Center for Epidemiologic Studies–Depression Scale, with a score of 5 or greater indicative of depressive symptoms and 16 or greater indicative of high depressive symptoms.
[c]Measured by the Pittsburgh Sleep Quality Index, with a score of 5 or greater indicative of poor sleep quality.

Reprinted with permission from Bail, J., et al. (2020). Cancer-related symptoms and cognitive intervention adherence among breast cancer survivors: A mixed methods study. *Cancer Nursing*, 43(5), 354–365.

among BCSs indicate significant associations among sleep quality, depressive symptoms, and cognitive function.[42-45] Recently, Johns and colleagues[46] reported that baseline sleep quality was significantly correlated with depressive symptoms and perceived cognitive impairment among BCSs (mean age, 57 years; 94% female; 77% Caucasian) in their mindfulness-based stress reduction intervention. Vance et al[47] describe sleep, mood, and cognition as having a dynamic relationship and posit that their interactions influence daily functioning and ability to perform tasks. Consistent with this idea, Prigozin and colleagues[48] found sleep, mood, and cognitive function were significantly associated with interference in daily activities (eg, housework, employment, socializing, and physical activity) among BCSs. Qualitative studies confirm this finding through BCSs' descriptions of concurrent cancer-related symptoms interfering with their ability to perform activities of daily living.[3-5] In addition, concurrent cancer symptoms have been shown to interfere with intervention participation among BCSs. Derry and colleagues[49] found BCSs who dropped out of their 12-week yoga intervention reported greater perceived cognitive impairment and depressive symptoms and poorer sleep quality at baseline compared with those who completed the study. McChargue and colleagues[50] found sleep quality and depressive symptoms significantly impacted BCSs' adherence to their behavioral therapy sleep intervention. Yet, the influence of concurrent cancer-related symptoms on CT adherence among BCSs has not been reported. Findings from this study suggest that concurrent cancer-related symptoms hindered CT adherence among BCSs. In addition, this study illuminated that poor sleep quality tends to exacerbate depressive symptoms and perceived cognitive impairment among some BCSs, indicating that sleep quality may be pivotal in CT adherence among BCSs.

■ Implications for Clinical Practice

Two considerations for clinical practice emerged. First, the National Comprehensive Cancer Network survivorship guidelines[2] can be applied. These guidelines recommend routinely assessing cognitive function, sleep, mood, and distress and encouraging healthy living strategies for self-management.[2] In assessing cognitive function, it is advised to (a) ask BCSs if they are experiencing any cognitive difficulties and validate BCSs' self-reported cognitive concerns; (b) screen for depression, pain, fatigue, poor sleep quality, and distress; (c) review current medications and discuss those that interfere with cognition; (d) provide strategies for healthy living (eg, physical activity, nutrition, good sleep hygiene, and stress reduction); and (e) refer BCSs with signs of cognitive impairment for neuropsychological assessment and CT if available.[2] Second, clinicians need to be aware that cancer-related symptoms may exacerbate cognition. Education on and resources for self-management of cancer-related symptoms can be provided.[2] Reviewing and reinforcing education materials and resources are vital. Findings from this study suggest that concurrent cancer-related symptoms hindered CT among BCSs. Applying the National Comprehensive Cancer Network survivorship guidelines and providing symptom self-management education and resources may support BCSs to attend (mentally and physically) to cognitive interventions.

■ Strengths and Limitations

This study had both strengths and limitations. African American (53%) and Caucasian (47%) BCSs were nearly equally represented, allowing the researchers to fully explore perspectives of both groups. A meaningful integration of quantitative and qualitative methods in the study design provided an in-depth understanding of the relationship between selected cancer-related symptoms and adherence and the different ways they contributed to adherence to the SOAR intervention among BCSs. While the small sample size (30 participants) was a limitation, still data saturation was met.

■ Conclusion

This study is the first to document an understanding of cancer-related symptoms and CT among BCSs. Experiences of and responses to CT and cancer-related symptoms shape adherence to CT among BCSs. Breast cancer survivors in this study who continued CT reported experiencing improved sleep, mood, and cognition. Clinicians can routinely assess cognition and provide education and resources for management of cancer-related symptoms. To aid in cognitive intervention adherence among BCSs, future studies may consider applying a comprehensive approach aimed at addressing concurrent cancer-related symptoms.

References

1. American Cancer Society. *Cancer Facts & Figures 2018*. Vol. 2018. Atlanta, GA: American Cancer Society, Inc.

2. National Comprehensive Cancer Network (NCCN). Survivorship Guidelines (version 3.2017); 2017. http://www.nccn.org/professionals/physician_gls/pdf/survivorship.pdf. Accessed February 18, 2019.

3. Von Ah D, Habermann B, Carpenter JS, Schneider BL. Impact of perceived cognitive impairment in breast cancer survivors. *Eur J Oncol Nurs*. 2013;17(2): 236–241.

4. Becker H, Henneghan A, Mikan SQ. When do I get my brain back? Breast cancer survivors' experiences of cognitive problems. *Clin J Oncol Nurs*. 2015; 19(2):180–184.

5. Boykoff N, Moieni M, Subramanian SK. Confronting chemobrain: an in-depth look at survivors' reports of impact on work, social networks, and health care response. *J Cancer Surviv*. 2009;3(4):223–232.

6. Vance DE, Frank JS, Bail J, et al. Interventions for cognitive deficits in breast cancer survivors treated with chemotherapy. *Cancer Nurs*. 2017; 40(1):E11–E27.

7. Von Ah D, Jansen CE, Allen DH. Evidence-based interventions for cancer- and treatment-related cognitive impairment. *Clin J Oncol Nurs*. 2014;18 (suppl):17–25.

8. Edwards JD, Xu H, Clark DO, Ross LA, Unverzagt FW. Speed of processing training results in lower risk of dementia. *Alzheimers Dement*. 2017;3(4): 603–611.

9. Kesler SR, Watson CL, Blayney DW. Brain network alterations and vulnerability to simulated neurodegeneration in breast cancer. *Neurobiol Aging*. 2015;36(8):2429–2442.

10. Meneses K, Azuero A, Su X, Benz R, McNees P. Predictors of attrition among rural breast cancer survivors. *Res Nurs Health*. 2014;37(1):21–31.

11. Wang JB, Pierce JP, Ayala GX, et al. Baseline depressive symptoms, completion of study assessments, and behavior change in a long-term dietary intervention among breast cancer survivors. *Ann Behav Med*. 2015;49(6):819–827.

Reprinted with permission from Bail, J., et al. (2020). Cancer-related symptoms and cognitive intervention adherence among breast cancer survivors: A mixed methods study. *Cancer Nursing, 43*(5), 354–365.

12. Henneghan A. Modifiable factors and cognitive dysfunction in breast cancer survivors: a mixed-method systematic review. *Support Care Cancer*. 2016;24(1): 481–497.

13. Meneses K, Benz R, Bail JR, et al. Speed of processing training in middle-aged and older breast cancer survivors (SOAR): results of a randomized controlled pilot. *Breast Cancer Res Treat*. 2018;168(1):259–267.

14. Lenz ER, Pugh LC, Milligan RA, Gift A, Suppe F. The middle-range theory of unpleasant symptoms: an update. *Adv Nurs Sci*. 1997;19(3):14–27.

15. Ivankova NV, Creswell JW, Stick SL. Using mixed-methods sequential explanatory design: from theory to practice. *Field Method*. 2006;18(1):3–20.

16. Creswell JW, Creswell JD. *Research Design: Qualitative, Quantitative, and Mixed Methods Approaches*. Thousand Oaks, CA: Sage Publications; 2017.

17. Broadbent DE, Cooper PF, FitzGerald P, Parkes KR. The Cognitive Failures Questionnaire (CFQ) and its correlates. *Br J Clin Psychol*. 1982; 21(pt 1):1–16.

18. Vom Hofe A, Mainemarre G, Vannier L-C. Sensitivity to everyday failures and cognitive inhibition: are they related? *Exp Brain Res*. 1998;48(1):49–56.

19. Buysse DJ, Reynolds CF3rd, Monk TH, Berman SR, Kupfer DJ. The Pittsburgh Sleep Quality Index: a new instrument for psychiatric practice and research. *Psychiatry Res*. 1989;28(2):193–213.

20. Akman T, Yavuzsen T, Sevgen Z, Ellidokuz H, Yilmaz AU. Evaluation of sleep disorders in cancer patients based on Pittsburgh Sleep Quality Index. *Eur J Cancer Care*. 2015;24(4):553–559.

21. Radloff LS. The CES-D scale: a self-report depression scale for research in the general population. *Appl Psychol Meas*. 1977;1(3):385–401.

22. Hann D, Winter K, Jacobsen P. Measurement of depressive symptoms in cancer patients: evaluation of the Center for Epidemiological Studies Depression Scale (CES-D). *J Psychosom Res*. 1999;46(5):437–443.

23. Aggarwal A, Freund K, Sato A, et al. Are depressive symptoms associated with cancer screening and cancer stage at diagnosis among postmenopausal women? The Women's Health Initiative observational cohort. *J Womens Health*. 2008;17(8):1353–1361.

24. RStudio Team. *RStudio: Integrated Development for R*. Boston, MA: RStudio, Inc; 2015: www.rstudio.com. Accessed February 18, 2019.

25. Cohen J. *Statistical Power Analysis for the Behavioral Sciences*. New York, NY: Routledge Publishing; 1988.

26. DiCicco-Bloom B, Crabtree BF. The qualitative research interview. *Med Educ*. 2006;40(4):314–321.

27. Turner DWIII. Qualitative interview design: a practical guide for novice investigators. *Qual Rep*. 2010;15(3):754.

28. Lincoln YS, Guba EG. But is it rigorous? Trustworthiness and authenticity in naturalistic evaluation. *New Dir Eval*. 1985;1986(30):73–84.

29. QSR International. NVivo Qualitative Data Analysis Software. 2017. www.qsrinternational.com/nvivo. Accessed February 18, 2019.

30. Fetters MD, Curry LA, Creswell JW. Achieving integration in mixed methods designs-principles and practices. *Health Serv Res*. 2013;48(6 pt 2):2134–2156.

31. Werheid K, Ziegler M, Klapper A, Kühl KP. Awareness of memory failures and motivation for cognitive training in mild cognitive impairment. *Dement Geriatr Cogn Disord*. 2010;30(2):155–160.

32. Flashman LA, McAllister TW. Lack of awareness and its impact in traumatic brain injury. *Neurorehabilitation*. 2002;17(4):285–296.

33. Hill NL, Kolanowski AM, Fick D, Chinchilli VM, Jablonski RA. Personality as a moderator of cognitive stimulation in older adults at high risk for cognitive decline. *Res Gerontol Nurs*. 2014;7(4):159–170.

34. Becker H, Henneghan AM, Volker DL, Mikan SQ. A pilot study of a cognitive-behavioral intervention for breast cancer survivors. *Oncol Nurs Forum*. 2017;44(2):255–264.

35. Von Ah D, Carpenter JS, Saykin A, et al. Advanced cognitive training for breast cancer survivors: a randomized controlled trial. *Breast Cancer Res Treat*. 2012;135(3):799–809.

36. Damholdt MF, Mehlsen M, O'Toole MS, Andreasen RK, Pedersen AD, Zachariae R. Web-based cognitive training for breast cancer survivors with cognitive complaints: a randomized controlled trial. *Psychooncology*. 2016.

37. Kesler S, Hadi Hosseini SM, Heckler C, et al. Cognitive training for improving executive function in chemotherapy-treated breast cancer survivors. *Clin Breast Cancer*. 2013;13(4):299–306.

38. Courneya KS, Segal RJ, Gelmon K, et al. Predictors of supervised exercise adherence during breast cancer chemotherapy. *Med Sci Sports Exerc*. 2008; 40(6):1180–1187.

39. Somerset SM, Graham L, Markwell K. Depression scores predict adherence in a dietary weight loss intervention trial. *Clin Nutr*. 2011;30(5):593–598.

40. Wolinsky FD, Vander Weg MW, Martin R, et al. Does cognitive training improve internal locus of control among older adults? *J Gerontol B Psychol Sci Soc Sci*. 2010;65(5):591–598.

41. Wolinsky FD, Vander Weg MW, Martin R, et al. The effect of speed-of-processing training on depressive symptoms in ACTIVE. *J Gerontol A Biol Sci Med Sci*. 2009;64(4):468–472.

42. Chen ML, Miaskowski C, Liu LN, Chen SC. Changes in perceived attentional function in women following breast cancer surgery. *Breast Cancer Res Treat*. 2012;131(2):599–606.

43. Cheung YT, Tan EH, Chan A. An evaluation on the neuropsychological tests used in the assessment of postchemotherapy cognitive changes in breast cancer survivors. *Support Care Cancer*. 2012;20(7):1361–1375.

44. Myers JS, Wick JA, Klemp J. Potential factors associated with perceived cognitive impairment in breast cancer survivors. *Support Care Cancer*. 2015;23(11):3219–3228.

45. Von Ah D, Tallman EF. Perceived cognitive function in breast cancer survivors: evaluating relationships with objective cognitive performance and other symptoms using the Functional Assessment of Cancer Therapy–Cognitive Function Instrument. *J Pain Symptom Manage*. 2015;49(4):697–706.

46. Johns SA, Von Ah D, Brown LF, et al. Randomized controlled pilot trial of mindfulness-based stress reduction for breast and colorectal cancer survivors: effects on cancer-related cognitive impairment. *J Cancer Surviv*. 2016;10(3): 437–448.

47. Vance DE, Heaton K, Eaves Y, Fazeli PL. Sleep and cognition on everyday functioning in older adults: implications for nursing practice and research. *J Neurosci Nurs*. 2011;43(5):261–271; quiz 272-263.

48. Prigozin A, Uziely B, Musgrave CF. The relationship between symptom severity and symptom interference, education, age, marital status, and type of chemotherapy treatment in israeli women with early-stage breast cancer. *Oncol Nurs Forum*. 2010;37(6):E411–E418.

49. Derry HM, Jaremka LM, Bennett JM, et al. Yoga and self-reported cognitive problems in breast cancer survivors: a randomized controlled trial. *Psychooncology*. 2015;24(8):958–966.

50. McChargue DE, Sankaranarayanan J, Visovsky CG, Matthews EE, Highland KB, Berger AM. Predictors of adherence to a behavioral therapy sleep intervention during breast cancer chemotherapy. *Support Care Cancer*. 2012;20(2):245–252.

Reprinted with permission from Bail, J., et al. (2020). Cancer-related symptoms and cognitive intervention adherence among breast cancer survivors: A mixed methods study. *Cancer Nursing*, *43*(5), 354–365.

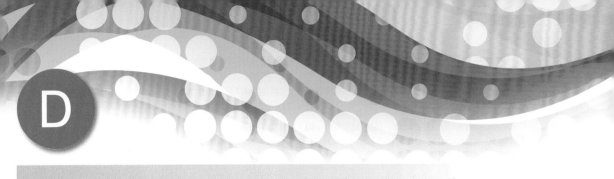

A Randomized Controlled Trial of an Individualized Preoperative Education Intervention for Symptom Management After Total Knee Arthroplasty

Rosemary A. Wilson ▼ Judith Watt-Watson ▼ Ellen Hodnett ▼ Joan Tranmer

Pain and nausea limit recovery after total knee arthroplasty (TKA) patients. The aim of this study was to determine the effect of a preoperative educational intervention on postsurgical pain-related interference in activities, pain, and nausea. Participants ($n = 143$) were randomized to intervention or standard care. The standard care group received the usual teaching. The intervention group received the usual teaching, a booklet containing symptom management after TKA, an individual teaching session, and a follow-up support call. Outcome measures assessed pain, pain interference, and nausea. There were no differences between groups in patient outcomes. There were no group differences for pain at any time point. Respondents had severe postoperative pain and nausea and received inadequate doses of analgesia and antiemetics. Individualizing education content was insufficient to produce a change in symptoms for patients. Further research involving the modification of system factors affecting the provision of symptom management interventions is warranted.

Introduction

In Canada, more than 42,000 total knee arthroplasty (TKA) surgeries were performed from 2012 from 2013 (Canadian Institute for Health Information, 2014). TKA is a common, successfully performed joint replacement procedure for pain and immobility associated with knee joint compromise. Arthritis is the most common preoperative diagnosis (95.4% osteoarthritis and 2.2% rheumatoid arthritis). The purpose of joint replacement for these patients is to reduce pain and knee joint stiffness, and thereby increase mobility and function.

Pain and nausea are common symptoms for patients after this procedure. Moderate to severe pain on movement and at rest has been documented during the first 3 postoperative days (Brander et al., 2003; Salmon, Hall, Perrbhoy, Shenkin, & Parker, 2001; Strassels, Chen, & Carr, 2002; Wu et al., 2003). Similarly, nausea has been found to be worse on postoperative day 1, but has the greatest impact on patients on day 2 (Wu et al., 2003).

Previous research (Beaupre, Lier, Davies, & Johnston, 2004; Bondy, Sims, Schroeder, Offord, & Narr, 1999; Lin, Lin, & Lin, 1997; McDonald, Freeland, Thomas, & Moore, 2001; McDonald & Molony, 2004; McDonald, Thomas, Livingston, & Severson, 2005; Roach, Tremblay, & Bowers, 1995; Sjoling, Nordahl, Olofsson, & Asplunf, 2003) has explored education interventions for pain prevention and treatment in the TKA population. These trials used a variety of delivery methods for the intervention including video, pamphlets, and classroom sessions, and the impact on pain outcomes was variable. Three studies reported that the education intervention resulted in moderately lower pain scores (McDonald & Molony, 2004, McDonald et al., 2001, Sjoling et al., 2003). Despite the relationship between pain and nausea and their prevalence after TKA, none of the studies addressed analgesic pain management or antiemetic therapy.

Many factors may impact the effectiveness of the preoperative education intervention, including timing and content. Stern and Lockwood (2005), in a systematic review of 15 randomized controlled trials (RCTs), concluded that preadmission written material combined with verbal instruction was more effective and resulted in better performance of postoperative exercises or skills than information provided postoperatively. A systematic review of 13 studies (Louw, Diener, Butler, & Puentedura, 2013) indicated that preoperative education, which focused on pain communication and

Rosemary A. Wilson, RN(EC), PhD, Assistant Professor, School of Nursing, Queen's University, Kingston, Ontario, Canada.

Judith Watt-Watson, RN, PhD, Professor Emeritus, Lawrence S. Bloomberg Faculty of Nursing, Senior Fellow, Massey College, University of Toronto, Toronto, Ontario, Canada.

Ellen Hodnett, RN, PhD, Professor Emeritus, Lawrence S .Bloomberg Faculty of Nursing, University of Toronto, Toronto, Ontario, Canada.

Joan Tranmer, RN, PhD, Professor, School of Nursing, Queen's University, Kingston, Ontario, Canada.

This original research was partially funded by an award from the Kingston General Hospital Women's Auxiliary Millennium Fund.

The authors declare that there are no conflicts of interest.

DOI: 10.1097/NOR.0000000000000210

management strategies, may result in better patient outcomes than education focused on pathophysiology. Preoperative education for patients with TKA had a significant, positive effect in one study (McDonald et al., 2001). The authors hypothesized that this was due to the difference in educational content of the intervention: a focus on pain management and communication rather than the anatomy and physiology of the surgery. Louw et al. (2013) advised more investigation regarding the content of educational interventions associated with TKA. Further, Wallis and Taylor (2011) conducted a systematic review and meta-analysis of 23 RCTs involving both patients with hip and knee replacement. The meta-analysis ($n = 2$) included 99 participants and provided minimal quality evidence that preoperative exercise combined with education leads to quicker return to mobility and activity after joint replacement, compared with standard preoperative care (standard mean difference = 0.50 [0.10, 0.90]).

Education that includes ways for patients to communicate pain and underlines the use of pain management strategies, including analgesics, has been used in other patient groups. Watt-Watson et al. (2004) addressed common patient concerns with taking analgesics in addition to reviewing the importance of pain relief and pain communication in a study of 406 patients with coronary artery bypass. Patients in the intervention group reported fewer concerns about taking analgesics (22.6 ± 14.7 vs. 18.5 ± 14.1, $p < .05$) and fewer concerns about addiction (3.7 ± 3.6 vs. 4.8 ± 3.8). The finding that most patients would not ask for analgesics, despite having fewer concerns about addiction and taking analgesics because they expected clinicians to know when these were needed, suggested that discussion of these beliefs about postoperative symptom management would be important for TKA patients, as well.

An individualized preoperative education approach has been used successfully to reduce symptoms in patients with cancer (Benor, Delbar, & Krulik, 1998; DeWit et al., 2001; Sherwood et al., 2005; Velji, 2006; Yates et al., 2004). Further, systematic reviews have recommended individualization of preoperative educational content (Johansson, Nuutila, Virtanen, Katajisto, & Salantera, 2005; McDonald, Page, Beringer, Wasiak, & Sprowson, 2014). However, no studies were found that used an individualized approach to preoperative patient education for patients with TKA.

Therefore, the intervention used in this trial was designed to be an individualized, preoperative approach to patient education and was informed by an adaptation of Wilson and Cleary's (1995) conceptual model of patient outcomes (Figure 1). The intervention focused on patient communication for pain management, analgesic use, and antiemetic use (see Table 1). This study aimed to investigate the impact of an individually delivered preoperative education intervention on pain-related interference, pain, and nausea for patients undergoing unilateral TKA.

Research Questions

- *Primary research question:* What is the effect of an individualized preoperative education intervention for patients with TKA on pain-related interference with usual activities on postoperative day 3?
- *Secondary research question:* What is the effect of an individualized preoperative education intervention for patients with TKA on nausea, pain, and analgesic and antiemetic administration on postoperative days 1, 2, and 3?

Methods

TRIAL DESIGN

An RCT design was used to evaluate outcomes on the first, second, and third days after TKA surgery (see Figure 2). This trial was conducted at an academic health sciences center in Southeastern Ontario. Ethics approval was obtained from the associated university's Research Ethics Board and the Trial Site Hospital's Research Ethics Board.

TABLE 1. PRE-KNEE SYMPTOM EDUCATION INTERVENTION CONTENT

Topic	Supporting Evidence
Pain, importance of pain management	McDonald et al. (2001); Chang et al. (2005); Johnson, Rice, Fuller, and Endress (1978); Lin et al. (1997); McDonald et al. (2004); Melzack and Wall (1996); Sjoling et al. (2003); Watt-Watson et al. (2004)
Importance of pain management to promote activity	McDonald et al.; Lin et al.; Sjoling et al.; Watt-Watson et al.
Communicating pain to health professionals	McDonald et al.; Johnson et al.; McDonald et al.; Sjoling et al.; Watt-Watson et al.
Asking for analgesics	McDonald et al.; Johnson et al.; Sjoling et al.; Lin et al.; Watt-Watson et al.
Asking for antiemetics	Gan et al. (2003); Melzack and Wall
Preventing dehydration (fluids)	Hodgkinson et al. (2003); Phillips, Johnston, and Gray (1993)
Misbeliefs about taking medication	Chang et al.; Watt-Watson et al.; Wilson, Goldstein, VanDenKerkhof, and Rimmer (2005)
Nonpharmacological measures	Melzack and Wall; Watt-Watson et al.

Wilson, R., et al. (2016). A randomized controlled trial of an individualized preoperative education intervention for symptom management after total knee arthroplasty. *Orthopaedic Nursing, 35,* 20–29.

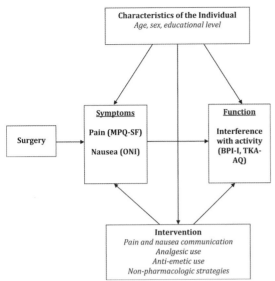

Figure 1. Conceptual framework: adaptation of Wilson and Cleary's (1995) model.

Study Participants

Patients were included if they were scheduled for elective unilateral primary TKA using planned intrathecal (spinal) anesthetic technique; had grade I–II American Society of Anesthesiologists Physical Status Classification (Larson, 1996); were able to speak and understand English; were able to be reached by telephone; were planned for home discharge; and consented to participate in this trial. Patients were excluded if they were not expected to be discharged home, or were booked for hemi, revision, or bilateral knee arthroplasty.

Recruitment took place at the weekly outpatient orthopaedic preadmission testing clinic at a facility affiliated with the trial center. Potential participants were identified by clinic staff, and eligible patients were asked for their permission by hospital staff to release their names to the investigator using a standardized script. The trial research assistant gave all willing patients a detailed verbal and written explanation of the trial during their preadmission appointment. Before randomization, written consent was gained by the trial research assistant, who then collected baseline demographic characteristics and clinical information.

Interventions

Intervention: The Pre-Knee Symptom Education Intervention

The Pre-Knee Symptom Education intervention was composed of three components: the booklet, an individual teaching session, and a follow-up support telephone call. Content used in this intervention was drawn from trials of preoperative education programs in surgical patients (McDonald et al., 2001; McDonald & Molony., 2004; Sjoling et al., 2003; Watt-Watson et al., 2004) and supported by focus groups' findings of indi-

vidual areas of concern for patients with TKA (Chang et al., 2005). To ensure concerns, found in the literature, were consistent with those of patients with TKA at the trial site, pilot interviews of 10 patients were conducted on day 2 or 3 post-TKA surgery. The Pre-Knee Symptom Education Booklet was reviewed with each consenting participant in an individualized, private teaching session during the preoperative patient visit to the Pre-Surgical Screening (PSS) Centre. This component was adapted from an educational tool used by Watt-Watson and colleagues (2004) for relevance to TKA postoperative recovery and the result of the pilot interviews done with local patients. The booklet was 12 pages long and included the content provided in Table 1 in addition to diagrams, pictures, and a space for recording questions for the investigator during the telephone follow-up call. The teaching session and booklet review were provided in a quiet examination room. The principal investigator delivered all intervention components during the PSS clinic appointment within 4 weeks of surgery. New concerns identified by trial participants as well as strategies presented were recorded on the Individualized Education Content Tool and reinforced during the follow-up support telephone call along with discussion of any questions raised by participants in the intervening time. The follow-up support telephone call occurred during the week before the scheduled surgical date.

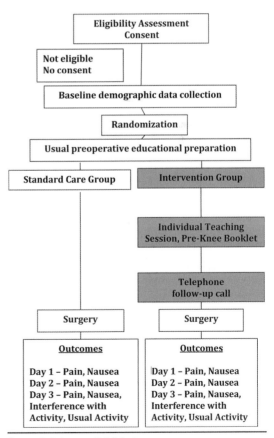

Figure 2. Schema of trial design.

Wilson, R., et al. (2016). A randomized controlled trial of an individualized preoperative education intervention for symptom management after total knee arthroplasty. *Orthopaedic Nursing, 35,* 20–29.

Questions asked by participants focused on (a) use of the intravenous patient-controlled analgesia (PCA-IV) pump, (b) concerns about the adverse effects of opioid analgesics, (c) physiotherapy timing, (d) home discharge analgesia, and (e) presurgical fasting guidelines and information regarding oral fluid intake.

STANDARD CARE

Participants in both groups received standard care, including an educational session provided by a physiotherapist outlining physiotherapy activities, a 30-minute video explaining the surgical procedure and postoperative orthopaedic routines, and a brief review of the use of PCA-IV by clinic nursing staff.

OUTCOMES

Baseline demographic data were collected using the self-reported Baseline Demographic Questionnaire before the intervention.

The primary outcome, pain interference, was measured using the Brief Pain Inventory, Interference (BPI-I) subscale on postoperative day 3 (Cleeland & Ryan, 1994). Pain-related interference, as measured by the BPI-I, refers to the extent to which pain interferes with general activities, sleep, mood, walking, movement from bed to chair, and relationships with others. This measure has well-established construct validity (Mendoza et al., 2004b, 2004a; Tan, Jensen, Thornby, & Shanti, 2004; Watt-Watson et al., 2004). Psychometric testing of postoperative use of the BPI-I demonstrates a consistent subscale structure between acute and chronic pain states (Mendoza et al., 2004a, 2004b; Watt-Watson et al., 2004; Zalon, 1999) as well as sensitivity to change (Mendoza et al., 2004a) and sex differences (Watt-Watson et al., 2004). The use of the BPI-I in the immediate postoperative period (Zalon, 1997) and beyond postoperative day 3 has been demonstrated (Mendoza et al., 2004a; Watt-Watson et al., 2004). Two items were deleted: "normal work" and "enjoyment of life" as these items were not relevant to the early postoperative period. The addition of one item addressing the activity of transferring from bed to chair was added, and the modified tool was pilot tested on the third postoperative day in a group of TKA patients ($n = 14$). The additional item, transferring from bed to chair, was easily answered by all participants and similarly judged to be an appropriate item for the administration time. Similar adaptation of the BPI-I items took place in a study by Watt-Watson et al. (2004) where both "normal work" and "enjoyment of life" were deleted and "deep breathing and coughing" was inserted for use in a postoperative patient population. Cronbach's α for this change was reported as .71.

Secondary outcomes included levels of pain and nausea, and analgesic and antiemetic use. Pain and pain quality were measured using the Short Form McGill Pain Questionnaire (MPQ-SF) (Melzack, 1987; Melzack et al., 1987). Nausea was measured using the Overall Nausea Index (ONI), one component of the Nausea Questionnaire (Melzack, 1989), used previously by Parlow et al. (2004) in a trial of postoperative anti-ematic therapies.

Antiemetic and opioid administration data were recorded from the chart for each of postoperative days 1 to 3.

SAMPLE SIZE

Sample size for this trial was based on group means from another study ($n = 406$) using the BPI-I as a primary outcome (Watt-Watson et al., 2004). Using a moderate effect size of .5 based on between standard deviation and within standard deviation (Cohen, 1988), the sample size required was 64 per arm (α = .05, power = 80%). A reduction of half the standard deviation of the general population, as reported by Watt-Watson et al. (2004), is a reasonable estimate of the clinically important effect of this intervention. Minimal trial attrition was expected as all measurements were taken during the inpatient hospital stay. A conservative estimate of 10% was used. As a result the sample size required for this trial was 140 in total, with an α level of .05 and power of 80%.

RANDOMIZATION AND BLINDING

Participants were randomly assigned to the intervention plus standard care group or the standard care group using a randomization service provided by a research program not connected to this trial. Personnel at the research office used a computer-generated block randomization table provided by statistical services. The research assistant called the research office number, provided the participant number, and received group assignment information. Group assignment was recorded on the Baseline Demographics Questionnaire and was stored in a location separate from all postoperative data collection forms.

The intervention was initiated immediately after randomization for participants in the experimental group in a private room in the presurgical screening area. Although participants could not be unaware of group allocation, the research assistants collecting postoperative outcome data were blinded to group allocation, reducing the potential for cointervention or the introduction of bias by trial personnel during data collection.

STATISTICAL ANALYSIS

Results were analyzed using an intention-to-treat approach. Baseline data were analyzed using descriptive statistics. A two-tailed level of significance of .05 was used for all analyses. Data were analyzed using the SPSS/PASW software package, version 18.

Independent samples t test was used to determine differences in pain-related interference with activity between the intervention and standard care groups on postoperative day 3 on total and component scores. Repeated measures-analysis of covariance was used to determine differences between groups and over the measurement periods in pain scores (MPQ-SF, Numeric Rating Scale [NRS] questions), nausea scores (ONI), and total 24-hour analgesic administration. Differences in antiemetic administration between the two groups were determined using χ^2. Linear-by-linear χ^2 was also used to detect differences in frequency of postoperative activities completed (TKA-AQ). Separate analyses were conducted using participants, rating moderate to severe worst pain and nausea—scores of 4 to 10 (Jones et al., 2005)—in the last 24 hours with antiemetic and analgesic administration.

Wilson, R., et al. (2016). A randomized controlled trial of an individualized preoperative education intervention for symptom management after total knee arthroplasty. *Orthopaedic Nursing, 35*, 20–29.

Results

A total of 337 patients were screened for participation in this trial (see Figure 3). Of these, 162 were eligible and only 19 of these declined to participate.

Therefore, 143 were randomized after baseline demographic data collection in the preadmission phase of surgery preparation. One participant in the standard care group did not meet eligibility criteria at the time of surgery as a result of a change of procedure type (bilateral vs. unilateral TKA), and one participant in each group had the procedure cancelled indefinitely. As a result, the total number for the analysis of baseline characteristics was 143 and 140 for postoperative outcomes. No participants withdrew from the trial during data collection. Baseline demographic data are included in Table 2.

Baseline characteristics were similar between groups with a mean age of 67 ± 8 years in the intervention group and 66 ± 8 years in the standard care group, consistent with many studies of patients with TKA and national TKA data. The primary diagnosis requiring surgery was osteoarthritis in both groups, with approximately one third of participants requiring opioid analgesics for arthritic pain preoperatively.

PRIMARY RESEARCH QUESTION

Day 3 measurements of the BPI-I are presented in Table 3. Total scores for the standard care group (22.4 ± 15.1) and the intervention group (24.4 ± 14.4) were not significantly different ($p = .45$). Independent sample t tests were nonsignificant for all BPI-I items. Highest interference scores for both groups at day 3 were in the moderate range and included general activity (standard care: 5.6 ± 3.2; intervention: 5.8 ± 3.2) and transfer from bed to chair (standard care: 5.0 ± 3.4; intervention: 4.6 ± 2.9). It is important to note that these pain-related interference scores were measured on the third postoperative day, 1 day before the expected discharge date for this group of patients.

SECONDARY RESEARCH QUESTIONS

Pain

Postoperative pain was measured using the MPQ-SF on each of postoperative days 1, 2, and 3 (see Table 4). There were no significant group differences on any of the three postoperative days in either pain right now at rest, pain now with movement, or worst pain in last 24 hours. There was, however, a significant effect for time in pain

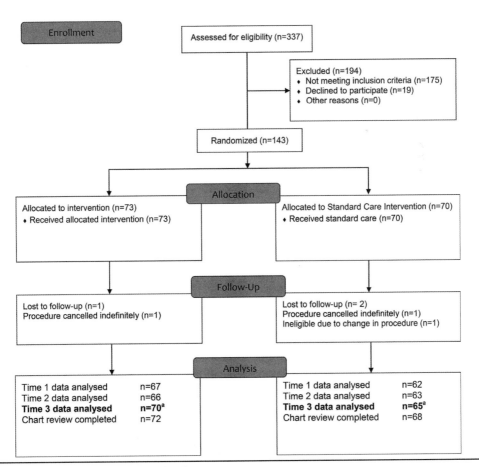

FIGURE 3. Flow of participants through the trial. [a]Primary outcome.

Wilson, R., et al. (2016). A randomized controlled trial of an individualized preoperative education intervention for symptom management after total knee arthroplasty. *Orthopaedic Nursing, 35,* 20–29.

TABLE 2. BASELINE DEMOGRAPHICS OF PARTICIPANTS

Demographics	Intervention (n = 73) n (%)	Standard Care (n = 70) n (%)
Sex		
Female	46 (63)	43 (61)
Home status		
Live alone	13 (18)	15 (21)
Highest education level		
Less than high school	34 (47)	36 (51)
Postsecondary	39 (53)	34 (49)
Home pain medication		
None	13 (18)	18 (26)
Opioid	21 (29)	24 (34)
Nonopioid	39 (53)	28 (40)
Preoperative diagnosis		
Osteoarthritis	70 (96)	67 (96)
Rheumatoid arthritis	3 (4)	3 (4)

TABLE 4. PAIN ON POSTOPERATIVE DAYS 1, 2, AND 3

NRS (0–10)	Intervention (n = 62) M (SD)	Standard Care (n = 55) M (SD)
Pain right now at rest[a]		
Postoperative day 1	4.1 (2.9)	3.7 (2.8)
Postoperative day 2	3.3 (3.0)	2.9 (2.2)
Postoperative day 3	2.8 (2.5)	2.8 (2.7)
Pain right now when moving[b]		
Postoperative day 1	6.4 (2.6)	6.4 (2.7)
Postoperative day 2	6.2 (2.8)	5.9 (2.4)
Postoperative day 3	5.4 (3.0)	6.1 (2.5)
Worst pain last 24 hours[c]		
Postoperative day 1	7.5 (2.5)	7.2 (2.8)
Postoperative day 2	7.7 (2.4)	7.5 (2.1)
Postoperative day 3	7.0 (2.4)	7.0 (2.3)

Note. NRS = Numeric Rating Scale.
[a]$F = 0.36, p = .70.$
[b]$F = 1.61, p = .20.$
[c]$F = 0.14, p = .87.$

right now at rest ($p = .0002$) and worst pain last 24 hours ($p = .013$), with pain decreasing over time but not for the item, pain right now when moving ($p = .06$). Similarly, there was a significant effect for time in the Present Pain Intensity (PPI) global pain rating (0–5) ($p = .001$) but no group difference across time ($p = .70$). As with the NRS and PPI, there was a significant effect of time for both the PRI-S ($p = .02$), the PRI-A ($p = .05$) and the PRI-T ($p = .02$), but there were no significant group differences across the three measurement times. Across both groups, the average rating of worst pain in the last 24 hours was 7 ± 2.4, in the severe range on each of the three postoperative days. Seventy-three percent of the total sample reported moderate to severe pain on movement on day 3, whereas 81% of the sample reported having experienced moderate to severe pain in the last 24 hours.

TABLE 3. PAIN-RELATED INTERFERENCE WITH ACTIVITY ON POSTOPERATIVE DAY 3

Interference Scores BPI-I	Intervention (n = 70) M (SD)	Standard Care (n = 65) M (SD)
Total (scores 0–60)[a]	24.4 (14.4)	22.4 (15.1)
Subscales (scores 0–10)		
General activity	5.6 (3.2)	5.8 (3.2)
Walking	4.8 (3.0)	4.4 (3.5)
Mood	3.3 (3.2)	2.4 (3.2)
Transfer from bed to chair	4.8 (2.9)	5.0 (3.4)
Sleep	3.8 (3.5)	3.3 (3.1)
Relationships with others	1.9 (2.9)	1.6 (2.7)

Note. BPI-I = Brief Pain Inventory, Interference.
[a]$t = -0.76; p = .45.$

NAUSEA

The impact of the intervention on nausea was measured using the six-point ONI. There was no difference between groups in nausea scores (previous 24 hours) over time ($F = 0.02; p = .88$); however, there was a difference within groups in nausea scores (previous 24 hours) over time ($F = 50.9; p < .01$) with nausea decreasing over the 3-day period.

ANALGESIC AND ANTIEMETIC ADMINISTRATION

PCA-IV opioids prescribed for participants postoperatively during the 3-day study period were morphine (82%) and hydromorphone (18%). Oral opioids prescribed on day 3 were morphine, hydromorphone, or oxycodone (67%, 14%, and 18% of participants, respectively) and one participant received oral codeine. Repeated-measures analysis of variance demonstrated no difference between groups in daily 24-hour opioid administration, but for the total sample there was a significant main effect for time as analgesic administration in both groups declined over the 3 postoperative days ($F = 36.1; p = .000$). For patients consistently reporting moderate to severe pain on each day, opioid analgesic administration also declined over their hospital stay (see Table 5). Overall, 7 participants did not receive any opioid analgesic doses on postoperative day 3, two of whom did not receive any doses on postoperative day 2. One participant did not receive any opioid over the 3-day period.

The routine dosing protocol ordered for all patients with TKA reporting even mild nausea was three doses of a prescribed antiemetic (ondansetron). Overall, 79 (56%) participants were administered at least one dose of antiemetic over the 3-day trial period. However, for those reporting moderate to severe nausea on the first postoperative day, 29% in the intervention group and 25% in the standard care group received no antiemetics

Wilson, R., et al. (2016). A randomized controlled trial of an individualized preoperative education intervention for symptom management after total knee arthroplasty. *Orthopaedic Nursing, 35*, 20–29.

TABLE 5. TOTAL OPIOID ANALGESIC ADMINISTRATION FOR ALL PARTICIPANTS IN MILLIGRAMS OF ORAL MORPHINE EQUIVALENTS FOR 24 HOURS ON EACH OF THE 3-DAY TRIAL PERIOD

	Intervention (n = 72) Median (Interquartile Range)	Standard Care (n = 68) Median (Interquartile Range)
Postoperative day 1	78 (69)	78 (87)
Postoperative day 2	62 (65)	56 (55)
Postoperative day 3	40 (45)	40 (42)

in the previous 24-hour period. For those reporting either no or mild nausea in each group, 17% received at least one dose of antiemetic during the same period.

Discussion

There were no significant group differences in any of the outcomes in this trial. However, the results of the total sample are important to highlight. There were no differences in total or component scores for pain-related interference with activity as measured by the BPI-I Interference with general activity, walking, and transfer from bed to chair were in the moderate to severe range and consistent with results reported by Akyol, Karayurt, and Salmond (2009). A major emphasis of the education content within all three components of intervention delivery was the importance of appropriately timed analgesic use to increase opioid administration and improve pain and pain-related interference with activity. In the context of similar opioid use on postoperative day 3 in both groups—median daily oral morphine equivalents: intervention 40 mg (interquartile range = 45 mg), standard care 40 mg (interquartile range = 42 mg)—moderate to severe BPI-I scores in the intervention group illustrate that placing the focus on the patient alone to ensure pre-activity analgesia administration is not sufficient to improve pain-related interference. Watt-Watson and colleagues (2004) reported that only 33% of prescribed analgesics were administered in 53% of patients reporting moderate to severe pain in their study of 406 patients with cardiac surgery. These authors identified a lack of understanding of opioid analgesia among health professionals, and recommended that future trials include focus groups with nursing staff in particular to discuss issues affecting pain management in the postoperative setting.

The education provided by all three components of the intervention that focused on strategies to prevent resting pain and pain on movement, including appropriate communication of pain to healthcare providers, failed to produce a difference in pain ratings and qualitative aspects of pain description. Moderate to severe pain, in the context of declining and inadequate opioid analgesic administration, is troubling and raises important questions about the postoperative environment in terms of clinical care. Components of the intervention that reinforced analgesic use before movement in an interval appropriate to the type of analgesic administered

were intended to maximize pain relief and improve mobility to prevent further complications, but the intervention focused on the patients and ignored the roles of the care providers. Additionally, data were not collected that discriminated between surgical pain and other pain. Wittig-Wells, Shapiro, and Higgins (2013) found that other or nonsurgical pain, present in 37% of their sample, interfered with walking, mood, sleep, and relationships with other people. Kearney et al. (2011) reported a similar lack of effect on postoperative pain or activity in a trial of structured preoperative information in joint replacement patients.

Opioid analgesic administration (see Table 5) declined over the 3-day study period ($F = 36.1$; $p = .000$), whereas pain ratings on movement stayed in the moderate range in both groups across all 3 postoperative days. It is important to note that the median oral morphine equivalent administration was 40 mg for patients in both trial groups, only one third of the opioid doses that were prescribed. This finding is similar to the 33% of prescribed doses administered in the study by Watt-Watson and colleagues (2004).

Unrelieved pain and stress response as a result of acute, surgical injury can have psychological and physiological consequences for patients (Apkarian, Bushnell, Treede, & Zubieta, 2005; Carr & Thomas, 1997; Kehlet, 1997). The phenomenon of central sensitization of dorsal horn neurons by prolonged and repetitive nociceptive input can create the physiology for a longer-term pain problem (Bausbaum & Jessell, 2000) predisposing patients to related comorbidities. Patients with TKA with persistent, unrelieved pain are less likely to do specific physiotherapy activities (i.e., range of motion and weight bearing) that may result in delayed rehabilitation and knee stiffness.

Concomitant moderate to severe nausea rates in this trial may reflect the established interrelationship between pain and nausea. Twenty-eight percent of the intervention and 24% of the standard care groups reported experiencing moderate to severe nausea in the previous 24 hours on postoperative day 3. The attenuation of the pain experience by the presence of nausea and the production of nausea by the pain experience (Fields, 1999; Julius & Bausbaum, 2001; Kandel, Schwartz, & Jessell, 2000) reinforces the need to address both of these symptoms simultaneously.

This trial presents clear evidence that there are significant system issues influencing postoperative symptom management after TKA. Participants in both groups who were reporting moderate to severe nausea or pain frequently did not receive the antiemetic therapy or analgesics ordered. Evidenced-based protocols for nausea management were in place at the trial site, but data show that they were not followed consistently and in some cases, not at all. Antiemetic agents used in these protocols, ondansetron and prochlorperazine, are effective for postoperative nausea when given appropriately (Dzwonczyk, Weaver, Puente, & Bergese, 2012). In this trial, 25% of participants who reported moderate to severe nausea had no antiemetics administered at all. Similarly, participants who reported moderate to severe pain received approximately one third of the prescribed doses of oral analgesic on postoperative day 3 despite hospital-wide programs that support the need for effective pain

Wilson, R., et al. (2016). A randomized controlled trial of an individualized preoperative education intervention for symptom management after total knee arthroplasty. *Orthopaedic Nursing, 35,* 20–29.

management (e.g., Pain, the 5th Vital Sign). Other research has suggested that this is not an unusual finding; nursing staff education and attitude may be contributing factors. Gordon and colleagues (2008), in a study of practice-associated pro re nata (PRN) administration of opioids in 602 registered nurses, found that comfort with dose titration was directly and positively related to years of practice experience.

At the trial site, the pain management service is available for consultation by the nursing staff at all times to modify or increase analgesic doses. Although patients reporting scores in the moderate to severe range on pain assessment should, by institutional policy, be reviewed either by the attending service or the pain service, they were not. Although an inadequate explanation for deficiencies in care, staffing resources and patient acuity may have contributed to fewer pain and nausea assessments, placing the onus on the patient to report symptoms requiring treatment.

It appears that the current postoperative environment does not support best practice for nursing staff in terms of symptom management regardless of the measures put in place. This finding is not unique to orthopaedic patient care. In a systematic review of 16 trials of labor support during childbirth in institutional settings, Hodnett, Gates, Hofmeyr, and Sakala (2009) concluded that the effectiveness of labor support interventions was mediated by the environment in which the interventions were provided. Although this clinical group has different requirements than patients with TKA, findings of the review in terms of environmental factors were similar. The ability of interventions with patients to overcome barriers present in the environment is limited if strategies to address these barriers are not also included.

Limitations of this trial are primarily related to support for the implementation of the educational material in the postoperative setting. As the intervention for this trial was directed only at the participants with no component for staff education or protocol development or monitoring, the influence of the healthcare environment on the ability of the participants to engage in the associated behaviors was not reinforcing. Systems issues such as staff lack of adherence to established protocols for symptom management may have resulted in more pain and nausea and greater functional interference.

Institutional accountability reflecting hospital accreditation standards in the clinical environment for the provision of symptom management and early identification and investigation of activity and mobility concerns needs to be established. A consistent approach used by disciplines involved in the care of patients with TKA needs to span from initial assessment for surgery to postoperative care and includes all points of contact between. In the preoperative setting, nursing staff caring for orthopaedic patients must take the lead in ensuring surgical preparation, which includes education that is reinforced by all team members, regardless of their role. Postoperatively, orthopaedic nursing staff must attend to the need for temporally appropriate symptom assessment and pharmacologic and nonpharmacologic interventions for patients. As this trial demonstrates that the delivery of individualized educational content with reinforcement provided by booklet and telephone follow-up was not sufficient to impact postoperative symptoms after TKA surgery, the nursing role as a symptom management provider and patient advocate is essential to the recovery after TKA. Further trials that also include standardized information provided to patients by preadmission, surgical scheduling and postoperative nursing and medical staff would be beneficial in supporting learned behaviors and knowledge uptake. Consistent with the recommendations of Watt-Watson and colleagues (2004), a qualitative research approach using focus groups of orthopaedic nursing, medical, and physiotherapy staff could be undertaken to determine the environmental and patient-related characteristics, affecting the provision of analgesics and antiemetics and the relationship to postoperative activity.

Conclusion

The numbers of Canadians requiring primary TKA has increased 140% over the last 10 years (CIHI, 2013). The highest rate of TKA surgery is in the 75- to 84-year-age range (65%). There are no published guidelines for the preoperative preparation or postoperative care of these relatively older aged patients. Inadequate management of symptoms such as pain and nausea in the early postoperative period may result in increased morbidity for patients and increased costs for the healthcare system. The purpose of the trial was to examine the impact of individualizing preoperative patient education as a means to address postoperative symptoms affecting recovery from TKA.

Providing information to patients alone was not sufficient to address the need for postoperative symptom prevention and management after TKA. A broader, consistent approach that includes healthcare providers at all levels of patient contact is required to support recovery and rehabilitation after this type of surgery. Further research is required to delineate the barriers in the healthcare environment to appropriate pain and nausea management and to provide more evidence for the relationship between pain and nausea and functional outcomes for patients who have had TKA.

REFERENCES

Akyol, O., Karayurt, O., & Salmomd, S. (2009). Experiences of pain and satisfaction with pain management in patients undergoing total knee replacement. *Orthopedic Nursing, 28*, 79–85.

Apkarian, A., Bushnell, M., Treede, R., & Zubieta, J. (2005). Human brain mechanisms of pain perception and regulation in health and disease. *European Journal of Pain, 9*(4), 463–484.

Bausbaum, A. I., & Jessell, T. M. (2000). The perception of pain. In E. Kandel, J. Schwartz, & Jessell, T. (Eds.), *Principles of neural science* (4th ed., pp. 472–491). New York: McGraw-Hill.

Beaupre, L. A., Lier, D., Davies, D. M., & Johnston, D. B. C. (2004). The effect of a preoperative exercise and education program on functional recovery, health related quality of life, and health service utilization following primary total knee arthroplasty. *Journal of Rheumatology, 31*, 1166–1173.

Benor, D.E., Delbar, V., & Krulik, T. (1998). Measuring the impact of nursing interventions on cancer patients' ability to control symptoms. *Cancer Nursing, 21*, 320–334.

Wilson, R., et al. (2016). A randomized controlled trial of an individualized preoperative education intervention for symptom management after total knee arthroplasty. *Orthopaedic Nursing, 35*, 20–29.

Bondy, L. R., Sims, N., Schroeder, D. R., Offord, K. P., & Narr, B. J. (1999). The effect of anesthetic patient education on preoperative patient's anxiety. *Regional Anesthesia and Pain Medicine, 24*, 158–164.

Brander, V. A., Stulberg, S. D., Adams, A. D., Harden, R. N., Bruehl, S., Stanos, S. P., & Houle, T. (2003). Ranawat Award Paper: Predicting total knee replacement pain: A prospective, observational study. *Clinical Orthopaedics and Related Research, 416*, 27–36.

Canadian Institute for Health Information. (2014). *Hip and knee replacements in Canada 2012–2013 quick stats.* Canadian Institute for Health Information. Retrieved from http://www.cihi.ca

Canadian Institute for Health Information. (2013). *Hip and knee replacements in Canada—Canadian Joint Replacement Registry 2013 Annual Report.* Ottawa: CIHI; 2013.

Carr, E., & Thomas, V. (1997). Anticipating and experiencing post-operative pain: The patient's perspective. *Journal of Clinical Nursing, 6*, 191–201.

Chang, H. J., Mehta, P. S., Rosenberg, A., & Scrimshaw, S. C. (2004). Concerns of patients actively contemplating total knee replacement: Differences by race and gender. *Arthritis and Rheumatism, 51*(1), 117–123.

Cleeland, C., & Ryan, K. (1994). Pain assessment: Global use of the Brief Pain Inventory. *Annals of Academic Medicine Singapore, 23*, 129–138.

Cohen, J. (1988). *Statistical power analysis for the behavioral sciences* (2nd ed.). Hillsdale: Earlbaum Associates.

De Wit, R., & Van Dam, F. (2001). From hospital to home care: A randomized controlled trial of a Pain Education Programme for cancer patients with chronic pain. *Journal of Advanced Nursing, 36*(6), 742–754.

Dzwonczyk, R., Weaver, T., Puente, E., & Bergese, S. (2012). Postoperative nausea and vomiting prophylaxis from an economic point of view. *American Journal of Therapeutics, 19*(1), 11–15.

Fields, H. (1999). Pain: An unpleasant topic. *Pain, Supplement, 6*, S61–S69.

Gan, T. J., Meyer, T., Apfel, C. C., Chung, F., Davis, P. J., Eubanks, S., ... Tramèr, M. R. (2003). Consensus guidelines for managing postoperative nausea and vomiting. *Anesthesia & Analgesia, 97*(1), 62–71.

Gordon, D., Pellino, T., Higgins, G., Pasero, C., & Murphy-Ende, K. (2008). Nurses' opinions of administration of PRN range opioid oral orders for acute pain. *Pain Management Nursing, 9*(3), 131–140.

Hodnett, E., Gates, S., Hofmeyr, G.J., & Sakala, C. (2009). Continuous support for women during childbirth. *Cochrane Database of Systematic Reviews, 3*, CD003766.

Hodgkinson, B., Evans, D., & Wood, J. (2003). Maintaining oral hydration status in older adults: A systematic review. *International Journal of Nursing Practice, 9*, S19–S28.

Johansson, K., Nuutila, L., Virtanen, H., Katajisto, J., & Salantera, S. (2005). Preoperative education for orthopaedic patients: Systematic review. *Journal of Advanced Nursing, 50*, 212–223.

Johnson, J., Rice, V., Fuller, S., & Endress, P. (1978). Sensory information, instruction in a coping strategy, and recovery from surgery. *Research in Nursing and Health, 1*(1), 4–17.

Jones, D., Westby, M., Griedanus, N., Johanson, N., Krebs, D., Robbins, L., Rooks, D., & Brander, V. (2005). Update on hip and knee arthroplasty: Current state of evidence. *Arthritis and Rheumatism, 53*(5), 772–780.

Julius, D., & Bausbaum, A. (2001). Molecular mechanisms of nociception. *Nature, 413*, 203–210.

Kandel, E., Schwartz, J., & Jessell, T. (2000). The perception of pain. *Principles of neural science* (4th ed., pp. 472–491). New York: McGraw-Hill.

Kearney, M., Jennrich, M. K., Lyons, S., Robinson, R., & Berger, B. (2011). Effects of preoperative education on patient outcomes after joint replacement surgery. *Orthopaedic Nursing, 30*(6), 391–6

Kehlet, H. (1997). Multimodal approach to control postoperative pathophysiology and rehabilitation. *British Journal of Anaesthesia, 78*, 606–617.

Larson, C. P. (1996). Evaluating the patient and preoperative preparation. In P. G. Barash, B. F. Cullen, & Stoelting, R. K. (Eds.), *Handbook of clinical anesthesia* (2nd ed., pp. 3–15). Philadelphia: Lippincott-Raven.

Lin, P. C., Lin, L. C., & Lin, J. J. (1997). Comparing the effectiveness of different educational programs for patients with total knee arthroplasty. *Orthopedic Nursing, 16*, 43–49.

Louw, A., Diener, I., Butler, D. S., & Puentedura, E. J. (2013). Preoperative education addressing postoperative pain in total joint arthroplasty: Review of content and educational delivery methods. *Physiotherapy Theory and Practice, 29*(3), 175–194. doi:10.3109/0959 3985.2012.727527

McDonald, D. D., Freeland, M., Thomas, G., & Moore, J. (2001). Testing a preoperative pain management intervention for elders. *Research in Nursing and Health, 24*, 402–409.

McDonald, D. D., & Molony, S. L. (2004). Postoperative pain communication skills for older adults. *Western Journal of Nursing Research, 26*, 836–852.

McDonald, D., Thomas, G., Livingston, K., & Severson, J. (2005). Assisting older adults to communicate their postoperative pain. *Clinical Nursing Research, 14*(2), 109–126. doi:10.1177/1054773804271934

McDonald, S., Page, M. J., Beringer, K., Wasiak, J., & Sprowson, A. (2014). Pre-operative education for hip and knee replacement (Review). *Cochrane Database of Systematic Reviews, 5*, 10.1002/14651858.CD003526. pub3.

Melzack, R. (1989). Measurement of Nausea. *Journal of Pain and Symptom Management, 4*, 157–160.

Melzack, R. (1987). The short form McGill Pain Questionnaire. *Pain, 30*, 191–197.

Melzack, R., Abbott, F., Zackon, W., Mulder, D., & Davis, W. (1987). Pain on a surgical ward: a survey of the duration and intensity of pain and the effectiveness of medication. *Pain, 29*, 67–72.

Melzack, R., & Wall, P. (1996). *The challenge of pain* (2nd ed.). London: Penguin.

Mendoza, T. R., Chen, C., Brugger, A., Hubbard, R., Snabes, M., & Palmer, S. N., ...Cleeland, C. S. (2004a). The utility and validity of the modified brief pain inventory in a multiple-dose postoperative analgesic trial. *The Clinical Journal of Pain, 20*(5), 357–362.

Mendoza, T. R., Chen, C., Brugger, A., Hubbard, R., Snabes, M., & Palmer, S. N., ...Cleeland, C. S. (2004b). Lessons learned from a multiple-dose post-operative analgesic trial. *Pain, 109*(1), 103–109.

Parlow, J., Costache, I., Avery, N., & Turner, K. (2004). Single-does haloperidol for the prophylaxis of postoperative nausea and vomiting after intrathecal morphine. *Anesthesia and Analgesia, 98*, 1072–1076.

Phillips, P. A., Johnston, C. I., & Gray, L. (1993). Disturbed fluid and electrolyte homeostasis following dehydration in elderly people. *Age and Aging, 22*, S26–S33.

Roach, J. A., Tremblay, L. M., & Bowers, D. L. (1995). A preoperative assessment and education program:

Wilson, R., et al. (2016). A randomized controlled trial of an individualized preoperative education intervention for symptom management after total knee arthroplasty. *Orthopaedic Nursing, 35*, 20–29.

implementation and outcomes. *Patient Education and Counseling, 25,* 83–88.

Salmon, P., Hall, G., Perrbhoy, D., Shenkin, A., & Parker, C. (2001). Recovery from hip and knee arthroplasty: Patients' perspective on pain, function, quality of life, and well-being up to 6 months post-operatively. *Archives of Physical Medicine and Rehabilitation, 82,* 360–366.

Sherwood, P., Given, B., Given, C., Champion, V., Doorenbos, A., Azzouz, F., ... Monahan, P. O. (2005). A cognitive behavioural intervention for symptom management in patients with advanced cancer. *Oncology Nursing Forum, 32,* 1190–1198.

Sjoling, M., Nordahl, G., Olofsson, N., & Asplund, K. (2003). The impact of preoperative information on state anxiety, postoeprative pain and satisfaction with pain management. *Patient Education and Counseling, 51,* 169–176.

Stern, C., & Lockwood, C. (2005). Knowledge retention from preoperative patient information. *International Journal of Evidence-Based Healthcare, 3,* 45–63.

Strassels, S. A., Chen, C., & Carr, D. (2002). Postoperative analgesia: Economics, resource use, and patient satisfaction in an urban teaching hospital. *Anesthesia and Analgesia, 94,* 130–137.

Tan, G., Jensen, M. P., Thornby, J. L., & Shanti, B. F. (2004). Validation of the Brief Pain Inventory for chronic non-malignant pain. *Journal of Pain, 5,* 133–137.

Velji, K. (2006). Effect of an individualized symptom education program on the symptom distress of women receiving radiotherapy for gynecological cancer. Available from ProQuest database (AAT NR21992).

Wallis, J., & Taylor, F. (2011). Pre-operative interventions (non-surgical and non-pharmacological) for patients with hip or knee osteoarthritis awaiting joint replacement surgery—a systematic review and meta-analysis. *Osteoarthritis and Cartilage, 19*(12), 1381–1395. doi:10.1016/j.joca.2011.09.001

Watt-Watson, J., Stevens, B., Katz, J., Costello, J., Reid, G., & David, T. (2004). Impact of pre-operative education on pain outcomes after coronary artery bypass graft surgery. *Pain, 109,* 73–85.

Wilson, I. B., & Cleary, P. D. (1995). Linking clinical variables with Health-Related Quality of Life: A conceptual model of patient outcomes. *Journal of the American Medical Association, 273,* 59–65.

Wilson, R., Goldstein, D., VanDenKerkhof, E., & Rimmer, M. (2005). APMS clinical dataset. October 1, 2004, to October 1, 2005. Kingston, Ontario, Unpublished.

Wittig-Wells, D. R., Shapiro, S. E., & Higgins, M. K. (2013). Patients' experiences of pain in the 48 hours following total knee Arthroplasty. *Orthopaedic Nursing, 32*(1), 39–44.

Wu, C., Naqibuddin, M., Rowlingson, A., Lietman, S., Jermyn, R., & Fleisher, L. (2003). The effect of pain on health-related quality of life in the immediate postoperative period. *Anesthesia and Analgesia, 97,* 1078–1085.

Yates, P., Edwards, H., Nash, R., Aranda, S., Purdie, D., & Najman, J., ...Walsh, A. (2004). A randomized controlled trial of a nurse-administered educational intervention for improving cancer pain management in ambulatory settings. *Patient education and counseling, 53*(2), 227–237.

Zalon, M. L. (1997). Pain in frail, elderly women after surgery. *Image: Journal of Nursing Scholarship, 29*(1), 21–26.

Wilson, R., et al. (2016). A randomized controlled trial of an individualized preoperative education intervention for symptom management after total knee arthroplasty. *Orthopaedic Nursing, 35,* 20–29.

Critical Appraisal of Wilson et al.'s Study: "A Randomized Controlled Trial of an Individualized Preoperative Education Intervention for Symptom Management After Total Knee Arthroplasty"

OVERALL SUMMARY

This report provided a well-written description of a strong quantitative study that used a rigorous randomized controlled trial (RCT) design that included appropriate randomization and blinding procedures. The preoperative education intervention for patients undergoing total knee arthroplasty (TKA) was designed on the basis of earlier research and a broad conceptual model. The authors provided good information about the intervention's educational components and a rationale for the content. Although the intervention versus control group differences were not statistically significant, the findings were credible—that is, the results are unlikely to reflect problems with inadequate statistical power or biases in the design. The authors concluded that a patient education approach to pain management for patients undergoing TKA might not be effective without changing overall systems of pain management in hospitals. Their conclusions could perhaps have been strengthened by data from a qualitative component that might have told them *why* patients in the intervention group did not get more pain medication than they received.

TITLE

The title of this report effectively communicated the nature of the study design (an RCT), the nature of the intervention (individualized preoperative education), the outcomes (symptom management), and the population (patients undergoing TKA).

ABSTRACT

The abstract for this paper was written as a traditional abstract, without subheadings. The abstract was succinct but conveyed critical information about the study aim, the nature of the intervention, the RCT study design, and the sample size ($N = 143$). Key outcomes were identified (pain, pain interference, and nausea). The abstract also reported the findings, i.e., the absence of significant differences between the intervention and control group on key outcomes. Finally, the authors provided a brief interpretation of their findings and suggestions for future research. The abstract provided information that readers would need in deciding whether to read the full report.

INTRODUCTION

The introduction provided a reasonable rationale for this study. The authors explained the nature and scope of the problem (i.e., pain and nausea as symptoms for patients undergoing TKA, with many such procedures being undertaken annually). They also noted that several trials to address this problem through educational interventions have been tested, using a variety of delivery methods, and that some had been found to result in lower pain scores. However, the results of these trials were mixed, and no trials had addressed issues relating to nausea following the TKA procedure.

The authors acknowledged that they were guided in the design of their intervention by several systematic reviews. The researchers also were guided by the positive results of individualized preoperative interventions tested with other patient groups (e.g., patients with cancer). Based on earlier studies and using a broad conceptual model (a conceptual map for which was provided in Fig. 1), the researchers developed a multicomponent intervention. The model itself does not appear to have been the foundation for specific intervention components, however. For example, it was not a model that purported to explain the mechanisms through which the intervention would lead to positive effects (e.g., by decreasing anxiety about potential addiction by using opioids, by enhancing patients' self-efficacy, by improving patients' communication skills).

The content for the intervention was derived from several earlier studies; topics and supporting evidence were nicely summarized in their Table 1. The introduction concluded with a statement of the study purpose: "This study aimed to investigate the impact of an individually delivered preoperative education intervention on pain-related interference, pain, and nausea for patients undergoing unilateral TKA."

RESEARCH QUESTIONS

The researchers specified two questions. The primary question asked about the effect of the intervention on pain-related interference on postoperative day 3. The secondary question asked about effects of the intervention on pain, nausea, and analgesic and antiemetic administration on postoperative days 1, 2, and 3. The researchers did not formally state hypotheses, but the implication was that the researchers predicted that the intervention would reduce pain, nausea, and pain interference.

The researchers did not test the effects of the intervention on possible mechanisms through which the intervention might have had positive effects. For example, if the researchers had expected lower pain levels among those in the intervention group because the educational content was expected to decrease fears of addiction, they might have asked study participants about such fears as an additional outcome. Several other factors might be expected to *mediate* the effect of the intervention on the outcomes, and questions about these mediators could have been addressed.

METHODS

The "Method" section was well organized into several subsections.

Trial Design

Wilson and colleagues used a strong two-group randomized controlled design to evaluate the effectiveness of the educational intervention. Their Figure 2 nicely summarized schematically the progression of activities and events in the trial, from eligibility assessment to the measurement of outcomes. The design was well suited to testing the effects of an intervention and was excellent in terms of internal validity. The trial was conducted at a single academic health sciences center in Ontario, Canada, however, which could limit the generalizability of the results.

Study Participants

The researchers clearly described the inclusion and exclusion criteria for participation in the trial. Participants had to be scheduled for elective TKA using intrathecal anesthetics. Participants also had to be English speakers with telephone access and had to be planned for discharge to home. Patients who were booked for hemi, revision, or bilateral knee arthroplasty were excluded. The report provided adequate information about the recruitment and enrollment process.

Interventions

Wilson and colleagues presented the details about the three components of the intervention (a special booklet, an individualized teaching session, and a follow-up support telephone call). The researchers provided information about who delivered the intervention (the principal investigator in every case) and the timing of the delivery of intervention components (within 4 weeks before surgery for the teaching session and review of the booklet and during the week before the scheduled surgery date for the telephone follow-up). The report did not describe the researchers' rationale for this schedule (for instance, why the follow-up was not within a day or two of the surgery).

The report also presented information about standard care, which is commendable. Patients in both the intervention and control group received an educational session by a physiotherapist, a 30-minute video explaining the surgical procedure, and a brief review of using the intravenous patient-controlled analgesia pump by clinic nursing staff. The timing of providing these supports was not indicated.

Outcomes

In a section labeled "Outcomes," the researchers described the instruments they used to collect baseline and outcome data. They used existing self-report scales to measure pain, nausea, and pain interference. The measure of pain interference was the Brief Pain Inventory, Interference (BPI-I), a scale with items tapping the extent to which pain interferes with general activities, sleep, mood, movements, and relationships with others. The researchers adapted the BPI-I slightly by deleting two items and adding a new item (transferring from bed to chair) to enhance the relevance of the scale to patients in the study. The researchers noted that the original measure has well-established construct validity and sensitivity to change. The researchers did a small pilot test of the adapted scale, but they did not compute its internal consistency. They did note that a similarly adapted scale had an internal consistency reliability of .71, which is modest. The researchers stated that secondary outcomes were measured using the Short Form McGill Pain Questionnaire (MPQ-SF) and the Overall Nausea Index. No information was provided about the reliability and validity of these scales. Ideally, the researchers should have computed and reported a coefficient alpha to indicate the internal consistency of all of their scales, using data from their sample. Also, the authors did not provide readers with information about how the BPI-I scale was scored. Readers cannot be sure if higher scores on the BPI-I are associated with greater or lesser degrees of interference from pain, making it difficult to interpret the results (although it seems likely that higher scores correspond to greater interference). Data regarding the secondary outcomes of analgesic and antiemetic administration were recording from the patients' charts.

Sample Size

The researchers did a power analysis to estimate the sample size they would need in this study. They based their estimate of the effect size ($d = .5$) on a previous study by one of the team members. The power analysis indicated that a sample of 64 patients in each group would be required, but they built in a cushion of 10% for attrition. Thus, the researchers sought a sample size of 140 patients. Commendably, the researchers further justified their effect size estimate by noting that a d of .50 would be a clinically significant amount of improvement.

Randomization and Blinding

The researchers used an excellent randomization method—they relied on a randomization service not connected to the trial. Such a service is preferred to randomization by the team members because it minimizes the risk of bias. Although neither the patients nor the person delivering the intervention could be blinded because of the nature of the intervention, the research assistants who collected the postoperative outcome data were blinded to group assignment.

Statistical Analysis

The researchers provided a good description of the statistical tests and the statistical software they used to analyze their data. For the primary question relating to pain interference, which was measured only once on postoperative day 3, they used an independent groups t-test to compare the two study groups. For the secondary questions relating to pain and nausea, a repeated measures analysis of covariance was used, which was appropriate because these outcomes were measured three times. Finally, for the data on administration of analgesics and antiemetic medication, chi-squared tests were used to compare proportions in the intervention and control groups.

RESULTS

The "Results" section began with a description of the study sample. A useful flow chart was included that showed how many patients were screened for eligibility ($N = 337$), how many were excluded for various reasons ($N = 194$), how many were randomized ($N = 143$), and how many actually received the treatment to which they were assigned. A total of 140 were measured for postoperative outcomes, which is the number the power analysis suggested the researchers needed. Background characteristics of the sample were presented in Table 2, which showed that the two groups were similar in terms of gender, education, use of pain medication, and preoperative diagnosis.

Primary Research Question

The researchers reported that group differences on the pain interference measure (the BPI-I scale) were not statistically significant ($p = .45$). The mean score for those in the intervention group was modestly (but not significantly) *higher* than the mean score for the control group. Table 3 also showed mean scores for six subscale scores on the BPI-I, and group differences were not significant for any of them.

Secondary Research Question

With regard to pain, the researchers stated that there were no group differences in levels of pain on any of the postoperative days. One potentially confusing aspect of the report is that the authors stated in their section labeled "Outcomes" that pain and pain quality were measured using the MPQ-SF. In the "Results" section, the authors mentioned another measure not previously described, the Present Pain Intensity (PPI) global pain rating. They also refer to other pain measures using acronyms without any explanation (PRI-S, PRI-A, and PRI-T). Information about these measures should have been presented in the "Methods" section. Also, Table 4, which summarizes some of the results for pain outcomes, refers to a "Numeric Rating Scale" (NRS) without indicating whether these scores are for the MPQ-SF. In any event, for several of these measures, the researchers reported significant declines in pain scores over time but not significant differences between patients in the intervention and the control groups.

With regard to nausea, the researchers reported that differences between the intervention and control group on the measure of nausea was not significant ($p = .88$). In both groups, nausea declined over the 3-day period.

Similarly, there were no significant differences between the intervention and control groups with regard to daily opioid administration, but there were significant declines over time in both groups. The "Results" section also presented interesting descriptive information about the use of medications in this sample. For example, the researchers reported that seven participants received no opioid analgesic doses on day 3, and that only 56% of patients were administered at least one dose of antiemetic over the 3-day period.

DISCUSSION

The researchers concluded that their intervention was not effective in reducing pain, nausea, and pain interference in patients undergoing TKA. With nonsignificant results, it is sometimes risky to draw such conclusions because of the possibility of a Type II error, but the authors' conclusions seem appropriate because they used a powerful RCT design, their analysis appears to have had adequate power, and the results were consistent across all outcomes.

The researchers' main conclusion was that patient education was ineffective because the problem of appropriately timed and appropriately dosed medication reflected a systems-wide problem. They noted that the trial presented "clear evidence that there are significant systems issues influencing postoperative symptom management after TKA." They pointed out that the patients often did not receive the medications ordered, that evidence-based protocols for nausea management were not followed, and that the pain service in the hospital did not review cases with high levels of pain, as mandated by institutional policy.

Although these conclusions are very likely to be legitimate, the researchers do not appear to have considered alternative or supplementary explanations for the disappointing results, such as deficiencies with the intervention itself, or barriers to symptom management stemming from the patient population (in addition to system barriers). It likely would have been useful if this study had been designed as a mixed methods project—that is, if patients had been asked to provide in-depth information about their symptom experiences, their requests for medication, or their reluctance to request analgesics. The researchers did, however, suggest that a future trial should include a qualitative component targeting orthopedic nursing, medical, and physiotherapy staff. The study might also have benefited by including measures of some proximal outcomes of the intervention—such as patients' knowledge of and attitudes toward pain management strategies.

The researchers noted in their discussion that a limitation of this study was that staff education should have been included as a supplementary component. However, this would not have been feasible with the existing research design because staff education would have benefited members of both the intervention and the control group. To test whether a combined patient–staff education effort would result in better symptom management, the trial would have to be conducted in multiple sites, with some sites randomly assigned to either receive or not receive the multiprong intervention.

One final comment is that the researchers did not discuss their findings within the context of earlier research. Prior intervention trials, such as studies by McDonald, were described in the introduction as having positive impacts on pain. The authors did not present an explanation of why their results might be at odds with those of previous studies that helped to guide this research.

OTHER COMMENTS

Presentation

This report was clearly written and well organized. Except for a few areas of confusion regarding pain outcomes, the report provided excellent information about what was done, why it was done, and what was discovered. The report included several excellent figures and tables.

Ethical Aspects

The authors stated that ethical approval for this study was obtained from the Research Ethics Board of both the university where the researchers worked and the hospital where the data were collected. Potential participants were asked for their permission by hospital staff to release their names to the investigator, using a standardized script. Written informed consent was obtained before randomization. Nothing in the description of this study suggested ethical transgressions.

Note: A few entries in this glossary were not explained in this book but are included here because you might come across them in the research literature. These entries are marked with an asterisk (*).

5 As Five steps that are undertaken in an evidence-based practice project: Ask a well-worded question; Acquire best evidence; Appraise the evidence; Apply the evidence to clinical practice; and Assess the outcome.

5 Whys A process involving rounds of successive questioning; used in some quality improvement projects to gain insight into the root cause of a problem.

Absolute risk (AR) The proportion of people in a group who experienced an undesirable outcome.

Absolute risk reduction (ARR) The difference between the absolute risk in one group (e.g., those exposed to an intervention) and the absolute risk in another group (e.g., those not exposed).

Abstract A brief description of a study, usually located at the beginning of a report.

Accessible population The population available for a study; often a nonrandom subset of the target population.

Acquiescence response set A bias in self-report instruments, especially in psychosocial scales, that occurs when participants characteristically agree with statements ("yea-say"), independent of item content.

AGREE instrument A widely used instrument (Appraisal of Guidelines Research and Evaluation) for assessing clinical practice guidelines.

***Allocation concealment** The process used to ensure that the people who enroll participants into a clinical trial are unaware of upcoming assignments to treatment conditions.

Alpha (α) (1) In tests of statistical significance, the significance criterion—the risk the researcher is willing to accept of making a Type I error (a false positive); (2) in measurement, an index of internal consistency, i.e., Cronbach's alpha.

Analysis The organization and synthesis of data so as to answer research questions or test hypotheses.

Analysis of covariance (ANCOVA) A statistical procedure used to test mean group differences on an outcome variable while controlling for one or more covariates.

Analysis of variance (ANOVA) A statistical procedure for testing mean differences among three or more groups by comparing variability between groups to variability within groups, yielding an F-ratio statistic.

Ancestry approach In literature searches, using citations in relevant studies to track down earlier research on which the studies were based (the "ancestors").

Anonymity Protection of participants' confidentiality such that even the researcher cannot link individuals with the data they provided.

Applicability The degree to which research evidence can be applied to individuals, small groups of individuals, or local contexts (as opposed to broad populations).

***Applied research** Research conducted to find a solution to an immediate practical problem.

Argument An explanation of what a researcher wants to study, with supportive evidence and background material linked in a manner that provides a rationale.

*__Arm__ A particular treatment group to which participants are allocated (e.g., the control *arm* or treatment *arm* of a controlled trial).

Ascertainment bias Systematic differences between groups being compared in how outcome variables are measured, verified, or recorded when data collectors have not been blinded; also called *detection bias*.

Assent The affirmative agreement of a vulnerable person (e.g., a child) to participate in a study, typically to supplement formal consent by a parent or guardian.

Associative relationship An association between two variables that cannot be described as causal.

Assumption A principle that is accepted as being true based on logic or reason, without proof.

Asymmetric distribution A distribution of data values that is skewed, with two halves that are not mirror images of each other.

Attention control group A control group that gets a similar amount of attention as those in the intervention group, without receiving the "active ingredients" of the treatment.

Attrition The loss of participants over the course of a study, which can create bias by changing the composition of the sample initially drawn.

Audit trail In a qualitative study, the systematic documentation of decisions, procedures, and data that allows an independent auditor to draw conclusions about trustworthiness.

Authenticity The extent to which qualitative researchers fairly and faithfully show a range of different realities in the collection, analysis, and interpretation of their data.

Autoethnography An ethnographic study in which researchers study their own culture or group.

Axial coding The second level of coding in a grounded theory study using the Corbin and Strauss approach, involving the process of categorizing, recategorizing, and condensing first level codes by connecting a category and its subcategories.

Baseline data Data collected at an initial measurement (e.g., prior to an intervention) to enable an assessment of changes.

*__Basic research__ Research designed to enhance knowledge in a discipline for the sake of knowledge production rather than for solving an immediate problem.

Basic social process (BSP) The central social process emerging through analysis of grounded theory data; a type of *core variable*.

Benchmark In measurement, a threshold value on a measure that corresponds to an important value, such as a threshold for interpreting whether a change in scores is meaningful or clinically significant.

Beneficence An ethical principle that involves maximizing benefits for study participants and preventing harm.

*__Beta (β)__ (1) In statistical testing, the probability of a Type II error; (2) in multiple regression, the standardized coefficients indicating the relative weights of the predictor variables in the equation.

Bias Any influence that distorts the results of a study and undermines validity or trustworthiness.

Bibliographic database Data files containing bibliographic (reference) information that can be accessed electronically to conduct a literature search.

Bimodal distribution A distribution of data values with two peaks (high frequencies).

Biomarker An objective, quantifiable characteristic of biological processes.

Bivariate statistics Statistical analysis of two variables to assess the empirical relationship between them.

Blind review The review of a manuscript or proposal such that neither the author nor the reviewer is identified to the other party.

Blinding The process of preventing those involved in a study (participants, intervention agents, data collectors, or health care providers) from having information that could lead to a bias, particularly information about which treatment group a participant is in; also called *masking*.

Bracketing In descriptive phenomenological inquiries, the process of identifying and holding in abeyance any preconceived beliefs and opinions about the phenomena under study; also called *epoché*.

Carryover effect The influence that one treatment (or measurement) can have on subsequent treatments/measurements, notably in crossover designs or test–retest reliability assessments.

Case-control design A nonexperimental design that compares "cases" (people with a specified condition, such as lung cancer) to matched controls (similar people without the condition), to examine differences that could have contributed to "caseness."

Case study A method involving a thorough, in-depth analysis of an individual, group, or other social unit.

Categorical variable A variable with discrete categories (e.g., blood type) rather than values along a continuum (e.g., weight).

Category system In studies involving observation, the prespecified plan for recording behaviors and events; in qualitative studies, the system developed from the narrative information to organize the data.

Causal (cause-and-effect) relationship A relationship between two variables wherein the presence or value of one variable (the "cause") determines the presence or value of the other (the "effect").

Cause-probing research Research designed to illuminate the underlying causes of phenomena.

*Ceiling effect An effect resulting from restricted variation above a certain point on a measurement continuum, which constrains true variability and reduces the amount of upward change that is detectable.

Cell The intersection of a row and column in a table with two dimensions, such as a crosstabs table.

Central category The main category or pattern of behavior in grounded theory analysis; sometimes called the *core category*.

Central tendency A statistical index of what is "typical" in a set of scores, derived from the center of the score distribution; indices of central tendency include the mode, median, and mean.

Certificate of Confidentiality A certificate issued by the National Institutes of Health in the United States to protect researchers against forced disclosure of confidential research information.

Change score A person's score difference between two measurements on the same measure, calculated by subtracting the value at one point in time from the value at the second point.

Checklist An instrument used to record observations, typically with a list of behaviors from a category system in the left column and a space for tallying frequency or duration in the right column.

Chi-squared test A statistical test used in various contexts, most often to assess group differences in proportions; symbolized as χ^2.

Clinical nursing research Research designed to generate knowledge to guide nursing practice and to improve the health and quality of life of nurses' clients.

Clinical practice guidelines Practice guidelines that are evidence-based, combining a synthesis and appraisal of research evidence with specific recommendations for clinical decisions.

Clinical significance The practical importance of research results in terms of whether they have genuine, palpable effects on the daily lives of patients or on the health care decisions made on their behalf.

Clinical trial A study designed to assess the safety, efficacy, and effectiveness of a new clinical intervention, often involving several phases (e.g., Phase III typically is a *randomized controlled trial* using an experimental design).

Closed-ended question A question that offers respondents a set of specified response options.

Cluster randomization The random assignment of intact units or organizations (e.g., hospitals), rather than individuals, to treatment conditions.

Cochrane Collaboration An international organization that aims to facilitate well-informed decisions about health care by preparing systematic reviews of the effects of health care interventions.

Code of ethics The fundamental ethical principles established by a discipline or institution to guide researchers' conduct in research with human (or animal) participants.

Coding The process of transforming raw data into standardized form for data processing and analysis; in quantitative research, the process of attaching numbers to categories; in qualitative research, the process of identifying recurring words, themes, or concepts within the data.

Coefficient alpha The most widely used index of internal consistency that indicates the degree to which the items on a multi-item scale are measuring the same underlying construct; also referred to as *Cronbach's alpha.*

Coercion In a research context, the explicit or implicit use of threats (or excessive rewards) to gain people's cooperation in a study.

Cohen's kappa See *kappa.*

Cohort design A nonexperimental design in which a defined group of people (a cohort) is followed over time to study outcomes for subsets of the cohorts; also called a *prospective design.*

Comparative effectiveness research (CER) A patient-centered research approach that focuses on comparisons of alternative treatments to identify which leads to the greatest health improvements.

Comparison group A group of study participants whose scores on outcomes are used to evaluate the outcomes of the group of primary interest (e.g., nonsmokers as a comparison group for smokers); term often used in lieu of *control group* when the study is not a randomized experiment.

Complex intervention An intervention in which complexity exists along one or more dimensions, including number of components, number of targeted outcomes, and the time needed for the full intervention to be delivered.

Composite scale A measure of an attribute, involving the aggregation of responses from multiple items into a single numerical score that places people on a continuum with respect to the attribute.

Concealment A tactic involving the unobtrusive collection of research data without participants' knowledge or consent, used to obtain an accurate view of naturalistic behavior when the behavior would be distorted if participants knew they were being observed.

Concept An abstraction based on observation or self-reporting of behaviors or characteristics (e.g., fatigue, pain).

Concept analysis A systematic process of analyzing a concept or construct, with the aim of identifying the boundaries, definitions, and dimensionality for that concept.

Conceptual definition The abstract or theoretical meaning of a concept of interest.

Conceptual files A manual method of organizing qualitative data, by creating file folders for each category in the coding scheme and inserting relevant excerpts from the data.

Conceptual framework See *framework*.

Conceptual map A schematic representation of a theory or conceptual model that graphically represents key concepts and linkages among them; also called a *schematic model*.

Conceptual model Interrelated concepts assembled in a rational and often explanatory scheme to illuminate relationships but less formally than a theory; sometimes called a *conceptual framework*.

Concurrent design A mixed methods study design in which the qualitative and quantitative strands of data collection occur simultaneously; symbolically designated with a plus sign (e.g., QUAL + QUAN).

Concurrent validity A type of criterion validity that concerns the degree to which scores on a measure are correlated with an external criterion, measured at the same time.

Confidence interval (CI) The range of values within which a population parameter is estimated to lie, at a specified probability (e.g., 95% CI).

Confidentiality Protection of study participants' privacy, such that data they provide are never publicly identified and divulged.

Confirmability A criterion for trustworthiness in a qualitative inquiry, referring to the objectivity or neutrality of the data and interpretations.

Confounding variable A variable that is extraneous to the research question and that confounds the relationship between the independent and dependent variables; confounding variables can be controlled in the research design or through statistical procedures.

Consecutive sampling The recruitment of *all* people from an accessible population who meet the eligibility criteria over a specific time interval or for a specified sample size.

Consent form A written agreement signed by a study participant and a researcher concerning the terms and conditions of voluntary participation in a study.

CONSORT guidelines Widely adopted guidelines (Consolidated Standards of Reporting Trials) for reporting information for a randomized controlled trial, including a checklist and a flow chart for tracking participants through the trial.

Constant comparison A procedure used in qualitative analysis (especially in grounded theory) wherein newly collected data are compared in an ongoing fashion with data obtained earlier, to refine theoretically relevant categories.

Construct An abstraction or concept that is invented (constructed) by researchers based on inferences from human behavior or human traits (e.g., health locus of control).

Construct validity The degree to which evidence about study particulars supports inferences about the higher order constructs they are intended to represent; in measurement, the degree to which a measure truly captures the focal construct.

Constructivist grounded theory An approach to grounded theory, developed by

Charmaz, in which the grounded theory is constructed from shared experiences and relationships between the researcher and study participants and interpretive aspects are emphasized.

Constructivist paradigm An alternative paradigm to the positivist paradigm that holds that there are multiple interpretations of reality, and that the goal of research is to understand how individuals construct reality within their context; associated with qualitative research; also called *naturalistic paradigm*.

Contamination of treatments The inadvertent, biasing influence of one treatment on another treatment condition, e.g., when control group members unintentionally receive all or part of the intervention being tested.

Content analysis An approach to extracting, organizing, and synthesizing material from written materials, including transcripts of narrative data from a qualitative study, according to key concepts and themes.

Content validity The degree to which a multi-item measure has an appropriate set of relevant items reflecting the full content of the construct domain being measured.

Content validity index (CVI) An index of the degree to which an instrument is content valid, based on ratings of a panel of experts; content validity for individual items and the overall scale can be assessed.

Continuous quality improvement An approach to health care that involves an environment in which management and staff strive to constantly improve quality.

Continuous variable A variable that can take on an infinite range of values along a specified continuum (e.g., height); less strictly, a variable measured on an interval or ratio scale.

Control, research Procedures used to hold constant confounding influences on the dependent variable (the outcome) under study.

Control group Participants in a clinical trial who do not receive the experimental intervention and whose performance provides a counterfactual against which the effects of an intervention can be measured.

Controlled trial A trial of an intervention that includes a control group, with or without randomization.

Convenience sampling Selection of the most readily available persons as participants in a study.

Convergent design A concurrent, equal-priority mixed methods design in which different but complementary data, qualitative and quantitative, are gathered about a central phenomenon under study; symbolized as QUAL + QUAN.

Core category (variable) In a grounded theory study, the central phenomenon that is used to integrate all categories of the data.

Correlation A bond or association between variables, such that variation in one variable is systematically related to variation in another.

Correlation coefficient An index summarizing the degree of relationship between variables, typically ranging from $+1.00$ (for a perfect positive relationship) through 0.0 (for no relationship) to -1.00 (for a perfect negative relationship).

Correlation matrix A two-dimensional display showing the correlation coefficients between all pairs of variables in a set of three or more variables.

Correlational research Nonexperimental research that explores the interrelationships among variables of interest, with no researcher intervention.

Cost (economic) analysis An analysis of the relationship between costs and outcomes of nursing or other health care interventions.

*Counterbalancing The process of systematically varying the order of presentation of stimuli or treatments to control for ordering effects, especially in a crossover design.

Counterfactual The condition or group used as a basis of comparison in a study, embodying what would have happened *to the same people* exposed to a causal factor if they *simultaneously* were *not* exposed to it.

Covariate A variable that is statistically controlled in analysis of covariance; typically, a confounding influence on, or a preintervention measure of, the outcome.

Covert data collection The collection of information in a study without participants' knowledge.

Credibility A criterion for evaluating trustworthiness in qualitative studies, referring to confidence in the truth of the data; analogous to internal validity in quantitative research.

Criterion validity The extent to which scores on a measure are an adequate reflection of (or predictor of) a criterion that is considered a "gold standard" measure.

Critical appraisal An objective assessment of a study's strengths, limitations, and relevance, often to reach a conclusion about whether its evidence can be applied to practice.

Critical ethnography An ethnography that focuses on raising consciousness in the group or culture under study in the hope of effecting social change.

Critical theory An approach to viewing the world that involves a critique of society, with the goal of envisioning new possibilities and effecting social change.

Critique A critical appraisal that analyzes both weaknesses and strengths of a research report, often to assess its potential for publication; see also *critical appraisal*.

Cronbach's alpha A widely used index that estimates the internal consistency of a composite measure composed of several subparts (e.g., items); also called *coefficient alpha*.

Crossover design An experimental design in which one group of participants is exposed to more than one condition or treatment, in random order.

Cross-sectional design A study design in which data are collected at one point in time; sometimes used to infer change over time when data are collected from different age or developmental groups.

Crosstabs table A two-dimensional table in which the frequencies of two categorical variables are crosstabulated.

Crosstabulation A calculation of frequencies for two variables considered simultaneously—e.g., gender (male/female/other) crosstabulated with smoking status (smoker/nonsmoker).

***d* statistic** An effect size index for comparing two group means, computed by subtracting one mean from the other and dividing by the pooled standard deviation; also called *Cohen's d* or *standardized mean difference*.

Data The pieces of information obtained in a study (singular is *datum*).

Data analysis The systematic organization and synthesis of research data and, in quantitative studies, the testing of hypotheses using those data.

Data collection protocols The formal procedures researchers develop to guide the collection of data in a standardized fashion.

Data saturation The collection of qualitative data to the point where a sense of closure is attained because new data yield redundant information.

Data set The total collection of data on all variables for all study participants.

Data triangulation The use of multiple data sources for the purpose of validating conclusions.

Debriefing Communication with study participants after participation is complete regarding aspects of the study (e.g., explaining the study purpose more fully).

Deception The deliberate withholding of information, or the provision of false information, to study participants, usually to reduce potential biases.

Deductive reasoning The process of developing specific predictions from general principles; see also *inductive reasoning*.

Degrees of freedom (*df*) A statistical concept referring to the number of sample values free to vary (e.g., with a given sample mean, all but one value would be free to vary).

Delayed treatment design A design for an intervention study that involves putting control group members on a waiting list to receive the intervention after follow-up data are collected; also called a *wait-list design*.

Delphi survey A technique for obtaining judgments from an expert panel about an issue of concern; experts are questioned individually in several rounds, with a summary of the panel's views circulated between rounds, to achieve some consensus.

Dependability A criterion for evaluating integrity in qualitative studies, referring to the stability of data over time and over conditions; analogous to reliability in quantitative research.

Dependent variable The variable hypothesized to depend on or be caused by the independent variable; the outcome of interest.

Descendancy approach In literature searches, finding a pivotal early study and searching forward in citation indexes to find more recent studies ("descendants") that cited the key study.

Description question A question aimed at describing a health-related phenomenon.

Descriptive phenomenology An approach to phenomenology that focuses on the careful description of ordinary conscious experiences of everyday life.

Descriptive qualitative study An in-depth study that involves the collection of rich, qualitative data but does not have roots in a particular qualitative tradition; data are often analyzed using content analysis or thematic analysis.

Descriptive research Research that has as a primary objective the accurate portrayal of people's characteristics or circumstances and/or the frequency with which certain phenomena occur.

Descriptive statistics Statistics used to describe and summarize data (e.g., means, percentages).

Descriptive theory A broad characterization that thoroughly accounts for a phenomenon.

Determinism The belief that phenomena are not haphazard or random but rather have antecedent causes; an assumption in the positivist paradigm.

Diagnosis/assessment question A question about the accuracy and validity of instruments to screen, diagnose, or assess patients.

Dichotomous question A question with only two response alternatives (e.g., yes/no).

Directional hypothesis A hypothesis that makes a specific prediction about the direction of the relationship between two variables.

Disconfirming case In qualitative research, a case that challenges the researchers' conceptualizations; sometimes sought as part of a sampling strategy.

Domain In ethnographic analysis, a unit or broad category of cultural knowledge.

*Dose-response analysis An analysis to assess whether larger doses of an intervention are associated with greater benefits.

Double-blind study A clinical trial in which two sets of people are blinded with respect to the group that a study participant is in; often a situation in which neither the participants nor those administering the treatment know who is in the intervention or control group.

Economic (cost) analysis An analysis of the relationship between costs and outcomes of alternative health care interventions.

Effect size (ES) A statistical index expressing the magnitude of the relationship between two variables, or the magnitude of the difference between groups on an attribute of interest (e.g., Cohen's *d*); also used in meta-summaries of qualitative research to characterize the salience of a theme or category.

Effectiveness study A clinical trial designed to test the effectiveness of an intervention under ordinary conditions, usually for an intervention already found to be efficacious in an efficacy study.

Efficacy study A tightly controlled trial designed to establish the efficacy of an intervention under ideal conditions, using a design that maximizes internal validity; sometimes called an *explanatory trial.*

Element The most basic unit of a population for sampling purposes, typically a human being.

Eligibility criteria The criteria designating the specific attributes of the target population, by which people are selected for inclusion in a study or excluded from it.

Emergent design A design that unfolds in the course of a qualitative study as the researcher makes ongoing design decisions reflecting what has already been learned.

Emergent fit A concept in grounded theory that involves comparing new data and new categories with previous conceptualizations.

Emic perspective An ethnographic term referring to the way members of a culture view their own world; the "insider's view."

Empirical evidence Evidence rooted in objective reality and gathered using one's senses as the basis for generating knowledge.

Estimation of parameters Statistical procedures that estimate population parameters based on sample statistics.

Ethical dilemma A situation in which there is a conflict between ethical principles and the research methods needed to maximize the quality of study evidence.

Ethics In research, a system of moral values that concerns the degree to which research procedures adhere to professional, legal, and social obligations to study participants.

Ethnography A branch of human inquiry, associated with anthropology, that focuses on the culture of a group of people, with an effort to understand the worldview and customs of those under study.

Ethnonursing research A term coined by Leininger to denote the study of human cultures, with a focus on a group's beliefs and practices relating to nursing care and related health behaviors.

Etic perspective In ethnography, the "outsider's" view of the experiences of a cultural group.

Etiology (causation)/harm question A question about the underlying cause of a health problem, such as an environmental cause or personal behavior (e.g., smoking).

Evaluation research Research aimed at learning how well a program, practice, or policy is working.

Event sampling A type of observational sampling that involves the selection of integral behaviors or events to be observed.

Evidence hierarchy A ranked arrangement of the strength of research evidence based on the rigor of the method that produced it; traditional evidence hierarchies are appropriate primarily for cause-probing research.

Evidence-based practice (EBP) A practice that involves making clinical decisions based on clinical judgment, patient preferences, and on the best available evidence, usually evidence from disciplined research.

Exclusion criteria Criteria specifying characteristics that a target population does *not* have stipulated for the purpose of determining eligibility for a study sample.

Expectation bias The bias that can arise when participants (or research staff) have expectations about treatment effectiveness in intervention research; the expectation can result in altered behavior.

Experimental group The study participants who receive an experimental treatment or intervention.

Experimental research Research using a design in which the researcher controls (manipulates) the independent variable by randomly assigning people to different treatment groups; randomized controlled trials use experimental designs.

Explanatory design A sequential mixed methods design in which quantitative data are collected in the first phase and qualitative data are collected in the second phase to build on or explain quantitative findings.

Explanatory trial A traditional clinical trial, conducted under optimal conditions with carefully selected participants, to enhance internal validity.

Exploratory design A sequential mixed methods design in which qualitative data are collected in the first phase and

quantitative data are collected in the second phase based on the initial in-depth exploration.

External validity The degree to which study results can be generalized to people or settings other than the one studied.

Extraneous variable A variable that confounds the relationship between the independent and dependent variables and that needs to be controlled either in the research design or through statistical procedures; often called *confounding variable*.

Extreme response set A bias resulting from a respondent's consistent selection of extreme alternatives (e.g., *strongly agree* or *strongly disagree*) to scale items, regardless of item content.

F **ratio** The statistic obtained in several statistical tests (e.g., ANOVA) in which variation in the outcome that is attributable to different sources (e.g., between groups and within groups) is compared.

Face validity The extent to which an instrument looks as though it is measuring what it purports to measure.

Factor analysis A statistical procedure for disentangling complex interrelationships among items and identifying the items that "go together" as a unified dimension.

Feminist research Research that seeks to understand how gender and a gendered social order shape women's lives and their consciousness.

Field diary A daily record of events and conversations in the field; also called a *log*.

Field notes The notes recorded by researchers to document the unstructured observations made in the field and the interpretation of those observations.

Field research Research in which the data are collected "in the field," i.e., in naturalistic settings.

Fieldwork The activities undertaken by qualitative researchers (especially ethnographers) to collect data out in the field, i.e., in natural settings.

Findings The results of the analysis of research data.

Fit An element in Glaserian grounded theory analysis in which the researcher develops categories of a substantive theory that fit the data.

Fixed effects model In meta-analysis, a statistical model in which studies are assumed to be measuring the same overall effect; a pooled effect estimate is calculated under the assumption that observed variation between studies is attributable to chance.

Focus group interview An interview with a small group of individuals assembled to discuss a specific topic, usually guided by a moderator using a semi-structured topic guide.

Focused interview A loosely structured interview in which an interviewer guides the respondent through a set of questions using a topic guide; also called a *semi-structured interview*.

Follow-up study A study undertaken to assess the outcomes of individuals with a specified condition or who have received a specified treatment.

Forest plot A graphic representation of effects across studies in a meta-analysis, permitting a visual assessment of variation in effects across studies (i.e., heterogeneity).

Framework The conceptual underpinnings of a study—e.g., a *theoretical framework* in theory-based studies, or *conceptual framework* in studies based on a conceptual model.

Frequency distribution A systematic array of numeric values from the lowest to the highest, together with a count of the number of times each value was obtained.

Frequency effect size In a meta-summary of qualitative studies, the percentage of reports that contain a given thematic finding.

Full disclosure The communication of complete, accurate information about a study to potential study participants.

Functional relationship A relationship between two variables in which it cannot be assumed that one variable caused the other.

Gaining entrée The process of gaining access to study participants through the cooperation of key gatekeepers in a selected community or site.

Generalizability The degree to which the research methods justify the inference that the findings are true for a broader group than study participants; in particular, the inference that the findings can be generalized from the sample to the population.

GRADE The **G**rades of **R**ecommendation, **A**ssessment, **D**evelopment, and **E**valuation, an approach to grading confidence in findings from a systematic review.

Grand theory A broad theory aimed at describing and explaining large segments of the physical, social, or behavioral world; also called a *macrotheory*.

Grand tour question A broad question asked in an unstructured interview to gain a general overview of a phenomenon, on the basis of which more focused questions are subsequently asked.

Grey literature Unpublished and thus less readily accessible research reports (e.g., dissertations).

Grounded theory An approach to collecting and analyzing qualitative data that aims to develop theories about social psychological processes grounded in real-world observations.

Hawthorne effect The effect on the outcome resulting from people's awareness that they are participants under study.

Health services research The broad interdisciplinary field that studies how organizational structures and processes, health technologies, social factors, and personal behaviors affect access to health care, the cost and quality of health care, and, ultimately, people's health and well-being.

Hermeneutic circle In hermeneutics, the process in which, to reach understanding, there is continual movement between the parts and the whole of the text that is being analyzed.

Hermeneutics A qualitative research tradition, drawing on interpretive phenomenology, that focuses on the lived experiences of humans and on how they interpret those experiences.

Heterogeneity The degree to which objects are dissimilar (characterized by variability) on an attribute.

Heterogeneity of treatment effects (HTE) Variation in the effectiveness of an intervention across a population—i.e., the intervention's benefits (or harms) are not universal.

Historical research Systematic studies designed to discover facts and relationships about past events.

History threat The occurrence of events external to an intervention but concurrent with it, which can affect the outcome variable and threaten the study's internal validity.

Homogeneity The degree to which people or objects are similar (i.e., characterized by low variability) on an attribute; sometimes used as a design strategy used to control confounding variables.

Hypothesis A statement of predicted relationships between variables.

Hypothesis testing Statistical procedures for testing whether hypotheses should be accepted or rejected, based on the probability that hypothesized relationships in a sample exist in the population.

Hypothesis-testing validity The extent to which one can corroborate hypotheses regarding how scores on a measure function in relation to scores on measures of other variables; an aspect of construct validity.

*Implementation potential The extent to which an innovation is amenable to implementation in a new setting; implementation potential is sometimes assessed prior to evidence-based practice projects.

Implied consent Consent to participate in a study that a researcher assumes has been given based on participants' actions, such as returning a completed questionnaire.

Improvement science An emerging field that focuses on explorations of how to accelerate quality improvement and do it rigorously.

IMRAD format The organization of a research report into four main sections: the **I**ntroduction, **M**ethod, **R**esults, and **D**iscussion sections.

*Incidence The rate of new cases with a specified condition, determined by dividing the number of new cases over a given period of time by the number at risk for becoming a new case (i.e., free of the condition at the outset of the time period).

Inclusion criteria The criteria specifying characteristics of a population that a prospective participant must have to be considered eligible for a study.

Independent variable The variable that is believed to cause or influence the dependent variable; in experimental research, the manipulated (treatment) variable; the independent variable is both the "I" and the "C" in the PICO framework.

Inductive reasoning The process of reasoning from specific observations to more general rules (see also *deductive reasoning*).

Inference A conclusion drawn from limited information, using logical reasoning; in research, a conclusion drawn from study evidence, taking into account the methods used to generate that evidence.

Inferential statistics Statistics that are used to make inferences about whether results observed in a sample are likely to be reliable, i.e., found in the population.

Informant A person who provides information to researchers about a phenomenon under study; a term used mostly in qualitative studies.

Informed consent A process in the ethical conduct of a study that involves obtaining people's voluntary participation in a study, after informing them of possible risks and benefits.

Inquiry audit An independent scrutiny of qualitative data and relevant supporting documents by an external reviewer to determine their dependability and confirmability.

Insider research Research on a group or culture—usually in an ethnography—by a member of that group or culture; in ethnographic research, an *autoethnography*.

Institutional Review Board (IRB) A term used primarily in the United States to refer to the institutional group that convenes to review proposed and ongoing studies with respect to ethical considerations.

Instrument The device used to collect data (e.g., a questionnaire or observation checklist).

Intensity effect size In a qualitative meta-summary, the percentage of all thematic findings that are contained in any given report.

*Intention to treat The gold standard strategy for analyzing data in an intervention study that includes participants with the group to which they were assigned, regardless of whether they received or completed the treatment associated with the group.

Interaction effect The effect of two or more independent variables acting in combination (interactively) on an outcome.

Intercoder reliability The degree to which two coders, working independently, agree on coding decisions.

Internal consistency The degree to which items on a composite scale are interrelated and are measuring the same attribute, usually evaluated using coefficient alpha; a measurement property in the reliability domain.

Internal validity The degree to which it can be inferred that an intervention (the independent variable), rather than confounding factors, caused the observed effects on an outcome.

Interpretive phenomenology A type of phenomenology that stresses interpreting and understanding, not just describing, human experience sometimes referred to as *hermeneutics*.

Interrater (interobserver) reliability The degree to which two raters or observers, working independently, assign the same ratings or scores for an attribute being measured.

Interval estimation A statistical estimation approach in which the researcher computes a range of values that are likely, within a given level of confidence (e.g., a 95% confidence interval), to contain the true population parameter.

Interval measurement A measurement level in which an attribute is rank ordered on a scale that has equal distances between points on that scale (e.g., Fahrenheit degrees).

Intervention In experimental research (clinical trials), the treatment being tested; the "I" in the PICO framework.

Intervention fidelity The extent to which the implementation of a treatment is faithful to its plan.

Intervention protocol The specification of what the intervention and alternative (control) treatment conditions are, how they should be administered, and who should administer them.

Intervention research Research involving the development, implementation, and testing of an intervention.

Intervention theory The conceptual underpinning of a health care intervention, which articulates the theoretical basis for the achievement of desired outcomes.

Interview A data collection method in which an interviewer asks questions of a respondent, either face-to-face, by telephone, or over the Internet (e.g., via Skype).

Interview schedule The formal instrument that specifies the wording of all questions to be asked of respondents in studies in which structured self-report data are collected.

Intraclass correlation coefficient (ICC) A statistical index used to estimate the reliability (e.g., test–retest reliability) of a measure.

Inverse relationship A relationship characterized by the tendency of high values on one variable to be associated with low values on the second variable; also called a *negative relationship*.

Investigator triangulation The use of two or more researchers to analyze and interpret data, to enhance trustworthiness.

Iowa Model of Evidence-Based Practice A widely used framework that can be used to guide the development and implementation of a project to promote evidence-based practice.

Item A single question on an instrument, such as on a composite scale.

Journal article A report appearing in professional journals such as *Nursing Research* or *International Journal of Nursing Studies*.

Journal club A group that meets in clinical contexts to discuss and critically appraise research articles published in journals.

Kappa A statistical index of chance-corrected agreement or consistency between two nominal (or ordinal) measurements, often used to assess interrater reliability; also called *Cohen's kappa*.

Key informant A person knowledgeable about the phenomenon of research interest and who is willing to share information and insights with the researcher, most often in ethnographies.

Keyword An important term used to search for references on a topic in bibliographic databases, identified by authors or indexers to enhance the likelihood that the report will be found.

Knowledge translation (KT) The exchange, synthesis, and application of knowledge by relevant stakeholders within complex systems to accelerate the beneficial effects of research aimed at improving health care.

Known-groups validity A type of construct validity that concerns the degree to which a measure can discriminate between groups known or expected to differ with regard to the construct of interest.

Lean approach In quality improvement, a model whose aim is to improve quality and efficiency at lower costs; also called the *Toyota Production System*.

Level of evidence (LOE) scale A scale that rank orders evidence for cause-probing questions in terms of risk of bias, based on evidence hierarchies; Level I evidence is typically systematic reviews of randomized controlled trials.

Level of measurement A system of classifying measurements according to the nature of the measurement and the type of permissible mathematical operations; the levels are nominal, ordinal, interval, and ratio.

Level of significance The risk of making a Type I error in a statistical analysis, with the criterion (alpha) established by the researcher beforehand (e.g., $\alpha = .05$).

Likert scale Traditionally, a type of scale to measure attitudes, involving the summation of scores on a set of items that respondents rate for their degree of agreement or disagreement; more loosely, the name often used for summated rating scales.

Literature review A summary of research on a topic, often prepared to put a research problem in context or to summarize existing evidence; typically, less rigorously conducted than a systematic review.

Log In participant observation studies, the observer's daily record of events and conversations.

Logistic regression A multivariate regression procedure that analyzes relationships between one or more independent (predictor) variables and a categorical dependent variable.

Longitudinal design A study design in which data are collected at more than one point in time, in contrast to a cross-sectional design.

Macrotheory A broad theory aimed at describing large segments of the physical, social, or behavioral world; also called a *grand theory*.

Manifest effect size In meta-summaries, an effect size index calculated from the manifest content represented in the findings of primary qualitative studies; includes *frequency effect sizes* and *intensity effect sizes*.

Manipulation The introduction of an intervention or treatment in an experimental or quasi-experimental study to assess its impact on outcomes of interest.

MANOVA See *multivariate analysis of variance*.

Masking See *blinding*.

Matching The pairing of participants in one group with those in a comparison group based on their similarity on one or more attributes, to enhance group comparability.

Maturation threat A threat to the internal validity of a study that results when changes to the outcome variable result from the passage of time.

Maximum variation sampling A sampling approach used by qualitative researchers involving the purposeful selection of cases with wide variation on key attributes.

Mean A measure of central tendency, computed by summing all scores and dividing by the total number of cases.

Meaning/process question A question about what health-related phenomena mean to people or about how a process or experience unfolds.

Measure A device whose purpose is to obtain numerical information to quantify an attribute or construct (e.g., a scale).

Measurement The assignment of numbers to objects according to specified rules to characterize quantities of some attribute.

Measurement error The systematic and random error associated with a person's score on a measure, reflecting factors other than the construct being measured and resulting in an observed score that is different from a hypothetical true score.

Measurement property A characteristic reflecting a distinct aspect of a measure's quality (e.g., reliability, validity).

Median A measure of central tendency; the point in a score distribution above and below which 50% of the cases fall.

Mediating variable A variable that mediates or acts like a "go-between" in a causal chain linking two other variables.

Member check A method of validating the credibility of qualitative data through debriefings and discussions with study participants.

MeSH Medical Subject Headings, the system used to index articles in MEDLINE.

Meta-aggregation An approach to the synthesis of qualitative evidence in which findings are categorized and summarized rather than transformed, as in a metasynthesis.

Meta-analysis A technique for quantitatively integrating the results of multiple studies addressing the same or highly similar research question.

Meta-ethnography An approach to integrating findings from qualitative studies by translating and interpreting concepts and metaphors across studies; developed by Noblit and Hare.

Metaphor A figurative comparison used by some qualitative analysts to evoke a visual or symbolic analogy.

Meta-summary A type of qualitative research synthesis that involves the development of a list of abstracted findings from primary studies and calculating manifest effect sizes.

Metasynthesis An interpretive translation of evidence produced by systematically integrating findings from multiple qualitative studies.

Method triangulation The use of multiple methods of data collection about the same phenomenon, to enhance credibility.

Methodological study A study designed to develop or refine methods of obtaining, organizing, or analyzing data.

Methods, research The steps, procedures, and strategies for designing a study and gathering and analyzing study data.

Middle-range theory A theory that attempts to explain a piece of reality or human experience, focusing on a limited number of concepts (e.g., a theory of stress).

Minimal important change (MIC) A benchmark for interpreting change scores that represents the smallest change that is meaningful to patients or clinicians and thus establishes clinical significance.

Minimal risk Anticipated risks from study participation that are no greater than those ordinarily encountered in daily life or during the performance of routine tests or procedures.

Mixed methods (MM) research Research in which both qualitative and quantitative data are collected and analyzed to address different but related questions.

Mixed studies review A systematic review that integrates and synthesizes findings from qualitative, quantitative, and mixed methods studies on a topic.

Mode A measure of central tendency; the value that occurs most frequently in a distribution of scores.

Model A symbolic representation of concepts or variables and interrelationships among them.

Moderator variable A variable that affects (moderates) the strength or direction of a relationship between the independent variable and the outcome variable; can be detected through subgroup analyses.

Mortality threat A threat to the internal validity of a study, referring to differential attrition (loss of participants) from different groups.

Multimodal distribution A distribution of values with more than one peak (high frequency).

Multiple comparison procedures Statistical tests, normally applied after an analysis of variance indicates statistically significant group differences, that compare different pairs of groups; also called *post hoc tests*.

Multiple correlation coefficient An index that summarizes the degree of relationship between two or more independent (predictor) variables and a dependent variable; symbolized as *R*.

Multiple regression A statistical procedure for understanding the effects of two or more independent (predictor) variables on a dependent variable.

Multistage sampling A sampling strategy that proceeds through stages from larger to smaller sampling units (e.g., from states, to census tracts, to households).

Multivariate analysis of variance (MANOVA) A statistical procedure used to test the significance of differences between the means of two or more groups on two or more dependent variables, considered simultaneously.

Multivariate statistics Statistical procedures designed to analyze the relationships among three or more variables (e.g., multiple regression, analysis of covariance).

N The symbol designating the total number of participants (e.g., "the total *N* was 500").

n The symbol designating the number of subjects in a subgroup or cell of a study (e.g., "each of the four groups had an *n* of 125, for a total *N* of 500").

Narrative analysis A qualitative approach that focuses on a person's story as the object of the inquiry.

Naturalistic setting A setting for the collection of research data that is natural to those being studied (e.g., homes, places of work).

Naysayers bias A bias in self-report scales created when respondents characteristically disagree with statements ("naysay"), independent of item content.

Negative case analysis The refinement of a theory or description in a qualitative study through the inclusion of cases that appear to disconfirm earlier hypotheses.

Negative relationship A relationship between two variables in which there is a tendency for high values on one variable to be associated with low values on the other (e.g., as stress increases, quality of life decreases); also called an *inverse relationship*.

Negative skew An asymmetric distribution of data values with a disproportionately high number of cases at the upper end; when displayed graphically, the tail points to the left.

Nested sampling An approach to sampling in mixed methods studies in which some, but not all, of the participants from one strand are included in the sample for the other strand.

Network sampling The sampling of participants based on referrals from others already in the sample; also called *snowball sampling*.

Nominal measurement The lowest level of measurement involving the assignment of numbers to categories (e.g., 1 = married, 2 = not married).

Nondirectional hypothesis A research hypothesis that does not stipulate the expected direction of the relationship between variables.

Nonequivalent control group design A quasi-experimental design involving a comparison group that was not created through random assignment.

Nonexperimental research Studies in which the researcher collects data without introducing an intervention; also called *observational research*.

Nonparametric tests A class of statistical tests that do not involve stringent assumptions about the distribution of variables in the analysis.

Nonprobability sampling The selection of elements (e.g., participants) from a population using nonrandom methods (e.g., convenience sampling).

Nonresponse bias A bias that can result when a nonrandom subset of people invited to participate in a study decline to participate.

Nonsignificant result The result of a statistical test indicating that group differences or observed relationships could have occurred by chance, at a given probability level; sometimes abbreviated as *NS*.

Normal distribution A theoretical distribution that is bell-shaped, symmetrical, and not too peaked.

Null hypothesis A hypothesis stating the absence of a relationship between the variables under study; used primarily in statistical testing as the hypothesis to be rejected.

Number needed to treat (NNT) An estimate of how many people would need to receive an intervention to prevent one undesirable outcome, computed by dividing 1 by the value of the absolute risk reduction.

Nursing research Systematic inquiry designed to develop knowledge about issues of importance to the nursing profession.

Nursing sensitive outcome A patient outcome that improves if there is greater quantity or quality of nursing care.

Objectivity The extent to which two independent researchers would arrive at similar judgments or conclusions (i.e., judgments not biased by personal values or beliefs).

Observation A method of collecting information and/or measuring constructs by directly watching and recording behaviors and characteristics.

Observational study A study that does not involve an intervention—i.e., nonexperimental research in which phenomena are merely observed.

Odds An index that summarizes the probability of an event occurring to the probability that it will not occur, calculated by dividing the number of people who experienced an event by the number who did not.

Odds ratio (OR) The ratio of one odds to another odds, e.g., the ratio of the odds of an event in one group to the odds of an event in another group; an odds ratio of 1.0 indicates no difference between groups.

Open coding The first level of coding in a grounded theory study, referring to the basic descriptive coding of the content of narrative materials.

Open-access journal A journal that allows free online access to articles, without user subscription costs; traditional journals may include some articles that are open-access.

Open-ended question A question in an interview or questionnaire that does not restrict respondents' answers to predetermined response options.

Operational definition The definition of a concept or variable in terms of the procedures by which it is to be measured.

Operationalization The process of translating research concepts into measurable phenomena.

Ordinal measurement A measurement level that involves sorting people (or objects) based on their relative ranking on an attribute.

Outcome variable A term often used to refer to the dependent variable, i.e., the outcome (endpoint) of interest; the "O" in the PICO framework.

Outcomes research Research designed to document the effectiveness of health care services and the end results of patient care.

p **value** In statistical testing, the probability that the obtained results are due to chance; the probability of a Type I error.

Paradigm A way of looking at natural phenomena—a worldview—that encompasses a set of philosophical assumptions that guides one's approach to inquiry.

Paradigm case In Benner's hermeneutic analysis, a strong exemplar of the phenomenon under study, often used early in the analysis to gain understanding of the phenomenon.

Parameter A characteristic of a population (e.g., the mean age of all registered nurses [RNs]).

Parametric tests A class of statistical tests that involve assumptions about the distribution of the variables and the estimation of a parameter.

Participant See *study participant*.

Participant observation A method of collecting data through the participation in and observation of a group or culture, most often used in ethnographies.

Participatory action research (PAR) A research approach used with groups or communities that is based on the premise that the use and production of knowledge can be political and used to exert power.

***Path analysis** A regression-based procedure for testing causal models, typically using correlational data.

Patient-centered research Research that focuses on the development of evidence that is important and relevant to patients, especially about outcomes of special concern to them (e.g., quality of life).

Patient-centeredness A focus, in both health care and in research, on individual patients' needs and values, including involving patients in care decisions and research priorities.

Patient-reported outcome (PRO) A health outcome that is measured by directly asking patients for information.

Pearson's *r* A correlation coefficient designating the magnitude of relationship between two interval- or ratio-level variables; also called *the product-moment correlation*.

Peer debriefing A session with peers to review and explore various aspects of a study, often used to enhance trustworthiness in a qualitative study.

Peer reviewer A researcher who reviews and critiques a research report or proposal and makes a recommendation about publishing or funding the research.

***Per protocol analysis** Analysis of data from a randomized controlled trial that excludes participants who did not obtain the protocol to which they were assigned (or who received an incomplete dose of the intervention).

Perfect relationship A correlation between two variables such that the values of one variable can perfectly predict the values of the other; designated as 1.00 or -1.00.

Persistent observation A qualitative researcher's intense focus on the aspects of a situation that are relevant to the phenomena being studied.

Person triangulation The collection of data from different levels or types of persons, with the aim of validating data through multiple perspectives on the phenomenon.

Phenomenology A qualitative research tradition, with roots in philosophy and psychology, that focuses on the lived experience of humans.

Phenomenon The abstract concept under study; term often used by qualitative researchers in lieu of *variable*.

Photo elicitation An interview stimulated and guided by photographic images.

Photovoice A technique used in some qualitative studies that involves asking participants to take photographs of their culture or environment and then interpret the photos.

PICO format A framework for asking well-worded questions and for searching for evidence, where P = population, I = intervention or influence, C = comparison, and O = outcome.

Pilot study A small-scale study, or trial run, done in preparation for a major study or to assess feasibility.

Placebo A sham or pseudointervention, sometimes used as a control group condition.

*Placebo effect Changes in the outcome attributable to a placebo as a result of participants' expectations.

Plan-Do-Study-Act (PDSA) A quality improvement model that involves systematic, rapid cycles of activities; sometimes called *Plan-Do-Check-Act (PDCA)*.

Point estimation A statistical procedure that uses data from a sample (a statistic) to estimate the single value that best represents the population parameter.

Population The entire set of individuals or objects having some common characteristics (e.g., all RNs in California); the "P" in the PICO framework.

Positive relationship A relationship between two variables in which high values on one variable tend to be associated with high values on the other (e.g., as physical activity increases, heart rate increases).

Positive results Research results that are consistent with the researcher's hypotheses.

Positive skew An asymmetric distribution of values with a disproportionately high number of cases at the lower end; when displayed graphically, the tail points to the right.

Positivist paradigm The paradigm underlying the traditional scientific approach, which assumes that there is an orderly reality that can be objectively studied; often associated with quantitative research.

Post hoc test A test for comparing all possible pairs of groups following a significant test of overall group differences (e.g., in an analysis of variance).

Poster session A session at a professional conference in which several researchers simultaneously present visual displays summarizing their studies, whereas conference attendees circulate around the room perusing the displays.

Posttest data Data collected after introducing an intervention.

Posttest-only design An experimental design in which outcome data are collected from participants only after the intervention has been introduced.

Power The ability of a design or analysis to detect true relationships that exist among variables.

Power analysis A procedure used to estimate sample size requirements prior to undertaking a study or to estimate the likelihood of committing a Type II error.

Practice-based evidence Research evidence that is developed in real-world settings and is responsive to the needs and circumstances of specific patients and contexts.

Pragmatic clinical trial A trial that addresses practical questions about the benefits, risks, and costs of an intervention as it would unfold in routine clinical practice to enhance clinical decision making.

Pragmatism A paradigm on which mixed methods research is often said to be based, in that it acknowledges the practical imperative of the "dictatorship of the research question."

Precision The degree to which an estimated population value (a statistic) clusters closely around the estimate, usually expressed in terms of the width of the confidence interval.

Precision health care A model that proposes the customization of health care, with decisions and treatments tailored to individual patients based on their unique genetic, physiological, behavioral, lifestyle, and environmental profile.

Prediction The use of empirical evidence to make forecasts about how variables will perform in a new setting and with a different sample.

Predictive validity A type of criterion validity concerning the degree to which a measure is correlated with a criterion measured at a future point in time.

Predictor variable A variable (usually the independent variable) used to predict another variable (the outcome); term used primarily in the context of regression analysis.

Pretest (1) Data collected prior to an intervention; often called *baseline data*. (2) The trial administration of a newly developed instrument to identify potential weaknesses.

Pretest–posttest design A design in which data are collected from study participants both before and after introducing an intervention.

Prevalence The proportion of a population having a particular condition (e.g., fibromyalgia) at a given point in time.

Primary source Firsthand reports of facts or findings; in research, the original report prepared by the investigator who conducted the study.

Primary study In a systematic review, an original study whose findings are the data in the review.

Priority A feature of mixed methods designs, concerning which strand (qualitative or quantitative) is given more emphasis; in notation, the dominant strand is in all capital letters, as QUAL or QUAN, and the nondominant strand is in lower case, as qual or quan.

Probability sampling The selection of elements (e.g., participants) from a population using random procedures, such that each member has an equal probability of being selected.

Probing Eliciting more useful or detailed information from a respondent in an interview than was volunteered in the initial reply.

Problem statement The articulation of a dilemma or a disturbing situation that needs investigation.

Process analysis A descriptive analysis of the process by which a program or intervention gets implemented and used in practice.

Process consent In a qualitative study, an ongoing, transactional process of negotiating consent with participants, allowing them to collaborate in decision making about continued participation.

Product–moment correlation coefficient (r) A correlation coefficient designating the magnitude and direction of relationship between two variables measured on at least an interval scale; also called *Pearson's r*.

Prognosis question A question about the consequences or long-term outcomes of a disease or health problem.

Prolonged engagement In qualitative research, the investment of sufficient time during data collection to have an in-depth understanding of the phenomenon under study, thereby enhancing credibility.

Proposal A document communicating a research problem, its significance, proposed methods for addressing the problem, and, when funding is sought, how much the study will cost.

Prospective design A study design that begins with an examination of a presumed cause (e.g., cigarette smoking) and then goes forward in time to measure presumed effects (e.g., lung cancer); also called a *cohort design*.

Psychometric assessment An evaluation of the quality of an instrument, primarily in terms of its reliability and validity.

Psychometrics A field of inquiry concerned with the theory of measurement of abstract psychological constructs and the application of the theory in the development and testing of measures.

Publication bias A bias resulting from the fact that published studies overrepresent statistically significant findings, reflecting the tendency to not publish reports with nonsignificant results.

Purposive (purposeful) sampling A nonprobability sampling method in which the researcher selects participants based on personal judgment about who will be most informative.

Q sort A data collection method in which participants sort statements into piles (usually 9 or 11) according to some bipolar dimension (e.g., most helpful/least helpful).

Qualitative analysis The organization and interpretation of narrative data for the purpose of discovering important underlying themes, categories, and patterns.

Qualitative data Information in narrative (nonnumeric) form, such as the information provided in an unstructured interview.

Qualitative descriptive research Qualitative studies that yield rich descriptions of phenomena but that are not embedded in a qualitative tradition such as phenomenology.

Qualitative evidence synthesis (QES) A systematic review of qualitative evidence, typically using an aggregative approach to evidence synthesis; often focused on qualitative aspects of an intervention (e.g., barriers to participation).

Qualitative research The investigation of phenomena, typically in an in-depth and holistic fashion, through the collection of rich narrative materials using a flexible research design.

Quality improvement (QI) Systematic efforts to improve practices and processes within a specific organization or patient group.

Quantitative analysis The organization of numeric data through statistical procedures for the purpose of describing phenomena or testing the magnitude and reliability of relationships among them.

Quantitative data Information collected in a quantified (numeric) form.

Quantitative research The investigation of phenomena that lend themselves to precise measurement and quantification, often involving a rigorous and controlled design and statistical analysis of data.

Quasi-experiment A type of design for testing an intervention in which participants are not randomly assigned to treatment conditions; also called a *nonrandomized trial*.

Questionnaire A document used to gather self-report data via self-administration of questions.

Quota sampling A nonrandom sampling method in which "quotas" for certain subgroups, based on sample characteristics, are established to increase the representativeness of the sample.

r The symbol for a bivariate correlation coefficient (*Pearson's r*), summarizing the magnitude and direction of a relationship between two variables measured on an interval or ratio scale.

R The symbol for the multiple correlation coefficient, indicating the magnitude (but not direction) of the relationship between a dependent variable and multiple independent (predictor) variables, taken together.

R^2 The squared multiple correlation coefficient, indicating the proportion of variance in the dependent variable explained by a set of independent (predictor) variables.

Random assignment The assignment of participants to treatment conditions in a random manner (i.e., in a manner determined by chance alone); also called *randomization*.

Random effects model In meta-analysis, a model in which studies are not assumed to be measuring the same overall effect but rather reflect a distribution of effects; often preferred to a fixed effect model when variation of effects across studies is extensive.

Random number table A table displaying hundreds of digits (from 0 to 9) in random order; each number is equally likely to follow any other.

Random sampling The selection of a sample such that each member of a population has an equal probability of being included.

Randomization The assignment of participants to treatment conditions in a random manner (i.e., in a manner determined by chance alone); also called *random assignment*.

Randomized controlled trial (RCT) A full experimental test of an intervention, involving random assignment of participants to different treatment groups.

Randomness An important concept in quantitative research, involving having certain features of the study established by chance rather than by design or personal preference.

Range A measure of variability, computed by subtracting the lowest value from the highest value in a distribution of scores.

Rating scale A scale that requires ratings of an object or concept along a continuum.

Ratio measurement A measurement level with equal distances between scores and a true meaningful zero point (e.g., weight).

Raw data Data in the form in which they were collected, without being coded or analyzed.

Reactivity A measurement distortion arising from the study participant's awareness of being observed, or, more generally, from the effect of the measurement procedure itself.

Readability The ease with which written material (e.g., a questionnaire) can be read by people with varying reading skills, often determined through readability formulas.

Realist evaluation A theory-driven approach to evaluating complex programs, designed to examine "What works for whom and under what circumstances?"

Receiver operating characteristic curve (ROC curve) A method used in developing and refining a screening instrument to determine the best cutoff point for "caseness."

Reflective notes Notes that document a qualitative researcher's personal experiences, self-reflections, and progress in the field, especially when collecting observational data.

Reflexivity In qualitative studies, the researcher's critical self-reflection about his or her own biases, preferences, and preconceptions, often recorded in a reflexive journal.

Regression analysis A statistical procedure for predicting values of a dependent variable based on one or more independent (predictor) variables.

Relationship A bond or a connection between two or more variables.

Relative risk (RR) An estimate of the risk of "caseness" in one group compared to another, computed by dividing the absolute risk for one group (e.g., a treated group) by the absolute risk for another (e.g., the untreated group); also called the *risk ratio*.

Relevance In the context of patient-centered research, the degree to which evidence is meaningful and valuable to patients and other stakeholders and has the potential to be actionable.

Reliability The extent to which a measurement is free from measurement error; more broadly, the extent to which scores for people who have not changed are the same for repeated measurements.

Reliability coefficient A quantitative index, usually ranging in value from .00 to 1.00, that provides an estimate of how reliable an instrument is (e.g., the intraclass correlation coefficient).

Repeated measures ANOVA An analysis of variance used when there are multiple measurements of the outcome over time.

Replication The deliberate repetition of research procedures in a second investigation for the purpose of assessing whether earlier results can be confirmed.

Representative sample A sample whose characteristics are comparable to those of the population from which it is drawn.

Representativeness A key criterion for assessing the adequacy of a sample in quantitative studies, indicating the extent to which findings from the study can be generalized to the population.

Research Systematic inquiry that uses orderly, disciplined methods to answer questions or solve problems.

Research control Procedures used to hold constant confounding influences on the outcome under study.

Research design The overall plan for addressing a research question, including strategies for enhancing the study's integrity.

Research hypothesis The actual hypothesis a researcher wishes to test (as opposed to the *null hypothesis*), stating the expected relationship between two or more variables.

Research methods The techniques used to structure a study and to gather and analyze information in a systematic fashion.

Research problem A disturbing or perplexing condition that can be investigated through disciplined inquiry.

Research question A specific query the researcher wants to answer to address a research problem.

Research report A document (often a journal article) summarizing the main features of a study, including the research question, the methods used to address it, the findings, and the interpretation of the findings.

Research utilization The use of some aspect of a study in an application unrelated to the original research.

Researcher credibility The faith that can be put in a researcher, based on his or her training, qualifications, and experiences.

Respondent In a self-report study, the participant responding to questions posed by the researcher.

Responder analysis An analysis that compares people who are *responders* to an intervention, based on their having reached a benchmark on a change score (e.g., the minimal important change), to people who are nonresponders (have not reached the benchmark).

Response options The prespecified set of answers to a closed-ended question or item.

Response rate The rate of participation in a study, calculated by dividing the number of people participating by the number of people sampled.

Response set bias The measurement error resulting from the tendency of some individuals to respond to items in characteristic ways (e.g., always agreeing), independently of item content.

Results The answers to a researcher's questions or hypothesis tests, obtained through an analysis of the collected data.

Retrospective design A study design that begins with the manifestation of the outcome in the present (e.g., lung cancer), followed by a search for a presumed cause occurring in the past (e.g., cigarette smoking).

Risk/benefit assessment An assessment of the relative costs and benefits, to an individual study participant and to society at large, of participation in a study; also, the relative costs and benefits of implementing an innovation.

ROC curve See *receiver operating characteristic curve*.

Root cause analysis (RCA) In quality improvement, systematic efforts to identify the underlying causes of a problem that needs to be addressed.

Sample A subset of a population comprising those selected to participate in a study.

Sample size The number of people who participate in a study; an important factor in the *power* of statistical analyses and in statistical conclusion validity.

Sampling The process of selecting a portion of the population to represent the population.

Sampling bias Distortions that arise when a sample is not representative of the population from which it was drawn.

Sampling distribution A theoretical distribution of a statistic using the values of the statistic (e.g., the mean) from an infinite number of samples as the data points in the distribution.

Sampling error The fluctuation of the value of a statistic from one sample to another drawn from the same population.

Sampling frame A list of all the elements in the population from which a sample is drawn.

Sampling plan The formal plan specifying a sampling method, a sample size, and procedures for recruiting subjects.

Saturation The collection of qualitative data to the point where a sense of closure is attained because new data yield redundant information.

Scale A composite measure of an attribute or trait involving the aggregation of responses to multiple items into a single numerical score that places people on a continuum with respect to the trait.

Schematic model A graphic representation depicting concepts and linkages between them; also called a *conceptual map*.

Scientific merit The degree to which a study is methodologically and conceptually sound.

Scientific method A set of orderly, systematic, controlled procedures for acquiring dependable, empirical—and typically quantitative—information; the methodological approach associated with the positivist paradigm.

Scoping review A preliminary review of research findings to clarify the range and nature of the evidence base, often to refine the questions and protocols for a systematic review.

Score A numerical value derived from a measurement that communicates *how much* of an attribute is present in a person or whether the attribute is present or absent.

Screening instrument An instrument used to assess whether potential subjects for a study meet eligibility criteria, or for determining whether a person tests positive or is at risk for a specified condition.

Secondary analysis A form of research in which the data collected in one study are reanalyzed in another investigation to answer new questions.

Secondary source Secondhand accounts of events or facts; in research, a description of a study written by someone other than the original researcher.

Selection threat (self-selection) A threat to a study's internal validity resulting from preexisting differences between groups under study; the differences affect the outcome in ways extraneous to the effect of the independent variable (e.g., an intervention).

Selective coding A level of coding in a grounded theory study that begins once the core category has been discovered; involves limiting coding to only those categories related to the core category.

Self-determination A person's right to voluntarily decide whether to participate in a study.

Self-report A data collection method that involves direct verbal reporting by a study participant (e.g., in an interview or questionnaire).

Self-selection See *selection threat*.

Semi-structured interview An open-ended interview in which the researcher is guided by a list of topics to cover rather than specific questions to ask.

Sensitivity The ability of a screening or diagnostic instrument to correctly identify a "case" (true positives).

Sensitivity analysis An effort to test how sensitive the results of a statistical analysis are to changes in assumptions or in the way the analysis was done (e.g., in a meta-analysis, sometimes used to assess whether conclusions are sensitive to the quality of the studies included).

Sequential design A mixed methods design in which one strand of data collection (qualitative or quantitative) occurs prior to the other, informing the second strand; symbolically shown with an arrow (e.g., QUAL → QUAN).

Setting In a research context, the physical location in which data collection takes place in a study (e.g., clinics).

Significance level The probability that an observed relationship could be caused by chance; significance at the .05 level indicates the probability that a relationship of the observed magnitude would be found by chance only 5 times out of 100.

Simple random sampling Basic probability sampling involving the random selection of sample members from a sampling frame.

Site The overall location where a study is undertaken (e.g., Miami).

Skewed distribution An asymmetric distribution of data values around a central point, with two halves that are not mirror images of each other.

Snowball sampling The selection of participants through referrals from earlier participants; also called *network sampling*.

Social desirability response set A bias in self-report instruments created when participants tend to misrepresent their opinions in the direction of views consistent with prevailing social norms.

Space triangulation The collection of data on the same phenomenon in multiple sites to assess cross-site consistency and enhance trustworthiness of the findings.

Spearman's rho A correlation coefficient indicating the magnitude of a relationship between variables measured on the ordinal scale.

Specificity The ability of a screening or diagnostic instrument to correctly identify noncases (true negatives).

Stakeholder In the context of health care, a person or group that has a direct interest in a health care decision, action, or process.

Standard deviation A statistic that describes the "average" amount of variability in a set of scores.

Standard error The standard deviation of a theoretical sampling distribution, such as the sampling distribution of the mean.

Standardized mean difference (SMD) In meta-analysis, the effect size index for comparing two group means, computed by subtracting one mean from the other and dividing by the pooled standard deviation; also called Cohen's *d*.

Statement of purpose A declarative statement of the overall goals of a study.

Statistic An estimate of a population parameter, calculated from sample data.

Statistical analysis The organization and analysis of quantitative data using statistical procedures, including both descriptive and inferential statistics.

Statistical conclusion validity The degree to which inferences about relationships from a statistical analysis of the data are accurate.

Statistical control The use of statistical procedures to control confounding influences on the outcome variable.

Statistical heterogeneity Diversity of effects across primary studies included in a meta-analysis.

Statistical inference An inference about the population based on information from a sample, using laws of probability.

Statistical power The ability of a research design and analytic strategy to detect true relationships among variables.

Statistical significance A term indicating that the results from an analysis of sample data are unlikely to have resulted from chance at a specified level of probability.

Statistical test An analytic tool used to estimate the probability that results from a sample reflect true population values.

Stipend A monetary payment to individuals taking part in a study as an incentive for their participation and/or to compensate for time and expenses.

Strata Subdivisions of the population based on a specified characteristic (e.g., gender); singular is *stratum*.

Stratification The subdivision of a sample or a population into smaller units (e.g., married and unmarried), typically to enhance representativeness (e.g., in sampling).

Stratified random sampling The random selection of study participants from two or more strata of the population independently.

Study participant An individual who participates and provides information in a study.

Subgroup analysis Analytic efforts to understand whether intervention effects vary for defined groups of people (e.g., men vs. women); undertaken to disentangle heterogeneity of treatment effects (HTE).

Subject An individual who participates and provides data in a study; term used primarily in quantitative research.

Subscale A subset of items that measures one aspect or dimension of a multidimensional construct.

Summated rating scale A composite scale consisting of multiple items that are added together to yield a total score for an attribute (e.g., a Likert scale).

Survey research Nonexperimental research that involves gathering information about people's activities, beliefs, preferences, and attitudes via direct questioning.

Symmetric distribution A distribution of values with two halves that are mirror images of the each other.

Systematic review A rigorous synthesis of research findings on a particular research question, using systematic sampling, data collection, and data analysis procedures specified in a formal protocol.

Systematic sampling The selection of sample members such that every *kth* (e.g., every 10th) person or element in a sampling frame is chosen.

Tacit knowledge Information about a culture that is so deeply embedded that members do not talk about it or may not be consciously aware of it.

Target population The entire population in which a researcher is interested and to which he or she would like to generalize study results.

Taxonomy In an ethnographic analysis, a system of classifying and organizing terms and concepts, developed to illuminate a domain's organization and the relationship among the domain's categories.

Test statistic A statistic used to test the reliability of relationships between variables (e.g., t, chi-squared); sampling distributions of test statistics are known for circumstances in which the null hypothesis is true.

Test–retest reliability The type of reliability that concerns the extent to which scores for people who have not changed are the same when a measure is administered twice; an assessment of a measure's stability.

Thematic analysis A flexible approach to analyzing qualitative data from a descriptive qualitative study that follows an established process to identify and define themes.

Theme A recurring regularity emerging from an analysis of qualitative data.

Theoretical framework See *framework*.

Theoretical sampling In qualitative studies, especially in grounded theory studies, the selection of sample members based on emerging findings to ensure adequate saturation of important theoretical categories.

Theory An abstract generalization that presents a systematic explanation about relationships among phenomena or that thoroughly describes a phenomenon.

Therapy/intervention question A question about the effects of a treatment or intervention on patient outcomes.

Thick description A rich and thorough description of the research context, study participants, and the phenomenon of interest in a qualitative study.

Threats to validity In research design, reasons that an inference about the effect of an independent variable (e.g., an intervention) on an outcome could be wrong.

Time sampling In structured observations, the sampling of time periods during which observations will take place.

Time-series design A quasi-experimental design involving the collection of data over an extended time period, with multiple data collection points both before and after an intervention.

Time triangulation The collection of data on the same phenomenon or about the same people at different points in time to enhance trustworthiness.

Topic guide A list of broad question areas to be covered in a semi-structured interview or focus group interview.

Transferability The extent to which qualitative findings can be transferred to other settings or groups; an aspect of trustworthiness.

Translational science A discipline that focuses on how study findings can best be translated into practice.

Treatment An intervention; in experimental research (a clinical trial), the condition being manipulated.

Triangulation The use of multiple methods to collect and interpret data about a phenomenon to converge on an accurate representation of reality.

Trustworthiness The degree of confidence qualitative researchers have in their data and analyses, often assessed using the criteria of credibility, transferability, dependability, confirmability, and authenticity.

***t*-test** A parametric statistical test for testing the difference between two group means.

Type I error An error created by rejecting the null hypothesis when it is true (i.e., the researcher concludes that a relationship exists when in fact it does not—a false positive).

Type II error An error created by accepting the null hypothesis when it is false (i.e., the researcher concludes that *no* relationship exists when in fact it does—a false negative).

Underpowered A characteristic of a study that lacks sufficient statistical power to minimize the risk of a Type II error (i.e., the risk of concluding that a relationship does not exist when, in fact, it does).

Unimodal distribution A distribution of values with one peak (high frequency).

Unit of analysis The basic unit or focus of a researcher's analysis—typically individual study participants.

Univariate statistics Statistical analysis of a single variable for descriptive purposes (e.g., calculating a mean).

Unstructured interview An interview in which the researcher asks respondents questions without having a predetermined plan regarding the content or flow of information to be gathered.

Unstructured observation The collection of descriptive data through direct observation that is not guided by a formal, prespecified plan for observing, enumerating, or recording the information.

Validity A quality criterion referring to the degree to which inferences made in a study are accurate and well-founded; in measurement, the degree to which an instrument measures what it is intended to measure.

Variability The degree to which values on a set of scores are dispersed, i.e., are heterogeneous.

Variable An attribute that varies, that is, takes on different values (e.g., heart rate, anxiety).

*Variance A measure of variability or dispersion, equal to the standard deviation squared.

Vignette A brief description of an event, person, or situation to which respondents are asked to express their reactions.

Visual analog scale (VAS) A scaling procedure used to measure certain clinical symptoms (e.g., pain, fatigue) by having people indicate on a straight line the intensity of the symptom; usually measured on a 100-mm scale with values from 0 to 100.

Vulnerable groups Special groups of people whose rights in studies need special protection because of their inability to provide meaningful informed consent or because their circumstances place them at higher-than-average risk of adverse effects (e.g., children, unconscious patients).

Wait-list design A design for an intervention study that involves putting control group members on a waiting list for the intervention until follow-up data have been collected; also called a *delayed treatment design*.

Yea-sayers bias A bias in self-report scales created when respondents characteristically agree with statements ("yea-say"), independent of content.

Page numbers in bold indicate Glossary entries.
Entries in the chapter supplements are indicated by chapter number (e.g., an entry with Supp-1 is in the Chapter 1 Supplement on thePoint).

CCS1220